Hematology and Oncology Through Case Studies

Hematology and Oncology Through Case Studies

Editor: Cairo Clarke

AMERICAN
MEDICAL PUBLISHERS
www.americanmedicalpublishers.com

AMERICAN
MEDICAL PUBLISHERS
www.americanmedicalpublishers.com

Cataloging-in-Publication Data

Hematology and oncology through case studies / edited by Cairo Clarke.
p. cm.
Includes bibliographical references and index.
ISBN 979-8-88740-642-8
1. Hematology. 2. Oncology. 3. Blood--Diseases. 4. Cancer. 5. Leukemia. I. Clarke, Cairo.
RC636 .H46 2023
616.15--dc23

American Medical Publishers,
41 Flatbush Avenue,
1st Floor, New York,
NY 11217, USA

ISBN 979-8-88740-642-8 (Hardback)

Contents

Preface XI

Chapter 1 **A Rare Complication of Thymoma: Pure White Cell Aplasia in Good's Syndrome** 1
Kim Uy, Elizabeth Levin, Pawel Mroz, Faqian Li and Surbhi Shah

Chapter 2 **An Unusual Initial Presentation of Diffuse Large B-Cell Lymphoma as Recurrent Syncope** 5
Kunhwa Kim, Harpreet Kaur, Matthew Chan, Manju Balasubramanian, Sorab Gupta and Vinicius M. Jorge

Chapter 3 **A Rare Case of Midostaurin-Associated Sweet's Syndrome** 9
Hesham Yasin, Tessa Laytem, Grerk Sutamtewagul and Sabarish Ayyappan

Chapter 4 **Concurrent B Cell Acute Lymphoblastic Lymphoma/Leukemia and Monoclonal B Cell Lymphocytosis: A Case Report with Extensive Molecular Analysis** 13
Maryam Mehdipour Dalivand, Parastou Tizro, Julie Partain, Anita Aggarwal, Jack Lichy, Francisco Mot Ara and Victor E. Nava

Chapter 5 **Spontaneous Regression of Plasmablastic Lymphoma in an Immunocompetent Patient: Case Report and Review of the Literature** 18
Kee Tat Lee, Nurul Akmar Misron, Norasmidar Abdul Aziz, Chin Hau Wong and Hong Keng Liew

Chapter 6 **An Unusual Cause of Epistaxis: Paranasal Sinus Myeloid Sarcoma** 24
Karuna Dewan, John H. Baird and Courtney B. Shires

Chapter 7 **Multiple Myeloma in a Young Female Presenting with Neurological Symptoms** 29
Matthew Lee, Xinmin Zhang, Vinh Nguyen and Monique Hartley-Brown

Chapter 8 **A Western Case of Intravascular Large B-Cell Lymphoma as Unusual Cause of Persistent Fever** 36
Pier Paolo Piccaluga, Stefania Paolini, Cristina Campidelli, Nicola Vianelli and Luigi Bolondi

Chapter 9 **Durable Control of Mycosis Fungoides after Sepsis: "Coley's Toxin?" Case Report and Review of the Literature** 42
Benjamin Heyman, Chris R. Kelsey and Anne Beaven

Chapter 10 **CD7-Positive Diffuse Large B-Cell Lymphoma Presenting as an Intranasal Tumor** 46
Kazuaki Teshima, Masaaki Kume, Yasushi Kawaharada, Takashi Saito, Ko Abe, Sho Ikeda, Hideaki Ohyagi, Megumi Zuguchi, Masashi Zuguchi, Yosuke Kubota, Yoshitaka Enomoto, Masahito Miura, Satsuki Takahashi, Masahiro Saito, Ken Saito and Naoto Takahashi

Chapter 11 **Plasmablastic Lymphoma, a Rare Entity in Bone Marrow with Unusual Immunophenotype and Challenging Differential Diagnosis** 50
Majd Al Shaarani, Rodney E. Shackelford, Samip R. Master, Glenn M. Mills, Yasir AlZubaidi, Ahmed Mamilly and Eric X. Wei

Chapter 12 **Prolonged Myelosuppression due to Progressive Bone Marrow Fibrosis in a Patient with Acute Promyelocytic Leukemia** 59
Yuta Inagawa, Yukiko Komeno, Satoshi Saito, Yuji Maenohara, Tetsuro Yamagishi, Hiroyuki Kawashima, Taku Saito, Keiko Abe, Kuniko Iihara, Yasumasa Hatada and Tomiko Ryu

Chapter 13 **PD-1 Checkpoint Blockade in Patients for Acute Myeloid Leukemia after HSCT Relapse Resulted in Severe GVHD and sHLH** 66
Zhi zhuo Du, Mi Zhou, Jing Ling, Lan Cao, Lingjun Kong, Shengqin Cheng, Peifang Xiao and Shaoyan Hu

Chapter 14 **Efficacy of Inotuzumab Ozogamicin plus Ponatinib Followed by Allogeneic Stem Cell Transplantation in a Patient with Relapsed Philadelphia Chromosome-Positive Acute Lymphoblastic Leukemia** 70
Ilina Micheva, Vladimir Gerov, Stela Dimitrova and Merlin Efraim

Chapter 15 **The First Autopsy Case of Fatal Acute Cardiac Failure after Administration of Carfilzomib in a Patient with Multiple Myeloma** 74
Teruhito Takakuwa, Ippei Otomaru, Taku Araki, Akiko Miura, Yotaro Fujitani, Yasuhide Mochizuki, Yoshimi Miyagi, Hideto Senzaki and Ryosuke Yamamura

Chapter 16 **Central Nervous System Involvement by Small Lymphocytic Lymphoma after a Myxoma-Related Embolic Event** 79
Nicolas Gallastegui, Daniel P. Cassidy, Deborah O. Heros, Francisco Vega and Jonathan H. Schatz

Chapter 17 **Siltuximab-Related Favorable Clinical Outcome for a Patient Suffering from Idiopathic Multicentric Castleman Disease** 85
Stamatios Chrysochoou, Andreas Kreft and Eberhard Schneider

Chapter 18 **Successful Control of Hepatitis B Virus Reactivation following Restart of Ibrutinib in Chronic Lymphocytic Leukaemia** 89
Sara Kristina Viberg Tjønnfjord, Eirik Brekka Tjønnfjord, Zbigniew Konopski and Geir Erland Tjønnfjord

Chapter 19 **Aplastic Anemia and Good Syndrome in a Heavily Treated Stage IV Thymoma Patient: A Case Report and Review of the Literature** 93
Sofia Chiatamone Ranieri, Stefania Trasarti, Maria Antonietta Arleo, Luisa Bizzoni, Livia Bonanni, Valeria Di Battista, Maria Assunta Limongiello, Maria Grazia Nardacci, Giuseppe Gentile and Robin Foà

Chapter 20 **Symptomatic Hypoalbuminemia as an Indication for Treatment of Waldenström Macroglobulinemia: A Case Report and Review of the Literature** 99
Jeremy T. Larsen and Frederick D. Leonard

Chapter 21 **Ibrutinib Plus R-ICE Induces Remission in Blastoid Variant Mantle Cell Lymphoma with CNS Relapse** 103
Timothy S. Oh, Madelyn Burkart, Amir Behdad, Hatice Savas and Reem Karmali

Chapter 22 **Orbital Mucosa-Associated Lymphoid Tissue Lymphoma and Primary Cutaneous Classical Hodgkin Lymphoma: A Rare Case Report and Review of the Literature** 107
Nicole Yun, James Coggan, Ira Miller and Parameswaran Venugopal

Chapter 23 **Successful Treatment of Concomitant Pleural Mucosa-Associated Lymphoid Tissue Lymphoma and Monoclonal Gammopathy of Undetermined Significance with Lenalidomide, Rituximab, and Dexamethasone** 111
Yoshiki Uemura, Risa Maeda and Hiroyoshi Saegusa

Chapter 24 **Chronic Lymphocytic Leukemia Presenting as a Subcortical Watershed Infarct** 118
Mridul Gupta, Divita Singh, Patrick Lee and Sandhya Kadiyam

Chapter 25 **Combined Ruxolitinib and Venetoclax Treatment in a Patient with a *BCR-JAK2* Rearranged Myeloid Neoplasm** 123
Coen J. Lap, Samah Nassereddine, Min-Ling Liu, Victor E. Nava and Anita Aggarwal

Chapter 26 **Spontaneous Splenic Rupture and Rituximab-Induced Acute Thrombocytopenia in a Patient with High-Risk Mantle Cell Lymphoma** 129
Jared Williams and Shingi Chiruka

Chapter 27 **Prolonged Remission of Cancer of Unknown Primary following Initiation of Eculizumab Therapy for Paroxysmal Nocturnal Hemoglobinuria** 133
Ming Y. Lim, Keith E. Volmar and Nigel S. Key

Chapter 28 **Spontaneous Complete Remission of Acute Myeloid Leukemia in the Absence of Disease-Modifying Therapy following Severe Pulmonary Involvement by Coronavirus Infectious Disease-19** 136
Maryam Barkhordar, Fatemeh Tajic Rostami, Marjan Yaghmaie, Mehrdad Abbaszadeh, Bahram Chahardouli and Seied Asadollah Mousavi

Chapter 29 **Aggressive CD5-Positive Primary Bone Marrow Diffuse Large B-Cell Lymphoma with Leukemic Presentation** 142
Mark G. Evans, Sherif A. Rezk, Lauren C. Pinter-Brown and Xiaohui Zhao

Chapter 30 **A Case of Myeloid Sarcoma following Allogeneic HSCT Presenting as Localized Hip Pain** 145
Shannon Zhang, Casey Charlton, Akshay Amaraneni and Keri Maher

Chapter 31 **Age-Adjusted Schedules of Venetoclax and Hypomethylating Agents to Treat Extremely Elderly Patients with Acute Myeloid Leukemia** 148
Aaron M. Lee, Aaron M. Goodman and James K. Mangan

Chapter 32 **The Efficacy and Safety of Lenalidomide plus Rituximab in an Orbital Relapse of Diffuse Large B-Cell Lymphoma** 154
R. Palmieri, F. Esposito, F. Meconi, V. M. Rapisarda, L. Anemona, G. Paterno, S. Vaccarini, D. Nasso, L. Pupo and M. Cantonetti

Chapter 33 **A Rare Presentation of HIV-Negative Plasmablastic Lymphoma: A Diagnostic Dilemma** 158
Alaina J. Kessler, Bridget K. Marcellino, Scot A. Niglio, Bruce E. Petersen and Adriana K. Malone

Chapter 34 **A Rare Case of BCL2-Positive Multiple Myeloma Complicated with Follicular Lymphoma** ... 162
Yutaka Tsutsumi, Shinich Ito, Mirei Kobayashi and Takanori Teshima

Chapter 35 **Fatal Idiopathic Hyperammonemia after Induction Chemotherapy for Acute Myeloid Leukemia** ... 166
Christophe Angelo, Marie-Françoise Vincent, Mina Komuta, Philippe Hantson, Nicole Straetmans and Edwige Boulet

Chapter 36 **Hairy Cell Leukemia Masquerading as Pancytopenia in Pregnancy** ... 170
Louisa Shackleton, Stephen E. Langabeer, David O'Brien, Sarah L. McCarron, Bridgette Byrne, Rupert Barry, Richard Flavin, C. Larry Bacon and Catherine M. Flynn

Chapter 37 **Subdural Hygroma: A Morbid Complication of Intrathecal Chemotherapy in a Patient with B-Cell Acute Lymphocytic Leukemia** ... 173
Mina Shenouda, Madhulika Urella, Jennifer Dotson, Hassaan Yasin and Yehuda Lebowicz

Chapter 38 **Primary Cutaneous T-Cell Lymphoblastic Lymphoma: Case Report and Literature Review** ... 177
Sharad Khurana, Manuel Beltran, Liuyan Jiang, Ernesto Ayala and Vivek Roy

Chapter 39 **Paraneoplastic Pemphigus: A Striking Complication of Undiagnosed Lymphoma** ... 183
Blake O. Adnani, Kathleen O' Brien, Zaw W. Myint and Brandon L. Adler

Chapter 40 **Arsenic Trioxide Treatment during Pregnancy for Acute Promyelocytic Leukemia in a 22-Year-Old Woman** ... 187
Claire Cochet, Marion Simonet, Julie Cattin, Jean-Patrick Metz, Ana Berceanu, Eric Deconinck, Etienne Daguindau, Françoise Schillinger, Pierre Fenaux, Nicolas Mottet and Yohan Desbrosses

Chapter 41 **Myeloid Sarcomas Causing Unilateral Cranial Nerve Palsies in a Patient with Relapsed Acute Myeloblastic Leukemia** ... 192
A. Mendez-Hernandez, X. A. Andrade, S. Upadhyay, L. M. Parra-Rodriguez, E. Caldeira, L. H. Paz, H. Mann, M. Zia and L. Sumoza

Chapter 42 **Biological versus Clinical Risk Factors in Acute Myeloid Leukemia: Is There a Winner?** ... 197
M. Malagola, N. Polverelli, V. Cancelli, E. Morello, A. Turra, E. Borlenghi, F. Cattina, B. Rambaldi, S. Bernardi, C. Zanaglio, Elif Dereli Eke, L. Gandolfi, M. Farina and D. Russo

Chapter 43 **Primary Cutaneous Diffuse Large B-Cell Lymphoma of the Upper Limb: Double Hit/Double Expressor with CNS Involvement: From Hospice to Remission** ... 201
Brenda S. Castillo, Maria L. Rodriguez, Ju-Hsien John Chao and Behyar Zoghi

Chapter 44 **Central Nervous System Involvement by Waldenstrom Macroglobulinemia: A Case Report of the Bing-Neel Syndrome** ... 207
Ananth Arjunan and Hema Rai

Chapter 45 **A Case Report of Leptomeningeal Myelomatosis and Rapid Improvement with Regimen Consisting of Daratumumab, Pomalidomide, Vincristine, Procarbazine, and Dexamethasone** 210
Jew Win Kuan, Sing Ling Chai, Pathmanathan Rajadurai, Lee Gong Lau, Joseph Uchang and Sharifah Noor Akmal Syed Husain

Chapter 46 **Primary Bone Lymphoma: A Case Series and Review of Literature** 217
Poorva Bindal, Aakash Desai, Lukas Delasos, Sudhanshu Mulay and James Vredenburgh

Chapter 47 **Plasmablastic Lymphoma or Plasmablastic Myeloma: A Case of Post-Transplant Lymphoproliferative Disorder** 223
Poornima Ramadas, Michael Williams and David B. Duggan

Chapter 48 **Use of KRD-PACE as Salvage Therapy in Aggressive, Relapsed/Bortezomib-Refractory Extramedullary Multiple Myeloma: A Report of Two Cases and Literature Review** 228
Ricardo D. Parrondo, Vivek Roy, Taimur Sher, Victoria Alegria, Asher A. Chanan-Khan and Sikander Ailawadhi

Chapter 49 **An Unusually Short Latent Period of Therapy-Related Myeloid Neoplasm Harboring a Rare MLL-EP300 Rearrangement: Case Report and Literature Review** 234
Reina Takeda, Kazuaki Yokoyama, Seiichiro Kobayashi, Toyotaka Kawamata, Sousuke Nakamura, Tomofusa Fukuyama, Mika Ito, Nozomi Yusa, Eigo Shimizu, Nobuhiro Ohno, Rui Yamaguchi, Seiya Imoto, Satoru Miyano, Kaoru Uchimaru and Arinobu Tojo

Chapter 50 **Sarcoidosis and Multiple Myeloma: A Case Report and Literature Review** 240
Joao Tiago Serra, Aurelia Martinho, Fernanda Paixao Duarte and Fernando Aldomiro

Permissions

List of Contributors

Index

Preface

Hematology and oncology are closely related medical specialties that deal with the diagnosis, treatment, and management of blood disorders and cancer respectively. They are separate specialties, and they are combined for the treatment of hematologic malignancies. These malignancies refer to the cancers which originate in the blood forming tissue. Hematological malignancies are classified into three types, namely, multiple myeloma, leukemia and lymphoma. The cancer which develops in the bone marrow and affects plasma cells is known as multiple myeloma. Leukemia refers to a cancer that begins in the bone marrow or blood. On the other hand, lymphoma is a type of hematological malignancy which begins in a part of the immune system known as the lymphatic system. This book includes some of the vital pieces of works being conducted across the world, on various topics related to hematology and oncology. It presents researches and studies performed by experts across the globe. The book is appropriate for students seeking detailed information in this area of medicine as well as for experts.

Various studies have approached the subject by analyzing it with a single perspective, but the present book provides diverse methodologies and techniques to address this field. This book contains theories and applications needed for understanding the subject from different perspectives. The aim is to keep the readers informed about the progresses in the field; therefore, the contributions were carefully examined to compile novel researches by specialists from across the globe.

Indeed, the job of the editor is the most crucial and challenging in compiling all chapters into a single book. In the end, I would extend my sincere thanks to the chapter authors for their profound work. I am also thankful for the support provided by my family and colleagues during the compilation of this book.

Editor

1

A Rare Complication of Thymoma: Pure White Cell Aplasia in Good's Syndrome

Kim Uy,[1] **Elizabeth Levin**,[1] **Pawel Mroz**,[2] **Faqian Li**,[2] **and Surbhi Shah**[1]

[1]*University of Minnesota, Department of Medicine, Division of Hematology, Oncology and Transplantation, Minneapolis, MN, USA*
[2]*University of Minnesota, Department of Laboratory Medicine and Pathology, Minneapolis, MN, USA*

Correspondence should be addressed to Surbhi Shah; shahx090@umn.edu

Academic Editor: Pier P. Piccaluga

Pure white cell aplasia (PWCA) is a rare manifestation of thymoma. It is characterized by agranulocytosis with absent myeloid precursors in the bone marrow and normal hematopoiesis for other cell lines. Here we describe a 65-year-old female patient who presented with three days of fever and night sweat. Chest CT revealed an anterior mediastinal mass. A biopsy of the mass confirmed a diagnosis of thymoma mixed type A and B2. The patient developed a severe neutropenia, and her bone marrow revealed significantly decreased neutrophil-lineage cells, rare to absent B cells, and defective T cells, consistent with PWCA. Following thymectomy, a complete resolution of PWCA was achieved via multimodality therapy of intravenous immunoglobulins, granulocyte colony-stimulating factor, and immunosuppressant. This report highlights the care complexity regarding treatment choices and decision to perform thymectomy in patients presenting with PWCA.

1. Background

Primary tumors of the thymus gland are rare neoplasm [1]. If occurs, its most common type is benign thymoma. Thymus plays a central role in the development of adaptive immune system, particularly in the maturation process of T lymphocytes. Hence, patients with thymoma often present with a varying type of paraneoplastic syndromes [2, 3]. Good's syndrome or hypogammaglobulinemia is a recognized paraneoplastic syndrome of thymoma, and it is commonly associated with pure red cell aplasia. In contrast, pure white cell aplasia (PWCA) is a rare manifestation, particularly in setting of Good's syndrome. PWCA is characterized by agranulocytosis with absent myeloid precursors in the bone marrow and preserved hematopoiesis for other cell lines [4]. Here we report a thymoma patient presenting with Good's syndrome and PWCA.

2. Case Presentation

A previously healthy 65-year-old Caucasian woman presented with three days of fever and night sweats. On exam, she had oral thrush and truncal morbilliform rash. Laboratory workup showed severe neutropenia with WBC 1.5 K/μL, ANC 0 K/μL, and low serum immunoglobulin with IgA 54 mg/dL, IgM 83 mg/dL, and IgG 455 mg/dL. Other standard laboratory workup was unremarkable including detailed infectious and rheumatologic evaluations.

A bone marrow biopsy revealed decreased mature granulocytes and granulocytic precursors and increased CD3-positive T lymphocytes in small lymphoid aggregates (Figure 1). Flow cytometry showed rare to absent B cells and no aberrant immunophenotype on T cells. The patient was started on intravenous immunoglobulin (IVIg) and filgrastim without improvement in WBC. A skin biopsy of the rash revealed a dermatitis, suggestive of drug eruption but could not rule out viral exanthem.

Chest CT scan revealed an 8 cm circumscribed heterogeneously enhancing solid mass in the anterior mediastinum, suspicious for neoplastic process (Figure 2). It also showed multiple indeterminate nodules throughout the bilateral lungs. Given the severe neutropenia of unknown duration, these nodules were concerning for invasive fungal infection. Bronchoalveolar lavage was performed. Fungal cultures were

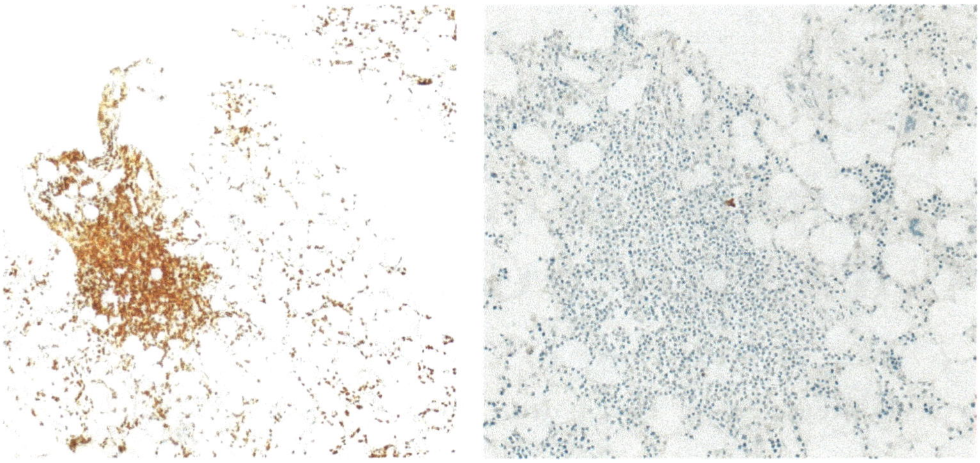

(a) (b)

FIGURE 1: Bone marrow biopsy: bone marrow aspiration of the posterior iliac crest revealed normocellular bone marrow 30–40% with granulocytopenia and increased CD3+ T lymphocytes some in aggregates (a). Flow cytometry showed rare to absent B cells and no aberrant immunophenotype on T cells (b).

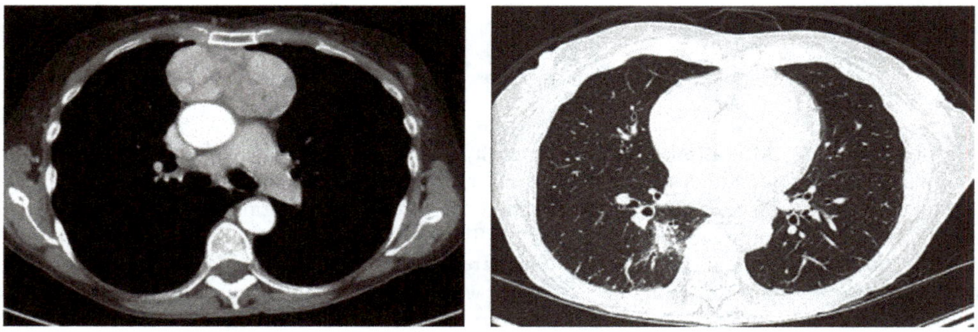

(a) (b)

FIGURE 2: Chest CT: a $4.1 \times 8.3 \times 7.9$ cm mass in the anterior mediastinum with lobulations and dense enhancement (a). Multiple indeterminate nodules throughout the bilateral lungs (b).

negative after four weeks. Serum beta-D-glucan, galactomannan antigen, Histoplasma antigen, and Cryptococcus antigens were also negative. The patient was empirically started on levofloxacin and voriconazole. A CT-guided mediastinal mass biopsy was pursued, revealing a network of cytokeratin AE1/AE3-positive epithelial cells mixed with CD3+, TdT+, and CD1a+ lymphocytes and rare CD20+ B cells. These were consistent with thymoma type B2. The biopsy also showed spindle cells consistent with thymoma type A (Figure 3). A diagnosis of thymoma mixed type A and B2 was given.

After multidisciplinary discussions, thymectomy was pursued despite concerns of poor wound healing in the setting of severe neutropenia. Pathology on the surgical specimen revealed encapsulated tumor consistent with thymoma, modified Masaoka stage I. Specimen had free tumor margins, and associated lymph nodes were benign. The patient recovered well following thymectomy, and filgrastim was discontinued due to its limited effect during the preoperative period. The patient was continued on prophylactic antibiotics as she remained neutropenic.

On postop follow-up, the patient had persistent neutropenia. Therefore, cyclosporine was initiated for immunomodulation, and filgrastim was reintroduced to boost myeloid stem cells. In one week, the WBC increased to 6.7 from 1.0 K/μL and ANC increased to 2.8 from 0.0 K/μL. However, when granulocyte colony-stimulating factor (G-CSF) was discontinued, WBC decreased to 2.2 K/μL and ANC decreased to 0.3 K/μL over a 3-day period. G-CSF was restarted for an additional one month until cyclosporine reached maintenance levels. In the next 4 months, the patient remained on a maintenance dose of cyclosporine with a target level of 200–400 ng/mL while monitoring toxicity. Subsequently, she was successfully weaned off all immune modulators with self-sustaining WBC after a total of 6-month therapy. Notably, the patient suffered multiple recurrent respiratory infections with CT showing an infiltrate in different lung fields and required short courses of antibiotics throughout her recovery. However, no major infectious complications were observed.

3. Discussion

In the United States, the overall incidence of thymoma is 0.13 per 100,000 person-years [1]. Thymoma equally affects

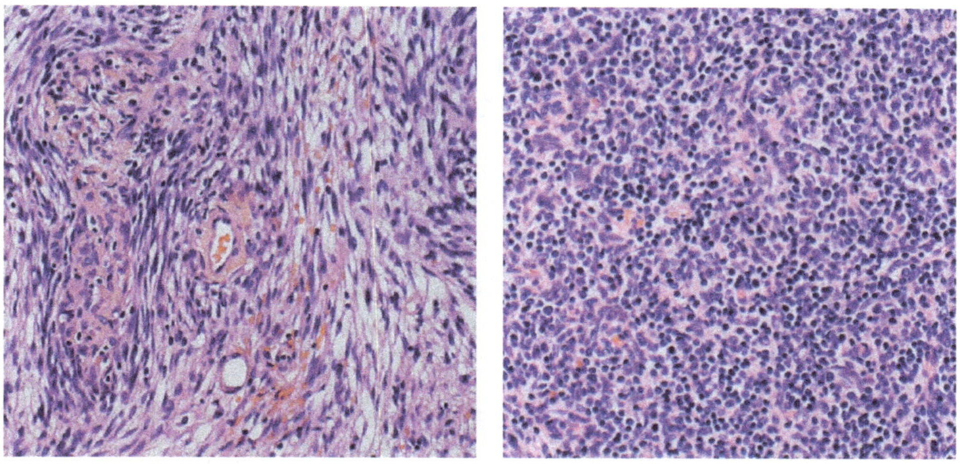

(a) (b)

FIGURE 3: Thymoma mixed type A and B2: grossly and microscopically encapsulated thymoma type A (a) showing spindle cells and type B2 (b) showing mixed epithelial cells and lymphocytes. The lymphocytes are positive for CD3 with rare CD20-positive B cells. These lymphocytes are also positive for TdT and CD1a.

males and females with a rising incident in the fourth or fifth decade and peak in the seventh decade of life [2]. Thymomas are neoplasms of thymic epithelial cells typically with mixed cortical and medullary properties. Its classifications are based on the non-neoplastic lymphocyte content and epithelial cell features, which are categorized into type A, AB, B1, B2, and B3 [5]. Surgical removal of thymoma is the mainstay of treatment, particularly for stage I and II thymoma [6].

Approximately, 6–11% of all thymoma cases present with hypogammaglobulinemia or Good's syndrome [2]. Principal findings of Good's syndrome include few or absent B cells, inverted CD4+ : CD8+ T cell ratio, CD4 T-cell lymphopenia, and impaired mitogenic function of T cells. Despite low immunoglobulin synthesis, up to 30% of Good's syndrome presentations are associated with hematologic disorders [2, 3]. The most common associations are pure red cell aplasia and myasthenia gravis [2]. Conversely, pure white cell aplasia (PWCA) in setting of Good's syndrome is a rare occurrence, accounting for 1.1% of patients with thymoma [2]. PWCA is a hematologic disorder characterized by agranulocytosis with absent neutrophil-lineage cells in the bone marrow and preserved erythropoiesis and megakaryocytopoiesis. Most PWCA are associated with type A and mixed type AB thymomas [7]. PWCA has also been found to be associated with drugs, viruses, and other autoimmune disorders [8–11].

Although the etiology of PWCA seen in thymoma remains elusive in the literature, it is consensus that PWCA is of autoimmune origin. Many speculate that presence of thymoma leads to a loss of autoimmune regulator, thus creating a "window of opportunity" for autoimmune disease to develop [3, 12]. Two mechanistic pathways had been proposed to support this theory. The first pathway proposes that dysregulated production of cytokines, possibly mediated by neoplastic thymic stromal cells, influences the growth and differentiation of both the thymus and precursor B cells in the bone marrow [3]. For example, thymic stromal lymphopoietin (TSLP), an IL-7-like cytokine produced mainly by thymic epithelial cells, has wide-ranging impacts on the development of pre-B cells in the bone marrow, as well as regulatory T and Th17 cells in the thymus. Wang et al. found that the levels of TSLP mRNA and protein expression were lower in patients with thymoma-associated myasthenia gravis than in thymoma patients without myasthenia gravis [13]. Other studies of patients with thymic neoplasia also detect autoantibodies against cytokines and a decrease in in vitro cytokine production in response to T-cell simulation [14, 15]. These findings suggested that decrease in the expression of cytokines contribute to T-cell imbalance in the thymus and affect precursor B-cell development in the bone marrow. The second pathway proposes that the abnormal environment of thymoma prevents non-neoplastic T cell to undergo appropriate thymic central tolerance and maturation, thus leading to activation of autoreactive T cells [16]. When these cells escape into the circulation, they could precipitate autoimmune reactions and contribute to abnormal activation of B cells, yielding lymphocytic- and antibody-mediated toxicities to myelomonocytic precursor cells [3]. Interestingly, our patient's bone marrow biopsy showed rare to absent B cells, lack of aberrant immunophenotype on T cells, and agranulocytosis in absence of positive rheumatological tests. These findings suggest that potential inhibitory factors diminish the growth of progenitor cells involving myelocyte and lymphoid lineages.

This case highlights the care complexity regarding treatment choices in patients presenting with PWCA, particularly surgical intervention in the setting of neutropenia and concerns for wound healing. While thymectomy does not necessarily reverse the immunological abnormalities in Good's syndrome, some have observed clinical improvement following resection [17]. Our case demonstrated that while G-CSF and IVIg were completely ineffective prior to thymectomy, the bone marrow was responsive postoperatively. With regards to immunomodulatory agents, the repertoire is broad due to limited literature describing the use of chemotherapeutic agents [18]. In this presented case, cyclosporine treatment at minimal doses was used with complete resolution of PCWA. Patients with PCWA and Good's syndrome are at increased risk of fatal infections due to concurrent leukopenia and immunodeficiency, thus suggesting the importance of supportive care with antibiotics and IVIg. Lastly, similar to other paraneoplastic presentations of thymoma these patients run a risk of recurrence; thereby, they should remain on surveillance.

Consent

Patient consent was obtained for the case report.

References

[1] E. A. Engels, "Epidemiology of thymoma and associated malignancies," *Journal of Thoracic Oncology*, vol. 5, no. 10, pp. S260–S265, 2010.
[2] T. Kelesidis and O. Yang, "Good's syndrome remains a mystery after 55 years: a systematic review of the scientific evidence," *Clinical Immunology*, vol. 135, no. 3, pp. 347–363, 2010.
[3] P. Kelleher and S. A. Misbah, "What is good's syndrome? Immunological abnormalities in patients with thymoma," *Journal of Clinical Pathology*, vol. 56, no. 1, pp. 12–16, 2003.
[4] L. Degos, A. Faille, M. Housset, L. Boumsell, C. Rabian, and T. Parames, "Syndrome of neutrophil agranulocytosis, hypogammaglobulinemia, and thymoma," *Blood*, vol. 60, no. 4, pp. 968–972, 1982.
[5] I. Dzhagalov and H. Phee, "How to find your way through the thymus: a practical guide for aspiring T cells," *Cellular and Molecular Life Sciences*, vol. 69, no. 5, pp. 663–682, 2012.
[6] F. C. Detterbeck, "Evaluation and treatment of stage I and II thymoma," *Journal of Thoracic Oncology*, vol. 5, no. 10, pp. S318–S322, 2010.
[7] J.-P. Dong, W. Gao, G.-G. Teng, Y. Tian, and H.-H. Wang, "Characteristics of good's syndrome in China," *Chinese Medical Journal*, vol. 130, no. 13, pp. 1604–1609, 2017.
[8] K. Akinosoglou, M. Melachrinou, D. Siagris et al., "Good's syndrome and pure white cell aplasia complicated by cryptococcus infection: a case report and review of the literature," *Journal of Clinical Immunology*, vol. 34, no. 3, pp. 283–288, 2014.
[9] H. Tamura, M. Okamoto, T. Yamashita et al., "Pure white cell aplasia: report of the first case associated with primary biliary cirrhosis," *International Journal of Hematology*, vol. 85, no. 2, pp. 97–100, 2007.
[10] F. Frattini, S. Crestani, P. P. Vescovi, and M. Franchini, "Pure white cell aplasia induced by mesalazine in a patient with ulcerative colitis," *Hematology*, vol. 18, no. 3, pp. 181-182, 2013.
[11] Z. Fumeaux, P. Beris, B. Borisch et al., "Complete remission of pure white cell aplasia associated with thymoma, autoimmune thyroiditis and type 1 diabetes," *European Journal of Haematology*, vol. 70, no. 3, pp. 186–189, 2003.
[12] M. Cheng and M. S. Anderson, "Thymic tolerance as a key brake on autoimmunity," *Nature Immunology*, vol. 19, no. 7, pp. 659–664, 2018.
[13] Z. Wang, Y. Chen, S. Xu et al., "Aberrant decrease of microRNA19b regulates TSLP expression and contributes to Th17 cells development in myasthenia gravis related thymomas," *Journal of Neuroimmunology*, vol. 288, pp. 34–39, 2015.
[14] S. Raschal, J. Siegel, J. Huml, and G. Richmond, "Hypogammaglobulinemia and anemia 18 years after thymoma resection," *Journal of Allergy and Clinical Immunology*, vol. 100, no. 6, pp. 846–848, 1997.
[15] P. D. Burbelo, S. K. Browne, E. P. Sampaio et al., "Anti-cytokine autoantibodies are associated with opportunistic infection in patients with thymic neoplasia," *Blood*, vol. 116, no. 23, pp. 4848–4858, 2010.
[16] M. R. Khawaja, R. P. Nelson Jr., N. Miller et al., "Immune-mediated diseases and immunodeficiencies associated with thymic epithelial neoplasms," *Journal of Clinical Immunology*, vol. 32, no. 3, pp. 430–437, 2012.
[17] A. Jansen, M. van Deuren, J. Miller et al., "Prognosis of good syndrome: mortality and morbidity of thymoma associated immunodeficiency in perspective," *Clinical Immunology*, vol. 171, pp. 12–17, 2016.
[18] Y. Jethava, J. Alamelu, S. Rangarajan, L. Lang-Lazdunski, J. van der Walt, and P. Fields, "Acquired agranulocytosis and factor XI deficiency in association with thymoma," *Journal of Clinical Oncology*, vol. 29, no. 20, pp. e604–e606, 2011.

2

An Unusual Initial Presentation of Diffuse Large B-Cell Lymphoma as Recurrent Syncope

Kunhwa Kim[1] **Harpreet Kaur,**[1] **Matthew Chan,**[1] **Manju Balasubramanian,**[2] **Sorab Gupta**[3] **and Vinicius M. Jorge**[3]

[1]*Department of Internal Medicine, Einstein Medical Center Philadelphia, Philadelphia, PA, USA*
[2]*Department of Pathology, Einstein Medical Center Philadelphia, Philadelphia, PA, USA*
[3]*Department of Hematology-Oncology, Einstein Medical Center Philadelphia, Philadelphia, PA, USA*

Correspondence should be addressed to Kunhwa Kim; kimkunhw@einstein.edu

Academic Editor: Dennis Galanakis

We describe a rare presentation of diffuse large B-cell Lymphoma (DLBCL) with recurrent episodes of syncope. During the workup for syncope, the patient was incidentally found to have an extensive mass in the left thorax, which was later diagnosed as stage 2 bulky disease DLBCL. This is the rare case of lymphoma presenting as recurrent syncope without cardiac involvement. The patient did not have any further episodes of syncope after her successful treatment of DLBCL.

1. Introduction

Diffuse large B-cell lymphoma (DLBCL) is the most common subtype of non-Hodgkin's lymphoma (NHL) that accounts for about 30% of adult lymphoma [1]. Patients with DLBCL can have a myriad of presentations from constitutional symptoms such as B symptoms to localized effects from a rapidly growing mass.

Malignancy presenting as syncope is rare, but a few numbers of cases have been reported in tumors involving the neck [2, 3]. So far, most of these reported cases were in patients with recurrent head and neck cancer. Syncope from DLBCL without cardiac involvement, despite its frequent cervical involvement, has been only reported in 3 cases thus far to our knowledge [4–6].

Here, we present an unusual case of a patient who presented with recurrent episodes of syncope without other complaints. During workup for syncope, the patient was incidentally found to have an extensive mass in the left thorax, which was later diagnosed as DLBCL. Other diagnostics for syncope were unremarkable. The patient did not have any further episodes of syncope after her successful treatment of DLBCL.

2. Case Presentation

A 52-year-old African-American female with a past medical history of type 2 diabetes mellitus, hypertension, and hyperlipidemia presented to the emergency department (ED) after a syncopal episode in her home. The patient was in her usual health state before the episode. She felt dizzy while standing up and collapsed within a few seconds resulting in unconsciousness. She regained consciousness shortly afterward with residual dizziness, but otherwise did not report any symptoms before or after this episode. No seizure-like activity or incontinence was reported. Her medications included insulin, amlodipine, lisinopril, and escitalopram. The blood glucose level was normal prior to arrival. She has been adherent to all medications as prescribed. She denied weight loss, night sweats, or fatigue. She denied trauma, alcohol abuse, or drug intake. Interestingly, a week before this event, the patient had presented to the ED after a similar near syncopal episode. During her first encounter, she was discharged home with a recommendation to be followed-up by her primary care physician (PCP) with initial workup to be negative at the time. She unfortunately did not follow with her PCP.

On presentation, her vital signs were normal: heart rate was 98 beats/minute, blood pressure was 126/60 mmHg without orthostatic changes, respiratory rate was 16, and the oxygen saturation on room air was 98%. On the initial physical exam, she was well in appearance and not in any distress. The cardiac, pulmonary, and neurologic exams were unremarkable. The laboratory evaluation was within normal range: white blood count of 9,370/μL, hemoglobin of 12.8 g/dL, and platelet count of 245,000/μL. Routine blood chemistries panel were normal: BUN/Cr 19/0.8 mg/dL, sodium 141, potassium 4.6, glucose 109 mg/dL, AST/ALT 12/13 units/L, LDH 173 mg/dL, and uric acid 5.0 mg/dL.

Her EKG showed normal sinus rhythm without ST changes. Her 2 d echocardiogram was normal with preserved ejection fraction at 55% without increased pulmonary arterial pressure. Her chest X-ray with a lateral view had a questionable enhancement in the mediastinum. The following CT head and angiography of head and neck obtained as a part of the recurrent syncope workup revealed widely patent cervical and intracranial circulation without abnormality (Figure 1). Incidentally, a soft tissue mass was found in the superior and the posterior mediastinum.

The patient was admitted to the general medical floor for further workup for the mediastinal mass and syncope. She underwent CT chest with contrast and MRI with and without contrast which showed an anterior and left posterior mediastinum mass measuring $4.4 \times 5.7 \times 13.5$ cm encasing the descending aorta and multiple left-sided intercostal vessels with epidural extension into the left-sided neural foramina from T4-5 through T6-7 (Figure 2). There was no invasion or mechanical compression of aorta. There were bilateral bulky axillary lymph nodes measuring up to 5 cm. There were no findings of pulmonary embolism or compromised vascularity. The patient did not have any prominent neurologic deficit but was started on dexamethasone empirically due to concerns for possible cord compression.

After a biopsy of an axillary lymph node, the patient was diagnosed with diffuse large B-cell lymphoma (Figure 3). Her FISH test was negative for double hit/triple hit lymphoma. She underwent bone marrow biopsy and lumbar puncture for CSF cytology. Results from both tests were negative for tumor infiltration into the bone marrow and CSF. Her PET/CT was negative for disease in the spleen and below the diaphragm. She was staged as stage II bulky lymphoma by Lugano modification of Ann Arbor staging system with NCCN-IPI score of 2.

The patient received 6 cycles of chemotherapy with cyclophosphamide, doxorubicin, vincristine, and prednisone plus rituximab (R-CHOP) and monthly intrathecal methotrexate infusion with each cycle of chemotherapy. Repeated PET/CT after completion of treatment showed no evidence of disease. She had one more repeat syncopal episode before treatment initiation, and her telemetry monitor more than 24-hour was uneventful. She had no further episodes since treatment. She denied any episode of dizziness, vertigo, or near syncopal episode during follow-up. The patient is currently awaiting consolidative therapy with radiation.

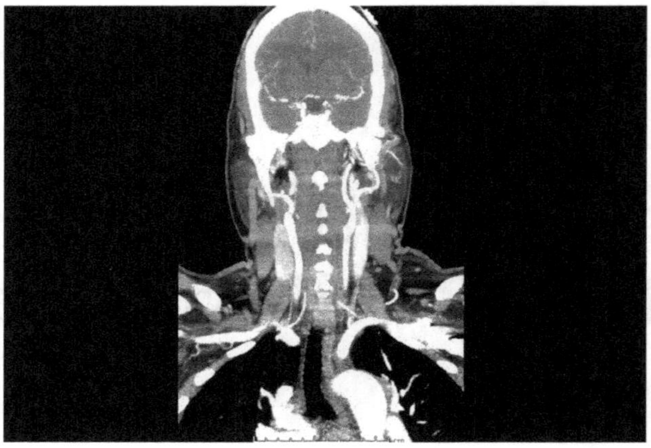

FIGURE 1: CT angiography shows patient blood circulation without tumor infiltration or encasement of the carotid body or the carotid sinus.

3. Discussion

Syncope is one of the most common presentations accounting for 1–3% of the total ED visits and admissions [7]. The differential diagnosis for syncope is broad, and making a diagnosis is often challenging. Syncope presentation as the first and the only symptom in malignancies is exceedingly rare. Only a few cases have been reported, and most of these cases were from patients with recurrent head and neck cancer [2, 3] or lung cancer [8].

Our case highlights an atypical presentation of DLBCL as recurrent syncope. The patient presented with episodes of syncope associated with fast recovery and no symptoms in between these episodes. Her syncope was initially confused with vasovagal syncope because of its similar characteristics and no other symptoms at baseline. The patient also did not have derangement in vital signs or electrolytes at presentation. Her further syncope workup including orthostatic vital signs, EKGs, later hospitalization under telemetry monitor, 2D echo, or CT brain and angiography was all normal.

To our knowledge, there are 7 reported cases of lymphoma presenting as syncope without direct cardiac involvement (3 cases of diffuse large B-cell lymphoma [4–6], 2 of primary mediastinal lymphoma [9, 10], and 2 of Hodgkin's lymphoma [11, 12]). All previously reported cases were found to have mechanical infiltrates or vascular compromise from the mass. Our case was interesting that the patient had an extensive mass in the anterior and the posterior mediastinum surrounding the descending aorta; however, both her CT angiography of head and neck and CT chest with contrast showed intact vasculature in the head and neck and also in the aorta. She did not have persistent bradycardia or hypotension, and there was also no apparent infiltration around the carotid body or around the aorta.

Many of the previously reported cases of malignancies presenting as syncope described similarities to vasovagal syncope as our case. The exact etiology of vasovagal-like syncope arising from underlying malignancies remains unknown. Literature review from previous similar case

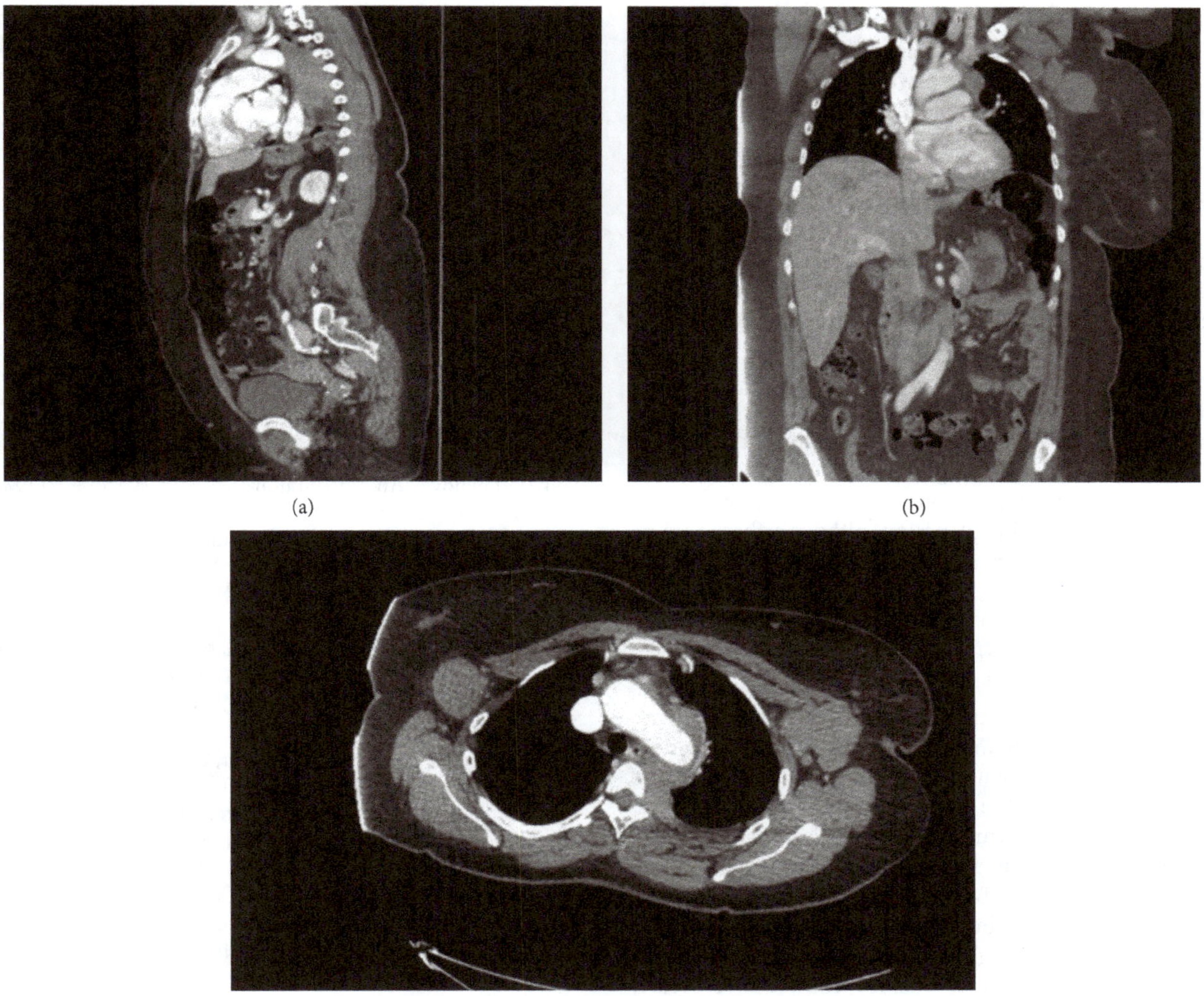

(a) (b) (c)

FIGURE 2: Sagittal (a), coronal (b), and axial (c) images of CT chest with contrast shows posterior mediastinal mass that encases descending aorta and extensively infiltrates to epidural space.

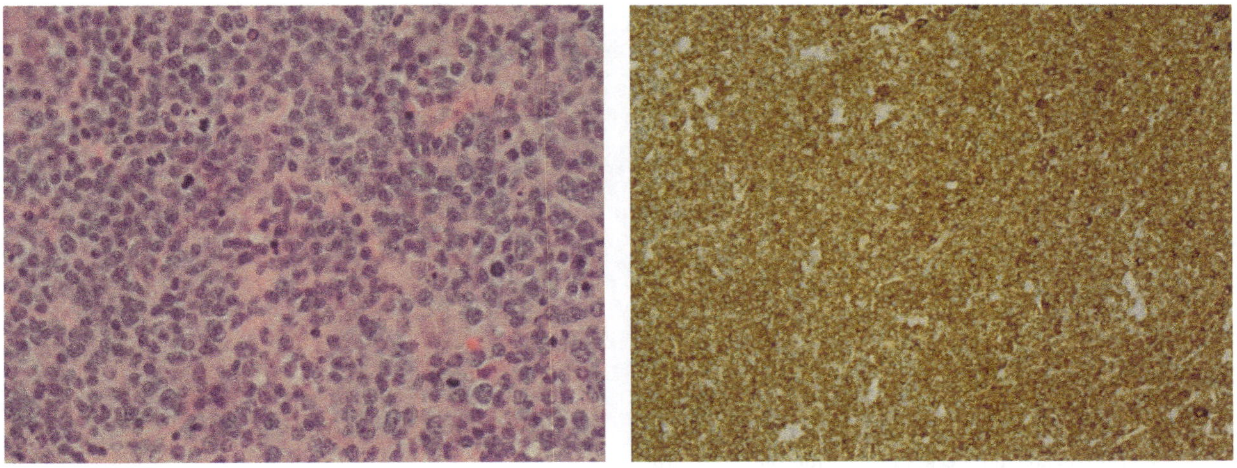

(a) (b)

FIGURE 3: Immunohistological staining of the axillary lymph node: hematoxylin and eosin stain ×60 (a) and CD20 stain ×20 (b).

reports postulated that "irritation" of the vagus nerve might be the cause. A case series of syncope in lung cancer patients interestingly found that there was a higher incidence of syncope in patients with tumors located in the left hilum like our case [8]. This irritation also might explain that syncope is more prominent in patients with head and neck cancer with recurrence [13]. Our case had nonspecific lymphadenopathy along the left-sided carotid artery, which could be a potential explanation of the cause of syncope. Another possible explanation of etiology in our case could be syncope as an atypical, paraneoplastic, and systemic presentation as diffuse large B-cell lymphoma is known for, like B-cell lymphoma symptoms. A few cases have reported syncope as paraneoplastic neurologic syndromes in the past including Hodgkin's lymphoma, manifesting as autonomic failure [14, 15]. Then, this case might illustrate that syncope in malignancy, especially in lymphoma patients, may not have an obvious anatomical explanation, although there was no obvious electrolytes or hormonal derangement in the workup studies.

Our patient had no further episodes of syncope after her successful treatment with R-CHOP and 6 times of intrathecal methotrexate treatment, and she achieved full remission for her lymphoma. Case series of head and neck cancer patients with syncope showed that treatment of malignancy improved the syncope from 13 out of 17 cases [2]. Most of reported lymphoma cases also described successful treatment of syncope after treatment. Notably, our patient had a comparatively good short-term prognosis, despite extensive tumor burden from stage 2 bulky disease. In our case, syncope might be considered as a rare mass effect from DLBCL, which enables comparatively early presentation.

Here, we described a rare presentation of diffuse large B-cell lymphoma which was incidentally diagnosed while on workup for recurrent syncope. Syncope as the presentation of malignancy is rare and challenging to make as a clinical-anatomic correlation. We suggest that malignancy might be considered as a cause of recurrent syncope in the case of patients who have unexplained etiology, despite multiple investigations and of patients with significant history that raises concerns for cancers in thorax including lymphoma.

References

[1] S. H. Swerdlow, E. Campo, N. L. Harris et al., "WHO classification of tumours of haematopoietic and lymphoid tissues," in *IARC WHO Classification of Tumours*, vol. 2, International Agency for Research on Cancer (IARC), Lyon, France, 4th edition, 2017.

[2] D. R. Macdonald, E. Strong, S. Nielsen, and J. B. Posner, "Syncope from head and neck cancer," *Journal of Neuro-Oncology*, vol. 1, no. 3, pp. 257–267, 1983.

[3] C. A. Bauer, M. I. Redleaf, M. G. Gartlan, T. T. Tsue, and T. M. McColloch, "Carotid sinus syncope in head and neck cancer," *The Laryngoscope*, vol. 104, no. 4, pp. 497–503, 1994.

[4] B. Chen, C. Zou, and J. Wu, "Diffuse large B-cell non-Hodgkin lymphoma involving the unilateral carotid space in an elderly man: a case report," *Molecular and Clinical Oncology*, vol. 6, no. 1, pp. 115–118, 2017.

[5] K. Yoshifuku, K. Nishimoto, T. Matsuzaki, and M. Ushikai, "A case of neurally mediated syncope caused by cervical malignant lymphoma," *Journal of Otolaryngology of Japan*, vol. 118, no. 6, pp. 776–781, 2015.

[6] A. Li, A. Bandali, S. Ghani, and C. Reid, "Neurocardiogenic syncope: a rare presentation of pharyngeal lymphoma," *BMJ Case Reports*, vol. 2012, p. bcr2012007333, 2012.

[7] W. N. Kapoor, "Evaluation and outcome of patients with syncope," *Medicine*, vol. 69, no. 3, pp. 160–175, 1990.

[8] X. Jiang, J. Zhao, C. Bai, E. Xu, Z. Chen, and Y. Han, "Small-cell lung cancer with recurrent syncope as the initial symptom: a case report and literature review," *Molecular and Clinical Oncology*, vol. 5, no. 5, pp. 545–549, 2016.

[9] C. Shenoy, "An uncommon cause of syncope," *QJM: An International Journal of Medicine*, vol. 101, no. 3, p. 241, 2008.

[10] J. Dúbrava, L. Drgoňa, and R. Kadlečík, "An unusual cause of recurrent syncope: mediastinal lymphoma diagnosed with transesophageal echocardiography," *European Journal of Internal Medicine*, vol. 16, no. 3, pp. 204–206, 2005.

[11] R. Félix, A. Fonseca, and A. Góis, "Carotid sinus syndrome in a patient with Hodgkin's lymphoma," *International Journal of Case Reports in Medicine*, vol. 2015, Article ID 620549, 4 pages, 2015.

[12] I. Arapakis, M. Fradis, J. Schipper, G. J. Ridder, and W. Maier, "Recurrent syncope as presenting symptom of Burkitt's lymphoma at the carotid bifurcation," *Annals of Otology, Rhinology and Laryngology*, vol. 113, no. 5, pp. 373–377, 2004.

[13] M. Nakahira, H. Nakatani, and T. Takeda, "Syncope as a sign of occult malignant recurrence in the retropharyngeal and parapharyngeal space: CT and MR imaging findings in four cases," *American Journal of Neuro Radiology*, vol. 23, no. 7, pp. 1257–1260, 2002.

[14] C. Shibao, P. Muppa, M. W. Semler, and I. Biaggioni, "A standing dilemma: autonomic failure preceding Hodgkin's lymphoma," *The American Journal of Medicine*, vol. 127, no. 4, pp. 284–287, 2014.

[15] M. Ghadiri-Sani, M. Waqar, D. Smith, and M. Doran, "Paraneoplastic neurological syndromes: severe neurological symptoms resulting from relatively benign or occult tumours—two case reports," *Case Reports in Oncological Medicine*, vol. 2013, Article ID 458378, 5 pages, 2013.

3

A Rare Case of Midostaurin-Associated Sweet's Syndrome

Hesham Yasin, Tessa Laytem, Grerk Sutamtewagul, and Sabarish Ayyappan

University of Iowa Health Care, Iowa City, Iowa, USA

Correspondence should be addressed to Hesham Yasin; hishamyassin@gmail.com

Academic Editor: Stephen E. Langabeer

Acute febrile neutrophilic dermatosis which is referred as Sweet's syndrome (SS) is a dermatological condition characterized by fever, erythematous rash, and leukocytosis. SS can be idiopathic or associated with malignancies or medications. We present a rare case of SS which developed shortly after starting midostaurin in a patient with acute myelogenous leukemia (AML).

1. Introduction

Acute febrile neutrophilic dermatosis, known as Sweet's syndrome (SS), is a dermatological condition characterized by abrupt appearance of erythematous rash, accompanied frequently by the presence of fever and leukocytosis. Majority of cases are idiopathic or malignancy-associated but rarely can be drug-induced. Midostaurin, a recently FDA-approved agent, has shown improved outcomes in FLT3-mutated acute myeloid leukemia (AML). To date, there are three reported cases in which midostaurin administration had a temporal association with the onset of SS. We are presenting here another similar case.

2. Case Presentation

A 60-year-old Caucasian male with no significant medical history presented to his primary care physician with a one-month history of fatigue, decreased appetite, 15-pound weight loss, and easy bruising and bleeding. Physical exam at that time was remarkable only for moderately pale conjunctiva. Laboratory evaluation was remarkable for a hemoglobin level of 8.3 g/dL, WBC count of 2.6 k/mm^3, and platelet count of 28 k/mm^3. The peripheral blood differential was remarkable for occasional blasts and elevated lactate dehydrogenase (LDH) at 402 U/L. The kidney and liver function tests were normal. Given the pancytopenia and presence of blasts in the peripheral smear, a bone marrow aspiration and biopsy were obtained, which showed acute myeloid leukemia (AML) with genetic studies showing mutated TP53, NPM1, PTPN11, and FLT3. The patient was admitted to the hospital and started on induction chemotherapy with cytarabine and daunorubicin (7 + 3 regimen). He tolerated the initial course and had no significant events except for expected gradual decrement in blood cell count. On day eight of hospitalization, the patient was started on midostaurin due to positive FLT3 mutation and high-risk disease. Within 12 hours of starting midostaurin (day 9), he developed intermittent fevers. Routine infectious workup was sent, and cefepime was started empirically. The patient's fevers continued, and given the persistent fever, cefepime was discontinued two days later (day 11) and antibiotics were escalated to piperacillin-tazobactam and vancomycin. No source of infection was found at that time. On the same day (day 11), the patient reported a mildly painful and nonpruritic rash. He first noticed it on both arms, and subsequently, the rash spread to bilateral lower extremities. On exam, the patient had bilateral pink-to-erythematous, scattered, edematous papules with very few hemorrhagic changes (Figure 1). There was no other rash seen on his bilateral upper and lower extremities. Blood work at that time was notable for a hemoglobin level of 6.4 g/dL, WBC count of 0.4 k/mm^3, platelets of 21 k/mm^3, and neutrophil count of 250/mm^3. The patient then underwent punch biopsy of a single skin lesion on the upper arm. Results showed findings of spongiosis with focal intraepidermal vesiculation as well as papillary dermal edema with upper dermal neutrophilic and lymphocytic inflammation with extravasated

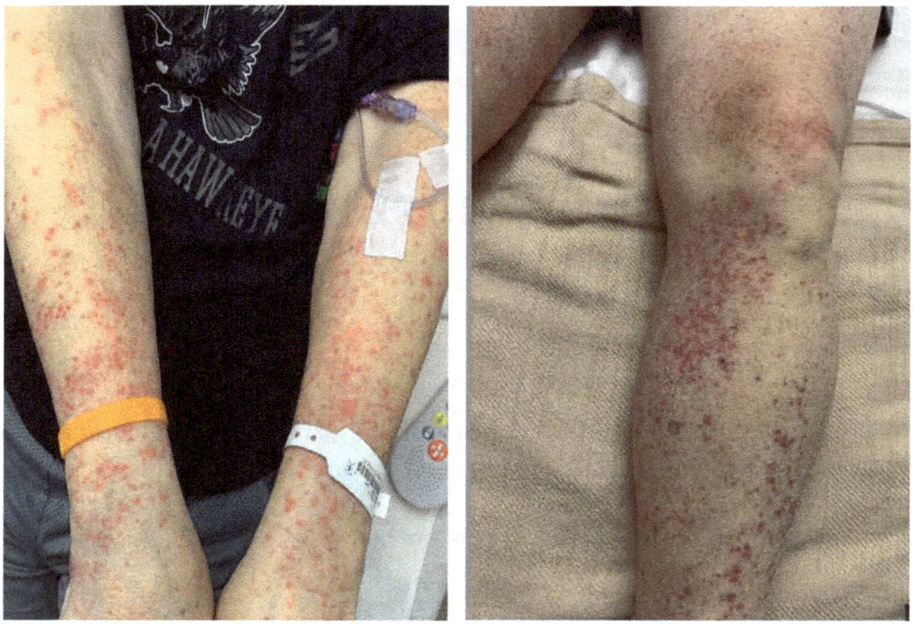

FIGURE 1: Maculopapular rash in the patient's bilateral upper and lower extremities.

erythrocytes. These findings, in the context of the clinical picture, were consistent with SS (Figure 2). The patient was then started on prednisone 60 mg daily. Over the next few days, the patient demonstrated rapid improvement of the rash. Prednisone tapering was started after seven days with planned incremental decrease by 10 mg every four days until discontinuation. The patient continued to spike fevers for seven days after the prednisone was started. Repeat infectious workup did not localize any source of infection, and therefore, it was presumed the fever was due to SS. Midostaurin was continued after the diagnosis of SS. The patient was continued to follow up with the leukemia clinic on a regular basis. The patient went into remission and then started AML consolidation therapy. To date, he has not had recurrence of the rash. The list of the drugs the patient was taking 30 days prior to the development of rash is presented in Table 1.

3. Discussion

Acute febrile neutrophilic dermatitis, first described by Sweet in 1964 and hence named "Sweet's syndrome" after him [1], is an inflammatory dermatological disease caused by extensive infiltration of the dermis and epidermis by neutrophils [2]. It is characterized by fever, neutrophilia, and tender erythematous skin lesions that can be papules, nodules, or plaques [3]. Sweet's syndrome is classified into three subtypes: classical (or idiopathic) SS, malignancy-associated SS, and drug-associated SS [3]. Classical SS is diagnosed when malignancy is ruled out and no temporal association with a drug can be established. It is more common in women and often associated with recent upper respiratory tract or gastrointestinal infection, pregnancy, and inflammatory bowel disease [4–6]. Hematological malignancies account for the largest proportion of malignancy-associated SS, and in a review, AML was the commonest malignancy to be associated with this subtype [7, 8]. There are multiple agents that have been reported to be associated with development of drug-associated SS. Frequently reported medications associated with SS include granulocyte-colony stimulating factor, trimethoprim-sulfamethoxazole, azathioprine, minocycline, and all-trans retinoic acid [9–11]. Fever is the most common extracutaneous symptom which can precede the rash by several days to weeks [3]. Dermatological manifestations are usually painful, red-to-purple-colored papules or nodules which may coalesce into larger plaques. Lesions are usually asymmetrically distributed and commonly occur on the face, upper extremities, and neck [12]. There are several reports of extracutaneous manifestations such as arthralgia and arthritis, encephalitis, and ocular manifestations in the literature [13–15]. Diagnostic criteria are summarized in Table 2. To make a diagnosis, presence of two major criteria and at least two minor criteria is required. To establish the diagnosis of malignancy-associated SS, temporal relationship must occur between malignancy and symptoms in addition to meeting the criteria for diagnosis of classical SS. Diagnostic criteria for drug-induced SS are summarized in Table 3, and all of the five criteria must be present to establish the diagnosis [3, 9]. Histological examination will reveal a characteristic diffuse infiltrate predominantly consisting of mature neutrophils typically located in the upper dermis [2]. Lesions left untreated can persist for weeks to months [16]. Treatment of malignancy or discontinuation of the offending drug can result in subsequent improvement and disappearance of symptoms [3]. Topical or intralesional corticosteroids can be used to treat patients who have a small number of lesions [17]. Systemic corticosteroids are the mainstay for therapy and usually result in dramatic improvement of symptoms within 72 hours. The starting prednisone dose ranges from 0.5 to 1.5 mg/kg/day which is slowly tapered over several weeks [2, 17]. Potassium iodide

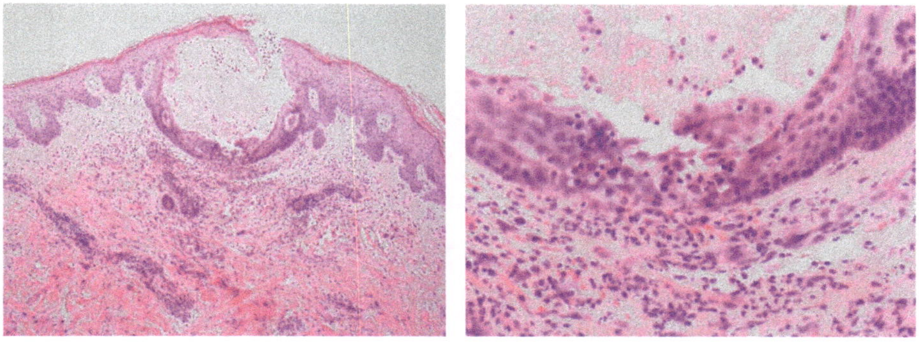

Figure 2: Microscopic view of the pathological specimen from skin biopsy: spongiosis with focal intraepidermal vesiculation as well as papillary dermal edema with upper dermal neutrophilic and lymphocytic inflammation with extravasated erythrocytes.

Table 1: Drug administered to the patient prior to the onset of rash (none has been reported to be associated with Sweet's syndrome except midostaurin).

Medication	Days the medication was administered prior to the onset of rash
Amoxicillin-clavulanic acid	30
Cytarabine	11
Daunorubicin	11
Allopurinol	11
Ciprofloxacin	11
Isavuconazonium	3
Midostaurin	3
Piperacillin-tazobactam	1
Cefepime	2
Vancomycin	1

Table 2: Diagnostic criteria for Sweet's syndrome.

Major criteria	Minor criteria
Abrupt onset of painful erythematous papules, nodules, or plaques	Fever >38°C
Histopathological findings of dense neutrophilic infiltrates without evidence of leukocytoclastic vasculitis	Association with hematologic or visceral malignancy, inflammatory disease, or pregnancy, or preceded by upper respiratory tract infection, gastrointestinal infection, or vaccination
	Dramatic response to treatment with systemic steroids or potassium iodide
	Abnormalities in laboratory tests (three of four): erythrocyte sedimentation rate >20 mm/h; high C-reactive protein; leukocytes >8000, with >70% neutrophils

Table 3: Diagnostic criteria for drug-induced Sweet's syndrome.

Diagnostic criteria	Presence in our patient
Abrupt onset of painful erythematous papules, nodules, or plaques	Yes
Histopathological findings of dense neutrophilic infiltrates without evidence of leukocytoclastic vasculitis	Yes
Fever >38°C	Yes
Temporal relation between use of medication and clinical presentation or relapse with readministration	Yes
Disappearance of lesions after discontinuation of drug or treatment with systemic steroids	Yes

has been previously reported but can be difficult to titrate and safely administer [18]. There are many reports of steroid-sparing agents including colchicine, dapsone, and cyclosporine [17, 19, 20].

Midostaurin, a tyrosine kinase inhibitor, is a targeted drug therapy for FLT3-mutated AML [21]. The most common side effects for this agent are cytopenia, neutropenic fever, and gastrointestinal and pulmonary complaints. Rash was reported as a side effect, but there are no reports of SS in clinical trials [22]. To the best of our knowledge, there are three case reports of patients who developed Sweet's syndrome while being treated with midostaurin [23–25]. Our patient developed SS just three days after starting the treatment. Among all the listed medications that the patient was taking in the last 30 days (Table 1), none of these medications were reported in the literature to be associated with SS. The patient's underlying AML is very likely to be the causative inducer of SS, but the temporal association with midostaurin administration was assumed to contribute to the pathogenesis. Our patient met the five criteria required for drug-induced SS (Table 3), and the patient had resolution with steroid treatment. In conclusion, midostaurin is an effective agent against FLT3-mutated AML, and it has been increasingly used in clinical practice. It is important to consider midostaurin as a culprit medication in the setting of SS.

References

[1] R. B. Sweet, "AN acute febrile neutrophtlic dermatosts," *British Journal of Dermatology*, vol. 76, no. 8-9, pp. 349–356, 1964.

[2] C. D. Villarreal-Villarreal, J. Ocampo-Candiani, and A. Villarreal-Martínez, "Sweet syndrome: a review and update," *Actas Dermo-Sifiliográficas*, vol. 107, no. 5, pp. 369–378, 2016.

[3] P. R. Cohen, "Sweet's syndrome—a comprehensive review of an acute febrile neutrophilic dermatosis," *Orphanet Journal of Rare Diseases*, vol. 2, no. 1, 2007.

[4] A. Lallas, T. G. Tzellos, M. Papageorgiou, and I. Mandekou-Lefaki, "Sweet's syndrome associated with upper respiratory tract streptococcal infection: "wait-and-see" strategy or anecdotal use of corticosteroids?" *Hippokratia*, vol. 15, no. 3, p. 283, 2011.

[5] H. Ytting, I. Vind, D. Bang, and P. Munkholm, "Sweet's syndrome—an extraintestinal manifestation in inflammatory bowel disease," *Digestion*, vol. 72, no. 2-3, pp. 195–200, 2005.

[6] P. R. Cohen, A. Zalka, and M. E. Grossman, "Sweet's syndrome and pregnancy," *Journal of the American Academy of Dermatology*, vol. 30, no. 2, pp. 297–300, 1994.

[7] S. Raza, R. S. Kirkland, A. A. Patel, J. R. Shortridge, and C. Freter, "Insight into sweet's syndrome and associated-malignancy: a review of the current literature," *International Journal of Oncology*, vol. 42, no. 5, pp. 1516–1522, 2013.

[8] C. A. Nelson, M. H. Noe, C. M. McMahon et al., "Sweet syndrome in patients with and without malignancy: a retrospective analysis of 83 patients from a tertiary academic referral center," *Journal of the American Academy of Dermatology*, vol. 78, no. 2, pp. 303–309, 2018.

[9] D. C. Walker and P. R. Cohen, "Trimethoprim-sulfamethoxazole-associated acute febrile neutrophilic dermatosis: case report and review of drug-induced sweet's syndrome," *Journal of the American Academy of Dermatology*, vol. 34, pp. 918–923, 1996.

[10] B. Arun, B. Berberian, N. Azumic, S. R. Frankela, H. Luksenburga, and C. Fretera, "Sweet's syndrome during treatment with all-trans retinoic acid in a patient with acute promyelocytic leukemia," *Leukemia and Lymphoma*, vol. 31, no. 5-6, pp. 613–615, 1998.

[11] M.-J. Thibault, R. C. Billick, and H. Srolovitz, "Minocycline-induced sweet's syndrome," *Journal of the American Academy of Dermatology*, vol. 27, no. 5, pp. 801–804, 1992.

[12] C. Hofmann, O. Braun-Falco, and D. Petzoldt, "Akute febrile neutrophile dermatose (sweet-syndrom)," *DMW—Deutsche Medizinische Wochenschrift*, vol. 101, no. 30, pp. 1113–1118, 1976.

[13] M. Cugno, R. Gualtierotti, P. L. Meroni, and A. V. Marzano, "Inflammatory joint disorders and neutrophilic dermatoses: a comprehensive review," *Clinical Reviews in Allergy and Immunology*, vol. 54, no. 2, pp. 269–281, 2018.

[14] Y. Nobeyama and R. Kamide, "Sweet's syndrome with neurologic manifestation: case report and literature review," *International Journal of Dermatology*, vol. 42, no. 6, pp. 438–443, 2003.

[15] B. Baartman, P. Kosari, C. C. Warren et al., "Sight-threatening ocular manifestations of acute febrile neutrophilic dermatosis (sweet's syndrome)," *Dermatology*, vol. 228, no. 3, pp. 193–197, 2014.

[16] P. R. Cohen, L. Almeida, and R. Kurzrock, "Acute febrile neutrophilic dermatosis," 1989, https://europepmc.org/article/med/2646883.

[17] P. R. Cohen and R. Kurzrock, "Sweet's syndrome," *American Journal of Clinical Dermatology*, vol. 3, no. 2, pp. 117–131, 2002.

[18] T. Horio, S. Imamura, K. Danno, F. Furukawa, and S. Ofuji, "Treatment of acute febrile neutrophilic dermatosis (sweet's syndrome) with potassium iodide," *Dermatology*, vol. 160, no. 5, pp. 341–347, 1980.

[19] H. Aram, "Acute febrile neutrophilic dermatosis (sweet's syndrome)," *Archives of Dermatology*, vol. 120, no. 2, pp. 245–247, 1984.

[20] H. Maillard, C. Leclech, P. Peria, M. Avenel-Audran, and J. L. Verret, "Colchicine for sweet's syndrome. a study of 20 cases," *British Journal of Dermatology*, vol. 140, no. 3, pp. 565-566, 1999.

[21] M. Levis, "Midostaurin approved for FLT3-mutated AML," *Blood*, vol. 129, no. 26, pp. 3403–3406, 2017.

[22] R. M. Stone, S. J. Mandrekar, B. L. Sanford et al., "Midostaurin plus chemotherapy for acute myeloid leukemia with aFLT3mutation," *New England Journal of Medicine*, vol. 377, no. 5, pp. 454–464, 2017.

[23] A. Kaur, M. S. Jacobs, and S. Raza, "Characteristics of sweet's syndrome associated with novel acute myeloid leukemia targeted drugs-midostaurin and enasidenib," *Advances in Cell and Gene Therapy*, vol. 2, no. 4, 2019.

[24] S. Alkassis, A. Rizwan, L. Daoud, and J. Chi, "Midostaurin-induced sweet syndrome in a patient with FLT3-ITD-positive AML," *BMJ Case Reports*, vol. 14, no. 8, Article ID e243615, 2021.

[25] S. Chiewchanvit, S. Jamjanya, T. Rattanathammethee, P. Mahanupab, N. Tovanabutra, and M. Chuamanochan, "Bullous sweet syndrome in a patient with acute myeloid leukemia treated with midostaurin. rapid response to acitretin and colchicine: a case report," *Dermatologic Therapy*, vol. 34, Article ID e15171, 2021.

4

Concurrent B Cell Acute Lymphoblastic Lymphoma/Leukemia and Monoclonal B Cell Lymphocytosis: A Case Report with Extensive Molecular Analysis

Maryam Mehdipour Dalivand,[1] **Parastou Tizro**,[1] **Julie Partain**,[2] **Anita Aggarwal**,[3,4] **Jack Lichy**,[1,5] **Francisco Mot Ara**,[6] **and Victor E. Nava**[1,5,6]

[1]*The George Washington University, Department of Pathology, Washington, DC, USA*
[2]*Oregon Health and Science University, Portland, OR, USA*
[3]*The George Washington University, Department of Medicine, Hematology and Oncology, Washington, DC, USA*
[4]*Veterans Health Administration, Department of Internal Medicine, Oncology and Hematology, Washington, DC, USA*
[5]*Veterans Health Administration, Department of Pathology, Washington, DC, USA*
[6]*Hospital J.M. de Los Rios, Department of Pathology, Caracas, Venezuela*

Correspondence should be addressed to Victor E. Nava; victor.nava@va.gov

Academic Editor: Sudhir Tauro

Although acute lymphoblastic leukemia (ALL) and monoclonal B cell lymphocytosis (MBL) are common neoplasia, a simultaneous presentation is very unusual. Here, we present two different B cell clones, MBL and B-ALL, cocirculating in a 78-year-old African American male. Detailed molecular characterization revealed an unusual MPL (T487I) point mutation and unmutated VH4-39. After nonstandard chemotherapy, the patient remains in morphologic remission. These findings may stimulate further research to clarify the pathogenesis of hematologic neoplasms.

1. Introduction

Acute lymphoblastic leukemia (ALL) is the second most common acute leukemia in adults [1] and the most common in children. The average lifetime risk of developing ALL is approximately 1 in 1000 and higher in white males older than 70 years with prior exposure to genotoxic stimuli [2].

This malignancy of unknown etiology has not been reported in association with monoclonal B cell lymphocytosis (MBL), which is defined as the presence of less than 5×10^9/L clonal B cells in peripheral blood (PB) of asymptomatic patients without lymphadenopathy, organomegaly, or cytopenia, has been reported in up to 12% of the healthy individuals older than 40 years of age, and may be a precursor of chronic lymphocytic leukemia (CLL). MBL is divided into three subtypes: CLL-type (75% of cases) sharing immunophenotypic characteristics of CLL: CD19+, dim CD20+, CD5+, CD23+, dim surface immunoglobulin (Ig) light chain+, and FMC7−; atypical CLL-type: harboring atypical CLL immunophenotypic features, such as bright CD20, lack of CD23, and/or expression of FMC7; and non-CLL-type: CD5-negative and usually also lacking CD10 expression, as seen in marginal zone B cell lymphoma, lymphoplasmacytic lymphoma, and hairy cell leukemia. The epidemiology of MBL has strong parallels with CLL being associated with age older than 60 years, male gender, and family history of the disease. However, as with CLL or ALL, the exact etiology is unknown [3].

Here, we present a novel coexistence of B-ALL and CLL-type MBL with extensive molecular characterization.

2. Case Report

A 78-year-old African American male with the medical history of Agent Orange exposure, hypertension, diabetes mellitus, benign prostatic hyperplasia, asthma, colon polyps, and sleep apnea presented to a primary care physician with intermittent back pain and fatigue for a month. A computed tomography scan revealed diffuse subtle mixed sclerotic/lytic bone lesions in the axial skeleton/iliac bones, which appear to be increasing in size over a period of 10 years. No relevant family history was identified. Clinical or radiological evidence of lymphadenopathy or organomegaly was absent. Multiple myeloma work up was negative (including normal serum and urine protein electrophoresis, serum kappa/lambda free light chains, beta2-microglobulin, and immunoparesis of IgA (<500 mg/L) and IgM (<50 mg/L)). However, an elevated lactate dehydrogenase (266 units/L) was noted. Complete blood counts showed normal white blood cell count (6700/mm^3) with absolute lymphocytosis (4600/mm^3, normal range 0.8–3.1/mm^3), mild normocytic anemia (hemoglobin of 11.3 mg/dl), and normal platelets count (188000/mm^3). PB smear review showed mild polychromasia, mild left shift (few myelocytes), few nucleated red blood cells, and atypical lymphocytosis comprised of two morphologically distinct populations (Figure 1). Most atypical lymphocytes represented mature small forms with subtle nuclear irregularities and clumpy chromatin, suggestive of low-grade lymphoproliferative disorder. However, a few undifferentiated blasts with fine chromatin, high nuclear: cytoplasmic ratio, and prominent nucleoli were also noted, concerning for high-grade hematopoietic malignancy (Figure 1).

Flow cytometry (FC) analysis using standard CD45 vs. side scatter gating (Figure 1) revealed approximately 17% lymphoblasts positive for CD19, CD22, CD10, CD34, HLA-DR, and TdT and negative for CD20, CD5, CD23, CD25, CD103, CD11c, CD36, CD56, MPO, CD13, CD33, and CD14, compatible with evolving B-ALL. In addition, approximately 35% of lymphocytes (23% of total cells gated, 1600 lymphocytes/mm^3) represented monoclonal surface kappa-restricted mature B cells (positive for CD19, CD20, CD5, CD23, CD25, and CD11c and negative for CD38, CD10, CD34, CD103, CD56, and FMC7), immunophenotypically consistent with CLL but at the level of monoclonal B cell lymphocytosis/monoclonal B cell lymphocytosis of uncertain significance (MBL/MLUS). Bone marrow (BM) examination confirmed the diagnosis of precursor B-ALL with approximately 76% lymphoblasts (Figure 2). Interestingly, only sparse reactive lymphoid aggregates composed by a mixture of CD3-positive T cells and approximately equal amounts of CD20 polyclonal B cells with no aberrant coexpression of CD5 or CD23 were identified by histopathology. However, FC analysis performed on BM also detected the MBL clone, which accounted for 8% of lymphocytes (8% of the total viable cells) and could represent a PB contaminant or more likely minimal involvement by MBL (below the level of detection by immunohistochemistry).

In an attempt to confirm biclonality, DNA isolated from the PB specimen was analyzed by polymerase chain reaction (PCR) for clonal rearrangements of the immunoglobulin heavy chain (IgH) gene. This assay yielded five distinct PCR products with the FR1 and FR2 primer sets and four with FR3 (Figure 3). Only minimal polyclonal background was detected in an unsorted sample.

BM karyotyping of unstimulated cells revealed triclonal abnormal complexity, 46XY, add (20) (q11.2), add (21) (q1.1) [4], 47xy + 12 [3], and 46xy del (13) [2], in addition to normal background (46xy [5]). Clone 1 with an unbalanced rearrangement of 20q and 21q [4] was more compatible with acute leukemia or an underlying or evolving myelodysplastic syndrome/myeloproliferative neoplasm (MDS/MPN). In contrast, clone 2 (isolated trisomy of chromosome 12) and clone 3 (isolated deletion 13q) were more in keeping with a mature B cell lymphoid process, such as CLL. Fluorescent in situ hybridization (FISH) detected trisomy 10 and gain of an additional signal for RUNX1 at 21q22.12 (RUNX1/ETV6 probe) in 16% and 71% of cells examined, respectively. Additional FISH using a probe specific for 20q12 (DS0S108, Abbot Molecular) identified deletion of 20q12 in 57% of interphases, confirming the unbalance rearrangement of chromosome 20. No deletions of 6q, ATM (11q), 13q, or TP53 (17p) were found. These findings would indicate a neutral prognostic profile in CLL. Other aberrancies included in an ALL panel (BCR-ABL1 and KMT2A/MLL rearrangements) were not detected. Unexpectedly, DNA sequencing of IgVH revealed unmutated status in VH4-39, which has been associated with adverse prognosis, including transformation in CLL [5].

For further molecular characterization, we performed next generation sequencing (NGS) in the BM aspirate, using a custom designed Qiagen QIAseq v3 amplicon based targeted DNA comprehensive heme panel with genomic DNA run on an Illumina platform. Sequencing data were aligned against reference genome (hg19), and variants were called on an OHSU designed bioinformatics pipeline using multiple established variant callers (including FreeBayes, MuTect2, and Scalpel). The lower limit of detection for the assay is 2%.

A T487I point mutation was found in the thrombopoietin receptor gene (myeloproliferative leukemia protein/MPL/CD110), which is a known variant of uncertain significance according to ClinVar [4] and could represent a heterozygous germline variant, given the observed allelic frequency of 52%. Interestingly, this genetic alteration has not been reported in lymphoid neoplasms.

After obtaining cytologic confirmation that the cerebrospinal fluid was uninvolved by lymphoma, the patient was started on appropriate chemotherapy as per nonstandard B-ALL protocol. Because of his age, he was treated with MD Anderson B-ALL protocol with 1 cycle of hyperfractionated cyclophosphamide, vincristine, doxorubicin, dexamethasone (HCVD) and inotuzumab (Ino), mini-methotrexate, and cytarabine, followed by 4 cycles of consolidation and 4 cycles of maintenance with blinatumomab. Eight doses of prophylactic intrathecal methotrexate were also administered. The patient achieved remission, as demonstrated by BM and PB examination including FC analysis. Of note, the MBL clone was also undetectable. PB and BM marrow examination (including flow cytometry, IgH PCR, and karyotyping) demonstrated remission two

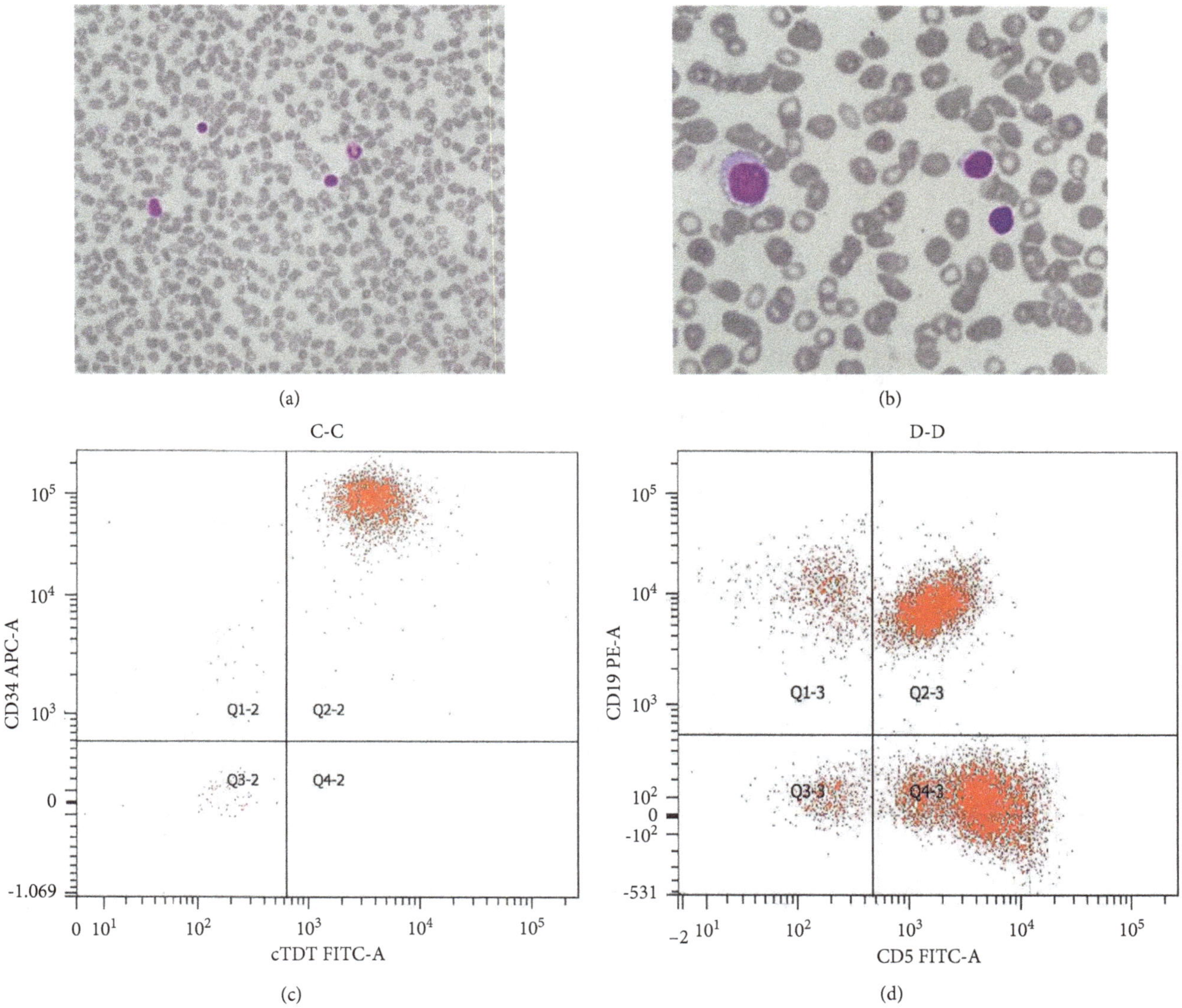

Figure 1: Peripheral blood smears (Wright-Giemsa stained) showing dimorphic lymphoid population at low magnification ((a), 400x) with a lymphoblast (arrow), two atypical small mature lymphocytes, and a band. (b) Lymphoblasts at higher magnification (1000x). Flow cytometric analysis of peripheral blood demonstrating B acute lymphoblastic leukemia with blasts coexpressing CD34 and TdT (c) and cocirculating monoclonal B cell lymphocytosis with aberrant coexpression of CD5 and CD23 (d).

months after treatment. However, BM cytogenetic analysis performed 1-year posttherapy demonstrated the original abnormal karyotype.

3. Discussion

CLL is the most frequent leukemia in adults, has been incidentally found in association with diverse solid tumors [6], and may be preceded by MBL. However, coexistence of CLL or MBL and other hematologic neoplasms is less frequent. Huang reported cocirculating B-ALL and CLL in an elderly woman [7].

Similarly, we report here for first time concurrent B-ALL and MBL with extensive molecular characterization.

Using PCR, at least four distinct peaks of IgH rearrangement were detected in PB which together with the observed dimorphic cell morphology strongly suggested a biclonal process. In addition, VH gene somatic mutation analysis revealed unmutated VH4-39 status, which has been reported in Richter's transformation [5] but not in association with acute leukemia.

NGS from a BM specimen identified a MPL (T487I) point mutation, which may be associated with congenital amegakaryocytic thrombocytopenia (CAMT), awaits further investigation in regard to ALL/MBL collision, and remains a VUS in ClinVar [4]. Various MPL mutations have been identified in myeloid neoplasms, including CAMT, hereditary thrombocythemia, MPN, refractory anemia with ringed sideroblasts associated with marked thrombocytosis, and acute myeloid leukemia [8]. Furthermore, a very similar MPL mutation (T487 A) was observed in a patient with acute megakaryoblastic leukemia, which induces a myeloproliferative disorder in mice through a cytokine-independent cell growth mechanism [9].

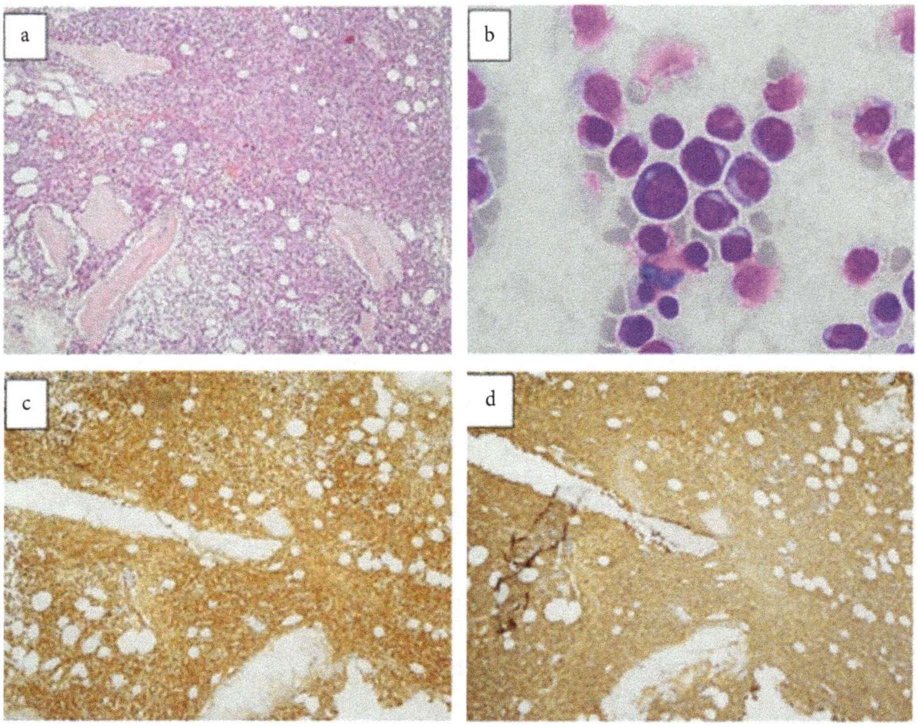

FIGURE 2: Bone marrow sections (hematoxylin and eosin stained) with sheets of lymphoblasts ((a), 100x). Heterogeneous lymphoblasts in bone marrow aspirates (Wright-Giemsa stained) at high magnification ((b), 1000x). Immunohistochemistry demonstrating positivity for TdT (c) and CD34 (d) on lymphoblasts in bone marrow sections (100x).

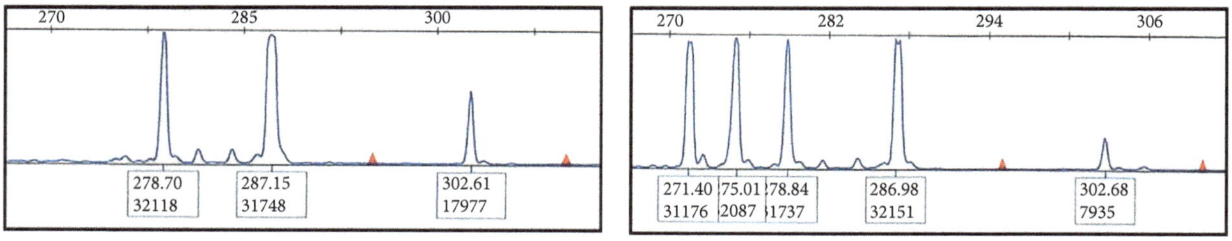

(a) (b)

FIGURE 3: DNA isolated from the bone marrow aspirate and peripheral blood was analyzed for clonal rearrangements of the immunoglobulin heavy chain gene using the BIOMED-2 primer sets in the IGH Gene Clonality Assay Kit (InVivoScribe). Three PCR reactions were carried out with upstream primers in the FR1, FR2, and FR3 regions of the IGH gene and a downstream primer in the JH region. The images show results with the FR2-JH primer set.

The MPL (T487I), we identified, has also been reported in nonhematopoietic malignancies (ovarian carcinoma and cervical pleomorphic liposarcoma) [10]; however, it is unreported in the unique setting of collision hematologic malignancy.

4. Conclusion

We present a novel coexistence of MBL and B-ALL with detailed molecular characterization, including a MPL (T487I) point mutation and VH4-39 unmutated usage, which may stimulate research to better understand the pathogenesis of hematologic neoplasms.

References

[1] T. Terwilliger and M. Abdul-Hay, "Acute lymphoblastic leukemia: A comprehensive review and 2017 update," *Blood Cancer Journal*, vol. 7, no. 6, p. e577, 2017.

[2] D. A. Arber, "The 2016 WHO classification of acute myeloid leukemia: What the practicing clinician needs to know," *Seminars in Hematology*, vol. 56, no. 2, pp. 90–95, 2019.

[3] L. R. Goldin, M. L. McMaster, and N. E. Caporaso, "Precursors to lymphoproliferative malignancies," *Cancer Epidemiology Biomarkers and Prevention*, vol. 22, no. 4, pp. 533–539, 2013.

[4] National Center for Biotechnology Information: https://www.ncbi.nlm.nih.gov/clinvar/variation/VCV000576110.1.

[5] P. Jain and S. O'Brien, "Richter's transformation in chronic lymphocytic leukemia," *Oncology*, vol. 26, no. 12, pp. 1146–1152, 2012.
[6] A. Mellemgaard, C. H. Geisler, and H. H. Storm, "Risk of kidney cancer and other second solid malignancies in patients with chronic lymphocytic leukemia," *European Journal of Haematology*, vol. 53, no. 4, pp. 218–222, 1994.
[7] Q. Huang, "Cocirculating precursor B acute lymphoblastic leukemia and chronic lymphocytic leukemia," *Blood*, vol. 122, no. 13, p. 2148, 2013.
[8] J. Ding, H. Komatsu, A. Wakita et al., "Familial essential thrombocythemia associated with a dominant-positive activating mutation of the c-MPL gene, which encodes for the receptor for thrombopoietin," *Blood*, vol. 103, no. 11, pp. 4198–4200, 2004.
[9] S. Malinge, C. Ragu, V. Della-Valle et al., "Activating mutations in human acute megakaryoblastic leukemia," *Blood*, vol. 112, no. 10, pp. 4220–4226, 2008.
[10] B. Tandon, I. S. Hagemann, H. M. Maluf, J. D. Pfeifer, and H. Al-Kateb, "Association of Li-fraumeni syndrome with small cell carcinoma of the ovary hypercalcemic type and concurrent pleomorphic liposarcoma of the cervix," *International Journal of Gynecological Pathology*, vol. 36, no. 6, pp. 593–599, 2017.

5

Spontaneous Regression of Plasmablastic Lymphoma in an Immunocompetent Patient: Case Report and Review of the Literature

Kee Tat Lee,[1] **Nurul Akmar Misron**,[2] **Norasmidar Abdul Aziz**,[1] **Chin Hau Wong**,[1] **and Hong Keng Liew**[1]

[1]*Department of Medicine, Hospital Sultanah Bahiyah, Langgar, Kedah, Malaysia*
[2]*Department of Pathology, Hospital Sultanah Bahiyah, Langgar, Kedah, Malaysia*

Correspondence should be addressed to Kee Tat Lee; keetat.lee@gmail.com

Academic Editor: Pier Paolo Piccaluga

Plasmablastic lymphoma (PBL) is a rare and highly aggressive type of lymphoma, which is commonly associated with human immunodeficiency virus (HIV) infection. Spontaneous regression of aggressive lymphomas is rare as they typically require administration of chemotherapy and radiotherapy for treatment. Here, we describe a case of a spontaneous regression of PBL after nasal biopsy and computed tomography (CT) guided biopsy of paravertebral mass in an immunocompetent patient. We postulate that the patient's immune system may be activated as a result of the stress and physical trauma brought on by nasal and paravertebral mass biopsy. Our case highlights the rare phenomenon of spontaneous regression of lymphoma which needs to be further studied on to establish its underlying pathophysiology.

1. Introduction

Plasmablastic lymphoma is a rare and aggressive B cell lymphoproliferative disorder. Delecluse et al. first described this rare disease in the oral cavity of patients with HIV in 1997 [1]. Since the original report, PBL has been more widely recognized and has been incorporated as a new entity in the latest World Health Organization (WHO) classification of lymphoma [2].

However, the diagnosis of PBL remains a diagnostic challenge due to its overlapping features between lymphoma and myeloma. PBL is a high-grade B cell lymphoma that expresses plasma cell markers (CD38, CD138, CD79a, and MUM-1), but typically tests negative for B cell markers (CD19, CD20, and PAX-5). The Ki-67 proliferation index of these tumours is usually high [3].

Despite the advancement in the therapy of aggressive lymphoma, the prognosis of patients with PBL remains dismal with short overall survival. Due to its rarity, it is difficult to establish a standard of care for this disease. Several case reports and case studies show that spontaneous regression can sometimes occur in low-grade lymphomas, but rarely in cases of aggressive lymphomas. Here, we report a case of a 61-year-old gentleman with PBL that spontaneously regressed after CT-guided biopsy of paravertebral mass. Relevant literature is reviewed.

2. Case Report

A 61-year-old gentleman with no significant medical history presented with the three weeks history of intermittent epistaxis, nasal block, and loss of weight. Physical examination was unremarkable, and he did not have lymphadenopathy or hepatosplenomegaly. Rigid nasal endoscopy revealed a smooth surface mass covering the entire left nasal cavity, pushing the nasal septum to the right and bleeds easily on contact. Subsequently, a CT scan of the paranasal sinus, neck, and thorax revealed a mass over left frontal and ethmoid sinuses which occupied almost the entire left nasal

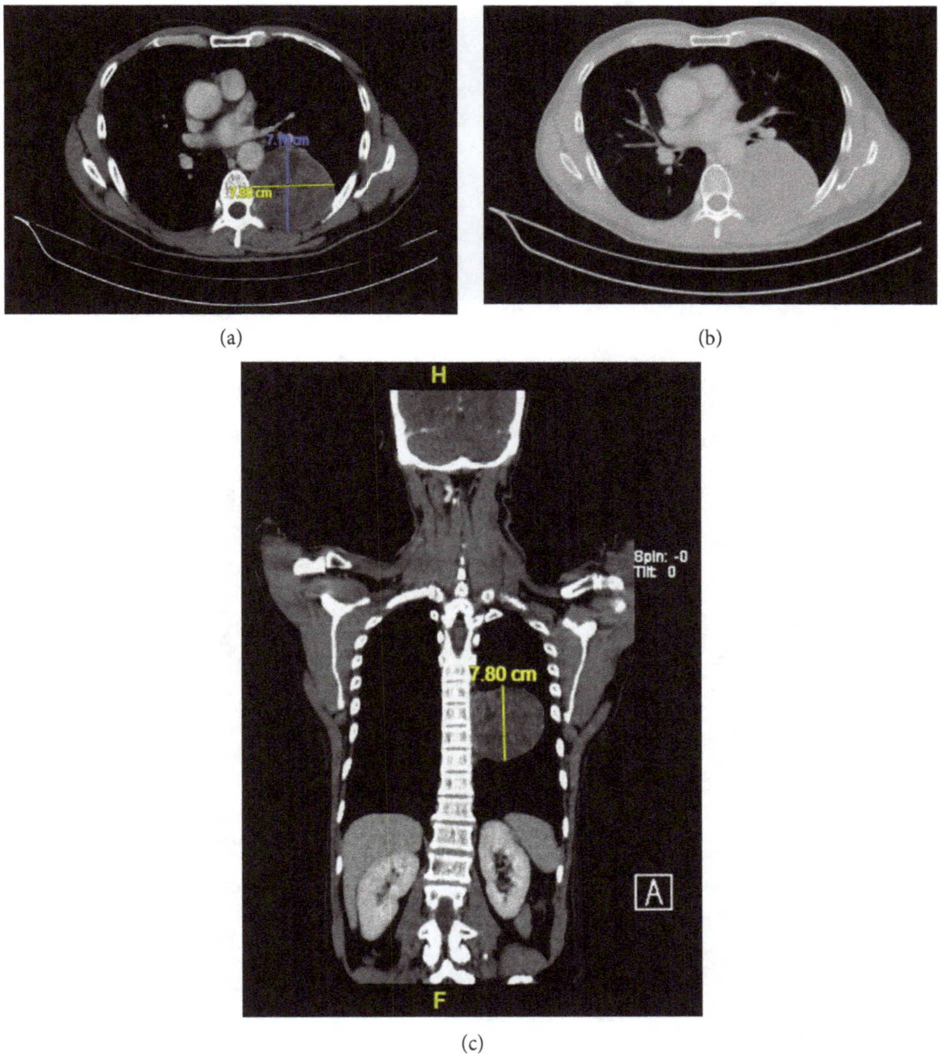

FIGURE 1: CT showing a well-defined heterogeneously enhancing mass at the left paravertebral region with extension into left T7/8 neural foramina. (a)-(b) Axial view; (c) coronal view.

cavity. Incidentally, there was a well-defined heterogeneously enhancing mass at the left paravertebral region ($7.1 \times 7.8 \times 7.8$ cm) with extension into left T7/8 neural foramina (Figure 1). Initial laboratory investigation showed white blood cell (WBC) count of 14.2×10^3/uL, hemoglobin (Hb) of 13.8 g/dL, and platelet count of 377×10^3/uL, with normal renal and hepatic function. His lactate dehydrogenase (LDH) was 141 U/L (upper limit of normal: 246). Hepatitis B, hepatitis C, and HIV serologies were nonreactive. Nasopharyngeal mass biopsy was performed, and histological examination highlighted diffuse infiltration by the atypical medium to large lymphoid cells and exhibited multiple membrane bound nucleoli. Immunohistochemistry (IHC) showed that the neoplastic cells were diffusely positive for CD79a, MUM-1, and CD56 and focally positive for PAX-5 (Figure 2). These cells were negative for CD20, CD30, ALK-1, CD3, CD5, CD10, Bcl-2, Bcl-6, CD138, HMB45, and S-100. Nuclear proliferation as assessed by Ki-67 was almost 100%. Unfortunately, Epstein-Barr virus (EBV) encoded RNA by IHC was not performed. Based on the morphological and IHC characteristics, diagnosis of PBL was made. Bone marrow biopsy did not show any marrow infiltration. CT-guided biopsy of the paraveterebral mass was done to rule out possible neurogenic tumour as PBL has rarely been associated with a paravertebral mass. However, the results were inconclusive due to the inadequate sample. He was scheduled for a repeated CT-guided biopsy of the paravertebral mass, and his histopathological examination results came back later which revealed ancient schwannoma. Surprisingly, he reported resolution of his symptoms after the first biopsy of the paravertebral mass, and hence, treatment for PBL was not initiated. Spontaneous regression of his PBL was further confirmed by a repeat rigid nasal endoscopy, which showed good patency of both nasal cavities, and a repeat CT scan of the paranasal sinuses, which revealed spontaneous regression of his left nasal mass (Figure 3). A watch-and-wait approach was employed, and he was followed up closely to look for any evidence of recurrence. He remained in remission during his last follow up after 4 years from diagnosis.

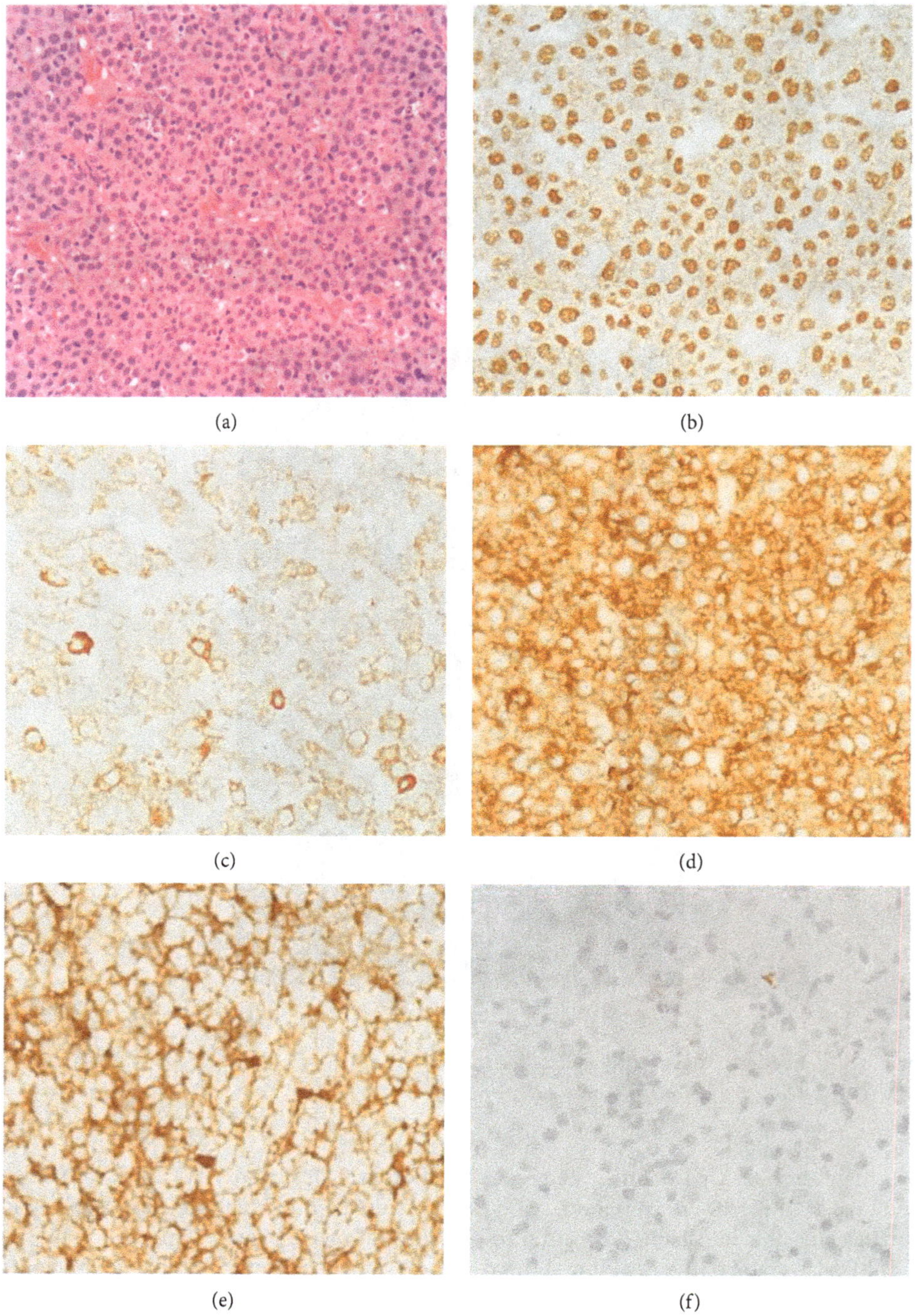

(a) (b) (c) (d) (e) (f)

FIGURE 2: Nasopharyngeal mass biopsy. Hematoxylin and eosin staining ((a) original magnification ×40) and immunohistochemical staining were positive for MUM-1 ((b) original magnification ×40), CD79a ((c) original magnification ×40), kappa ((d) original magnification ×40), and lambda ((e) original magnification ×40) and negative for CD20 ((f) original magnification ×40).

3. Discussion

PBL is an aggressive lymphoma which is strongly associated with immunosuppression. In the past decade, there are increasing numbers of PBL case report or series being published worldwide. Some of the reported cases include immunocompetent patients and involve extraoral sites [4–9]. PBL is found predominantly in males (75%), and median age of diagnosis is 50 years old [10]. HIV-negative PBL affects relatively older patients with median age of 71 years as compared to 46 years old in HIV-positive patients [5].

The prognosis of patients with PBL is poor with median overall survival (OS) of 8–15 months [3, 4]. There is no clear concensus on the optimal treatment of PBL. However, chemotherapy such as CHOP (cyclophosphamide, hydroxydaunorubicin, vincristine, and prednisone) or more aggressive chemotherapy regimens such as DA-EPOCH (dose-adjusted etoposide, prednisone, vincristine, cyclophosphamide, and doxorubicin), CODOX-M/IVAC

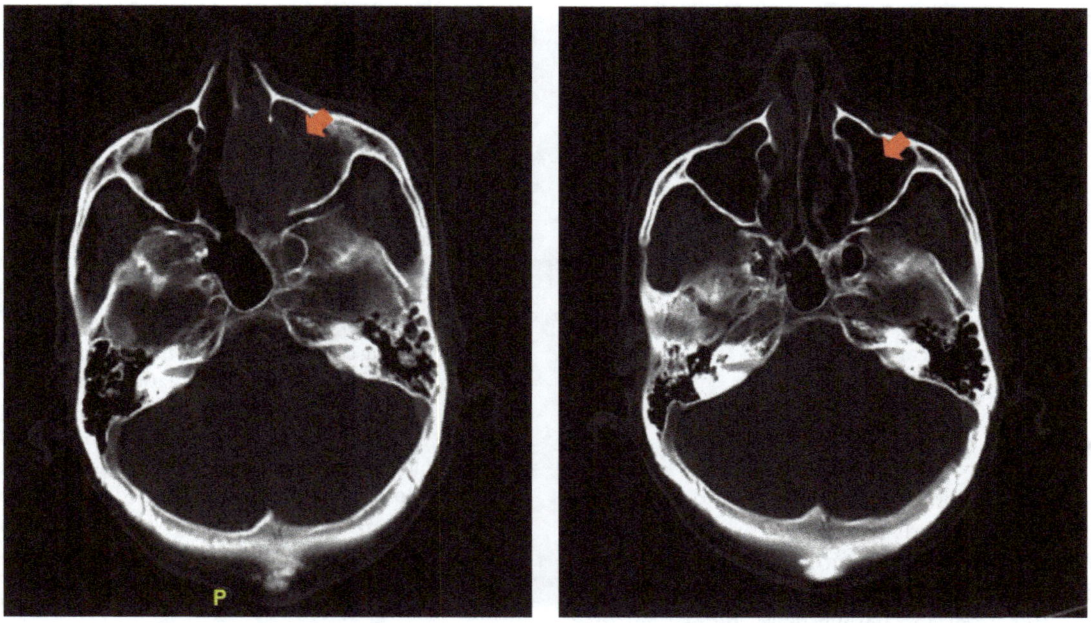

(a) (b)

FIGURE 3: Initial CT showing a mass over left frontal and ethmoid sinuses which occupied almost the entire left nasal cavity (a). Repeated CT showing regression of left nasal mass (b).

TABLE 1: Summary of clinical characteristic of spontaneous regression of PBL cases without antineoplastic therapy.

No.	Age/sex	Immune status	B symptom	Stage[a]	Primary site	Nodal	Therapy	Follow up	Recurrence
1 [16]	35/male	Yes/HIV	No	I	Maxilla	No	HAART	1 month	No
2 [17]	55/ female	Yes/HIV	N/A	N/A	Oral cavity	N/A	HAART	10 months	No
3 [18]	78/ female	Yes/MTX treatment	N/A	II	Buccal mucosa	Yes (cervical)	Decrease dose of MTX	2 years	No
4 [19]	80/male	No	No	I	Maxilla	No	No	5 months	No
5 [20]	80/male	No	No	I	Gingiva	No	No	N/A	No
6 [21]	66/ female	Yes/HIV	No	I	Maxilla	No	HAART	12 months	No
7 [22]	69/male	Yes/MTX[b] treatment	No	IV	N/A[c]	No	Stop MTX	12 weeks	No
8 [23]	69/male	No	No	I	Gingiva	N/A	No	2 years	No
9	61/male	No	No	I	Nasal	No	No	4 years	No

[a]Assessed using Ann Arbor staging. [b]MTX, methotrexate. [c]N/A, not available.

(cyclophosphamide, vincristine, doxorubicin, high-dose methotrexate/ifosfamide, etoposide, and high-dose cytarabine), or hyper-CVAD (hyperfractionated cyclophosphamide, vincristine, doxorubicin, and dexamethasone alternating with methotrexate and cytarabine) have been used with various success rates. Currently, there is no evidence of significant survival benefits with intensive chemotherapy over CHOP regimes [3, 4, 10].

Spontaneous regression of aggressive lymphoma is very uncommon and has rarely been reported in literature. Here, we report a case of sinonasal PBL that spontaneously regressed without chemotherapy. The exact mechanism of spontaneous regression remains unknown, but several hypotheses have been proposed previously. Immune stimulation secondary to active infection is one of the proposed mechanisms that can lead to tumour regression. This was first described by Dr. William Coley 100 years ago, where he reported spontaneous regression of inoperable sarcoma after being infected with *Streptococcus pyogenes* erysipelas [11]. Other proposed hypotheses include the augmented host immune response via humoral and cellular effector mechanisms, which can lead to tumour regression [12].

In this case, our patient reported resolution of his symptoms after biopsy of the paravertebral mass. We postulate that the patient's immune system may be activated as a result of the stress and physical trauma brought on by nasal and paravertebral mass biopsy. This was consistent with findings of several case reports where aggressive lymphomas undergo spontaneous remission after tumour biopsy, suggesting that biopsy might stimulate an antitumour immunity [13–15].

In addition to our present case, we identified and reviewed another eight similar cases of PBL with spontaneous regression (Table 1) [16–23]. The median age of the study cohort was 69 years old (range 35–80). Most of the patients were in Ann Arbor stage I (89%), and only one of them had nodal involvement. Three of them were HIV positive, and PBL regressed after highly active antiretroviral therapy (HAART), which may be related to immune restoration secondary to HAART. In particular, three of the previously reported cases (cases 4, 5, and 8) of PBL were similar to our case, all of them were above 60 years old without significant medical illness, and PBL regressed without chemotherapy or specific treatment.

4. Conclusion

Our case highlights the rare phenomenon of spontaneous regression of PBL in an elderly patient. The exact mechanism of this phenomenon remains unknown. However, we postulate that this could be triggered by activation of his immune system after nasal and paravertebral biopsy. Further research is needed to help better understand the pathophysiology behind this phenomenon as this could potentially have major therapeutic implications.

Consent

Written consent has been obtained from patient.

Acknowledgments

The authors thank the Director General of Health Malaysia for the permission to present these findings.

References

[1] H. J. Delecluse, I. Anagnostopoulos, F. Dallenbach et al., "Plasmablastic lymphomas of the oral cavity: a new entity associated with the human immunodeficiency virus infection," *Blood*, vol. 89, no. 4, pp. 1413–1420, 1997.

[2] S. H. Swerdlow, E. Campo, S. A. Pileri et al., "The 2016 revision of the world health organization classification of lymphoid neoplasms," *Blood*, vol. 127, no. 20, pp. 2375–2390, 2016.

[3] J. J. Castillo, M. Bibas, and R. N. Miranda, "The biology and treatment of plasmablastic lymphoma," *Blood*, vol. 125, no. 15, pp. 2323–2330, 2015.

[4] J. Morscio, D. Dierickx, J. Nijs et al., "Clinicopathologic comparison of plasmablastic lymphoma in HIV-positive, immunocompetent, and posttransplant patients: single-center series of 25 cases and meta-analysis of 277 reported cases," *American Journal of Surgical Pathology*, vol. 38, no. 7, pp. 875–886, 2014.

[5] E. Tchernonog, P. Faurie, P. Coppo et al., "Clinical characteristics and prognostic factors of plasmablastic lymphoma patients: analysis of 135 patients from the LYSA group," *Annals of Oncology*, vol. 28, no. 4, pp. 843–848, 2017.

[6] Y. J. Li, J. W. Li, K. L. Chen et al., "HIV-negative plasmablastic lymphoma: report of 8 cases and a comprehensive review of 394 published cases," *Blood Research*, vol. 55, no. 1, pp. 49–56, 2020.

[7] H. W. Wang, W. Yang, J. Z. Sun, J. Y. Lu, M. Li, and L. Sun, "Plasmablastic lymphoma of the small intestine: case report and literature review," *World Journal of Gastroenterology*, vol. 18, no. 45, pp. 6677–6681, 2012.

[8] F. Tavora, L. F. Gonzalez-Cuyar, C. C. J. Sun, A. Burke, and X. F. Zhao, "Extra-oral plasmablastic lymphoma: report of a case and review of literature," *Human Pathology*, vol. 37, no. 9, pp. 1233–1236, 2006.

[9] A. Matikas, G. Kanellis, C. Papadimitriou et al., "Plasmablastic lymphoma of the breast in an immunocompetent patient: long-lasting complete response induced by chemotherapy and autologous stem cell trasplantation," *Anticancer Research*, vol. 34, no. 9, pp. 5111–5115, 2014.

[10] J. J. Castillo, E. S. Winer, D. Stachurski et al., "Clinical and pathological differences between human immunodeficiency virus-positive and human immunodeficiency virus-negative patients with plasmablastic lymphoma," *Leukemia and Lymphoma*, vol. 51, no. 11, pp. 2047–2053, 2010.

[11] S. A. Hoption Cann, J. P. van Netten, and C. van Netten, "Dr William Coley and tumour regression: a place in history or in the future," *Postgraduate Medical Journal*, vol. 79, no. 938, pp. 672–680, 2003.

[12] W. R. Drobyski and R. Qazi, "Spontaneous regression in non-hodgkin's lymphoma: clinical and pathogenetic considerations," *American Journal of Hematology*, vol. 31, no. 2, pp. 138–141, 1989.

[13] M. Kumamoto, H. Nakamine, T. Hara et al., "Spontaneous complete regression of high grade non-hodgkin's lymphoma. Morphologic, immunohistochemical, and gene amplification analyses," *Cancer*, vol. 74, no. 11, pp. 3023–3028, 1994.

[14] M. Koga, J. Kusukawa, and N. Hayabuchi, "Spontaneous regression of extranodal malignant lymphoma occurred in the gingiva," *Oral Oncology*, vol. 39, no. 3, pp. 323-324, 2003.

[15] R. Abe, K. Ogawa, Y. Maruyama, N. Nakamura, and M. Abe, "Spontaneous regression of diffuse large B-cell lymphoma harbouring epstein-barr virus: a case report and review of the literature," *Journal of Clinical and Experimental Hematopathology*, vol. 47, no. 1, pp. 23–26, 2007.

[16] R. Armstrong, J. Bradrick, and Y. C. Liu, "Spontaneous regression of an HIV-associated plasmablastic lymphoma in the oral cavity: a case report," *Journal of Oral and Maxillofacial Surgery*, vol. 65, no. 7, pp. 1361–1364, 2007.

[17] M. Corti, L. De Carolis, A. Campitelli, M. Narbaitz, and P. Baré, "Response of human immunodeficiency virus–associated oral plasmablastic lymphoma to highly active antiretroviral therapy without chemotherapy," *Infectious Diseases in Clinical Practice*, vol. 20, no. 1, pp. 79–81, 2012.

[18] A. García-Noblejas, A. Velasco, J. Cannata-Ortiz, and R. Arranz, "Spontaneous regression of immunodeficiency associated plasmablastic lymphoma related to methotrexate after decrease of dosage," *Medical Clinics of North America*, vol. 140, no. 12, pp. 569-570, 2013.

[19] T. Igawa, Y. Sato, H. Kawai et al., "Spontaneous regression of plasmablastic lymphoma in an elderly human immunodeficiency virus (HIV)-negative patient," *Diagnostic Pathology*, vol. 10, no. 1, p. 183, 2015.

[20] M. Yao, N. Yoshioka, K. Hasegawa, T. Shimo, and A. Sasaki, "A case of spontaneous regression of plasmablastic lymphoma in the upper gingiva," *International Journal of Oral and Maxillofacial Surgery*, vol. 46, no. 1, p. 315, 2017.

[21] N. B. Daroit, V. Silva, B. J. Maraschin et al., "Spontaneous regression of an oral manifestation of plasmablastic

lymphoma: literature review and commentary about the phenomena," *British Journal of Medicine and Medical Research*, vol. 21, no. 11, pp. 1–7, 2017.

[22] K. Yordanova, S. Stilgenbauer, R. M. Bohle et al., "Spontaneous regression of a plasmablastic lymphoma with MYC rearrangement," *British Journal of Haematology*, vol. 186, no. 6, pp. e203–e207, 2019.

[23] K. Ono, T. Okui, S. Ibaragi et al., "A case of intraoral plasmablastic lymphoma spontaneously regressed after biopsy in HIV-negative patient," *Journal of Oral and Maxillofacial Surgery, Medicine, and Pathology*, vol. 31, no. 4, pp. 280–283, 2019.

6

An Unusual Cause of Epistaxis: Paranasal Sinus Myeloid Sarcoma

Karuna Dewan[1], **John H. Baird**[2], **and Courtney B. Shires**[3]

[1]*Department of Otolaryngology Head and Neck Surgery, Stanford University, Stanford, USA*
[2]*Division of Hematology, Department of Medicine, Stanford University, Stanford, USA*
[3]*Department of Otolaryngology Head and Neck Surgery, The University of Tennessee Health Sciences Center, Memphis, USA*

Correspondence should be addressed to Karuna Dewan; karunadoc@gmail.com

Academic Editor: Sylvain Choquet

We report a case of a 65-year-old female who presented with right-sided headaches, blurring of vision in the right eye, cold-induced epistaxis, and facial numbness in the trigeminal nerve distribution. Laboratory studies revealed a significant number of myeloblasts on peripheral smear with granulated cytoplasm, irregular nuclei, and prominent vacuoles. Magnetic resonance imaging (MRI) of the brain demonstrated a T1-enhancing 1.5 cm right-sided dural-based lesion involving the medial sphenoid wing, cavernous sinus, infratemporal fossa, and sphenoid sinus region. An endoscopic biopsy of the lesion within the sphenoid sinus confirmed the diagnosis of myeloid sarcoma, with myeloblasts comprising 30% of cellularity by flow cytometry. A subsequent bone marrow biopsy revealed a hypercellular marrow with 23% blasts by flow cytometry that demonstrated a similar immunophenotypic pattern to those seen in the sinus mass. Fluorescence in situ hybridization (FISH) testing revealed the balanced translocation t(8;21)(q22;q22.1), consistent with a diagnosis of acute myeloid leukemia with *RUNX1-RUNX1T1*-balanced translocation by WHO 2016 criteria. Myeloid sarcoma represents a rare extramedullary presentation of acute myeloid leukemia (AML), either alone or in conjunction with blood or bone marrow involvement. This case emphasizes the need for a broad differential diagnosis and an aggressive work-up for any unusual paranasal sinus mass.

1. Introduction

Myeloid sarcoma (also known as granulocytic sarcoma or chloroma) is a rare extramedullary clinical presentation of acute myeloid leukemia (AML) seen in less than 10% of patients [1], in which a discrete mass of myeloblasts infiltrate and efface normal tissue architecture. Designated as a separate entity in the WHO 2016 classification [2], this extramedullary disease often presents concurrently or subsequent to systemic or bone marrow involvement with any subtype of AML, but in rare instances, can occur in isolation. These tumors may be found in any location including bone, periosteum, soft tissues, and lymph nodes, and less commonly the orbit, intestine, mediastinum, epidural region, uterus, and ovary [3–5]. Myeloid sarcoma is most often associated with AML with a monocytic differentiation (French-American-British (FAB) M4 or M5 classifications) or with AML harboring the cytogenetic abnormality t(8;21) [5] (also known as core binding factor (CBF) AML). With greater understanding of genetic and molecular risk factors, the prognosis of AML is now represented across a diverse spectrum, with favorable risk subtypes such as CBF AML achieving long term survival with intensive chemotherapy alone, and adverse risk subtypes often requiring more intensive therapy with allogeneic stem cell transplant [6–8].

We describe here a 65-year-old woman presenting with headache and cold-induced epistaxis. On subsequent work-up, she was found to have a sphenoid sinus myeloid sarcoma as the presenting sign of underlying AML.

2. Case Presentation

A 65-year-old female presented to the emergency room with a complaint several weeks of worsening of right-sided headache, nausea, vomiting, cold-induced epistaxis, and blurring of vision from the right eye. Over the previous two months, the patient developed right facial numbness, 25-pound weight loss, and increasing right tongue swelling. On physical examination, the patient was noted to have disconjugate gaze to the right, as well as a right cranial nerve VII and XII palsy. Laboratory studies reveled 10% circulating blasts; there was no evidence of coagulopathy or tumor lysis syndrome. On review of the peripheral blood smear, there was a mixture of myeloblasts and promonocytes with granulated cytoplasm, irregular nuclei, and prominent vacuoles. Computed tomography (CT) imaging of the head performed in the emergency department demonstrated a large focus of edema involving the right temporal lobe as well as hyperdense dural thickening in the right medial petrous apex with 6 mm of midline shift (Figure 1). Magnetic resonance imaging (MRI) [9] demonstrated abnormal T1-intense signal along the dural surface of the right medial petrous region and paraclinoid region as well as sphenoid bone and cavernous sinus with upper sphenoid tumor extension, also extending to the foramen ovale and into the upper margins of the right infratemporal fossa (Figure 2). Imaging performed 2 months prior as part of surgical planning for a right mastoidectomy for chronic mastoiditis showed no evidence of this mass.

The patient was taken to the operating room for endoscopic biopsy of tissue in the sphenoid sinus, which subsequently demonstrated a myeloperoxidase- (MPO-) positive blast population infiltrating the sinus mucosal and bony tissue, positive for CD34, CD117, HLA-DR, CD33, CD11b, and partial CD13 by flow cytometry, consistent with a myeloid sarcoma. Positron emission tomography-computed tomography (PET-CT) was performed that showed intense fluorodeoxyglucose (FDG) avidity in the right temporal lobe, paraclinoid region, sphenoid bone, cavernous sinus, and infratemporal fossa on the right. A subsequent bone marrow biopsy demonstrated a hypercellular marrow with 23% myeloblasts with similar morphologic and immunophenotypic characteristics to the sinus myeloid sarcoma tissue. FISH analysis showed a t(8;21)(q22; q22.1) in all myeloblasts on metaphase analysis, without any additional cytogenetic abnormalities, consistent with a diagnosis of acute myeloid leukemia (AML) with a balanced translocation of *RUNX1-RUNX1T1*. Subsequent PCR-based testing demonstrated no mutations in *c-KIT*.

The patient was transferred to the inpatient hematology service and initiated induction chemotherapy with cytarabine and daunorubicin (7 + 3 regimen). Her induction course was complicated by hyperbilirubinemia, likely drug-induced. A repeat bone marrow biopsy obtained on day 12 demonstrated no increase in blasts but residual positivity for t(8;21) by FISH in 9 out of 20 metaphases; however, this resolved on repeat biopsy 1 week later. Repeat MRI showed residual tumor involving the right Meckel cave and cavernous sinus. Because of this, she went on to receive consolidative radiotherapy involving the whole brain, with follow-up MRI confirming complete resolution of the mass.

Given the patient's favorable risk disease, she proceeded to consolidative chemotherapy with high-dose cytarabine (HiDAC) alone. After 1 cycle, she presented with increasing fatigue and generalized weakness, and repeat bone marrow biopsy confirmed a relapse of AML, with 23% blasts negative for any evidence of the prior t(8;21), but demonstrating a new isolated del(20)(q11.2) in 9 out of 20 metaphases on karyotypic analysis. Lumbar puncture was performed and was negative for any leukemic involvement. She received salvage chemotherapy with G-CLAM, with her subsequent course complicated by neutropenic enterocolitis and recurrent drug-induced hyperbilirubinemia. She experienced delayed count recovery, with a repeat bone marrow biopsy demonstrating no residual disease. She was

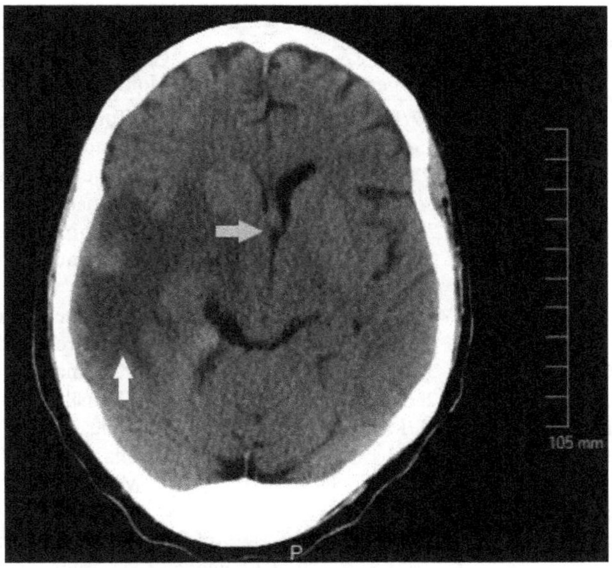

Figure 1: Computed tomography (CT) head imaging demonstrating a large focus of edema involving the right temporal lobe (white arrow) as well as hyperdense dural thickening in the right medial petrous apex with 6 mm of midline shift (grey arrow).

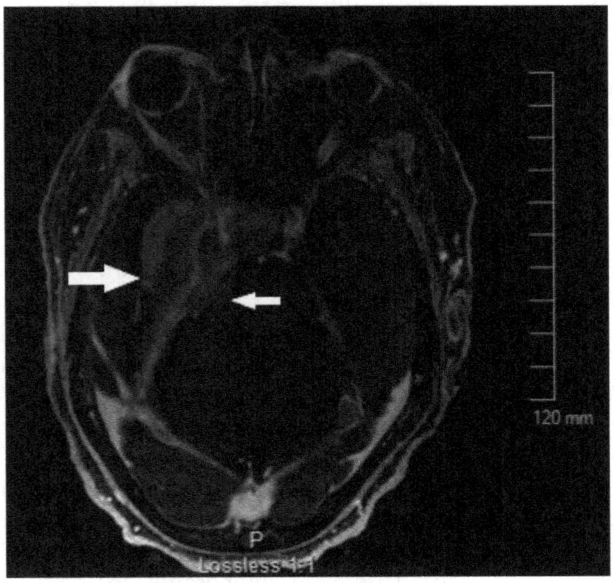

Figure 2: T1-weighted magnetic resonance imaging (MRI) of the head demonstrating abnormal signal along the dural surface of the right medial petrous region (smaller arrow) and paraclinoid region as well as sphenoid bone and cavernous sinus with upper sphenoid tumor extension (larger arrow), also extending to the foramen ovale and into the upper margins of the right infratemporal fossa.

TABLE 1: Known cases of head and neck myeloid sarcoma reported within the literature. There are no reported cases with disease confined to the paranasal sinuses [10].

Case no.	Age (yr)/gender	Myeloid sarcoma site	Presentation	Bone marrow disease
1	77/F	Tongue	Tongue lesion	Yes
2	55/M	Mandible	Jaw pain	Yes
3	47/F	Tonsils, base of tongue	Sore throat	Yes
4	6/1M	Tonsil	Throat pain	Yes
5	25/M	Eye, parotid and submandibular gland	Bulging of right eye	Yes
6	79/M	Cutaneous cheek and eyelid lesion	Skin lesions	Yes
7	65/F	Lip	Lip mass	Yes
8	63/M	Cutaneous cheek lesion	Pimple	Yes
9	80/M	Cutaneous eyelid, forehead lip lesion	Skin rash	No
10	55/M	Gingiva, maxilla	Gingival mass	Yes
11	21/M	Tonsil	Enlarged tonsil	Yes
12	48/M	Mandible, maxilla	Unknown	Yes
13	77/M	Maxilla, alveolus	Mouth pain, dyspnea, fatigue	Yes
14	56/M	Mandible	Blasts in blood	Yes
15	85/F	Lip	Lip and skin lesion	Yes
16	69/M	Middle turbinate (intranasal)	Sinus pain and pressure	Yes
17	17/M	Cutaneous cheek lesions, breast mass	Skin lesion and breast mass	No

started on growth factor support and discharged home, where 1 week later, she experienced altered mental status and a fall. Her initial CT scan demonstrated left frontal trauma with associated intraparenchymal hemorrhage in the left frontal and right temporal lobes in the setting of thrombocytopenia. After a slow and incomplete recovery in the neurologic critical care unit, the family elected to take the patient home on hospice care, and she subsequently passed away.

3. Discussion

To our knowledge, there are fewer than 20 reported cases of nasopharyngeal myeloid sarcoma reported in the literature (Table 1), with a majority occurring concurrently with systemic disease and having contiguous orbital involvement [3, 10]. None of the previously reported cases describe disease contained entirely within the paranasal sinuses as in the current case.

Myeloid sarcoma has an association with several cytogenetic abnormalities, most commonly *MLL* rearrangements and t(8;21) and to a lesser degree monosomy 7, trisomy 8, inv(16), trisomy 4, monosomy 16, del(16q), del(5q), del(20q), and trisomy 11 [11–13]. Although myeloid sarcoma may occur at any age, it is more common in younger patients likely owing to the prevalence of *MLL* rearrangements and splitting. Approximately 16% of myeloid sarcoma cases carry concurrent NPM mutations, which are often associated with normal cytogenetics and FAB M4 or M5 morphologic classification. The accurate diagnosis of these cases can be challenging, particularly when there is no evidence of systemic disease, and imaging features are not sufficiently specific to distinguish myeloid neoplasm from other tumors including lymphoid and nonhematopoietic tumors.

PET-CT scan can be useful in the diagnosis and monitoring of disease progression in myeloid sarcoma. Cribe et al. noted PET-CT resolution of disease in organs correlated with resolution of bone marrow disease [14]. While two other author groups, Stozel et al. and Ravulapati et al., have noted that bone marrow can appear cleared of disease, PET-CT scan demonstrates remaining organ disease [15, 16]. In the case presented here, PET-CT scan was done initially for staging purposes and was not repeated.

There is a lack of definitive data regarding what prognostic significance extramedullary disease has in the context of concurrent systemic disease, if any. Early retrospective cohort studies suggested that the presence of concurrent extramedullary disease conferred an adverse impact; in one larger study, the 2-year event-free survival rate and overall survival rate was 32% and 43% versus 18% and 29% in isolated myeloid sarcoma and in concurrent systemic disease, respectively [10]. However, similar cohorts have also shown that, in isolated myeloid sarcoma, AML will almost inevitably arise with a median time to development of 5–12 months from diagnosis. Thus, the current consensus is that while patients with myeloid sarcoma have an overall poor prognosis with 5-year survival rates between 20 and 30% [4, 17–19], this appears only mildly and perhaps nonsignificantly worsened compared to age- and risk-matched survival in AML without extramedullary disease.

Given the high prevalence of concurrent systemic disease, most patients with myeloid sarcoma require conventional intensive induction chemotherapy combining an anthracycline and cytarabine at the time of diagnosis. Complete response rates to this conventional AML-type treatment vary significantly, from 94.4% to 67.4% [20] in favorable and adverse risk groups, respectively. The impact of extramedullary disease on treatment response and survival in favorable risk AML, in particular, those with t(8;21) treated with chemotherapy alone, remains unclear after several conflicting studies [21–23]. For patients who experience an incomplete response to this initial therapy or in those patients who have isolated myeloid sarcoma, some studies have shown excellent locoregional control with the use of consolidative radiotherapy [24, 25] though it remains unclear whether this intervention has an impact on overall survival.

In those patients who achieve a complete remission with their initial chemotherapy regimen, the uncertain prognostic implications of extramedullary disease in conjunction with the lack of randomized controlled studies comparing the optimal consolidative protocol often result in the use of allogeneic hematopoietic stem cell transplant (HCT) for eligible patients. The largest case series utilizing this approach in patients with myeloid sarcoma showed 5-year overall survival of 47% [26]. With the advent of routine testing for minimal residual disease (MRD), either through multiparametric flow cytometry or through PCR monitoring of targetable fusion transcripts (e.g., RUNX1-RUNX1T1 in AML with t(8;21)(q22;q22.1)), these results will likely be improved for selected patients with MRD-negative complete remissions.

While these tumors are quite rare, they can have unusual presentations in the head and neck region that result in symptoms such as exophthalmos, facial paralysis, or adenopathy [27]. It is important for the head and neck surgeon to consider this diagnosis as part of a wide differential so that a complete evaluation to evaluate for systemic disease can be undertaken. While the prognosis for myeloid sarcoma remains guarded, with the advent of more comprehensive genetic and molecular risk profiling and targeted treatment intensification based on these results, the results of early and aggressive treatment are likely to yield improved long-term outcomes.

References

[1] G. M. Dores, S. S. Devesa, R. E. Curtis, M. S. Linet, and L. M. Morton, "Acute leukemia incidence and patient survival among children and adults in the United States, 2001–2007," *Blood*, vol. 119, no. 1, pp. 34–43, 2011.

[2] D. A. Arber, A. Orazi, R. Hasserjian et al., "The 2016 revision to the World Health Organization classification of myeloid neoplasms and acute leukemia," *Blood*, vol. 127, no. 20, pp. 2391–2405, 2016.

[3] H. Shimizu, T. Saitoh, N. Hatsumi et al., "Clinical significance of granulocytic sarcoma in adult patients with acute myeloid leukemia," *Cancer Science*, vol. 103, no. 8, pp. 1513–1517, 2012.

[4] K. Yamauchi and M. Yasuda, "Comparison in treatments of nonleukemic granulocytic sarcoma: report of two cases and a review of 72 cases in the literature," *Cancer*, vol. 94, no. 6, pp. 1739–1746, 2002.

[5] M. S. Tallman, D. Hakimian, J. M. Shaw, G. S. Lissner, E. J. Russell, and D. Variakojis, "Granulocytic sarcoma is associated with the 8;21 translocation in acute myeloid leukemia," *Journal of Clinical Oncology*, vol. 11, no. 4, pp. 690–697, 1993.

[6] H. Dohner, E. H. Estey, S. Amadori et al., "Diagnosis and management of acute myeloid leukemia in adults: recommendations from an international expert panel, on behalf of the European LeukemiaNet," *Blood*, vol. 115, no. 3, pp. 453–474, 2009.

[7] H. Döhner, E. Estey, D. Grimwade et al., "Diagnosis and management of AML in adults: 2017 ELN recommendations from an international expert panel," *Blood*, vol. 129, no. 4, pp. 424–447, 2016.

[8] E. Papaemmanuil, M. Gerstung, L. Bullinger et al., "Genomic classification and prognosis in acute myeloid leukemia," *New England Journal of Medicine*, vol. 374, no. 23, pp. 2209–2221, 2016.

[9] A. B. Shinagare, K. M. Krajewski, J. L. Hornick et al., "MRI for evaluation of myeloid sarcoma in adults: a single-institution 10-year experience," *American Journal of Roentgenology*, vol. 199, no. 6, pp. 1193–1198, 2012.

[10] J. Zhou, D. Bell, and L. J. Medeiros, "Myeloid sarcoma of the head and neck region," *Archives of Pathology & Laboratory Medicine*, vol. 137, no. 11, pp. 1560–1568, 2013.

[11] M. Breccia, F. Mandelli, M. C. Petti et al., "Clinico-pathological characteristics of myeloid sarcoma at diagnosis and during follow-up: report of 12 cases from a single institution," *Leukemia Research*, vol. 28, no. 11, pp. 1165–1169, 2004.

[12] C. Campidelli, C. Agostinelli, R. Stitson, and S. A. Pileri, "Myeloid sarcoma: extramedullary manifestation of myeloid disorders," *American Journal of Clinical Pathology*, vol. 132, no. 3, pp. 426–437, 2009.

[13] R. L. Bakst, M. S. Tallman, D. Douer, and J. Yahalom, "How I treat extramedullary acute myeloid leukemia," *Blood*, vol. 118, no. 14, pp. 3785–3793, 2011.

[14] A.-S. W. I. Cribe, M. Steenhof, C. W. Marcher, H. Petersen, H. Frederiksen, and L. S. Friis, "Extramedullary disease in patients with acute myeloid leukemia assessed by (18)F-FDG PET," *European Journal of Haematology*, vol. 90, no. 4, pp. 273–278, 2013.

[15] F. Stolzel, C. Rollig, J. Radke et al., "18F-FDG-PET/CT for detection of extramedullary acute myeloid leukemia," *Haematologica*, vol. 96, no. 10, pp. 1552–1556, 2011.

[16] S. Ravulapati, C. Siegel, A. Dara, and J. M. Lionberger, "Myeloid sarcoma without circulating leukemia mimicking gastrointestinal malignancy and lymphoma," *Hematology Reports*, vol. 10, no. 2, p. 7040, 2018.

[17] S. Paydas, S. Zorludemir, and M. Ergin, "Granulocytic sarcoma: 32 cases and review of the literature," *Leukemia & Lymphoma*, vol. 47, no. 12, pp. 2527–2541, 2009.

[18] T.-Y. Lan, D.-T. Lin, H.-F. Tien, R.-S. Yang, C.-Y. Chen, and K. Wu, "Prognostic factors of treatment outcomes in patients with granulocytic sarcoma," *Acta Haematologica*, vol. 122, no. 4, pp. 238–246, 2009.

[19] A.-M. Tsimberidou, H. M. Kantarjian, E. Estey et al., "Outcome in patients with nonleukemic granulocytic sarcoma treated with chemotherapy with or without radiotherapy," *Leukemia*, vol. 17, no. 6, pp. 1100–1103, 2003.

[20] Y. Harada, Y. Nagata, R. Kihara et al., "Prognostic analysis according to the 2017 ELN risk stratification by genetics in adult acute myeloid leukemia patients treated in the Japan Adult Leukemia Study Group (JALSG) AML201 study," *Leukemia Research*, vol. 66, pp. 20–27, 2018.

[21] G. J. Ruiz-Argüelles, A. Morales-Toquero, C. Manzano et al., "t(8;21)(q22;q22) Acute myelogenous leukemia in México: a single institution experience," *Hematology*, vol. 11, no. 4, pp. 235–238, 2013.

[22] J. C. Byrd, R. B. Weiss, D. C. Arthur et al., "Extramedullary leukemia adversely affects hematologic complete remission rate and overall survival in patients with t(8;21)(q22;q22): results from Cancer and Leukemia Group B 8461," *Journal of Clinical Oncology*, vol. 15, no. 2, pp. 466–475, 1997.

[23] A.-M. Tsimberidou, H. M. Kantarjian, S. Wen et al., "Myeloid sarcoma is associated with superior event-free survival and overall survival compared with acute myeloid leukemia," *Cancer*, vol. 113, no. 6, pp. 1370–1378, 2008.

[24] L. Y. Chak, M. D. Sapozink, and R. S. Cox, "Extramedullary lesions in non-lymphocytic leukemia: results of radiation therapy," *International Journal of Radiation Oncology*Biology*Physics*, vol. 9, no. 8, pp. 1173–1176, 1983.

[25] R. Bakst, S. Wolden, and J. Yahalom, "Radiation therapy for chloroma (granulocytic sarcoma)," *International Journal of Radiation Oncology*Biology*Physics*, vol. 82, no. 5, pp. 1816–1822, 2012.

[26] P. Chevallier, M. Mohty, B. Lioure et al., "Allogeneic hematopoietic stem-cell transplantation for myeloid sarcoma: a retrospective study from the SFGM-TC," *Journal of Clinical Oncology*, vol. 26, no. 30, pp. 4940–4943, 2008.

[27] I. A. Chaudhry, A. M. Alaraj, and H. M. Alkatan, "Unilateral eyelid swelling, proptosis and diplopia as initial manifestation of acute myeloid leukemia," *Saudi Journal of Ophthalmology*, vol. 26, no. 2, pp. 241–244, 2012.

7

Multiple Myeloma in a Young Female Presenting with Neurological Symptoms

Matthew Lee[1] **Xinmin Zhang,**[2] **Vinh Nguyen,**[3] **and Monique Hartley-Brown**[4]

[1]*Internal Medicine Resident, Donald and Barbara Zucker School of Medicine at Hofstra/Northwell, 300 Community Dr, Manhasset, NY 11030, USA*
[2]*Donald and Barbara Zucker School of Medicine at Hofstra/Northwell, Pathology Department at North Shore University Hospital-Long Island Jewish Medical Center, 300 Community Dr, Manhasset, NY 11030, USA*
[3]*Donald and Barbara Zucker School of Medicine at Hofstra/Northwell, Radiology Department at North Shore University Hospital-Long Island Jewish Medical Center, 300 Community Dr, Manhasset, NY 11030, USA*
[4]*Donald and Barbara Zucker School of Medicine at Hofstra/Northwell, Hematology-Oncology Department at North Shore University Hospital-Long Island Jewish Medical Center, 300 Community Dr, Manhasset, NY 11030, USA*

Correspondence should be addressed to Matthew Lee; mlee37@northwell.edu

Academic Editor: Marie-Christine Kyrtsonis

Background. Multiple myeloma is overall the 14th most common malignancy but is rarely seen in those younger than 35 years. Those in the younger age group have been shown to have a more aggressive course but reportedly have had similar responses to treatment compared to older cohorts. Extramedullary plasmacytomas are discrete soft tissue masses of neoplastic monoclonal plasma cells that often occur in patients with multiple myeloma. *Case.* This case entails a young female with new diagnosis of multiple myeloma and multiple extramedullary plasmacytomas presenting with neurological symptoms. She was treated with CyBorD regimen but was refractory and progressed. Treatment was changed to DCEP regimen, and daratumumab was added for primary refractory myeloma. The patient improved rapidly. *Conclusion.* This is a unique case of multiple myeloma in a young female that had failed first-line treatment but responded to targeted therapy of daratumumab. It highlights that multiple myeloma may present atypically in young patients. More research is needed on appropriate initial diagnosis and treatment of patients in this age group.

1. Introduction

Multiple myeloma is a malignant B-cell disorder that leads to proliferative plasma cells. It is the 14th most common malignancy accounting for 1.8% of all malignancies and 10% of hematologic malignancies [1]. However, multiple myeloma rarely occurs in those younger than 35 years (0.5%) [1]. Prior studies have shown a more aggressive presentation in this age group with higher rates of extramedullary plasmacytomas, plasma cell leukemias (11%), osteolytic lesions, renal failure (25%), and Bence Jones proteinuria (81%) [2–10]. This could be explained by either a delay in diagnosis or the inherent aggressive nature of disease in younger patients [11]. It has also been reported that this younger age group has had similar overall survival and remission to older cohorts [2–5, 11].

Here, we present a case of a young female newly diagnosed with multiple myeloma. She initially presented with significant neurological symptoms and multiple extramedullary plasmacytomas throughout the body including intracranially. She received first-line treatment with combined conventional chemotherapy and proteasome inhibitor (bortezomib), but was refractory. Second-line intensive chemotherapy initially failed, but with the addition of single agent daratumumab, the patient had a favorable disease response.

2. Case

A 24-year-old Egyptian female presents after a syncopal fall and head trauma. She reports having multiple falls for the past month prior to admission. Upon evaluation, the patient reported neurological symptoms including left-sided weakness in the upper and lower extremities, diplopia, and ataxia along with dysphagia. Most pertinent neurological exam findings were left abducens (CN VI) palsy, bilateral upper and lower extremity weakness of 2/5, and inability to stand due to pain with a 1 cm palpable left soft tissue pelvic mass.

Initial lab work revealed an elevated lactate dehydrogenase 375 U/L. The CBC and CMP findings were otherwise normal. Previous imaging from Egypt showed a fracture of her mandible with bilateral plate placement on X-ray. On our imaging, CT brain and maxillofacial showed several soft tissue masses present with contiguous bony erosion and destruction involving the central skull base and mandible (Figure 1(a)). At the skull base, the soft tissue mass eroded the basisphenoid and bordering maxilla, as well as the left greater wing of the sphenoid into the middle cranial fossa with infiltration of the left lateral rectus in the left orbit. CT of the spine showed paraspinal and epidural masses with bordering vertebral erosion (Figure 2(a)). CT of the chest, abdomen, and pelvis with contrast showed multiple lesions, with soft tissue infiltrating the chest wall, and left hemipelvis straddling the sacrum to involve the left gluteus musculature. These were superimposed on diffusely lytic lesions throughout thoracolumbar spine, some associated with mild compression fractures. MRI of the brain, cervical, thoracic, and sacral spine showed decreased T1 and T2 along with hyperintensive signals on diffusion of the calvarium, skull base, and facial bones with lytic lesions. Large expansile lesion involves L lateral orbital bony margin and zygoma 11 mm × 5 mm × 1.2 cm concerning for neoplasm. No new ischemic changes were observed in the brain. Cervical spine shows irregular T1 enhancement in clivus, C1, and C2, diffusely throughout C3-T1, and there was no central canal or foraminal compromise. Thoracic spine with extensive metastatic lesions with multiple compressions most pronounced at T4, T6, T8, and T11 and leptomeningeal involvement. Lumbar spine showing compression upon the cauda equina at the levels of L3-L4 and L4-L5 soft tissue in the left L3-L4, L4-L5, and L5-S1 neural foramina, encasing/compressing the left L3, L4, and L5 nerve root and bulky bilateral sacral masses.

At the time of initial evaluation, the main differential diagnosis was metastatic solid tumor malignancy, atypical neuroblastomas, and lymphoma. Decadron 4 mg every 6 hours was given for empiric treatment to reduce paraspinal inflammation. A fine needle aspiration/biopsy was done via CT guidance of a soft tissue sternal mass.

Flow cytometry on the biopsied specimen revealed an immunophenotype of monotypic plasma cells (11% of cells) positive for cytoplasmic lambda, CD38, CD56, dim CD45, and CD117 and negative for CD19 and CD20 with morphology showing atypical plasma cells with high nucleus-to-cytoplasm ratio, eccentric and irregular nucleuses, and frequent mitosis (Figures 3 and 4). Cytopathology immunohistochemical (CD20, CD117, cyclinD1, c-MYC, and p53) and in situ hybridization (EBR) stains showed neoplastic cells positive for c-MYC, CD56 and CD117 and negative for CD19, CD 20, cyclinD1, p53, and EBER. FISH using probe and location MYC (8q24) was negative for MYC rearrangement. A full multiple myeloma workup was then pursued. Serum free light chain analysis showed kappa light chain of 0.04 mg/dL, lambda light chain of 213 mg/dL, high IgG levels of 1840 mg/dL with an IgG lambda monoclonal band on urine and serum immunofixation, and low beta-2 microglobulin 0.5 mg/L.

According to the 2016 International Myeloma Working Group criteria, this patient met criteria for multiple myeloma with a biopsy proving soft tissue extramedullary plasmacytoma and multiple myeloma defining events with osteolytic lesions shown on imaging and a free light lambda chain ratio >100 mg/L and elevated LDH. The patient was diagnosed with stage III plasma cell IgG lambda multiple myeloma [12, 13]. The patient clinically had acute disease progression and severely worsening neurological symptoms; a bone marrow biopsy was deferred. A lumbar puncture was done and showed no malignant plasma cells in the CSF. She received palliative radiation therapy to the skull base, thoracic spine, and sacrum, and systemic treatment was started.

Cyclophosphamide 600 mg/m^2, bortezomib 1.3 mg/m^2, and dexamethasone 40 mg (CyBorD) regimen was initially given [14, 15]. An attenuated dose of cyclophosphamide was used with an attempt to quickly debulk the disease. Unfortunately, the disease continued to progress, the patient had worsening jaw pain, within 18 days after starting CyBorD. Repeat CT of the maxillofacial area revealed enlargement of the left masticator space lesion. Her treatment regimen was changed to second-line therapy with dexamethasone 40 mg, cyclophosphamide 400 mg/m^2, etoposide 40 mg/m^2, and cisplatin 10 mg/m^2(DCEP) [16]. Seven days later, with symptoms of dysphagia and lower extremity weakness, the decision was made to add daratumumab 16 mg/kg for primary refractory myeloma [17, 18].

After addition of daratumumab, she began to clinically improve. Subsequent CT of the maxillofacial showed a decrease in previously seen masticator space masses (Figure 1(b)). Furthermore, there were decreased size paraspinal and epidural lesions on CT lumbar and thoracic spine (Figure 2(b)). The Chest, abdomen, and pelvis CT scan also demonstrated substantial interval decreased size of right chest wall and left hemisacrum soft tissue masses. Based on the International Myeloma Workshop Group criteria [19], the patient had a partial response to one dose of daratumumab, with CT imaging showing ≥50% reduction in size of soft tissue plasmacytoma and marked reduction in lambda light chain levels from 213 to 3.02 mg/dL. The main toxicity during the hospital course was neutropenia with fever and a nadir ANC 500. Moreover, repeat MRI brain and spine 17 days later significantly decrease in enhancing soft tissue in the lumbar extradural space, with the resolution of

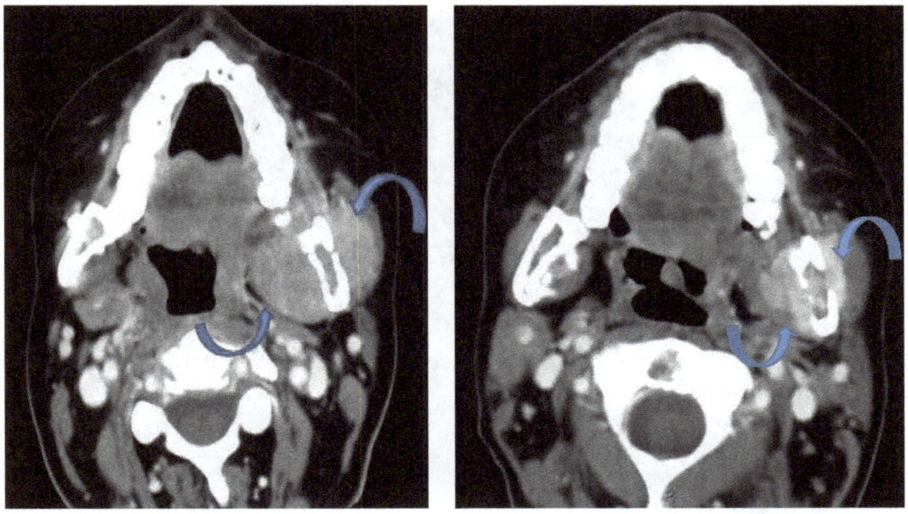

(a) (b)

FIGURE 1: Soft tissue masses of the left masticator space seen on admission is associated with adjacent mandibular erosion (a). This progressed and increased in size during admission, but finally showed response on CDEP and daratumumab (b).

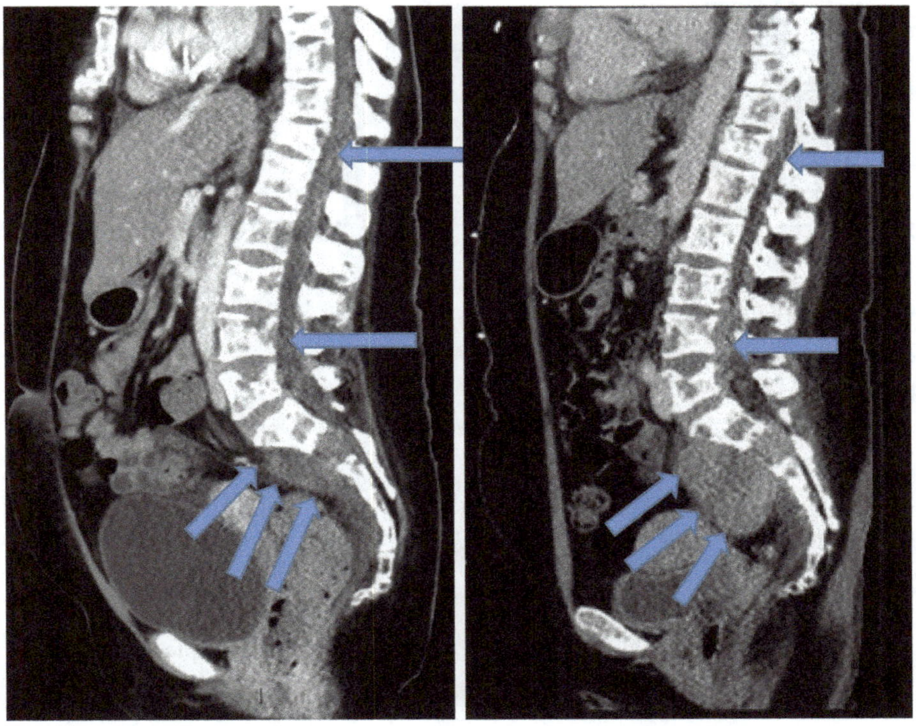

(a) (b)

FIGURE 2: Admission imaging (a) revealed multiple paraspinal and epidural masses (arrows) which decreased (b) following DCEP and daratumumab.

compression upon the cauda equina at the levels of L3-L4 and L4-L5 as described above. Persistent soft tissue in the left L3-L4, L4-L5, and L5-S1 neural foramina, encasing/compressing the left L3, L4, and L5 nerve roots was found. Slight improvement of large bulky bilateral sacral masses was observed, which extends to the left presacral and left sciatic foramen regions. Persistent obliteration of the left sacral foramina was observed. Stable mild superior endplate pathologic compression deformities at T12, L4 and L5 were also observed. In the brain MRI, the bony lesions overall appears smaller in size and less bulky, most consistent with a favorable response to treatment. No evidence for brain parenchymal metastatic disease, acute infarct, or acute hemorrhage. A repeat flow cytometry was done 30 days into her admission of her left iliac, but cytopathology analysis was done and showed from the core biopsy with paucicellular

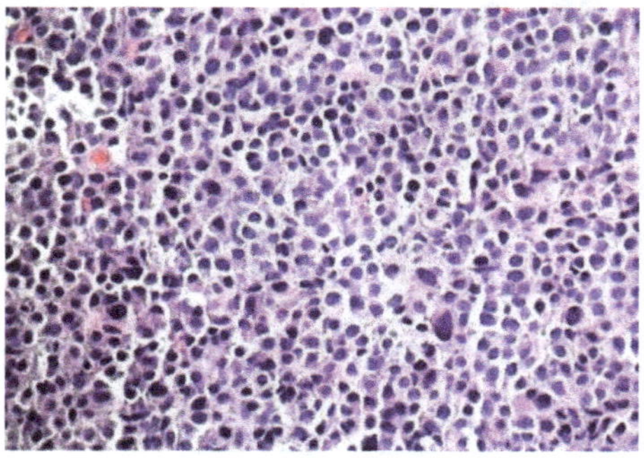

FIGURE 3: H&E (haematoxylin and eosin) stain of the biopsied soft tissue sternal mass shows soft tissue is diffusely infiltrated by large sheets of large cells with plasmacytoid morphology.

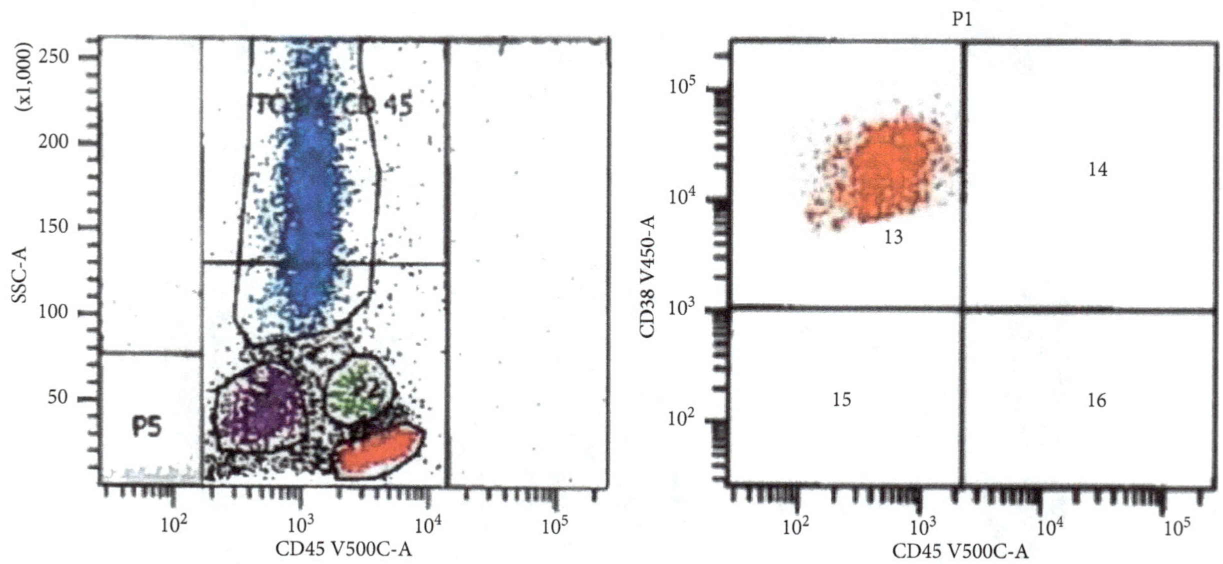

Population	#Events	%Par...	%Total
All events	10,000	####	100.0
P1	1,085	10.9	10.9
P2	364	3.6	3.6
P3	5,463	54.6	54.6
P4	1,021	10.2	10.2
P5	1,021	10.2	10.2

FIGURE 4: Flow cytometric analysis reveals a plasma cell population (P4) with higher side scatter (SSC). The plasma cells are positive for $CD38^{bright}$, cytoplasmic lambda, and CD56 and negative for CD 19.

and a few plasma cells and rare plasmacytoid cells of uncertain lineage (erythroid versus plasma cellular), amidst scattered bone marrow elements, fibrous tissue, and abundant blood. Immunostains were performed and show rare CD138 staining plasma cells, abundant CD3 staining T cells. Kappa and lambda are noncontributory due to depletion of the tissue upon deeper sectioning. Cam 5.2 is negative and excludes any epithelial cells. She continued to improve, and her ANC rose above 1000 over the next few days. She began moving her lower extremities and was able to walk with crutches at the time of discharge.

3. Discussion

This is a rare case of a very young patient presenting with neurological symptoms found to have multiple myeloma associated with multiple soft tissue extramedullary plasmacytomas. This case has multiple atypical aspects including the patient's age, presenting symptoms, and number and locations of extramedullary plasmacytomas. The median age of diagnosis of multiple myeloma is 69 years with only 15% of cases occurring in those less than 55 years [1]. Multiple myeloma occurs slightly more in men with typical symptoms of fatigue, anemia, bone pains, and/or hypercalcemia with renal insufficiency (CRAB features). The neurological complications, usually radiculopathy and peripheral neuropathies, are associated with spinal cord compression or neural compression secondary to bone damage.

The patient in this case however presented with atypical neurologic findings often seen in CNS disease. She had diplopia and ataxia along with paraplegia. The location of her plasmacytomas resulted in these unusual neurologic findings. In addition, given her high disease burden, her labs were not consistent with the typical CRAB features, and in fact the beta-2 microglobulin was low. Her IgG serum level was mildly elevated. The bulk of her measurable disease in the serum was noticed by the elevated serum lambda light chain of 213 mg/dL. Given the extent of bone damage, she had an oligosecretory myeloma, which is rare.

Another unique presentation of this case is the large number of soft tissue extramedullary plasmacytomas. Extramedullary plasmacytomas have an incidence of 0.04 cases per 100,000 individuals and usually are solitary masses with 80–90% arising from mucosal associated lymphoid tissue in the upper airways including nasopharynx and paranasal sinuses [20]. Furthermore, only 1-2% of patients at the time of initial diagnosis have extramedullary disease, and 8% develop extramedullary disease later on [21]. They also commonly present with obstruction of the nasal passages, masses in the palatal or maxillary, and with erosions leading to epistaxis and facial pain [20–22]. In this patient, she had multiple soft tissue masses throughout her chest wall, left pelvis, and thoracic spine along with a skull-base mass with intracranial and intraorbital extension. There have been only a few case reports of intracranial involvement with either multiple myeloma or intracranial plasmacytomas, but this level of intracranial involvement and associated chest and abdominopelvic involvement in one patient has not been reported in the literature [21–25]. The clinical scenario is suggestive of a possible aggressive form of oligosecretory myeloma which mainly progresses as plasmacytomas throughout the body, with minimal measurable disease present in the serum.

Despite progress in effective treatment, multiple myeloma remains incurable. The patient not only failed to respond to initial treatment with CyBorD regimen but also she progressed acutely while on therapy. Second-line therapy with DCEP regimen was ineffective acutely until daratumumab was added on and then she had a notable response.

The efficacy of daratumumab in treatment of multiple myeloma has been well documented over the past decade. Daratumumab is a monoclonal antibody to CD38 and widely expressed by several hematopoietic cells in the bone marrow, most notably plasma cells. Of note, it is also expressed on osteoclasts and bronchial epithelial cells [26]. It has been shown in preclinical studies that daratumumab kills myeloma cells by both antibody-dependent cellular cytotoxicity and phagocytosis by blocking the inhibitory signals from CD38, thus boosting cytotoxic T cells [27–29]. In its first clinical trial, SIRIUS, daratumumab was used in relapsed refractory myeloma in a multicentered phase 2 trial. A majority of these patients (80%) had received autologous stem-cell transplants and were refractory to proteasome inhibitors and immunomodulatory drugs (95%) and received a median of five previous lines of therapy. The 12-month overall survival was 64.8%, and median overall survival with 17.5 months was 29.2% showing overall response with 30% of the patients responding to daratumumab [18]. In 2015, it was initially approved by the FDA for treatment of patients with refractory multiple myeloma who had failed 3 or more prior lines of therapy [30]. In the CASTOR and POLLUX trial, both phase 3, randomized, multicenter, open label trials involving adding daratumumab for relapsed or refractory patients (who had already received one or more previous lines of therapy (autologous stem-cell transplant (ASCT), alkylating agents and proteasome inhibitors). Both trials showed significantly increased response rates and progression-free survival by more than 60% with the addition of daratumumab [31, 32].

Since then, daratumumab has been approved, in combination with proteasome inhibitors (PIs) and immunomodulatory drugs (IMiDs) in the upfront setting for newly diagnosed myeloma patients. These clinical trials have shown daratumumab to work synergistically with IMiDs and PIs with high potency and efficacy in killing myeloma cells with tolerable toxicity profiles [26, 31–36].

The ALCYONE trial was the first phase 3 daratumumab clinical trial to gain FDA approval for newly diagnosed multiple myeloma patients who were ineligible for autologous stem-cell transplantation. The patients were randomized to either nine cycles of bortezomib, melphalan, and prednisone alone (control arm) or with daratumumab (experimental arm) until disease progression. Patients in the daratumumab group had significantly longer progression-free survival at 18 months at 71.6% vs. 50.2% in the control group. The overall response in the daratumumab group was 91% with 22.3% negative for minimal residual disease (MRD) compared to 74% overall response and 6.2% negative for MRD in the control group [33]. MRD was defined by 1 tumor cell per 10^5 white cells.

Finally, the MAIA trial was done by comparing either daratumumab and lenalidomide with dexamethasone or lenalidomide with dexamethasone in multiple myeloma patients who were ineligible for autologous stem-cell transplant. Those in the daratumumab group had disease progression/death in 26.4% compared to 38.8% with lenalidomide and dexamethasone arm. Patients with daratumumab had 30 months without disease progression and were alive 70.6% in the experimental arm compared to 55.6% to the control arm [34]. A complete response or better was achieved in 47.6% of patients in the daratumumab group compared to 24.9% in the control group. In terms of MRD, 24.2% of patients in the daratumumab arm compared to 7.3% in the control arm had evidence of minimal residual disease [34]. Throughout all these trials the most common manageable toxicities of daratumumab were neutropenia, thrombocytopenia, increased respiratory infections, and infusion-related reactions.

Based on these clinical trials, daratumumab is highly potent and effective in the treatment of myeloma patients in combination with PIs and IMiDs, but for the advanced myeloma patient with high disease burden such as our patient, often the initial therapy for rapid disease control remains combination therapies such as CyBorD, DCEP, or other such heavy chemotherapy-based regimen. In this case, the availability of PIs and IMIDs was limited due to the inpatient setting. Additionally, at the time of the actual events, daratumumab was only FDA approved in the relapsed refractory multiple myeloma. Therefore, the choice for use of CyBorD induction with escalation to DCEP and daratumumab added once deemed refractory. This case suggests that not only would daratumumab be option for upfront therapy with PIs/IMiD combinations but also with multidrug chemotherapy regimens such as DCEP.

This case report shows a unique regimen of DCEP plus daratumumab resulting in a robust initial response, after the failure of CyBorD. This case report suggests that daratumumab in combination with DCEP may be another option to use for inpatient treatment of primary refractory and aggressive multiple myeloma disease. Especially, given the real world delays in obtaining IMiD/PI therapy for acutely ill hospitalized patients, this case also highlights how very different the presentation of multiple myeloma may be in a very young patient compared with older patients.

4. Conclusion

This provides insight into not only how young patients may present aggressively but also a potential way to manage it. The risk of multiple myeloma increases with age, but this is a case report of a patient who was diagnosed with a large amount of disease burden at a young age showing that young patients may present more aggressively. This case highlights that multiple myeloma should be included in the differential diagnosis of a young patient with neurological symptoms and mass lesions, after more common causes have been ruled out. Moreover, this patient has an aggressive form of multiple myeloma presenting with several plasmacytomas and neurological symptoms. She progressed and failed induction with CyBorD, and only after switching to DCEP with addition of daratumumab, did she have a partial response. The response was long enough to stabilize and discharge her from the hospital safely.

Further research is needed in this field to determine optimal treatment regimens for this subset of young patients. These cases are rare, thus hampering the use of clinical trials in these patients. Therefore, case reports and registries may be needed to help collect data for future analysis and studies. Ideally these patients would be most likely to benefit from a cure, given the young age and potential loss of life years.

Additional Points

Clinical Significance. It is important to recognize that multiple myeloma can occur in very young patients and may present and respond differently in this younger-aged cohort. Diagnosing and treating this group can be challenging, and it is crucial to identify optimal initial treatment regimens for these patients. A great way to gather this information would be by creating a registry.

Authors' Contributions

ML prepared the manuscript, and MB helped to edit and revise it. VN prepared the radiology pictures, and XZ prepared the pathology slides and flow cytometry. SS and JH provided the case material. All authors read and approved the final manuscript.

Acknowledgments

The authors would like to thank all members of the study team, the patient's family, and Northwell Health System and North Shore University Hospital for their support.

References

[1] A. M. Noone, N. Howlader, M Krapcho et al., Eds., *SEER Cancer Statistics Review, 1975-2015*, National Cancer Institute, Bethesda, MD, USA, 2018, https://seer.cancer.gov/csr/1975_2015/.

[2] R. A. Kyle, M. A. Gertz, T. E. Witzig et al., "Review of 1027 patients with newly diagnosed multiple myeloma," *Mayo Clinic Proceedings*, vol. 78, no. 1, pp. 21–33, 2003.

[3] J. Bladé, R. A. Kyle, and P. R. Greipp, "Multiple myeloma in patients younger than 30 years," *Archives of Internal Medicine*, vol. 156, no. 13, pp. 1463–1468, 1996.

[4] J. Bladé, R. A. Kyle, and P. R. Greipp, "Presenting features and prognosis in 72 patients with multiple myeloma who were younger than 40 years," *British Journal of Haematology*, vol. 93, no. 2, pp. 345–351, 1996.

[5] J. Bladé and R. A. Kyle, "Multiple myeloma in young patients: clinical presentation and treatment approach," *Leukemia & Lymphoma*, vol. 30, no. 5-6, pp. 493–501, 1998.

[6] S. Yohe, M. Luquette, T. C. Lund, L. M. Turcotte, M. Dolan, and R. W. McKenna, "Plasma cell myeloma in children and young adults: a report of 4 cases from a single institution and a review of the literature," *Journal of Pediatric Hematology/Oncology*, vol. 39, no. 6, pp. 452–457, 2017.

[7] H. Ludwig, B. G. M. Durie, V. Bolejack et al., "Myeloma in patients younger than age 50 years presents with more favorable features and shows better survival: an analysis of 10 549 patients from the International Myeloma Working Group," *Blood*, vol. 111, no. 8, pp. 4039–4047, 2008.

[8] P. K. Cheema, S. Zadeh, V. Kukreti et al., "Age 40 years and under does not confer superior prognosis in patients with multiple myeloma undergoing upfront autologous stem cell transmplant," *Biology of Blood and Marrow Transplantation*, vol. 15, no. 6, pp. 686–693, 2009.

[9] G. M. Hewell and R. Alexanian, "Multiple myeloma in young persons," *Annals of Internal Medicine*, vol. 84, no. 4, pp. 441–443, 1976.

[10] H. M. Lazarus, R. W. Kellermeyer, M. Aikawa, and R. H. Herzig, "Multiple myeloma in young men clinical course and electron microscopic studies of bone marrow plasma cells," *Cancer*, vol. 46, no. 6, pp. 1397–1400, 1980.

[11] N. Geetha, M. Jayaprakash, A. Rekhanair, K. Ramachandran, and B. Rajan, "Plasma cell neoplasms in the young," *The British Journal of Radiology*, vol. 72, no. 862, pp. 1012–1015, 1999.

[12] S. V. Rajkumar, "Multiple myeloma: 2016 update on diagnosis, risk-stratification, and management," *American Journal of Hematology*, vol. 91, no. 7, pp. 719–734, 2016.

[13] A. Palumbo, H. Avet-Loiseau, S. Oliva et al., "Revised international staging system for multiple myeloma: a report from international myeloma working group," *Journal of Clinical Oncology*, vol. 33, no. 26, pp. 2863–2869, 2015.

[14] C. B. Reeder, D. E. Reece, V. Kukreti et al., "Cyclophosphamide, bortezomib and dexamethasone induction for newly diagnosed multiple myeloma: high response rates in a phase II clinical trial," *Leukemia*, vol. 23, no. 7, pp. 1337–1341, 2009.

[15] S. Kumar, I. Flinn, P. G. Richardson et al., "Randomized, multicenter, phase 2 study (EVOLUTION) of combinations of bortezomib, dexamethasone, cyclophosphamide, and lenalidomide in previously untreated multiple myeloma," *Blood*, vol. 119, no. 19, pp. 4375–4382, 2012.

[16] S. Park, S. J. Lee, C. W. Jung et al., "DCEP for relapsed or refractory multiple myeloma after therapy with novel agents," *Annals of Hematology*, vol. 93, no. 1, pp. 99–105, 2014.

[17] H. M. Lokhorst, T. Plesner, J. P. Laubach et al., "Targeting CD38 with daratumumab monotherapy in multiple myeloma," *New England Journal of Medicine*, vol. 373, no. 13, pp. 1207–1219, 2015.

[18] M. Sagar Lonial Brendan, B. M. Weiss, S. Z. Usmani et al., "Single-agent daratumumab in heavily pre-treated patients with multiple myeloma: an open-label, international, multicentre phase 2 trial (Sirius)," *The Lancet*, vol. 387, no. 10027, pp. 1551–1560, 2016.

[19] S. V. Rajkumar, J.-L. Harousseau, B. Durie et al., "Consensus recommendations for the uniform reporting of clinical trials: report of the International Myeloma Workshop Consensus Panel 1," *Blood*, vol. 117, no. 18, pp. 4691–4695, 2011.

[20] Q. Zhu, X. Zou, R. You et al., "Establishment of an innovative staging system for extramedullary plasmacytoma," *BMC Cancer*, vol. 16, no. 1, p. 777, 2016.

[21] K. D. Short, S. V. Rajkumar, D. Larson et al., "Incidence of extramedullary disease in patients with multiple myeloma in the era of novel therapy, and the activity of pomalidomide on extramedullary myeloma," *Leukemia*, vol. 25, no. 6, pp. 906–908, 2011.

[22] A. Cerase, A. Tarantino, A. Gozzetti et al., "Intracranial involvement in plasmacytomas and multiple myeloma: a pictorial essay," *Neuroradiology*, vol. 50, no. 8, pp. 665–674, 2008.

[23] J. W. Hussong, S. L. Perkins, B. Schnitzer, H. Hargreaves, and G. Frizzera, "Extramedullary plasmacytoma: a form of marginal zone cell lymphoma?," *American Journal of Clinical Pathology*, vol. 111, no. 1, pp. 111–116, 1999.

[24] J. J. Pisano, R. Coupland, S.-Y. Chen, and A. S. Miller, "Plasmacytoma of the oral cavity and jaws," *Oral Surgery, Oral Medicine, Oral Pathology, Oral Radiology, and Endodontology*, vol. 83, no. 2, pp. 265–271, 1997.

[25] E. Wiltshaw, "The natural history of extramedullary plasmacytoma and its relation to solitary myeloma of bone and myelomatosis," *Medicine*, vol. 55, no. 3, pp. 217–238, 1976.

[26] T. Plesner and J. Krejcik, "Daratumumab for the treatment of multiple myeloma," *Frontiers in Immunology*, vol. 9, p. 1228, 2018.

[27] M. de Weers, Y.-T. Tai, M. S. van der Veer et al., "Daratumumab, a novel therapeutic human CD38 monoclonal antibody, induces killing of multiple myeloma and other hematological tumors," *The Journal of Immunology*, vol. 186, no. 3, pp. 1840–1848, 2011.

[28] M. S. van der Veer, M. de Weers, B. van Kessel et al., "The therapeutic human CD38 antibody daratumumab improves the anti-myeloma effect of newly emerging multi-drug therapies," *Blood Cancer Journal*, vol. 1, no. 10, p. e41, 2011.

[29] M. S. van der Veer, M. de Weers, B. van Kessel et al., "Towards effective immunotherapy of myeloma: enhanced elimination of myeloma cells by combination of lenalidomide with the human CD38 monoclonal antibody daratumumab," *Haematologica*, vol. 96, no. 2, pp. 284–290, 2011.

[30] K. McKeage, "Daratumumab: first global approval," *Drugs*, vol. 76, no. 2, pp. 275–281, 2016.

[31] A. Palumbo, A. Chanan-Khan, K. Weisel et al., "Daratumumab, bortezomib, and dexamethasone for multiple myeloma," *New England Journal of Medicine*, vol. 375, no. 8, pp. 754–766, 2016.

[32] M. A. Dimopoulos, A. Oriol, H. Nahi et al., "Daratumumab, lenalidomide, and dexamethasone for multiple myeloma," *New England Journal of Medicine*, vol. 375, no. 14, pp. 1319–1331, 2016.

[33] M.-V. Mateos, M. A. Dimopoulos, M. Cavo et al., "Daratumumab plus bortezomib, melphalan, and prednisone for untreated myeloma," *New England Journal of Medicine*, vol. 378, no. 6, pp. 518–528, 2018.

[34] T. Facon, S. Kumar, T. Plesner et al., "Daratumumab plus lenalidomide and dexamethasone for untreated myeloma," *New England Journal of Medicine*, vol. 380, no. 22, pp. 2104–2115, 2019.

[35] T. Plesner, H.-T. Arkenau, P. Gimsing et al., "Phase 1/2 study of daratumumab, lenalidomide, and dexamethasone for relapsed multiple myeloma," *Blood*, vol. 128, no. 14, pp. 1821–1828, 2016.

[36] A. Chari, A. Suvannasankha, J. W. Fay et al., "Daratumumab plus pomalidomide and dexamethasone in relapsed and/or refractory multiple myeloma," *Blood*, vol. 130, no. 8, pp. 974–981, 2017.

8

A Western Case of Intravascular Large B-Cell Lymphoma as Unusual Cause of Persistent Fever

Pier Paolo Piccaluga,[1,2,3,4] Stefania Paolini,[4] Cristina Campidelli,[5] Nicola Vianelli,[4] and Luigi Bolondi[6]

[1]*Department of Experimental, Diagnostic and Speciality Medicine, University of Bologna, Bologna, Italy*
[2]*Istituto Euro-Mediterraneo di Scienza e Tecnologia (IEMEST), Palermo, Italy*
[3]*Jomo Kenyatta University of Agriculture and Technology, Juja, Kenya*
[4]*S. Orsola-Malpighi Hospital, Hematology and Hematopathology Units, Bologna, Italy*
[5]*Azienda Ospedaliera Ospedali di Legnano, U. O. Anatomia Patologica, Legnao, Milan, Italy*
[6]*Department of Medical and Surgical Sciences, University of Bologna, Bologna, Italy*

Correspondence should be addressed to Pier Paolo Piccaluga; pierpaolo.piccaluga@unibo.it

Academic Editor: Kiyotaka Kawauchi

Fever of unknown origin (FUO) is a common and challenging clinical condition that can be referred, among others, to infections, drug's effects, various inflammatory disorders, and cancers. Among the latter, lymphomas can indeed cause fever, which is therefore accounted as a lymphoma-related sign in patients' staging. Intravascular large B-cell lymphoma (IVLBCL) is a very rare tumor, characterized by lymphoma cell accumulation within sinusoids and, despite a very aggressive course, the evidence of this disease is scarce. Two variants are currently recognized, respectively, occurring in either Western (mainly characterized by neurological symptoms and skin involvement) or Eastern countries (with hemophagocytic syndrome, bone marrow, spleen, and liver involvement). We describe an atypical and unprecedented IVLBCL patient, presenting with pronounced features of Eastern cases as well as skin involvement. Due to the scant amount of neoplastic cells, the diagnosis was very challenging, with FUO being the first and for a certain time unique clinical sign. Although lymphoma was suspected, the lack of evidence for neoplastic cells delayed the final diagnosis. Eventually, only autopsy revealed the extensive involvement of different organs and tissues.

1. Background

Fever of unknown origin (FUO) is a relatively common medical condition, more often related to unrecognized infections, autoimmune diseases, drug administration, and cancer [1]. As far as the latter is concerned, fever can represent the initial symptom at presentation. In particular, lymphomas are often associated with fever or other systemic symptoms, their presence defining a more advanced disease [2]. Intravascular large B-cell lymphoma (IVLBCL) is a rare, clinically aggressive lymphoma characterized by an almost exclusive growth of large cells within the lumen of all sized blood vessels [3]. Clinically, in its classical variant, IVLBCL presents with many nonspecific signs and symptoms such as FUO and involvement of the central nervous system (CNS) and skin [3]. The so-called cutaneous variant, in which only the skin is affected, has been more often described in Western countries and has a better prognosis. On the contrary, a hemophagocytic variant associated with hemophagocytic syndrome and often with hepatosplenic involvement and cytopenia can be encountered, more often in Asia [3]. The generally very poor prognosis of this disease has been substantially improved by immunochemotherapy, in particular with anti-CD20 monoclonal antibodies [3]. However, the majority of patients still experience relapse, especially when the CNS is involved. Furthermore, due to the puzzling presentation, the diagnosis is often delayed and not infrequently the disease is recognized *postmortem*.

We describe a patient who presented with persistent fever and died, unfortunately, before a conclusive diagnosis was made.

2. Case Report

A 58-year-old Caucasian woman was admitted to our hospital as a case of fever of unknown origin (FUO) after 2 weeks of continuous remittent fever without shivering, polyarthralgias, cervical pain, and headache. On admission, physical examination revealed oedema of the lower limbs with erythematous and painful skin and a temperature of 38°C, not responding to paracetamol and cephalosporin therapy. Laboratory investigations showed an erythrocyte sedimentation rate (ESR) of 120 mm/h, a C-reactive protein (CRP) level of 225 mg/L, a serum ferritin level of 2076 mg/L, and a fibrinogen level of 223 mg/dL. Liver enzymes (AST 83 U/L and ALT 114 U/L) and lactate dehydrogenase (LDH 746 U/L) levels were increased, with reduction of serum albumin and total plasmatic protein values (2.7 g/dL and 5.5 g/dL, respectively). Procalcitonin was not tested at this time, not being sensitive enough, in our opinion, to discriminate, in this case between infection and malignancy. All inflammatory markers, in fact, were altered.

Acute infectious diseases (hepatitis A, hepatitis B, hepatitis C, and hepatitis E virus, human immunodeficiency virus, cytomegalovirus, parvovirus B19, Epstein–Barr virus, echoviruses, poliovirus, coxsackieviruses, *Treponema pallidum*, *Coxiella burnetii*, *Toxoplasma*, *Salmonella typhi*, *Legionella pneumophila*, *Mycoplasma pneumoniae*, *Leishmania donovani*, *Chlamydya*, *Brucella*, *Leptospira*, *Rickettsia*, and *Borrelia* species IgM) were negative. In addition, Epstein–Barr virus, herpes zoster, herpes simplex, and *Cytomegalovirus* IgG were detected, revealing a previous exposition. Increased *B. burgdorferi* IgG titer was detected by indirect immunofluorescence assay (IIF), but this finding was not confirmed by western blot (WB) technique. Antistreptolysin-O titers results did not recover beta-haemolytic streptococcal infection. Nasopharyngeal and rectal swab results were negative for aerobic bacteria, pseudomonas, and fungi, while *Candida albicans* and *Candida glabrata* were isolated from oral cavity and vaginal swabs. Peripheral blood smears showed no evidence supporting malarial infection. Mantoux intradermic test failed to demonstrate an immune reaction against mycobacterial species. Bacterial (*Salmonella*, *Shigella*, and *Campylobacter*), mycobacterial, and parasitic culture obtained from blood, stool, and urinary samples were negative. Cerebrospinal fluid examination was performed, but again viral and bacterial involvement could not be proved. Similarly, galactomannan test was negative.

Serum protein electrophoresis presented a slight enlargement of the gamma zone; urine protein electrophoresis disclosed a nonspecific glomerular proteinuria. Immunoglobulin levels (IgG 763 mg/dL, IgA 319 mg/dL, and IgM 316 mg/dL), peripheral T- and B-cell subsets (CD4+CD3+ 59%, CD8+CD3+ 18%, CD3+ 77%, CD19+ 19%, CD16+CD56+ 3%, and CD4+CD8+ 0%), and autoantibodies were regular.

Transoesophageal echocardiography ruled out endocardial vegetations. Abdominal US scan displayed mild hepatomegaly and normal spleen diameters. Whole body computed tomography (CT), single-photon emission computed tomography with labelled leukocytes, bone and lung scintigraphy, and 18 (F)-fluorodeoxyglucose (FDG)-PET were normal. Cerebral magnetic resonance imaging was consistent with a nonspecific subacute inflammatory condition.

Esophagogastroduodenoscopy with duodenal biopsy was not conclusive for Whipple disease. Liver biopsy showed mild piecemeal necrosis with lobular spotty necrosis and cholestatic changes. Bone marrow trephine biopsy was hypocellular with a mild increase in granulopoietic and erythropoietic precursors and reactive plasmacytosis, and no evidence of leishmanial infection.

During the hospitalization, the patient did not respond to ciprofloxacin, imipenem, prednisone (initiated after admission to control fever and symptoms), and NSAID administration, maintaining an acceptable cenesthesis with an unchanged fever curve and persistence of the lower limb lesions. Subsequently, the patient developed an increasing normocytic anemia (RBC $2.51 \times 10^6/\mu L$, HGB 7.9 g/dL, HCT 20.8%, MCV 82.8 fL, MCH 31.5 pg, MCHC 38.0%, RDW 15.2%, and HDW 3.6 g/dL), with hypoalbuminemia (2.5 g/dL) and rising values of acute-phase proteins (CRP 38.6 mg/dL and fibrinogen 920 mg/dL) and liver enzymes: LDH (1131 U/L), alkaline phosphatase (617 U/L), bilirubin (11.87 mg/dL), and transaminase (ALT 129 U/L and AST 64 U/L). An empirical treatment with doxycyclin and AmBisome was commenced on suspicion of chlamydial or leishmania infection, without improvement.

Subsequently, the patient presented a worsening with intermittent delirant states, dyspnea with hypoxia, and thrombotic microangiopathy (TMA) associated with severe thrombocytopenia ($3 \times 10^9/L$). A second bone marrow trephine biopsy showed a mildly decreased hematopoiesis with a pronounced plasmocytosis and evidence of hemophagocytosis. Prednisone dose was increased (80 mg per day), and a plasma exchange treatment was started. By contrast, etoposide therapy was not initiated due to the suspect of cancer, in order not to compromise the following treatment. After a brief period of symptom improvement, the patient exhibited acute renal impairment, hyperbilirubinemia (18.26 mg/dL), respiratory failure with tachypnea, and severe metabolic acidosis. She was transferred to the intensive care unit (ICU) and developed progressive multiorgan failure, mental cloudiness, and massive nasogastric bleeding; afterwards, she quickly deteriorated and died.

Autopsy disclosed diffuse involvement by intravascular large B-cell lymphoma (IVLBCL) in several organs (heart, lungs, stomach, kidneys, adrenal glands, liver, and spleen). Multiple skin sampling revealed the presence of rare intraluminal neoplastic elements. Bone marrow specimens were massively infiltrated by neoplastic cells. Furthermore, the liver and spleen showed presence of hemophagocytosis (Figures 1 and 2). Immunophenotyping indicated that neoplastic cells were CD45+, CD20+, CD79a+, BCL2+/−

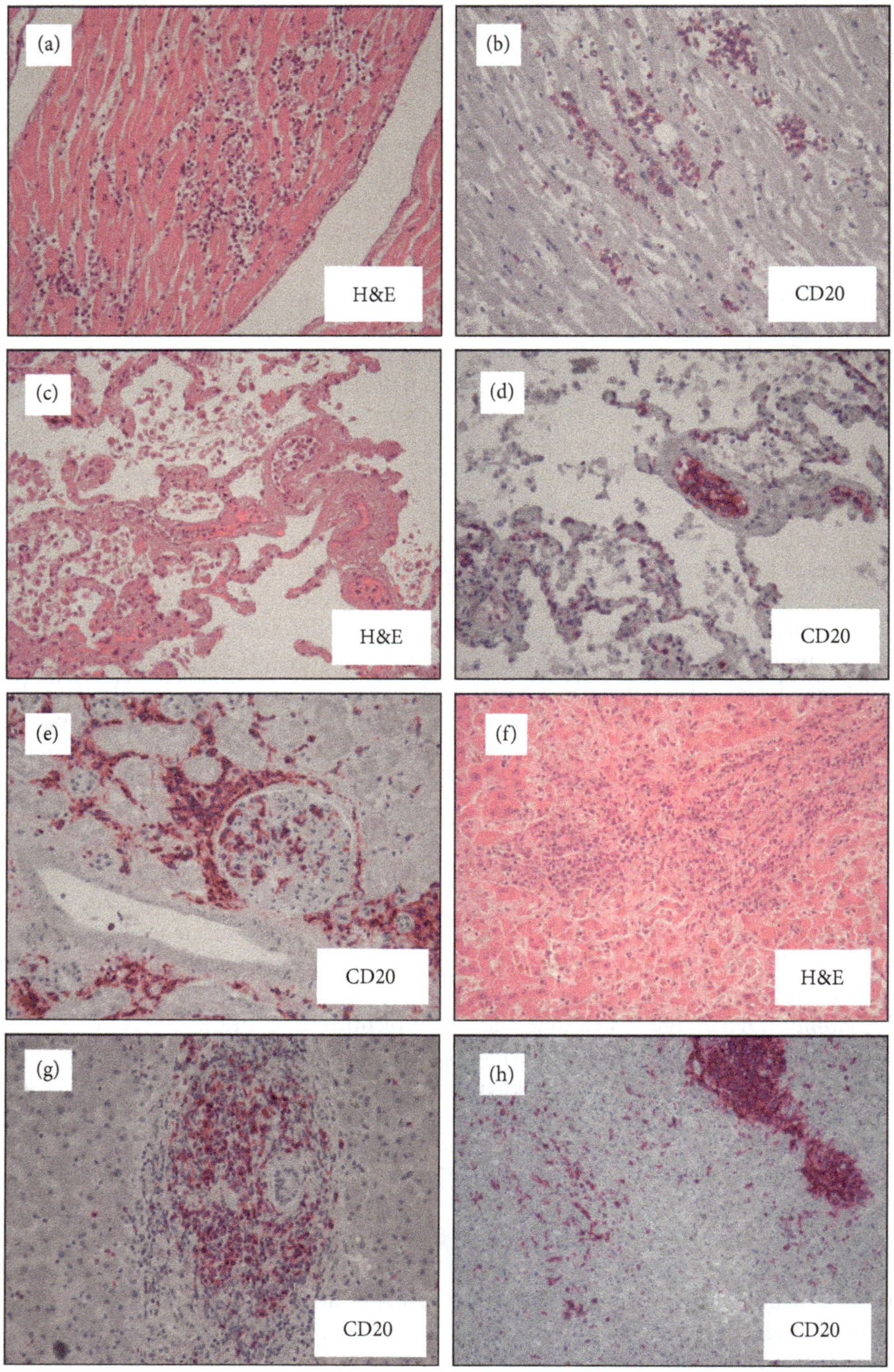

Figure 1: Microscopic appearance of IVLBCL infiltrating heart (a, b), lung (c, d), kidney (e), and liver (f and g) portal localization; (h) sinusoidal localization). H&E = hematoxylin and eosin.

(10–20% of the neoplastic population), CD3−, CD10−, CD5−, and BCL6−, with high Ki67 index (60%).

3. Discussion

Intravascular large B-cell lymphoma is an infrequent subtype of diffuse large B-cell lymphoma characterized by the selective growth of neoplastic cells within the lumina of small- to medium-sized blood vessels [2]. This condition was first described in 1959 by Pfleger and Tappeiner as angioendotheliomatosis proliferans systemisata [4]; only during the 1980s, the lymphoid nature of the disease was established [5–8]. IVLBCL has an aggressive behaviour with a poor outcome, and in many instances it is diagnosed postmortem; clinical presentation is extremely variable: B symptoms are the overriding presenting feature, and frequently it can manifest as FUO, which is more commonly reported than in other extranodal aggressive lymphomas (45% vs. 25% of cases at presentation) [9, 10].

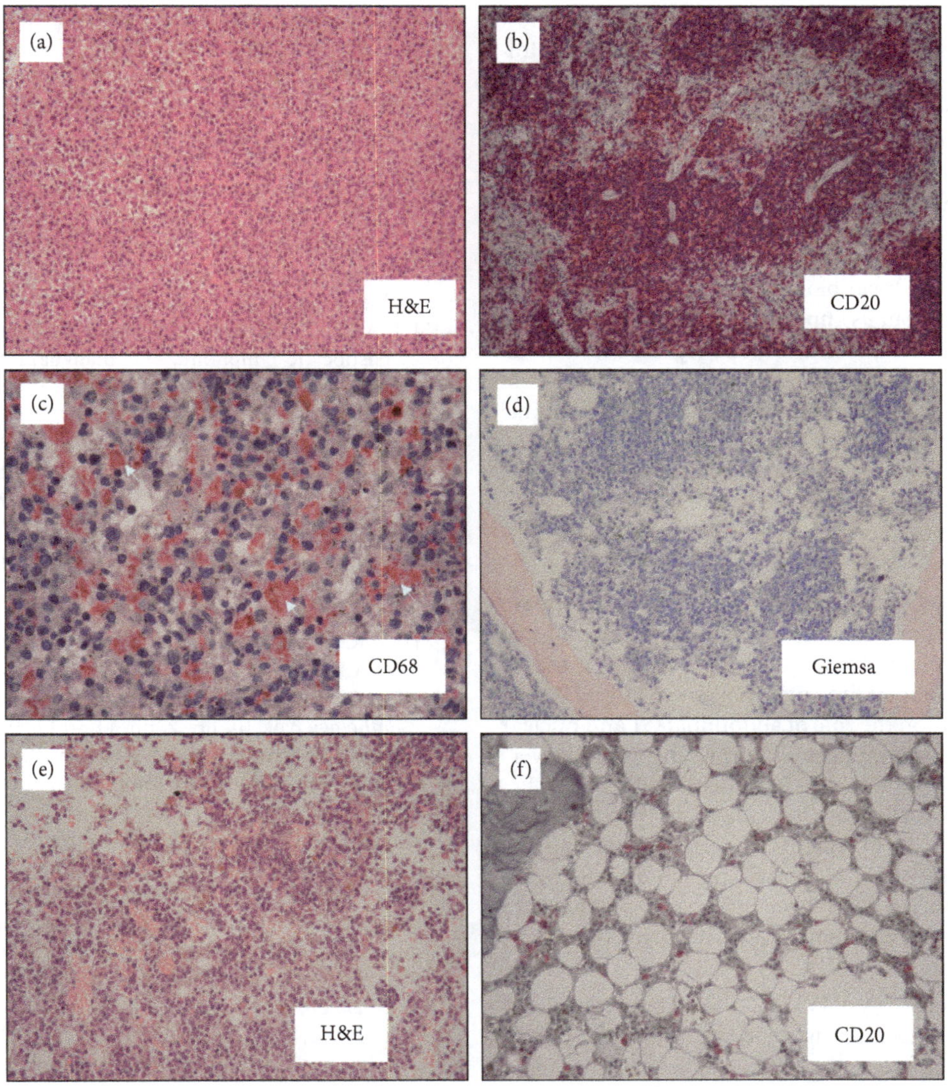

FIGURE 2: Microscopic appearance of IVLBCL infiltrating the spleen (a–c) and the bone marrow (d–f). Hemophagocytosis (light blue arrows) was observed in the spleen (c). H&E = hematoxylin and eosin.

Different clinical manifestations have been described depending on geographical origin [8, 9]. Interestingly, our patient showed features typical both of Asian series (HPS, fever, anemia with thrombocytopenia, and liver and bone marrow involvement) and of Western ones (neurological symptoms and skin involvement). In particular, HPS is the most frequent clinical manifestation of Asian-variant IVLBCL, while it is uncommon in European series [11, 12]. Ferreri and colleagues [12] suggested that differences in clinical-pathological features in IVLBCL might be more related to the co-occurrence of HPS rather than the geographical distribution of the disease; in fact, they reported that non-Japanese patients with IVLBCL and HPS showed features similar to those of Japanese HPS patients, while Japanese patients with IVL without HPS had a clinical picture similar to Western cases. Among all Western series of IVLBCL, histologically confirmed HPS has been demonstrated in only five cases [13–16] and two of them were of Caribbean and Vietnamese origin [12]. Our case, as other rare cases of Western HPS-associated IVLBCL, displayed significantly higher rates of advanced disease, fever, hepatosplenic involvement, bone marrow infiltration, fatigue, dyspnea, anemia, thrombocytopenia, and altered liver function tests. This admixed clinical picture probably contributed to mislead the diagnostic process. Unfortunately, it is impossible to assess whether an empiric treatment with etoposide, aimed to reduce HPS, might have allowed a more effective diagnosis.

Neurological disorders are present at initial diagnosis in 34% of European patients [17]; symptoms are miscellaneous, comprising alteration of conscience, peripheral nerves deficit, seizures, paresis, dementia, and extrapiramidal symptoms. Neuroimaging features are nonspecific: CT and MRI can mimic vasculitis, small-vessel ischemic disease, or demyelination [18]. In view of these considerations, suspecting IVLBCL on the basis of neurological symptoms is difficult; moreover, our patient developed delirant states only in the last part of the hospitalization. Skin lesions may present as erythematous eruption, plaques, cellulitis, ulcerated nodules, and, rarely, generalised telangiectasia [9].

Laboratory tests are altered in all cases of IVLBCL: the most represented is increased concentration of serum LDH, followed by hypoalbuminemia (<36 g/L), hyperbilirubinemia (>15 mg/L), hypercreatininemia (>15 mg/L), and increased C-reactive protein (>50 mg/L). Anemia is the most commonly observed blood cell count abnormality, followed by leukopenia and thrombocytopenia [19].

Up to now, no standard procedure for IVLBCL diagnosis has been established. Organ biopsy seems to be the most accurate diagnostic tool, but its importance strictly depends on the choice of the correct biopsy site. Several reports recommend random skin biopsies and repeated bone marrow biopsies in order to obtain a prompt diagnosis [19–24]. Conventional staging investigations (neuroimaging and total-body computed tomography and $_{18}$ (F)-FDG-positron emission tomography) show lower accuracy compared to conventional DLBCL in detecting the presence and the extent of the disease [25–27].

Mourad and colleagues [28] proposed a comprehensive algorithm for an approach to FUO (including abdominal CT, Tc-based nuclear scan, investigation for infective endocarditis, leg doppler imaging, and liver biopsy), with particular emphasis on the role of abdominal CT and nuclear imaging in detecting lymphoproliferative disorders; nevertheless, results may be negative in patients with IVLBCL.

Bone marrow evaluation is a standard procedure in patients affected by FUO. In this case, two bone marrow biopsies were performed, a hematological disease being suspected, but both were not conclusive; only postmortem revealed a massive lymphomatous involvement.

Last of all, the possibility of IVLBCL should be considered in unexplained reactive haemophagocytic syndrome and, even if the bone marrow is infrequently involved. Bone marrow biopsy seems to be the most useful tool when the clinical presentation is characterized by fever of unknown origin with anemia or thrombocytopenia [29]. In this regard, the recent advent of liquid biopsy might represent an attractive strategy [30].

The present case represents, to the best of our knowledge, the first example of IVLBCL, Asian variant, occurring in a European patient. Intensive diagnosis approaches are recommended in patients presenting with FUO, IVLBCL being in the spectrum of differential diagnosis.

Acknowledgments

This work was supported by Centro Interdipartimentale per la Ricerca sul Cancro "G. Prodi", BolognAIL, RFO (Prof. Piccaluga), AIRC (Prof. Piccaluga IG 2013 No. 14355), Strategico di Ateneo 2006 (Prof. Piccaluga), and FIRB Futura 2011 RBFR12D1CB (Prof. Piccaluga).

References

[1] C. Mulders-Manders, A. Simon, and C. Bleeker-Rovers, "Fever of unknown origin," *Clinical Medicine*, vol. 15, no. 3, pp. 280–284, 2015.

[2] S. Nakamura, M. Ponzoni, and E. Campo, "Intravascular large B-cell lymphoma," in *WHO Classification of Tumours of Haematopoietic and Lymphoid Tissues*, S. H. Swerdlow, E. Campo, N. L. Harris et al., Eds., pp. 252-253, IARC Press, Lyon, France, 2017.

[3] M. Ponzoni, E. Campo, and S. Nakamura, "Intravascular large B-cell lymphoma: a chameleon with multiple faces and many masks," *Blood*, vol. 132, no. 15, pp. 1561–1567, 2018.

[4] V. L. Pfleger and J. Tappeiner, "Zur Kenntnis der systemisierten endotheliomatose der cutanen blutgefa¨ße (reticuloendotheliose?)," *Hautarzt*, vol. 10, pp. 363–369, 1959.

[5] J. Ansell, J. Bhawan, S. Cohen, J. Sullivan, and D. Sherman, "Histiocytic lymphoma and malignant angioendotheliomatosis. One disease or two?," *Cancer*, vol. 50, no. 8, pp. 1506–1512, 1982.

[6] J. Bhawan, S. M. Wolff, A. A. Ucci, and A. K. Bhan, "Malignant lymphoma and malignant angioendotheliomatosis: one disease," *Cancer*, vol. 55, no. 3, pp. 570–576, 1985.

[7] U. Wrotnowski, S. E. Mills, and P. H. Cooper, "Malignant angioendotheliomatosis: an angiotropic lymphoma?," *American Journal of Clinical Pathology*, vol. 83, no. 2, pp. 244–248, 1985.

[8] M. R. Wick, S. E. Mills, B. W. Scheithauer, P. H. Cooper, M. A. Davitz, and K. Parkinson, "Reassessment of malignant "angioendotheliomatosis"," *The American Journal of Surgical Pathology*, vol. 10, no. 2, pp. 112–123, 1986.

[9] A. J. M. Ferreri, E. Campo, J. F. Seymour et al., "Intravascular lymphoma: clinical presentation, natural history, management and prognostic factors in a series of 38 cases, with special emphasis on the "cutaneous variant"," *British Journal of Haematology*, vol. 127, no. 2, pp. 173–183, 2004.

[10] M. Ponzoni, A. J. M. Ferreri, E. Campo et al., "Definition, diagnosis, and management of intravascular large B-cell lymphoma: proposals and perspectives from an international consensus meeting," *Journal of Clinical Oncology*, vol. 25, no. 21, pp. 3168–3173, 2007.

[11] T. Murase, S. Nakamura, K. Kawauchi et al., "An Asian variant of intravascular large B-cell lymphoma: clinical, pathological and cytogenetic approaches to diffuse large B-cell lymphoma associated with haemophagocytic syndrome," *British Journal of Haematology*, vol. 111, no. 3, pp. 826–834, 2000.

[12] A. J. M. Ferreri, G. P. Dognini, E. Campo et al., "Variations in clinical presentation, frequency of hemophagocytosis and clinical behavior of intravascular lymphoma diagnosed in different geographical regions," *Haematologica*, vol. 92, no. 4, pp. 486–492, 2007.

[13] J. P. Dufau, A. Le Tourneau, T. Molina et al., "Intravascular large B-cell lymphoma with bone marrow involvement at presentation and haemophagocytic syndrome: two Western cases in favour of a specific variant," *Histopathology*, vol. 37, no. 6, pp. 509–512, 2000.

[14] S. A. F. al-Hazzaa, W. R. Green, and R. B. Mann, "Uveal involvement in systemic angiotropic large cell lymphoma," *Ophthalmology*, vol. 100, no. 6, pp. 961–965, 1993.

[15] J. A. Snowden, C. A. Angel, D. A. Winfield, J. H. Pringle, and K. P. West, "Angiotropic lymphoma: report of a case with histiocytic features," *Journal of Clinical Pathology*, vol. 50, no. 1, pp. 67–70, 1997.

[16] D. Remotti, L. Insabato, A. De Renzo et al., "Intravascular B-cell lymphoma: report of two cases with different clinical presentation but rapid central nervous system involvement," *Leukemia & Lymphoma*, vol. 44, no. 8, pp. 1353–1359, 2003.

[17] D. K. Song, N. M. Boulis, P. E. McKeever, and D. J. Quint, "Angiotropic large cell lymphoma with imaging

characteristics of CNS vasculitis," *AJNR. American Journal of Neuroradiology*, vol. 23, no. 2, pp. 239–242, 2002.

[18] T. Murase, M. Yamaguchi, R. Suzuki et al., "Intravascular large B-cell lymphoma (IVLBCL): a clinicopathologic study of 96 cases with special reference to the immunophenotypic heterogeneity of CD5," *Blood*, vol. 109, no. 2, pp. 478–485, 2007.

[19] K. Shimada, T. Kinoshita, T. Naoe, and S. Nakamura, "Presentation and management of intravascular large B-cell lymphoma," *The Lancet Oncology*, vol. 10, no. 9, pp. 895–902, 2009.

[20] C. R. Barnett, S. Seo, S. Husain, and M. E. Grossman, "Intravascular B-cell lymphoma: the role of skin biopsy," *The American Journal of Dermatopathology*, vol. 30, no. 3, pp. 295–299, 2008.

[21] S. Srivatsa, J. Sharma, and S. Logani, "Intravascular lymphoma: an unusual diagnostic outcome of an incidentally detected adrenal mass," *Endocrine Practice*, vol. 14, no. 7, pp. 884–888, 2008.

[22] S. Gill, B. Melosky, L. Haley, and C. ChanYan, "Use of random skin biopsy to diagnose intravascular lymphoma presenting as fever of unknown origin," *The American Journal of Medicine*, vol. 114, no. 1, pp. 56–58, 2003.

[23] N. Asada, J. Odawara, S.-i. Kimura et al., "Use of random skin biopsy for diagnosis of intravascular large B-cell lymphoma," *Mayo Clinic Proceedings*, vol. 82, no. 12, pp. 1525–1527, 2007.

[24] E. N. Le, M. R. Gerstenblith, A. C. Gelber et al., "The use of blind skin biopsy in the diagnosis of intravascular B-cell lymphoma," *Journal of the American Academy of Dermatology*, vol. 59, no. 1, pp. 148–151, 2008.

[25] K. Shimada, H. Kosugi, S. Shimada et al., "Evaluation of organ involvement in intravascular large B-cell lymphoma by 18F-fluorodeoxyglucose positron emission tomography," *International Journal of Hematology*, vol. 88, no. 2, pp. 149–153, 2008.

[26] S. Al-Katib, R. Colvin, and F. Sokhandon, "Intravascular large B-cell lymphoma presenting with diffuse gallbladder wall thickening: a case report and literature review," *Case Reports in Radiology*, vol. 2018, Article ID 2494207, 5 pages, 2018.

[27] E. V. Khojeini and Y. J. Young Song, "Intravascular large B-cell lymphoma presenting as interstitial lung disease," *Case Reports in Pathology*, vol. 2014, Article ID 928065, 3 pages, 2014.

[28] O. Mourad, V. Palda, and A. S. Detsky, "A comprehensive evidence-based approach to Fever of Unknown Origin," *Archives of Internal Medicine*, vol. 163, no. 5, pp. 545–551, 2003.

[29] A. Hot, I. Jaisson, C. Girad et al., "Yield of bone marrow examination in diagnosing the source of fever of unknown origin," *Archives of Internal Medicine*, vol. 169, no. 21, pp. 2018–2023, 2009.

[30] Y. Suehara, M. Sakata-Yanagimoto, K. Hattori et al., "Liquid biopsy for the identification of intravascular large B-cell lymphoma," *Haematologica*, vol. 103, no. 6, pp. e241–e244, 2018.

9

Durable Control of Mycosis Fungoides after Sepsis: "Coley's Toxin?" Case Report and Review of the Literature

Benjamin Heyman,[1] **Chris R. Kelsey**,[2] **and Anne Beaven**[3]

[1]*Division of Regenerative Medicine, Department of Medicine, UC San Diego, Moores Cancer Center, San Diego, CA, USA*
[2]*Department of Radiation Oncology, Duke University, Durham, NC, USA*
[3]*Division of Hematology/Oncology, Department of Medicine, University of North Carolina, Chapel Hill, NC, USA*

Correspondence should be addressed to Benjamin Heyman; bheyman@ucsd.edu

Academic Editor: Masayuki Nagasawa

Mycosis fungoides, along with Sezary syndrome, is the most common subtype of cutaneous T-cell lymphoma. In this report, we present a patient with advanced-stage mycosis fungoides, who after successful treatment of methicillin-resistant *Staphylococcus aureus* bacteremia had prolonged disease control off systemic therapy. While this may have been due to single-agent gemcitabine, which can result in long remission, we hypothesize that our patient's durable response was in part due to the immune response elicited after treatment of her severe infection.

1. Introduction

Cutaneous T-cell lymphomas (CTCL) are a heterogeneous group of extranodal hematologic malignancies with diverse biology and clinical presentations. Mycosis fungoides (MF) is the most common subtype of CTCL, comprising approximately 50% of CTCLs [1]. Sezary syndrome (SS) is the leukemic form of MF, characterized by circulating abnormal α/β T lymphocytes with immunophenotype of memory cells, but with aberrant expression of common T-cell markers: $CD3^{dim}$, $CD4^+$, $CD45RO^+$, $CCR4^+$, $CD2^-$, $CD5^-$, $CD7^-$, and $CD8^-$ [2]. Patients present with persistent and progressive plaques, patches, cutaneous tumors, or erythroderma at isolated or multiple sites [3]. Sezary syndrome consists of an erythrodermic skin presentation in addition to leukemic involvement of MF [4]. Prognosis for early-stage disease MF is excellent, with normal survival for stage Ia. In contrast, patients with stage IV MF at diagnosis have a median OS of 1.5 years [5]. Currently, optimal treatment for MF is controversial as remissions are rare and are usually not durable [6]. We report a case of a patient with advanced-stage MF who after receiving a course of gemcitabine was hospitalized with sepsis and cervical diskitis, treated with antibiotics, and subsequently experienced a durable treatment-free remission of her CTCL after infection clearance.

2. Case

A 61-year-old African American woman with a past medical history of C6-7 spinal stenosis complained of a pruritic rash that began on her face one year prior. The rash appeared raised and erythematous and contained plaques and patches. Despite treatment with topical steroids and emollients, these lesions evolved into cutaneous tumors and spread to encompass >50% of her body surface. The largest tumor was located on her forehead and measured 5 cm (Figure 1(a)). Biopsy of a back lesion demonstrated a pandermal infiltrate of lymphocytes with epidermotropism and pautrier microabscesses in the epidermis. Immunohistochemical stains were positive for CD3, CD4, BF1, CD5, and CD45RA. T-cell clonality studies revealed a monoclonal T-cell receptor (TCR) gene rearrangement for the TCR-γ chain. A Sezary preparation demonstrated 73% of abnormal lymphocytes in the blood. Peripheral blood flow cytometry revealed that $CD4^+$/$CD7^-$ cells comprised 46% of lymphocytes, $CD4^+$/$CD26^-$ cells comprised 74% of lymphocytes, and the $CD4^+$/$CD8^+$

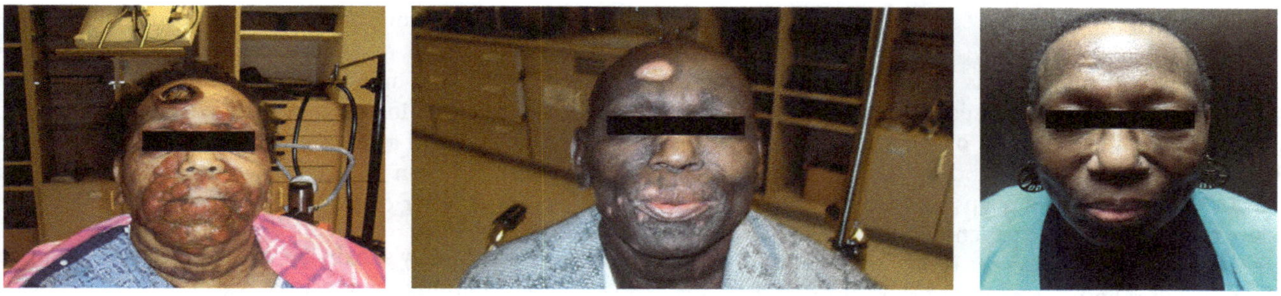

(a) (b) (c)

FIGURE 1: Photograph of cutaneous disease burden at diagnosis (a), after initial radiation therapy (b), and presently (c).

ratio was 18 : 1. CT scans demonstrated bilateral axillary and inguinal lymphadenopathy up to 2.9 × 2.5 cm in size, and node biopsy confirmed MF involvement ISCL/EORTC classification N3. Thus, at diagnosis, she had stage IVa (T3N3M0B2) disease.

Initial therapy consisted of interferon-α and concomitant total skin electron beam therapy (EBT) (36 Gy). The patient's nodules and tumors on her face, trunk, and back resolved; however, she continued to have significant pruritus and progressive lymphadenopathy (Figure 1(b)). Interferon was poorly tolerated; therefore, the treatment was changed to oral etoposide (50 mg/day). This resulted in temporary stabilization of her systemic disease. However, after four months, she had worsening cutaneous lesions and lymphadenopathy. She was subsequently started on single-agent gemcitabine. Initially, a dose of 1000 mg/m^2 on days 1, 8, and 15 of a 28-day cycle was planned, but it was decreased to 750 mg/m^2 every other week starting with cycle 3 due to neutropenia. She completed 13 cycles of gemcitabine with improvement in her cutaneous disease, as she was now found to have lichenification of the arms, abdomen, and lower extremities but continued cracking of hands and feet and she still suffered from pruritus.

After completing the 13th cycle, the patient presented to the emergency department with fever, hypotension, and new left-sided hemiparesis. She was diagnosed with sepsis, secondary to methicillin-resistant *Staphylococcus aureus* (MRSA) bacteremia. She was not neutropenic. Magnetic resonance imaging (MRI) of her spine revealed T2-hyperintense abnormalities involving the C5–C7 vertebral bodies and the C5-6 and C6-7 disc interspaces, concerning for cord edema/myelomalacia (Figure 2). She subsequently underwent an anterior cervical discectomy and fusion at C6-C7, from which cultures grew MRSA, confirming C6-7 diskitis. After surgery and completion of intravenous antibiotics, she was transitioned to a suppressive antibiotic regimen (rifampin and sulfamethoxazole/trimethoprim). With treatment of the infection and prolonged physical therapy, she regained almost complete use of her left side.

Following discharge, she was seen in follow-up where cutaneous physical exam revealed hyperkeratosis of upper and lower extremities, hypopigmentation of her face without any tumors, and 1 cm bilateral axillary lymphadenopathy. Further systemic treatment of her CTCL was held due to poor performance status, recent severe infection, and low burden of cutaneous disease. The patient was started on narrow-band ultraviolet light therapy for one month, but this was discontinued due to excellent skin symptom control with topical moisturizers. Eighteen months after the MRSA infection, she continued to have very mild cutaneous symptoms off systemic therapy. A Sezary preparation of her peripheral blood revealed 4% abnormal lymphocytes, and peripheral blood flow cytometry revealed CD4$^+$/CD7$^-$ T cells comprised 2.12% of lymphocytes, CD4$^+$/CD26$^-$ T cells comprised 1.88% of lymphocytes, and the CD4 : CD8 ratio of the T cells was 1.24 : 1. Restaging computed tomography (CT) scan demonstrated significantly decreased lymphadenopathy, with a left axillary lymph node now measuring 1.2 cm, which decreased from 2.9 cm at diagnosis. There was no evidence of disease progression until 33 months after her infection. At that time, the patient presented with new facial nodules on her left cheek and right forehead, concerning for relapse. Sezary preparation and peripheral blood flow cytometry were still negative for disease. A restaging CT scan revealed stable lymphadenopathy. She received focal RT (4 Gy × 2 to 8 Gy) to her nose, left cheek, and right temple, resulting in complete resolution of her nodules. After the completion of EBT, she has remained off further systemic therapy, which is now 46 months after gemcitabine was stopped for the development of MRSA bacteremia (Figure 1(c)).

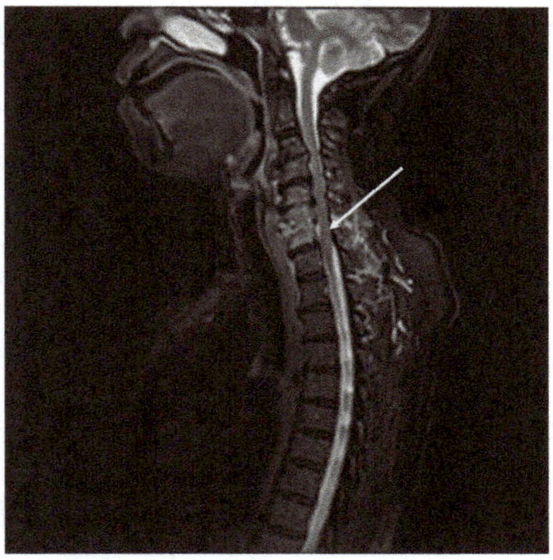

FIGURE 2: MRI of cervical spine demonstrating epidural abscess from MRSA.

3. Discussion

We present a patient who was diagnosed with advanced-stage MF and had a durable response off systemic treatment following a prolonged course of gemcitabine followed by MRSA bacteremia and cervical diskitis. The natural history of advanced-stage MF is of relapsing disease with remissions that are rarely durable. For patients with advanced-stage MF, there is no standard of care. Initial treatment for most patients requires both systemic and skin-directed therapies. Initial systemic therapies for advanced-stage MF include interferons, methotrexate, histone deacetylase inhibitors (romidepsin and vorinostat), brentuximab vedotin, psoralen and ultraviolet A, or single-agent cytotoxic chemotherapy [3]. Common chemotherapies include pegylated liposomal doxorubicin, pralatrexate, or gemcitabine [3].

Gemcitabine is a pyrimidine antimetabolite that inhibits DNA synthesis by blocking DNA polymerase and ribonucleotide reductase [7]. Our patient received 13 cycles of gemcitabine because of her aggressive initial presentation, failure to respond to initial therapies, improvement in symptoms, and lack of serious side effects until her infection. Zinzani et al. conducted a phase II clinical trial of single-agent gemcitabine in patients with relapsed or refractory (R/R) CTCLs, of which 30 patients had MF [8]. In patients with MF, the CR rate (CRR) was 10% and the partial response rate (PRR) was 60% [8]. For patients who obtained a CR, responses were ongoing at 6–22 months. Those with partial responses (PR) had a median duration of response ranging from 6 to 10 months [8]. A long-term updated analysis of 39 patients with R/R T-cell lymphoma treated with single-agent gemcitabine demonstrated an ORR of 48% and a CRR of 16%, in the 19 patients who had MF [9]. In the three patients with MF who developed CRs, responses were durable with remissions lasting 10, 18, and 120 months [9]. Lastly, Duvic et al. conducted a phase II clinical trial of single-agent gemcitabine in 33 patients with R/R cutaneous T-cell lymphomas, of which 8 patients were treated off protocol [10]. Thirty-one patients in the study had the diagnosis of MF, with 28 having advanced-stage disease. The ORR for protocol patients was 68%, with a CRR of 12%. The median duration of response for protocol patients achieving a PR was 4.1 months. The estimated median 3-year overall survival was 20.4 months [10]. Thus, single-agent gemcitabine can be effective in some patients, and, although rare, it can produce long-term remissions.

It is possible that our patient's durable response was due to single-agent gemcitabine; however, there is only one reported remission in the literature lasting >2 years. Therefore, we hypothesize that the immune response stimulated by her bacterial sepsis/diskitis may have contributed to the prolonged disease control. This idea was first proposed by William B. Coley in the early 1900s when he demonstrated that the exposure to bacteria/bacterial toxins hindered tumor growth. "Coley's toxins" were heat-killed combinations of *Streptococcus pyogenes* and *Serratia marcescens* that Dr. Coley injected into patients with advanced malignancies [11]. He reported that in 80% of the cases, for which no alternative treatment was available, survival was >5 years. Coley found that fever induction was the best predictor of patient response. The mechanism of action of "Coley's toxins" is not completely understood, but it is thought that the infection-stimulated tumor regression occurred because of an innate immune response, leading to increased expression of tumor necrosis factor (TNF), interferons, and other cytokines [11].

Although "Coley's toxin" never became part of standard care, cancer immunotherapy is a burgeoning area of research and, in the form of interferon alpha, has been a part of MF treatment for many years. Interferon alpha (IFN) was the first cancer immunomodulating agent approved by the FDA, in 1986, for use in hairy cell leukemia. Although not an FDA indication, it is an effective MF treatment with reports of objective responses in over 70% of patients [12, 13].

Since Coley's time, research has moved away from using bacterial vaccines to induce an antitumor response to the development of drugs that more specifically target tumor-immune cell interactions. These immunomodulating drugs target immune system checkpoints such as cytotoxic T lymphocyte antigen 4 (CTLA-4) and programmed cell death protein 1 (PD-1). A phase I trial of the anti-PD-1 monoclonal antibody, nivolumab, reported that in 13 patients with MF, the ORR was 15%, with a median progression-free survival (PFS) of 10 months [14]. A phase II trial of a similar agent, pembrolizumab, reported an ORR of 38% with one CR in 24 patients with MF. The one-year PFS was 69%, suggesting that checkpoint inhibitors may lead to durable responses in MF [15]. Currently, pembrolizumab in combination with radiotherapy is being investigated as a way to enhance the abscopal effect for the treatment of patients with R/R MF (NCT03385226).

4. Conclusion

We present data on a patient with advanced MF who had unusually prolonged disease control after single-agent gemcitabine with subsequent MRSA bacteremia and diskitis. Forty-six months after her infection, she has had excellent control of her disease without any systemic therapy since single-agent gemcitabine was stopped. Patients who receive single-agent gemcitabine typically do not achieve such impressive durable control of disease. Therefore, we suspect that her prolonged response was secondary to the severe bacterial infection, resulting in an antitumor immunity similar to Coley's toxin. Currently, there is a lack of reported cases in the literature regarding the role of infection and immune system stimulation on disease outcome in MF. Further reporting and investigation are required to better understand its role and significance in MF.

Authors' Contributions

Dr. Heyman conceived the idea for this work and wrote the manuscript. Drs. Beaven and Kelsey conceived the idea for this work, helped write the manuscript, provided critical feedback, edited, and contributed to the final manuscript.

References

[1] V. D. Criscione and M. A. Weinstock, "Incidence of cutaneous T-cell lymphoma in the United States, 1973–2002," *Archives of Dermatology*, vol. 143, no. 7, pp. 854–859, 2007.

[2] N. Yawalkar, K. Ferenczi, D. A. Jones et al., "Profound loss of T-cell receptor repertoire complexity in cutaneous T-cell lymphoma," *Blood*, vol. 102, no. 12, pp. 4059–4066, 2003.

[3] F. M. Foss and M. Girardi, "Mycosis fungoides and sezary syndrome," *Hematology/Oncology Clinics of North America*, vol. 31, no. 2, pp. 297–315, 2017.

[4] P. Virmani, S. H. Hwang, J. G. Hastings et al., "Systemic therapy for cutaneous T-cell lymphoma: who, when, what, and why?," *Expert Review of Hematology*, vol. 10, no. 2, pp. 111–121, 2017.

[5] Y. H. Kim, H. L. Liu, S. Mraz-Gernhard, A. Varghese, and R. T. Hoppe, "Long-term outcome of 525 patients with mycosis fungoides and Sézary syndrome: clinical prognostic factors and risk for disease progression," *Archives of Dermatology*, vol. 139, no. 7, pp. 857–866, 2003.

[6] P. Quaglino, M. Maule, H. M. Prince et al., "Global patterns of care in advanced stage mycosis fungoides/Sezary syndrome: a multicenter retrospective follow-up study from the cutaneous lymphoma international consortium," *Annals of Oncology*, vol. 28, no. 10, pp. 2517–2525, 2017.

[7] W. Plunkett, P. Huang, Y. Z. Xu, V. Heinemann, R. Grunewald, and V. Gandhi, "Gemcitabine: metabolism, mechanisms of action, and self-potentiation," *Seminars in Oncology*, vol. 22, pp. 3–10, 1995.

[8] P. L. Zinzani, G. Baliva, M. Magagnoli et al., "Gemcitabine treatment in pretreated cutaneous T-cell lymphoma: experience in 44 patients," *Journal of Clinical Oncology*, vol. 18, no. 13, pp. 2603–2606, 2000.

[9] P. L. Zinzani, F. Venturini, V. Stefoni et al., "Gemcitabine as single agent in pretreated T-cell lymphoma patients: evaluation of the long-term outcome," *Annals of Oncology*, vol. 21, no. 4, pp. 860–863, 2010.

[10] M. Duvic, R. Talpur, S. Wen, R. Kurzrock, C. L. David, and N. Apisarnthanarax, "Phase II evaluation of gemcitabine monotherapy for cutaneous T-cell lymphoma," *Clinical Lymphoma and Myeloma*, vol. 7, no. 1, pp. 51–58, 2006.

[11] S. A. Hoption Cann, J. P. van Netten, and C. van Netten, "Dr William Coley and tumour regression: a place in history or in the future," *Postgraduate Medical Journal*, vol. 79, no. 938, pp. 672–680, 2003.

[12] G. Papa, S. Tura, F. Mandelli et al., "Is interferon alpha in cutaneous T-cell lymphoma a treatment of choice?," *British Journal of Haematology*, vol. 79, no. s1, pp. 48–51, 1991.

[13] S. Rupoli, G. Goteri, S. Pulini et al., "Long-term experience with low-dose interferon-alpha and PUVA in the management of early mycosis fungoides," *European Journal of Haematology*, vol. 75, no. 2, pp. 136–145, 2005.

[14] A. M. Lesokhin, S. M. Ansell, P. Armand et al., "Nivolumab in patients with relapsed or refractory hematologic malignancy: preliminary results of a phase Ib study," *Journal of Clinical Oncology*, vol. 34, no. 23, pp. 2698–2704, 2016.

[15] M. Khodadoust, A. H. Rook, P. Porcu et al., "Pembrolizumab for treatment of relapsed/refractory mycosis fungoides and sezary syndrome: clinical efficacy in a citn multicenter phase 2 study," *Blood*, vol. 128, p. 181, 2016.

10

CD7-Positive Diffuse Large B-Cell Lymphoma Presenting as an Intranasal Tumor

Kazuaki Teshima,[1,2] Masaaki Kume,[1] Yasushi Kawaharada,[3] Takashi Saito,[4] Ko Abe,[1,2] Sho Ikeda,[2] Hideaki Ohyagi,[1,2] Megumi Zuguchi,[5] Masashi Zuguchi,[3] Yosuke Kubota,[3] Yoshitaka Enomoto,[3] Masahito Miura,[6] Satsuki Takahashi,[6] Masahiro Saito,[6] Ken Saito,[3] and Naoto Takahashi[2]

[1]*Department of Hematology, Hiraka General Hospital, Yokote, Japan*
[2]*Department of Hematology, Nephrology, and Rheumatology, Akita University Graduate School of Medicine, Akita, Japan*
[3]*Department of Surgery, Hiraka General Hospital, Yokote, Japan*
[4]*Department of Otolaryngology, Hiraka General Hospital, Yokote, Japan*
[5]*Department of Gastroenterology, Hiraka General Hospital, Yokote, Japan*
[6]*Department of Diagnostic Pathology, Hiraka General Hospital, Yokote, Japan*

Correspondence should be addressed to Kazuaki Teshima; green08kazuma@gmail.com

Academic Editor: Tatsuharu Ohno

We report a case of a 74-year-old man with a cluster of differentiation (CD) 7-positive diffuse large B-cell lymphoma (DLBCL) in the right nasal cavity. Flow cytometry analyses showed CD7 and CD20 positivity in tumor cells. The patient received 6 cycles of R-CHOP plus local radiation therapy because positron emission tomography-computed tomography after R-CHOP revealed an intranasal lesion. The patient achieved complete remission (CR) after radiation therapy. The frequency of CD7-positive DLBCL is rare, and only 11 cases with follow-up of clinical course have been reported thus far. CR or partial response was noted in 8 of 11 cases after receiving rituximab combined with chemotherapy. In total, 9 of 12 cases involved the development of extranodal lesions, which occurred as an intranasal tumor in 3 cases. It is important to examine the clinical features by accumulation of further cases.

1. Introduction

Aberrant expression of T-cell markers (CD2, CD3, CD4, CD5, CD7, and CD8) is occasionally observed in diffuse large B-cell lymphoma (DLBCL) [1]. In particular, expression of CD5 is noted in approximately 10% DLBCL cases, and it is related to a poor prognosis [2]. However, the clinical significance of the expression of other T-cell markers, including CD7, is unclear. Here, we report a rare case of CD7-positive DLBCL presenting as an intranasal tumor.

2. Case Presentation

A 74-year-old male patient with a history of left lung inferior lobe resection due to localized lung cancer who complained of rhinostenosis was diagnosed with a tumor in the right nasal cavity (Figure 1(a)). Positron emission tomography-computed tomography (PET-CT) showed intense focal uptake of SUVmax 18.3 in the right nasal cavity (Figure 1(b)). The tumor biopsy showed diffuse proliferation of large, atypical lymphoid cells. Flow cytometry (FCM) analyses showed clear CD7 and CD19 positivity in the tumor

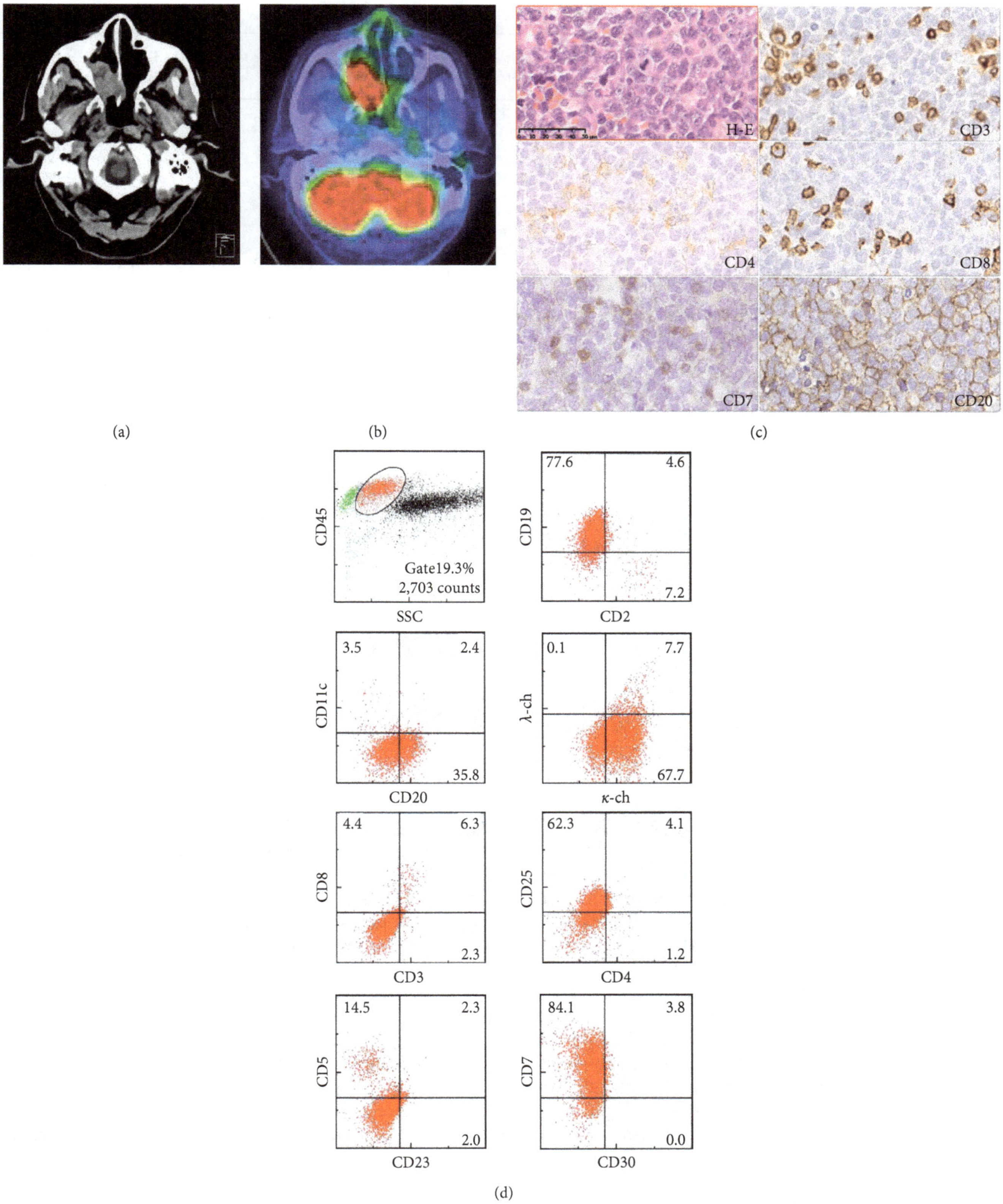

FIGURE 1: Imaging findings: (a) brain computed tomography scan at diagnosis; (b) positron emission tomography-computed tomography findings at diagnosis; (c) pathological findings at diagnosis (hematoxylin and eosin staining) and immunostaining with anti-CD3, anti-CD4, anti-CD8, anti-CD7, and anti-CD20; (d) flow cytometry analysis at diagnosis.

TABLE 1: Clinical characteristics of CD7-positive B-cell lymphoma.

Case No.	Age	Sex	Histology	Cell of origin	Main site(s) of involvement	Stage	Extranodal involvement	Treatment	Response	Status	Follow-up (months)	Detection method	References
Case 1	54	F	DLBCL	Non-GC	Inguinal LN	IIA	−	R-CHOP	CR	Alive, CR	NA	FCM, IHC	Sangle et al.
Case 2	66	M	DLBCL	NA	Thoracic cavity	IA	+	CHOP + RT	PR	Died of disease	NA	FCM, IHC	Tomita et al.
Case 3	47	M	Non-Hodgkin lymphoma	NA	Intra-abdominal mass	IVA	+	High dose CHOP	PD	Died of disease	5	FCM	Takahashi et al.
Case 4	64	M	DLBCL	GC	Cecum	IIA	+	Surgery + R-CHOP	CR	Alive, CR	68	IHC	Tsuyama et al.
Case 5	66	F	DLBCL	Non-GC	Axillary LN	IVB	+	R-CHOP + RT	PD	Died of disease, refractory	24	FCM, IHC	Tsuyama et al.
Case 6	62	F	DLBCL	GC	Nasal cavity	IIA	+	R-CHOP	PR	Alive with disease, relapse	34	FCM, IHC	Tsuyama et al.
Case 7	82	M	DLBCL	Non-GC	Nasal cavity	IA	+	R-CHOP	CR	Alive, CR	45	FCM, IHC	Tsuyama et al.
Case 8	64	M	DLBCL	Non-GC	Orbit	IB	+	R-CHOP	PD	Died of disease	2	FCM, IHC	Tsuyama et al.
Case 9	81	M	DLBCL	Non-GC	Soft tissue of leg	IVA	+	R-CHOP	CR	Died of disease, relapse	40	FCM, IHC	Tsuyama et al.
Case 10	55	M	DLBCL	Non-GC	Cervical LN	IVA	+	R-CHOP	CR	Died of disease, relapse	12	FCM, IHC	Tsuyama et al.
Case 11	65	M	DLBCL	Non-GC	Prostate	IVA	+	R-CHOP	CR	Alive, CR	49	FCM, IHC	Tsuyama et al.
Case 12	74	M	DLBCL	Non-GC	Nasal cavity	IA	+	R-CHOP + RT	CR	Alive, CR	18	FCM	Our case

M, male; F, female; DLBCL, diffuse large B-cell lymphoma; GC, germinal centre; LN, lymph node; CR, complete response; PR, partial response; PD, progressive disease; NA, not available; FCM, flow cytometry; IHC, immunohistochemistry.

cells, while CD20 was expressed at weak intensity (Figure 1(d)). These data were analyzed by FACSCanto II (BD Biosciences) using the antibody of CD7 (3A1-RD1; Beckman Coulter). These data were obtained from the SRL Laboratory (Hachioji city, Tokyo, Japan). Immunohistochemistry (IHC) results were positive for L26 (CD20), bcl-2, bcl-6, and MUM1 and negative for CD3, CD4, CD8, CD7 (LP15; Novocastra), CD10, and EBER (Figure 1(c)). Fluorescent in situ hybridization (FISH) did not reveal IgH/c-MYC rearrangement. Southern blotting revealed immunoglobulin heavy-chain gene rearrangement, however not T-cell receptor (TCR) gene rearrangement. Bone marrow biopsy was negative for the involvement of atypical large cells. The patient was diagnosed with stage IA DLBCL. The patient received 6 cycles of R-CHOP therapy; however, residual disease was found on the PET-CT. Therefore, the patient received local radiation therapy for the residual disease. He achieved complete remission after radiation therapy. At 18 months after chemoradiation therapy, there was no evidence of recurrence.

3. Discussion

CD7 is expressed on the surface of most thymocytes and T-cells preceding TCR-β-chain gene rearrangement and is the earliest differentiation antigen found during T-cell development [3]. Aberrant T-cell marker expression is occasionally observed in B-cell lymphoma [4]. Inaba et al. reported that CD7 was expressed in 5 (5%) of 101 DLBCL patients [5]. Table 1 describes the clinical characteristics of 12 cases, including the present case, of CD7-positive DLBCL reported thus far. Two cases were detected by FCM, 1 case was detected by IHC, and 9 cases were detected with both. In the present case, FCM showed CD7 positivity and IHC showed CD7 negativity. There are several possible causes for CD7-negative immunostaining results. One reason is that the antigenicity of CD7 may decline in the process of formalin fixation. Another reason is that epitope of lymphoma may be different from that of normal cells. FCM shows CD7 expressions despite no expression of CD3. Clonal immunoglobulin heavy-chain rearrangement was observed using Southern blotting, which detected no clonal TCR gene rearrangement. This means that clonally restricted B-cells in our DLBCL case express CD7. Suzuki et al. reported that aberrant T-cell marker expression detected by FCM could be confirmed in some, but not in all, cases detected by IHC [6]. They reported that among 6 CD7-positive cases by FCM, only 3 were confirmed to be positive for CD7 by IHC. They considered that it was important to employ FCM because the ability of IHC to detect aberrant T-cell marker expression is restrictive.

Inaba et al. reported that extranodal involvement and a higher international prognostic index are significantly more frequent in B-cell lymphomas positive for T-cell markers than in B-cell lymphomas negative for T-cell markers [5]. Tsuyama et al. reported the clinical examination of 223 DLBCL patients for T-cell marker antigen [7]. According to their report, the CD5-positive DLBCL group had a significantly poorer prognosis than the T-cell marker-negative group. In contrast, there was no significant difference in prognosis between T-cell marker-positive DLBCL other than CD5 and T-cell marker-negative DLBCL. Furthermore, Suzuki et al. reported 150 cases of DLBCL; however, the clinicopathological significance and prognosis of CD7 in DLBCL are still unknown [6].

As shown in Table 1, of the 11 previously reported cases of CD7-positive B-cell lymphoma, 9 cases involved the development of extranodal lesions, including 2 cases of intranasal tumor; 8 patients achieved complete response or partial response after receiving rituximab combined with chemotherapy. Similarly, the patient in the present case presented with an intranasal tumor and achieved complete remission with radiotherapy following R-CHOP therapy. Currently, there is no evidence of recurrence in the patient. According to the literature, CD2 or CD7 expression is associated with extranodal involvement in B-non-Hodgkin's lymphoma at diagnosis [5]. It is important to examine the clinical features by the accumulation of further cases.

Acknowledgments

The authors would like to thank Editage (http://www.editage.com) for English language editing.

References

[1] S. Swerdlow, E. Campo, and N. L. Harris, *WHO Classification of Hematopoietic and Lymphoid Tissue*, International Agency for Research on Cancer, Lyon, France, 2008.

[2] M. Yamaguchi, M. Seto, and M. Okamoto, "De novo CD5+ diffuse large B-cell lymphoma: a clinicopathologic study of 109 patients," *Blood*, vol. 99, no. 3, pp. 815–821, 2002.

[3] B. F. Haynes, S. M. Denning, K. H. Singer, and J. Kurtzberg, "Ontogeny of T-cell precursors: a model for the initial stages of human T-cell development," *Immunology Today*, vol. 10, no. 3, pp. 87–91, 1989.

[4] M. I. D. Rossi, T. Yokota, K. L. Medina et al., "B lymphopoiesis is active throughout human life, but there are developmental age-related changes," *Blood*, vol. 101, no. 2, pp. 576–584, 2003.

[5] T. Inaba, C. Shimazaki, T. Sumikuma et al., "Expression of T-cell-associated antigens in B-cell non-Hodgkin's lymphoma," *British Journal of Haematology*, vol. 109, no. 3, pp. 592–599, 2000.

[6] Y. Suzuki, T. Yoshida, G. Wang et al., "Incidence and clinical significance of aberrant T-cell marker expression on diffuse large B-cell lymphoma cells," *Acta Haematologica*, vol. 130, no. 4, pp. 230–237, 2013.

[7] N. Tsuyama, D. Ennishi, and M. Yokoyama, "Clinical and prognostic significance of aberrant T-cell marker expression in 225 cases of de novo diffuse large B-cell lymphoma and 276 cases of other B-cell lymphomas," *Oncotarget*, vol. 8, pp. 33487–33500, 2017.

11

Plasmablastic Lymphoma, a Rare Entity in Bone Marrow with Unusual Immunophenotype and Challenging Differential Diagnosis

Majd Al Shaarani,[1] Rodney E. Shackelford,[1] Samip R. Master,[2] Glenn M. Mills,[2] Yasir AlZubaidi,[1] Ahmed Mamilly,[3] and Eric X. Wei[1]

[1]*Department of Pathology and Translational Pathobiology, Louisiana State University Health Sciences Center, Shreveport, LA, USA*
[2]*Department of Hematology and Oncology, Louisiana State University Health Sciences Center, Shreveport, LA, USA*
[3]*Department of Radiology, Louisiana State University Health Sciences Center, Shreveport, LA, USA*

Correspondence should be addressed to Eric X. Wei; ericxwei@yahoo.com

Academic Editor: Marie-Christine Kyrtsonis

Plasmablastic lymphoma (PBL) is an aggressive malignancy that usually occurs in the setting of immunosuppression. The immunohistochemical profile of PBL is that of terminally differentiated B lymphocytes. CD138, CD38, and MUM1 are usually immunopositive. However, pan B-cell markers such as CD20 and PAX-5 are usually negative. *MYC* rearrangement is the most commonly encountered genetic alteration, with immunoglobulin (*IG*), especially immunoglobulin heavy (*IGH*) chain, being the most frequent partner. We report a case of PBL in a 48-year-old human immunodeficiency virus- (HIV-) positive male who was admitted to the hospital with signs and symptoms suspicious for tumor lysis syndrome. Bone marrow examination revealed hypercellular marrow with trilineage hypoplasia and sheets of intermediate to large neoplastic cells with basophilic vacuolated cytoplasm comprising the majority of cellular elements of the bone marrow. The neoplastic cells were negative for conventional B-cell, T-cell, plasma cell, and myeloid markers, while flow cytometric analysis revealed an abnormal CD45-dim population that was partially weakly positive for CD71 and CD79b. The diagnosis was initially thought to be a high-grade primitive hematopoietic neoplasm, possibly an acute undifferentiated leukemia. BOB-1, however, was immunopositive in the neoplastic cells, confirming its B-cell origin. MYC was positive by immunohistochemistry and break-apart FISH, as were CD45, MUM-1, and EMA immunostains. There was immunoglobulin kappa (*IGK*) light chain gene rearrangement by polymerase chain reaction (PCR). Additionally, Epstein–Barr virus- (EBV–) encoded small RNAs (EBER) were positive by in situ hybridization (ISH). The tumor proliferation index by Ki-67 immunostaining approached 95%. Although the tumor cells were negative for CD38 and CD138, the diagnosis of PBL was still rendered. We recommend using a broad spectrum of B-cell markers, including BOB-1 and OCT-2, in such challenging cases of B-cell lymphomas with no expression of conventional B-cell markers. We also emphasize that the negative CD38 and CD138 should not exclude PBL from the differential diagnosis.

1. Introduction

Plasmablastic lymphoma (PBL) is an aggressive postgerminal center, terminally differentiated B-cell malignancy that usually occurs in the setting of immunosuppression. Initially, PBL was considered a subtype of diffuse large B-cell lymphoma arising in the oral cavity of human immunodeficiency virus- (HIV–) positive patients, as was first described by Delecluse et al. [1–3]. It was later categorized by the WHO as a separate entity in 2008, and accumulative data have demonstrated cases at other anatomical sites and in immunocompetent patients [4]. Although the majority of cases are associated with HIV infection, other causes of immunosuppression such as posttransplantation can also be associated with this lymphoma. About 35% of the patients, however, are actually immunocompetent, indicating that PBL is not confined to the immunosuppressed status. In the majority of cases, the disease arises in the oral cavity of HIV-infected patients. However, other sites are also reported including the gastrointestinal (GI) system, soft tissue, skin, and much less frequently the lungs, bone, bone marrow, and central nervous system (CNS) [5, 6]. The immunohistochemical profile of PBL is that of terminally differentiated B lymphocytes or plasma cells, where CD138, CD38, and MUM1 are usually positive and pan B-cell markers including CD20 and PAX-5 are frequently negative. *MYC* rearrangements are common, often translocated with the immunoglobulin (*IG*) heavy chains (*IGH*), as the most commonly encountered genetic alteration [3, 7]. The rarity of such cases, the difficulty in making the diagnosis, and the very poor prognosis all make PBL a clinicopathological challenge [4].

2. Clinical History

The patient was a 48-year-old male with a past medical history of HIV, presenting with a historically lowest CD4+ T helper cell count at 73/μL and 190/μL during admission. The patient's past medical history also included HIV-associated immune complex-mediated proliferative glomerulonephritis, chronic kidney disease with multiple episodes of acute kidney injury, electrolyte abnormalities, myocardial infarction, congestive heart failure (ejection fraction of 15–20% two years prior to his most recent admission and then improved to 50–55%), hypertension, diabetes mellitus, anemia, thrombocytopenia, benign prostatic hyperplasia, and major depressive disorder with psychosis and suicidal ideation. He had previously been admitted on several occasions with chief complaints of shortness of breath, hematuria, electrolyte abnormalities, and psychiatric disorders. He eventually developed a subdural hemorrhage confirmed by magnetic resonance imaging (MRI), lactic acidosis, pancytopenia, hypercalcemia, and acute kidney injury (creatinine level of 3.4 mg/dL from 0.93 mg/dL). He reported having progressive dyspnea on exertion over the past few months, along with a chronic cough, productive of green to gray sputum, night sweats, and weight loss of 30 pounds. He denied, however, any hemoptysis, chest pain, paroxysmal nocturnal dyspnea, orthopnea, fever, or chills. He was transferred to the medical intensive care unit and was treated with hydration. His serum calcium level was 13.4 mg/dL, with lactate dehydrogenase levels more than 4000 U/L, and uric acid levels at 26.9 mg/dL. These findings were concerning for tumor lysis syndrome. Chest, abdomen, and pelvic computed tomography (CT) scans revealed hepatosplenomegaly (Figure 1(a)) and retroperitoneal, pelvic, and paracardial lymphadenopathy, with the largest lymph node measuring 2.4 × 1.4 cm (Figures 1(b)–1(d)). A bone marrow biopsy was performed. Initially, it was thought to be a high-grade primitive hematopoietic neoplasm, with acute undifferentiated leukemia in differential diagnosis. However, a diagnosis of plasmablastic lymphoma was later provided. Before chemotherapy could be initiated, the patient developed severe episodes of subdural hemorrhage, lost brain stem reflexes, and subsequently expired after extubation.

3. Pathological Findings

The bone marrow core biopsy and aspirate revealed a hypercellular marrow for the patient's age, at 90% cellularity, with trilineage hypoplasia and slight myelodysplastic changes. The neoplastic cells comprised approximately 75% of the cellular marrow and were arranged in clusters and sheets from intermediate to large cells (Figure 2(a)), with prominent nucleoli and irregular nuclear contours (Figure 2(b)). The bone marrow aspirate smears revealed discohesive neoplastic cells (Figure 2(c)), with a slightly open chromatin and basophilic vacuolated cytoplasm (Figure 2(d)). Flow cytometric analysis showed a distinct CD45-dim cell population, comprising about 15% of the total cells, which were partially positive for CD71 and CD79b and negative for CD34, CD38, CD138, CD117, myeloperoxidase (MPO), and all other B-cell and T-cell markers (Figures 3(a)–3(d)). Immunohistochemically, these tumor cells were positive for CD45 (dim partial), EMA, MUM-1, *MYC* (50%), and Epstein–Barr virus- (EBV-) encoded small RNAs (EBERs), measured by in situ hybridization (ISH) (Figures 4(a)–4(e)). A high proliferation index at 95% was identified by a Ki-67 immunostain (Figure 4(f)). The tumor cells were negative for ALK-1, BCL-1, BCL-2, BCL-6, CAM5.2, CD3, CD10, CD14, CD20, CD30, CD34, CD56, CD68, CD71, CD79a, CD117, CD138 (Figure 4(g)), E-cadherin, factor VIII, glycophorin, HHV-8, lysozyme, MPO, PAX-5, and TdT. There were virtually no normal B-cells by the CD20 and PAX-5 immunostains. The CD3 immunostain identified reactive T-cells. CD79a and CD138 demonstrated background plasma cells, which were polyclonal by kappa and lambda light chain ISH. It was initially considered a high-grade primitive hematopoietic neoplasm, with acute undifferentiated leukemia in the differential diagnosis. Additional immunostains revealed that the neoplastic cells were positive for BOB-1 (Figure 4(h)) and negative for OCT-2. Cytogenetic studies revealed a complicated karyotype 43~45,X,−Y, der(8)t(1;8)(q12;p22), dup(11)(q13q31), dup(14)(q24q32),−18,der(20)t(1;20)(q12; q13.3)[cp19]/46,XY [1] with a representative karyotype illustrated (Figure 5(a)). Seventeen of the twenty cells were absent for the Y chromosome. Ten cells had this abnormality and a loss of chromosome 18, with a number of unbalanced translocations and duplications, composing a highly complex karyotype carrying a poor prognosis. Two instances of unbalanced 1q translocations led to a quadrupling of this chromosomal arm. The distal portion of 14q was duplicated, as was practically the whole of 11q. Chromosome 18 was present in one copy. None of these abnormalities is known to be characteristic of lymphomas and likely reflect a general chromosomal instability. *MYC* break-apart fluorescent in situ hybridization (FISH) using a locus specific probe for the 8q24/*MYC* region was performed at our institution and was positive for *MYC* gene rearrangement in 9% (9/100) of the cells analyzed with adequate controls (Figure 5(b)). Additionally, a positive peak was detected in a single polymerase

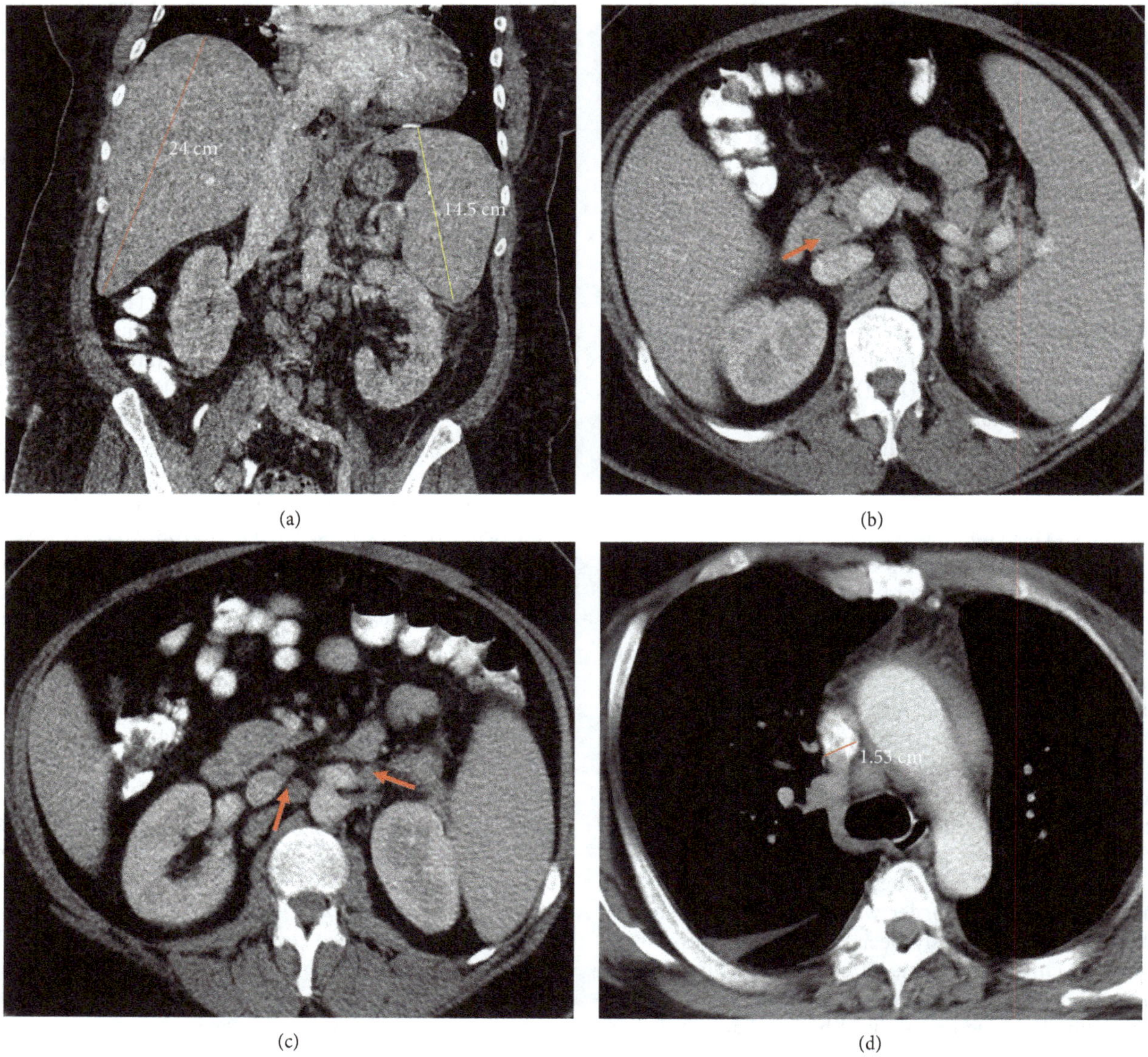

Figure 1: The abdomen and thoracic CT scan. (a) Coronal contrast-enhanced CT image of the abdomen with hepatosplenomegaly: the craniocaudal diameter of the right liver lobe is 24 cm (normal 12–17 cm); the craniocaudal diameter of the spleen is 14.5 cm (normal up to 13 cm). (b) Enlarged mesenteric lymph nodes (red arrow) measure 1.6 cm in short axis. (c) Para-aortic lymph nodes (red arrows) measure about 1.4 and 1.3 cm in short axis. (d) Lymph node in mediastinal station 4R measures about 1.5 cm in short axis.

chain reaction (PCR) for IG kappa (*IGK*) V-J gene segments, indicating a clonal immunoglobulin kappa light chain gene rearrangement and likely a B-cell lymphoproliferation. There was no evidence of clonal immunoglobulin heavy chain gene rearrangement. The diagnosis of a CD38-/CD138-negative plasmablastic lymphoma was made based on the clinical features of lymphadenopathy, hepatosplenomegaly, HIV and EBV status, B-cell marker BOB-1, CD45, MUM-1, and EMA expression, a high proliferative index, and *MYC* translocation. With this interesting IHC profile, we think it is highly recommended that using a broad spectrum of B-cell markers, including BOB-1, in such cases where other markers are negative or only focally and weakly positive. We also emphasize that a negative CD38 and CD138 expression pattern in tumor cells should not exclude PBL from the differential diagnosis and clinical management.

4. Discussion

4.1. Clinical Findings. PBL is a rare yet aggressive post-germinal center B-cell malignancy with morphologic and immunophenotypic features of terminal B-cell or plasma cell differentiation. PBL was first described by Delecluse et al. as a subtype of diffuse large B-cell lymphoma (DLBCL) [1]. In the 2008 WHO classification of tumors of hematopoietic and lymphoid tissues, PBL was described as a separate entity, rather than being included under DLBCL, NOS. This disease has a strong male preponderance with approximately seventy percent of cases occurring in males, and the median age of disease presentation is fifty years old [8]. Although, in the majority of cases, the disease arises in the oral cavity of HIV-infected patients, PBL has been reported in other sites including the GI system, soft tissue, skin, and much less frequently in the lungs, bone, bone marrow, and CNS

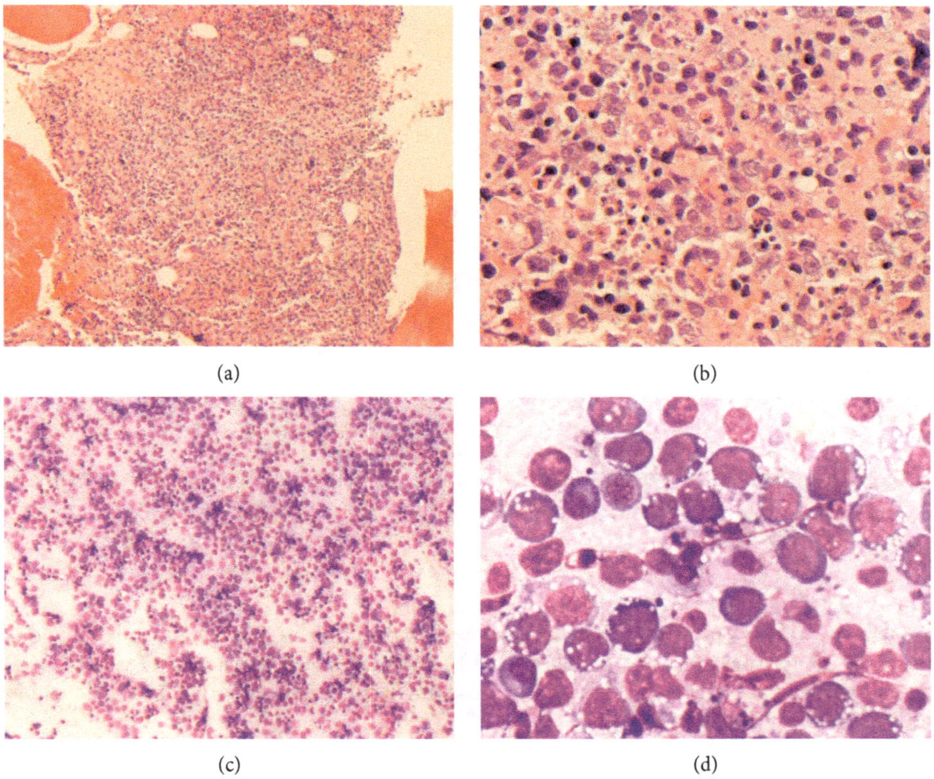

FIGURE 2: Bone marrow biopsy and aspirate smears show high-grade hematopoietic neoplasm. (a) The neoplasm has a diffuse growth pattern on core biopsy (H&E stain, ×100). (b) The neoplastic cells have irregular nuclear contours, conspicuous nucleoli, and abundant cytoplasm (H and E stain, ×400). (c) Bone marrow aspirate shows discohesive high-grade hematopoietic tumor cells (Wright-Giemsa, ×100). (d) The hematopoietic cells have slightly eccentric nuclei, prominent nucleoli, and deep blue vacuolated cytoplasm. Occasional plasma cells are seen in the background (Wright-Giemsa, ×600).

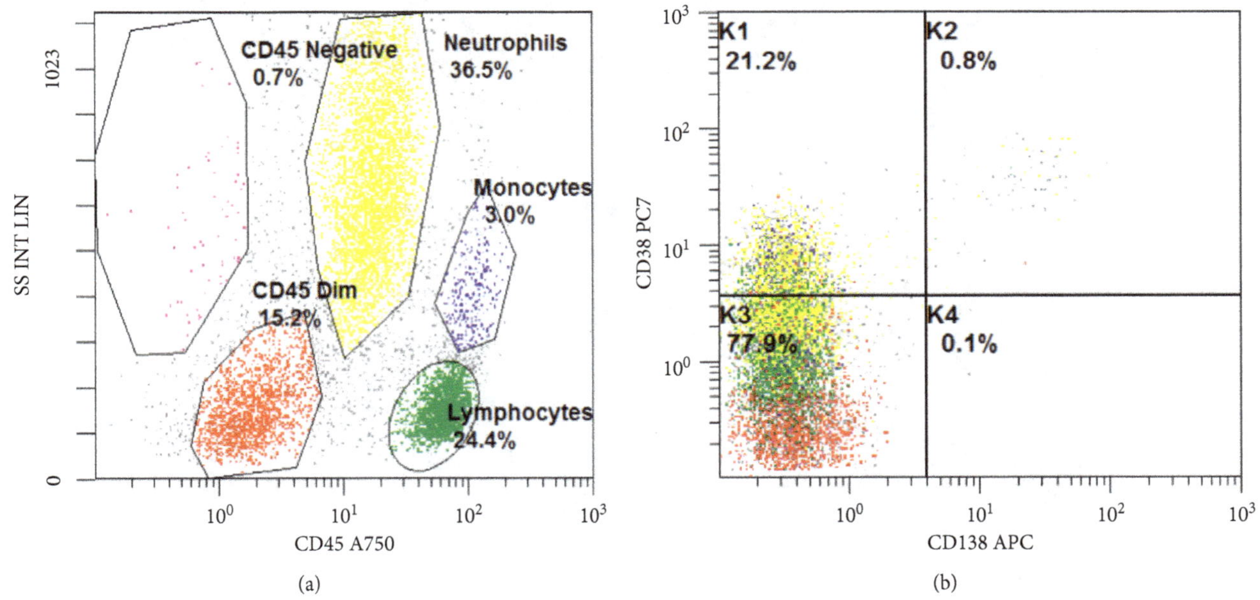

FIGURE 3: Continued.

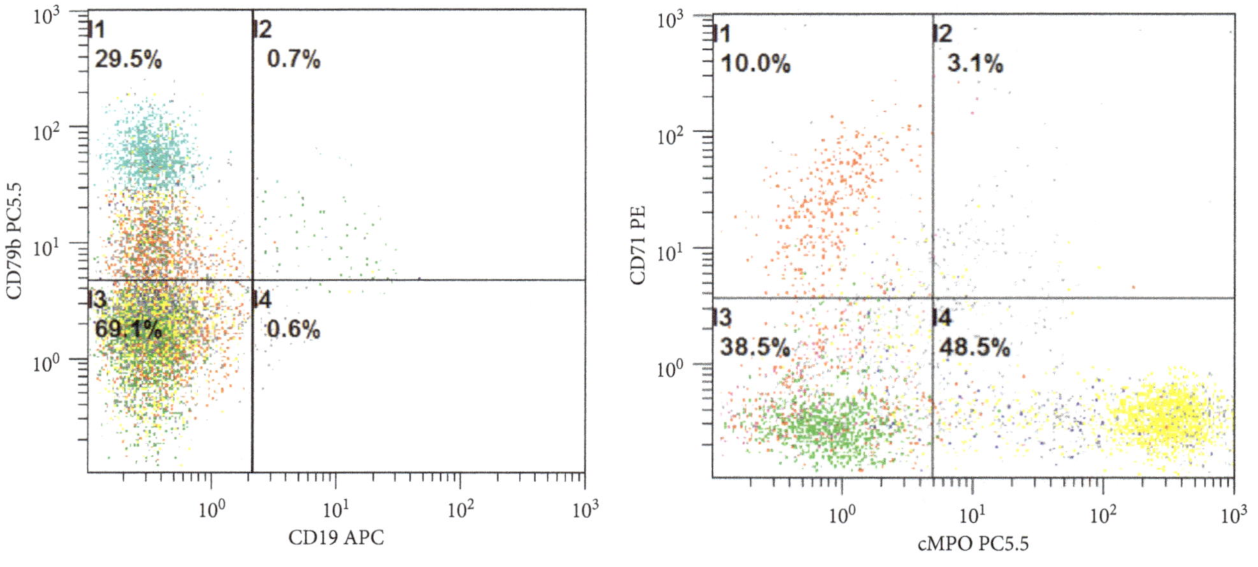

(c) (d)

Figure 3: Representative flow cytometric histograms of bone marrow aspirate. (a) There is a CD45-dim population of abnormal cells with low-side scatter (painted red), comprising about 15% of total cells. (b) The cells of interest are negative for CD38 and CD138. (c) These cells are negative for CD19, but partially positive for CD79b, with a subset moderately positive for CD79b (painted blue). (d) These cells are positive for CD71 and negative for cytoplasmic MPO.

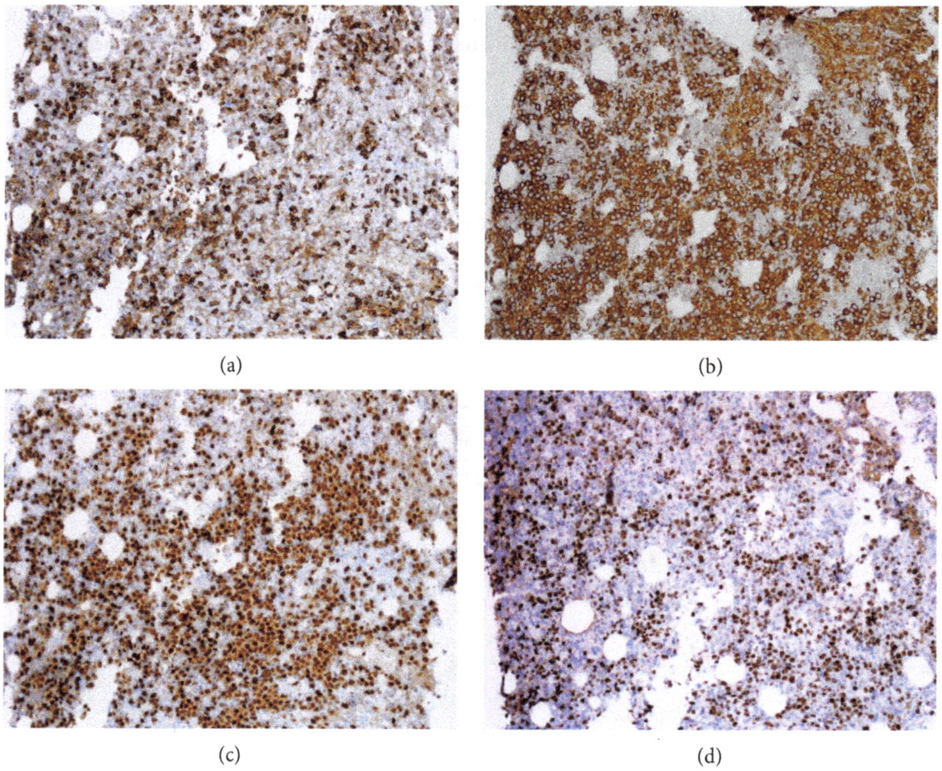

(a) (b)

(c) (d)

Figure 4: Continued.

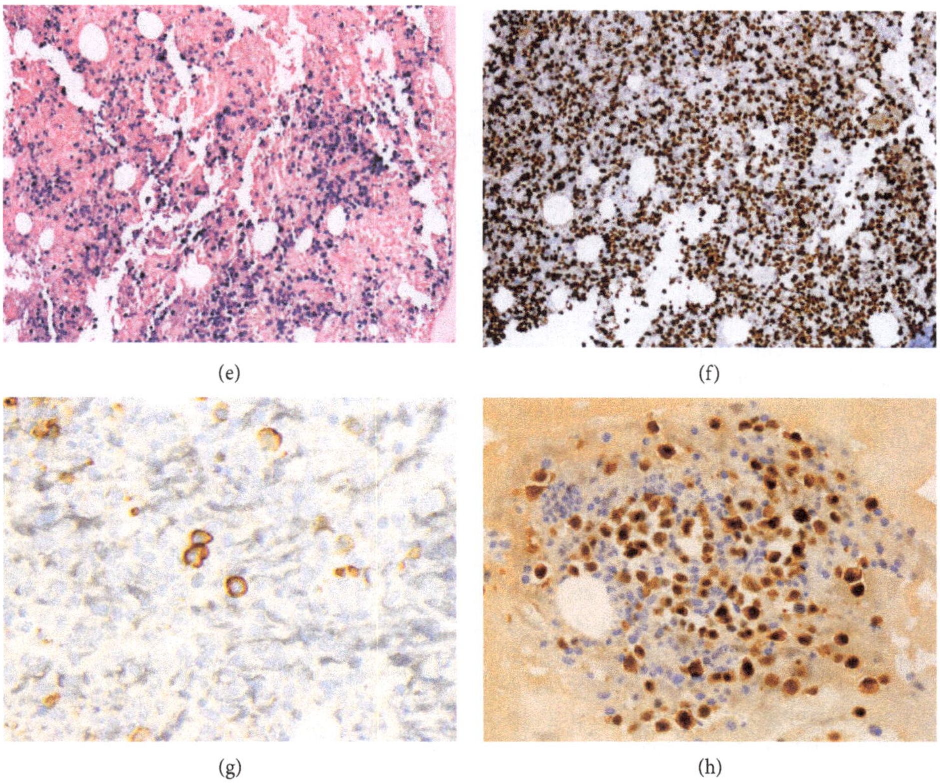

FIGURE 4: Immunohistochemistry and in situ hybridization study of the high-grade hematopoietic neoplasm. (a) CD45 (×100); (b) EMA (×100); (c) MUM-1 (×100); (d) MYC (×100); (e) EBER (×100); (f) Ki-67 (×100); (g) CD138 (×400); (h) BOB-1 (×200).

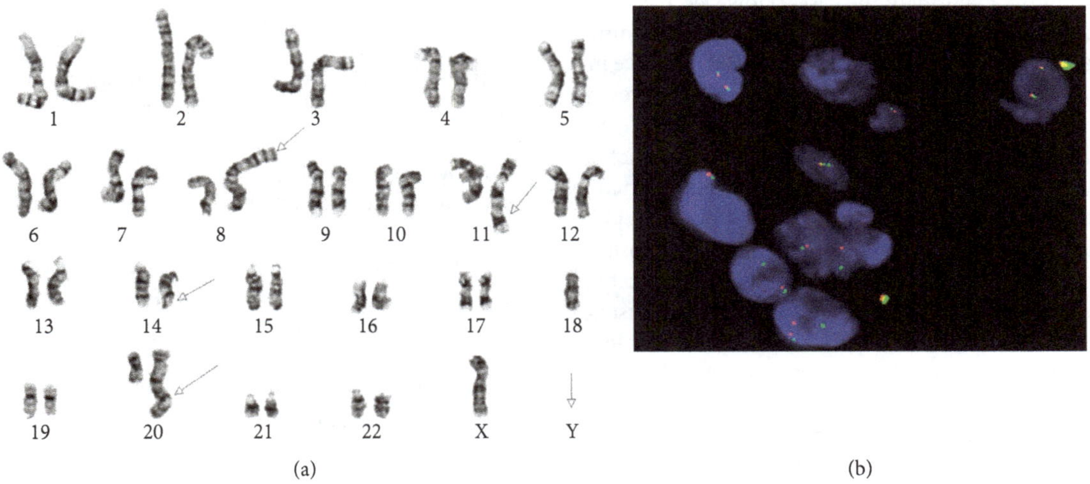

FIGURE 5: Cytogenetic analysis and FISH study of bone marrow aspirate. (a) The lymphoma cells exhibit complex karyotype, and a representative karyotype shows + der(1), t(1;8)(p13;p12), dup(11)(q13), add(14)(q32), and der(20)t(1;20)(q13.2;q21). (b) *MYC* break-apart FISH is positive for *MYC* gene rearrangement using a locus-specific probe for the 8q24/*MYC* region.

[2, 4, 8, 9]. Initially, the malignancy was thought to be only associated with immunosuppression, especially HIV infection, but later on it was identified in association with other causes of immunosuppression, including iatrogenic interventions such as transplant and autoimmune disorders, immunosenescence, and in immunocompetent patients [8–12]. HIV-positive or posttransplant patients tend to present at disseminated stage III/IV, including bone marrow involvement at presentation when compared to immunocompetent patients. It is possible that PBL may transform from a prior plasma cell myeloma. PBL may sometimes show paraproteins. The majority of PBL patients present with an intermediate-to-high risk international prognostic index. Our patient was a HIV-positive patient, presenting with pancytopenia, hepatosplenomegaly, general lymphadenopathy, possible tumor lysis syndrome, and a high clinical stage involving bone marrow. He did not have oral cavity involvement. Even though hepatosplenomegaly and general lymphadenopathy may suggest high-grade lymphoma, it may also be due to his HIV infection status. His pancytopenia and tumor lysis syndrome may implicate acute leukemia. Thus, accurate pathological diagnosis is essential for recognition of this disease entity and clinical management.

4.2. Histopathology. Morphologically, PBL may show variation depending on the sites and possibly the HIV status [6, 8]. Some of the common features include plasmablastic or immunoblastic morphology and plasmacytic differentiation. Mitoses, apoptosis, tingible body macrophages, and occasionally confluent necrosis are characteristic of different disease variations [4, 8, 13]. In HIV-positive patients and in oral and nasal mucosal areas, PBL usually reveals sheets of monomorphic plasmablastic or immunoblastic cell proliferations, with vesicular chromatin, large round- to oval-shaped nuclei, prominent centrally located nucleoli, and abundant cytoplasm. In HIV-negative patients, and in lymph nodes and extraoral cavities, it exhibits a more apparent plasmacytic differentiation with eccentric nuclei, inconspicuous nucleoli, and paranuclear hofs [6, 8, 14].

4.3. Immunophenotype. The immunophenotypic profile of PBL is that of terminally differentiated B lymphocytes. CD138, CD38, VS38c, MUM1, PRDMA, and XBP1 positivity is demonstrated in the majority of the cases. However, pan B-cell markers including CD20 and PAX-5 and leukocyte common antigen CD45 are usually negative or can be weakly positive in a minority of cases. CD79a, EMA, and CD30 are often expressed, as well as cytoplasmic immunoglobulin, commonly IgG, frequently with either kappa or lambda light chain restriction. CD4, CD10, CD43, CD45RO, and CD56 have been reported to be expressed in a subset of cases. BCL-1, BCL-2, and BCL-6 expression is usually absent. Ki-67 is usually diffusely positive, typically above 90% [2, 4, 10, 13, 15]. Although the majority of the cases are CD138- and CD38-positive, the diagnosis must not be overlooked if these stains are negative, such as in our case. In a clinical study of 60 Chinese PBL cases, it was found about 12% and 16% of cases were negative for CD38 and CD138, respectively [10]. Dittus and Sarosiek have recently reported an interesting case of PBL in the bone marrow that was positive for CD45, CD79a, CD117, and lambda immunoglobulin light chain but negative for CD38, CD138, PAX-5, and MUM1 [16]. Among the 12 PBL cases described by Teruya-Felstein et al., only one case of a 28-year-old HIV +ve male patient was negative for CD20, CD45, CD79a, CD138, and p63, with the bone and rectum involvement [5]. No other confirmatory B-cell markers were performed. Due to the similar immunohistochemical profile and anatomical locations between our case and reported cases in the literature, it is possible this lymphoma may exhibit different tumor markers when in different anatomical structures. The rarity of such cases and the lack of sufficient data prevent such generalizations. Rare types of B-cell lymphomas may not express conventional B-cell markers, and accurate diagnosis of such cases can be challenging. In an analysis among 34 cases of B-cell lymphomas with no expression of typical B-cell lymphomas, it was found that, in 13 such PBL cases, 9 cases expressed OCT-2, 10 cases had BOB-1 expression, and when combined together, 11 cases were positive for either OCT-2 or BOB-1 [17]. Compared to CD20, CD79a, and PAX-5, which on rare occasions can be found expressed in T-cell lymphomas, acute myeloid leukemia, or nonhematopoietic tumors, OCT-2 and BOB-1 are very sensitive and specific for confirmation of B-cell lymphoma or plasma cell neoplasm that are negative or equivocal for conventional B-cell antigen expression [17]. CD71, a transferrin receptor, is present on actively proliferative cells. It was partially positive in PBL tumor cells in our case by flow cytometry but was negative in bone marrow core biopsy by immunohistochemistry. CD71 expression has been detected by flow cytometry in B-cell lymphomas and acute leukemia [18, 19]. Although weak CD71 expression has been found in DLBCL and subset of acute leukemias, it is selectively expressed at high levels in early and late erythroid precursors and can be used as a lineage-specific marker for erythroid cells in bone marrow by immunohistochemistry [20]. Thus, CD71 partial expression in our PBL case by flow cytometry is nonspecific, and negative CD71 immunohistochemical stain confirms that tumor cells are not in erythroid lineage.

4.4. Cytogenetic and Molecular Studies. Our patient showed a complex karyotype with positive *MYC* break-apart FISH results. The dissociation between the karyotype and FISH data may be possibly due to a cryptic *MYC* translocation with an unknown partner gene, undetected by conventional cytogenetics. *MYC* gene rearrangements are the most commonly encountered PBL genetic alteration, with *IG*, particularly *IGH*, being the most frequent partner. These alterations are usually associated with several other complex heterogeneous cytogenetic alterations [3, 7, 8, 10, 21, 22]. Although the causality between EBV infection and *MYC* rearrangements has not been established, *MYC* alterations were more frequently detected when EBV infection was confirmed. Furthermore, Morcsio et al. have shown that EBV was detected in about 75% of AIDS patients' tumor cells but dropped down to 67% in transplant patients and further down to 50% in immunocompetent patients [11]. More studies are needed to clearly demonstrate the causative mechanism, if one actually exists. Al-Malki et al. have demonstrated that the presence of *MYC* gene rearrangement and HIV negativity were adverse prognostic factors [21]. In their review of 60 non-HIV-related PBL cases from Chinese patients, Han et al. found that *IGH* rearrangement was the most frequent alteration accounting for 33.3% of all 14 different types of genetic alterations they found. They also reported, for the first time, the presence of *PML/RARA* fusion in PBL [10].

4.5. Differential Diagnosis. The diagnosis of this rare entity depends not only on the histopathological features, but also on the integration of the clinical history, radiologic studies, and laboratory tests. The differential diagnosis encompasses lymphoid tumors with plasmacytic features, including plasmablastic myeloma, ALK-positive diffuse large B-cell lymphoma, Burkitt's lymphoma with plasmacytoid differentiation, immunoblastic DLBCL, and primary effusion lymphoma (PEL) [8, 13, 15]. Clinicopathological correlation appears to be most important factor when trying to differentiate PBL from a plasmablastic myeloma that shows an almost identical histopathological and immunophenotypical profile and is one of the most challenging differential diagnoses. The clinical and laboratory picture of plasmablastic myeloma includes serum and urine paraproteins, hypercalcemia, bone lytic lesions, anemia, and bone marrow involvement. In PBL, on the contrary, positive EBV staining in the tumor cells in the setting of immunosuppression, along with a high proliferative index, and *MYC* translocation supports the diagnosis [8, 23]. The presence of bone lytic lesions, however, should not be used to rule out PBL [16]. Another important diagnosis with similar morphology and immunophenotypical profile to be considered is ALK-positive large B-cell lymphoma [24]. ALK positivity with granular cytoplasmic staining and a t(2;17)(p23;q23) translocation in ALK-positive large B-cell lymphoma help differentiate these two entities [8, 23, 24]. PEL should also be in the differential diagnosis. In patients who are HIV-positive with the solid variant of PEL, differentiating these two entities can be a challenge. HHV-8 positivity is necessary to make the diagnosis for PEL [23, 25]. The expression of pan B-cell antigens (CD20, CD19, and PAX-5) in immunoblastic DLBCL and Burkitt's lymphoma helps differentiate from PBL that is only rarely positive for these markers [1, 8, 10].

4.6. Therapy and Prognosis. PBL is a real therapeutic challenge with a very aggressive course. The median overall survival ranges variably between different studies, but generally falls between 11 and 15 months in most cases [22, 26]. The prognostic factors are variable. There appears to be a correlation between survival and HIV status, with a better prognosis when the patient's HIV status is positive. This finding might stem from the administration of highly active antiretroviral therapy (HAART) that generally enhances the immunity in these patients [14]. Radiotherapy and surgery do not appear to have significant effects on patient survival. Currently, there is no consensus for a first-line medication regimen. Although CHOP (cyclophosphamide, doxorubicin, vincristine, and prednisone) and CHOP-like regimens are considered inadequate, other more aggressive regimens like CODOX-M/IVAC (cyclophosphamide, vincristine, doxorubicin, and high-dose methotrexate/ifosfamide, etoposide, and cytarabine), EPOCH (etoposide, cyclophosphamide, doxorubicin, vincristine, and prednisone), or hyper-CVAD (hyperfractionated cyclophosphamide, doxorubicin, vincristine, and dexamethasone) alternating with methotrexate and cytarabine do not confer better results [13, 26]. Bortezomib, especially in combination with either CHOP or EPOCH, has shown a durable remission in few case reports. These reports, however, are limited regarding the numbers of patients and the short follow-up times [26]. A review of the literature shows that brentuximab vedotin, an anti-CD30 antibody, was reported to have been used in only two patients. Either solely [27] or in combination with lenalidomide [26], brentuximab vedotin has demonstrated a very rapid response with significant reduction in the tumor sizes [26, 27]. Lenalidomide has also shown similar results in a few reported cases [26, 28, 29]. In a study of 82 PBL patients, Laurent et al. showed immune checkpoint expression (PD1/PD-L1) in the tumor microenvironment in the majority of cases and about 25% of the tumor cells expressed PD-L1. They could not find any correlation with survival, but they showed a rationale for testing anti-PD-L1 antibodies for the treatment of PBL [30].

Disclosure

The abstract of this case report was presented as a poster at the American Society of Clinical Pathology (ASCP) 2018 annual meeting and published in the *American Journal of Clinical Pathology*, Volume 150, Issue suppl_1, 21 September 2018, Page S94, https://doi.org/10.1093/ajcp/aqy097.226, https://academic.oup.com/ajcp/article/150/suppl_1/S94/5103277.

References

[1] H. J. Delecluse, I. Anagnostopoulos, F. Dallenbach et al., "Plasmablastic lymphomas of the oral cavity: a new entity associated with the human immunodeficiency virus infection," *Blood*, vol. 89, no. 4, pp. 1413–1420, 1997.

[2] G. Elyamany, E. Al Mussaed, and A. M. Alzahrani, "Plasmablastic lymphoma: a review of current knowledge and future directions," *Advances in Hematology*, vol. 2015, Article ID 315289, 9 pages, 2015.

[3] A. Valera, O. Balagué, L. Colomo et al., "IG/MYC rearrangements are the main cytogenetic alteration in plasmablastic lymphomas," *The American Journal of Surgical Pathology*, vol. 34, no. 11, pp. 1686–1694, 2010.

[4] S. H. Swerdlow, E. Campo, S. A. Pileri et al., "The 2016 revision of the World Health Organization classification of lymphoid neoplasms," *Blood*, vol. 127, no. 20, pp. 2375–2390, 2016.

[5] J. Teruya-Feldstein, E. Chiao, D. A. Filippa et al., "CD20-negative large-cell lymphoma with plasmablastic features: a clinically heterogenous spectrum in both HIV-positive and -negative patients," *Annals of Oncology*, vol. 15, no. 11, pp. 1673–1679, 2004.

[6] L. Colomo, F. Loong, S. Rives et al., "Diffuse large B-cell lymphomas with plasmablastic differentiation represent a heterogeneous group of disease entities," *The American Journal of Surgical Pathology*, vol. 28, no. 6, pp. 736–747, 2004.

[7] L. Taddesse-Heath, A. Meloni-Ehrig, J. Scheerle, J. C. Kelly, and E. S. Jaffe, "Plasmablastic lymphoma with MYC translocation: evidence for a common pathway in the generation of plasmablastic features," *Modern Pathology*, vol. 23, no. 7, pp. 991–999, 2010.

[8] C. M. Harmon and L. B. Smith, "Plasmablastic lymphoma: a review of clinicopathologic features and differential

diagnosis," *Archives of Pathology & Laboratory Medicine*, vol. 140, no. 10, pp. 1074–1078, 2016.
[9] J. J. Castillo, E. S. Winer, D. Stachurski et al., "HIV-negative plasmablastic lymphoma: not in the mouth," *Clinical Lymphoma Myeloma and Leukemia*, vol. 11, no. 2, pp. 185–189, 2011.
[10] X. Han, M. Duan, L. Hu, D. Zhou, and W. Zhang, "Plasmablastic lymphoma: review of 60 Chinese cases and prognosis analysis," *Medicine*, vol. 96, no. 9, p. e5981, 2017.
[11] J. Morscio, D. Dierickx, J. Nijs et al., "Clinicopathologic comparison of plasmablastic lymphoma in HIV-positive, immunocompetent, and posttransplant patients," *The American Journal of Surgical Pathology*, vol. 38, no. 7, pp. 875–886, 2014.
[12] C. Cattaneo, F. Facchetti, A. Re et al., "Oral cavity lymphomas in immunocompetent and human immunodeficiency virus infected patients," *Leukemia & Lymphoma*, vol. 46, no. 1, pp. 77–81, 2005.
[13] J. J. Castillo and J. L. Reagan, "Plasmablastic lymphoma: a systematic review," *The Scientific World Journal*, vol. 11, pp. 687–696, 2011.
[14] J. J. Castillo, E. S. Winer, D. Stachurski et al., "Clinical and pathological differences between human immunodeficiency virus-positive and human immunodeficiency virus-negative patients with plasmablastic lymphoma," *Leukemia & Lymphoma*, vol. 51, no. 11, pp. 2047–2053, 2010.
[15] G. Elyamany, A. M. Alzahrani, M. Aljuboury et al., "Clinicopathologic features of plasmablastic lymphoma: single-center series of 8 cases from Saudi Arabia," *Diagnostic Pathology*, vol. 10, no. 1, 2015.
[16] C. Dittus and S. Sarosiek, "A case of HIV-negative plasmablastic lymphoma of the bone marrow with a unique immunophenotype," *Clinical Case Reports*, vol. 5, no. 6, pp. 902–904, 2017.
[17] L. Yin, J. Xu, M. Li et al., "Oct2 and Bob1 are sensitive and specific markers in lineage determination of B cell lymphomas with no expression of conventional B cell markers," *Histopathology*, vol. 69, no. 5, pp. 775–783, 2016.
[18] J. M. Wu, M. J. Borowitz, and E. G. Weir, "The usefulness of CD71 expression by flow cytometry for differentiating indolent from aggressive CD10+ B-cell lymphomas," *American Journal of Clinical Pathology*, vol. 126, no. 1, pp. 39–46, 2006.
[19] Q. Liu, M Wang, Y Hu et al., "Significance of CD71 expression by flow cytometry in diagnosis of acute leukemia," *Leukemia & Lymphoma*, vol. 55, no. 4, pp. 892–898, 2014.
[20] H. Y. Dong, S. Wilkes, and H. Yang, "CD71 is selectively and ubiquitously expressed at high levels in erythroid precursors of all maturation stages: a comparative immunochemical study with glycophorin A and hemoglobin A," *The American Journal of Surgical Pathology*, vol. 35, no. 5, pp. 723–732, 2011.
[21] M. M. Al-Malki, J. J. Castillo, J. M. Sloan, and A. Re, "Hematopoietic cell transplantation for plasmablastic lymphoma: a review," *Biology of Blood and Marrow Transplantation*, vol. 20, no. 12, pp. 1877–1884, 2014.
[22] J. J. Castillo, M. Bibas, and R. N. Miranda, "The biology and treatment of plasmablastic lymphoma," *Blood*, vol. 125, no. 15, pp. 2323–2330, 2015.
[23] J. S. Ahn, R. Okal, J. A. Vos, M. Smolkin, A. S. Kanate, and F. G. Rosado, "Plasmablastic lymphoma versus plasmablastic myeloma: an ongoing diagnostic dilemma," *Journal of Clinical Pathology*, vol. 70, no. 9, pp. 775–780, 2017.
[24] Z. Pan, S. Hu, M. Li et al., "ALK-positive large B-cell lymphoma: a clinicopathologic study of 26 cases with review of additional 108 cases in the literature," *The American Journal of Surgical Pathology*, vol. 41, no. 1, pp. 25–38, 2017.
[25] H. Hashmi, D. Murray, S. Al-Quran, and W. Tse, "Primary effusion lymphoma without an effusion: a rare case of solid extracavitary variant of primary effusion lymphoma in an HIV-positive patient," *Case Reports in Hematology*, vol. 2018, Article ID 9368451, 5 pages, 2018.
[26] D. Pretscher, A. Kalisch, M. Wilhelm, and J. Birkmann, "Refractory plasmablastic lymphoma—a review of treatment options beyond standard therapy," *Annals of Hematology*, vol. 96, no. 6, pp. 967–970, 2017.
[27] B. M. Holderness, S. Malhotra, N. B. Levy, and A. V. Danilov, "Brentuximab vedotin demonstrates activity in a patient with plasmablastic lymphoma arising from a background of chronic lymphocytic leukemia," *Journal of Clinical Oncology*, vol. 31, no. 12, pp. e197–e199, 2013.
[28] J. M. Schmit, J. DeLaune, M. Norkin, and A. Grosbach, "A case of plasmablastic lymphoma achieving complete response and durable remission after lenalidomide-based therapy," *Oncology Research and Treatment*, vol. 40, no. 1-2, pp. 46–48, 2017.
[29] W. D. Marrero, A. Cruz-Chacón, C. Castillo, and F. Cabanillas, "Successful use of bortezomib-lenalidomide combination as treatment for a patient with plasmablastic lymphoma," *Clinical Lymphoma Myeloma and Leukemia*, vol. 18, no. 7, pp. e275–e277, 2018.
[30] C. Laurent, B. Fabiani, C. Do et al., "Immune-checkpoint expression in epstein-barr virus positive and negative plasmablastic lymphoma: a clinical and pathological study in 82 patients," *Haematologica*, vol. 101, no. 8, pp. 976–984, 2016.

12

Prolonged Myelosuppression due to Progressive Bone Marrow Fibrosis in a Patient with Acute Promyelocytic Leukemia

Yuta Inagawa,[1,2] Yukiko Komeno,[1] Satoshi Saito,[3] Yuji Maenohara,[4] Tetsuro Yamagishi,[5] Hiroyuki Kawashima,[5] Taku Saito,[4] Keiko Abe,[6] Kuniko Iihara,[6] Yasumasa Hatada,[3] and Tomiko Ryu[1]

[1]*Department of Hematology, Japan Community Healthcare Organization (JCHO) Tokyo Yamate Medical Center, Tokyo, Japan*
[2]*Department of Internal Medicine, JCHO Tokyo Yamate Medical Center, Tokyo, Japan*
[3]*Department of Gastroenterology, JCHO Tokyo Yamate Medical Center, Tokyo, Japan*
[4]*Department of Orthopaedic Surgery, Faculty of Medicine, The University of Tokyo, Tokyo, Japan*
[5]*Division of Orthopedic Surgery, Department of Regenerative and Transplant Medicine, Niigata University Graduate School of Medicine and Dental Sciences, Niigata, Japan*
[6]*Department of Pathology, JCHO Tokyo Yamate Medical Center, Tokyo, Japan*

Correspondence should be addressed to Yukiko Komeno; ykomeno-tky@umin.ac.jp

Academic Editor: Kazunori Nakase

A 34-year-old woman was diagnosed with acute promyelocytic leukemia. Chemotherapy was administered following the JALSG APL204 protocol. Induction therapy with all-trans retinoic acid resulted in complete remission on day 49. She developed coccygeal pain from day 18, which spread to the spine and cheekbones and lasted 5 weeks. She had similar bone pain on days 7–10 of the first consolidation therapy and on days 4–12 of the second consolidation therapy. Oral loxoprofen was prescribed for pain relief. On day 33 of the third consolidation, white blood cell and neutrophil counts were 320/μL and 20/μL, respectively. After she developed epigastralgia and hematemesis, she developed septic shock. Gastroendoscopy revealed markedly thickened folds and diffusely damaged mucosa with blood oozing. Computed tomography revealed thickened walls of the antrum and the pylorus. Despite emergency treatments, she died. Bacterial culture of the gastric fluid yielded *Enterobacter cloacae* and enterococci growth. Collectively, she was diagnosed with phlegmonous gastritis. Retrospective examination of serial bone marrow biopsy specimens demonstrated progressive bone marrow fibrosis, which may have caused prolonged myelosuppression. Thus, evaluation of bone marrow fibrosis by bone marrow biopsy after each treatment cycle might serve as a predictor of persistent myelosuppression induced by chemotherapy.

1. Introduction

Acute promyelocytic leukemia (APL) is a subtype of acute myelocytic leukemia (AML) with the most favorable outcome [1, 2]. APL prognosis has dramatically improved since the introduction of all-trans retinoic acid (ATRA), a molecular targeted therapy which induces differentiation of APL cells [3]. ATRA plus chemotherapy has now become the standard therapy. Recently, ATRA plus arsenic trioxide, another molecular targeted therapy, has also been administered with or without chemotherapy in both frontline and relapsed APL cases [2].

Bone marrow fibrosis (BMF) is a histopathological process characterized by an increased deposition of reticulin fibers, and in some cases collagen fibers, in the bone marrow [4]. A wide variety of malignant and nonmalignant disorders are associated with BMF. Nonmalignant conditions underlying BMF include endocrine disorders, autoimmune diseases, and infections [4]. Regarding malignant conditions, primary myelofibrosis and secondary myelofibrosis (arising from polycythemia vera or essential thrombocythemia) are classified as Philadelphia-negative myeloproliferative neoplasms (MPNs) which are often, but not always, accompanied by *JAK2*, *CALR*, or *MPL* mutations [1]. Acute megakaryoblastic leukemia is the most

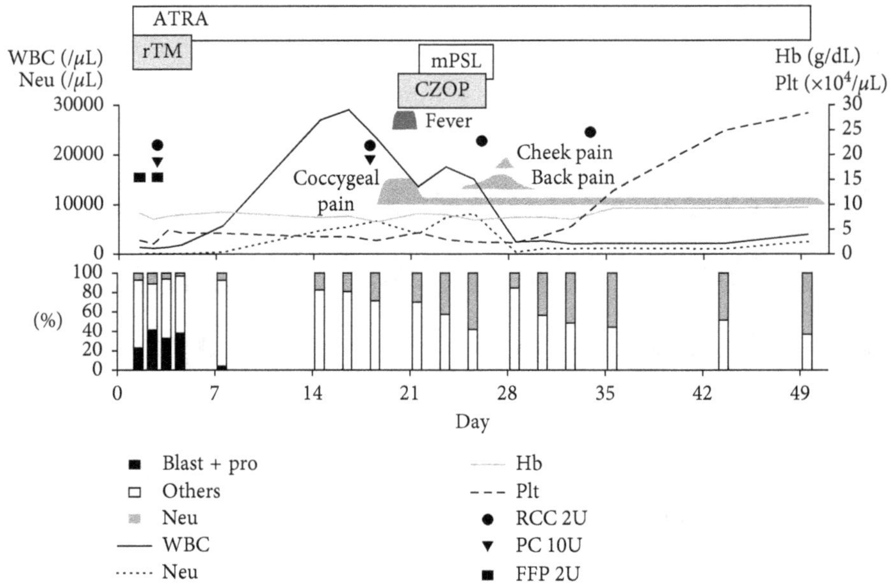

FIGURE 1: Clinical course of induction chemotherapy. On the horizontal axis, day 1 was set as the first day of induction chemotherapy. WBC, white blood cell; Neu, neutrophil; Hb, hemoglobin; Plt, platelet; Pro, promyelocyte; ATRA, all-trans retinoic acid; rTM, recombinant human thrombomodulin; mPSL, methylprednisolone; CZOP, cefozopran; RCC, red cell concentrate; PC, platelet concentrate; FFP, fresh frozen plasma.

common subtype of AML associated with BMF [1]. However, there are several previous reports of APL patients who presented with severe BMF at diagnosis [5–7].

Herein, we present details of a patient with APL, who suffered from fatal phlegmonous gastritis during prolonged myelosuppression caused by progressive BMF.

2. Case Presentation

A 34-year-old Japanese woman visited our hospital with purpura in the lower extremities. Blood tests showed pancytopenia (white blood cells (WBC) 1340/μL (blast 1.5%, promyelocyte 21.5%, and neutrophil (Neu) 7.0%), hemoglobin 8.4 g/dL, and platelets $2.8 \times 10^4/\mu$L) and disseminated intravascular coagulation (fibrinogen 67 mg/dL, fibrin degradation products 93 μg/mL, and D-dimer 32.7 μg/mL). She was emergently hospitalized. A bone marrow aspiration smear showed 1.8% blasts and 88.1% promyelocytes and myeloperoxidase strongly positive. Auer bodies and Faggot cells were also observed. The patient was diagnosed with acute promyelocytic leukemia (APL). Leukemic cells were CD13(+), CD33(+), CD34(−), CD117(+), and HLA-DR(−). Leukemic cell karyotype was 46,XX,der(15)t(15;17)(q22;q12), ider(17)(q10)t(15;17) [20/20]. *PML-RARA* fluorescence in situ hybridization (FISH) was positive in 98.0% of cells (fusion signal : 2/PML : 1/RARA : 1 = 2.0% and fusion signal : 3/PML : 1/RARA : 1 = 96.0%, where the PML probe binds to 15q24 and the RARA probe binds to 17q21). Quantitative polymerase chain reaction (qPCR) of *PML-RARA* fusion mRNA was 7.0×10^4 copies/μgRNA. Bone marrow biopsy demonstrated hypercellular marrow without an increase in argyrophilic fibers. Erythroid cells and megakaryocytes were severely decreased.

Induction chemotherapy was performed with oral all-trans retinoic acid (ATRA) at a dosage of 45 mg/m^2 as a single agent, following the JALSG APL204 protocol (Figure 1) [8]. On day 18, she experienced a sudden strong coccygeal pain while walking and became unable to walk. On day 20, she developed fever and cefozopran was administered. Since differentiation syndrome could not be ruled out, methylprednisolone 80 mg/day was administered for 4 days. Magnetic resonance imaging on day 21 demonstrated no obvious abnormality in the lower sacrum and coccyx. On day 24, she acquired back pain, which gradually worsened. On day 27, she had cheekbone pain, which disappeared the following day. Back pain disappeared on day 29, but coccygeal pain persisted. Oral loxoprofen was necessary for pain relief. On day 49, complete remission (CR) was confirmed by bone marrow examination and ATRA administration was discontinued. Bone marrow smear showed 0.6% blasts and 0.4% promyelocytes. Karyotype was normal. *PML-RARA* FISH was positive in 3.0% of cells (fusion signal : 2/PML : 1/RARA : 1 = 2.0% and fusion signal : 3/PML : 1/RARA : 1 = 1.0%). qPCR of *PML-RARA* fusion mRNA was 4.9×10^3 copies/μgRNA.

First consolidation chemotherapy involved cytarabine 200 mg/m^2 for 5 days and mitoxantrone 7 mg/m^2 for 3 days (Figure 2(a)). The patient had persistent coccygeal pain from the induction of chemotherapy until day 5. She experienced bone pain in the coccyx, spine, and costae on days 7–10. She again had back pain on days 14–15 and 18–19. Neutrophil count recovered on day 22 (WBC 7380/μL, Neu 5680/μL). Bone marrow aspiration/biopsy on day 35 demonstrated CR with 1.7% blasts and 0.5% promyelocytes. Karyotype was normal. *PML-RARA* FISH was negative. qPCR of *PML-RARA* fusion mRNA was undetectable.

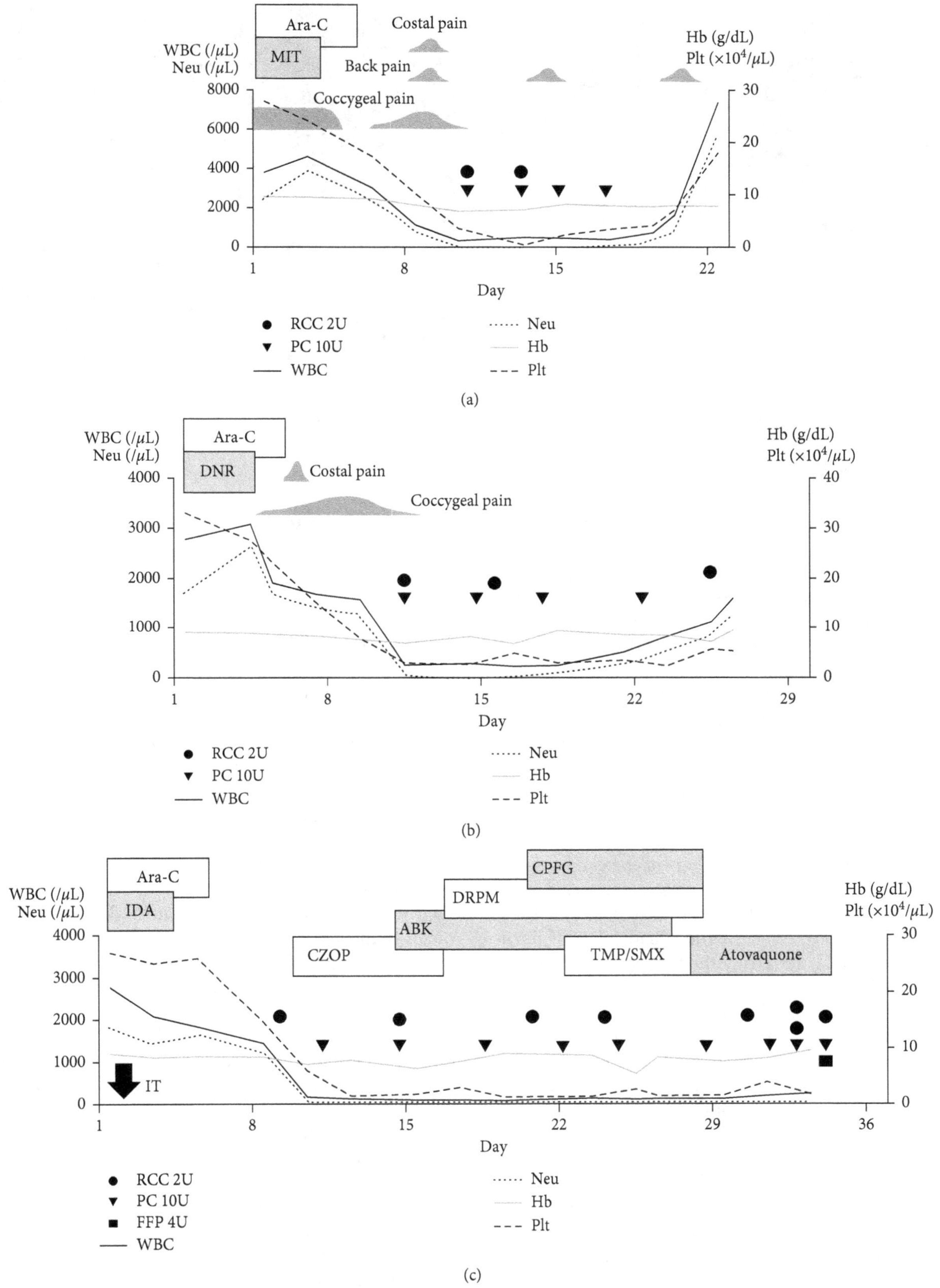

FIGURE 2: Prolonged myelosuppression during three courses of consolidation chemotherapy. (a) First course; (b) second course; (c) third course. As the consolidation therapy progressed, myelosuppression prolonged. Back pain and coccygeal pain became milder during the later course of consolidation therapy. On horizontal axis, day 1 was set as the first day of each course of chemotherapy. WBC, white blood cell; Neu, neutrophil; Hb, hemoglobin; Plt, platelet; RCC, red cell concentrate; PC, platelet concentrate; FFP, fresh frozen plasma; Ara-C, cytarabine; MIT, mitoxantrone; DNR, daunorubicin; IDA, idarubicin; CZOP, cefozopran; ABK, arbekacin; DRPM, doripenem; CPFG, caspofungin; TMP/SMX, trimethoprim/sulfamethoxazole; IT, intrathecal injection.

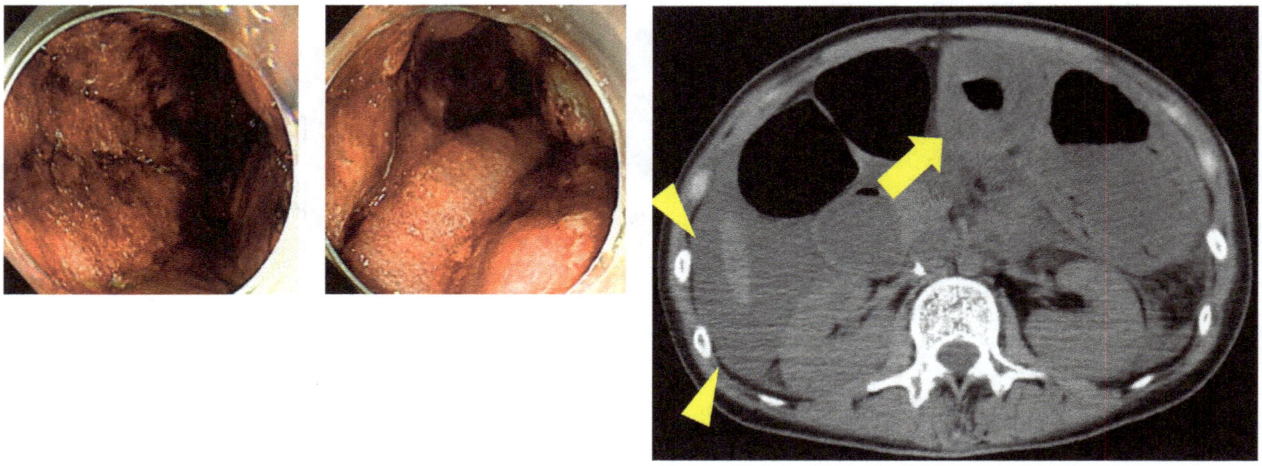

(a) (b) (c)

FIGURE 3: Phlegmonous gastritis. (a, b) Upper endoscopy. The gastric mucosa was reddish, and the folds were markedly thickened. (c) Abdominal CT. Fluid level was noted in the stomach. Arrow, thickened wall of the antrum and the pylorus with hypodense areas inside. Arrowheads, ascites.

Second consolidation chemotherapy involved cytarabine 200 mg/m^2 for 5 days with daunorubicin 50 mg/m^2 for 3 days (Figure 2(b)). The patient developed coccygeal bone pain on days 4–12 and costal pain on days 6–7. Neutrophil count recovered on day 25 (WBC 1600/μL, Neu 1280/μL). Bone marrow aspiration/biopsy on day 41 demonstrated CR with 1.2% blasts and 0.7% promyelocytes. Karyotype was normal. *PML-RARA* FISH was negative. qPCR of *PML-RARA* fusion mRNA was undetectable.

Third consolidation chemotherapy involved cytarabine 140 mg/m^2 for 5 days with idarubicin 12 mg/m^2 for 3 days (Figure 2(c)). On day 1, a peripherally inserted central venous catheter (PICC) was inserted. Intrathecal injection of methotrexate 15 mg, cytarabine 40 mg, and prednisolone 10 mg was also administered. Cytology of the cerebrospinal fluid was categorized as class I. To treat neutropenic fever, antibiotics were administered. Fever persisted and the PICC was removed. On day 25, the patient had bilateral pneumocystis pneumonia and trimethoprim-sulfamethoxazole was prescribed. Intravenous immunoglobulin was also administered. On day 28, she defervesced. Computed tomography on day 29 showed remission of ground-glass opacity. On day 30, due to abdominal discomfort, trimethoprim-sulfamethoxazole was replaced with atovaquone and other antibiotics were discontinued.

On the night of day 32, the patient vomited twice. During the early morning on day 33, she presented with epigastralgia and hematemesis and then became drowsy. She was afebrile. Blood pressure and oxygen saturation were unmeasurable. She was diagnosed with septic shock. Her abdomen was soft and flat on palpation, with epigastric tenderness. A central venous catheter was inserted. Intravenous dopamine, blood transfusion, and fluid therapy were administered. Laboratory data showed mild elevation of C-reactive protein (CRP) (3.1 mg/dL) and liver dysfunction. Echocardiography demonstrated hypovolemic state with normal ejection fraction. Upper endoscopy (Figures 3(a) and 3(b)) revealed dark-red bloody fluid in the stomach. Gastric folds were markedly thickened. Gastric mucosa was diffusely damaged, and blood was oozing from all areas. No ulcers or pulsatile bleeding were confirmed. The esophagus and the duodenum appeared normal. Phlegmonous gastritis was suspected. She was transferred to an intensive care unit. For pain relief, pentazocine was infused. Norepinephrine was also administered. At midnight, she became unconscious. Cardiopulmonary resuscitation was performed. She was intubated and connected to a respirator. Her abdomen was distended. Computed tomography (Figure 3(c)) revealed markedly thickened wall of the antrum and the pylorus with hypodense areas. Massive ascites was also observed. Gasses and fluid in the intestines were compatible with paralytic ileus. When a nasogastric tube was inserted, relatively fresh bloody fluid came out, which was used for bacterial culture. Laboratory data showed multiorgan failure and elevated CRP (10.0 mg/dL). Cefozopran was started. Blood pressure went down despite blood transfusion. Cardiopulmonary arrest was confirmed. The approval for autopsy was not obtained from the family.

Bacterial culture of the gastric fluid yielded *Enterobacter cloacae*, *Enterococcus* species, and methicillin-resistant *Staphylococcus*. Together with the results of imaging studies, the patient was diagnosed with phlegmonous gastritis (PG).

To investigate the cause of progressive myelosuppression, bone marrow biopsy samples were re-evaluated retrospectively (Figure 4). Each sample was classified as normocellular BM compatible with CR, and the number of megakaryocytes was within normal range. However, a silver stain demonstrated that BMF progressed rapidly after each cycle of consolidation chemotherapy, suggesting that prolonged myelosuppression was caused by progressive BMF. Argyrophilic fibers were increased. Intriguingly, at diagnosis, the bone trabecular border in contact with leukemic cells showed osteolysis-like appearance (Figures 5(a) and 5(b)). Immunostaining of PTH-related protein (PTH-rP)

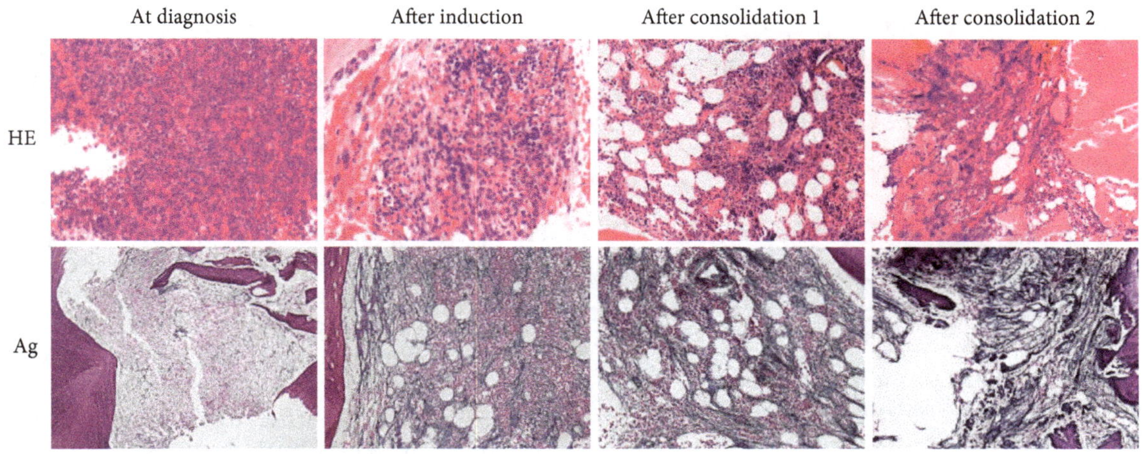

FIGURE 4: Serial bone marrow biopsies (hematoxylin-eosin (HE) and silver staining (Ag)). Only mild reticulin fibrosis was observed at the time of diagnosis. Fibrosis progressed as treatment progressed, and collagenous fibrosis was recognized. Magnification, 40x.

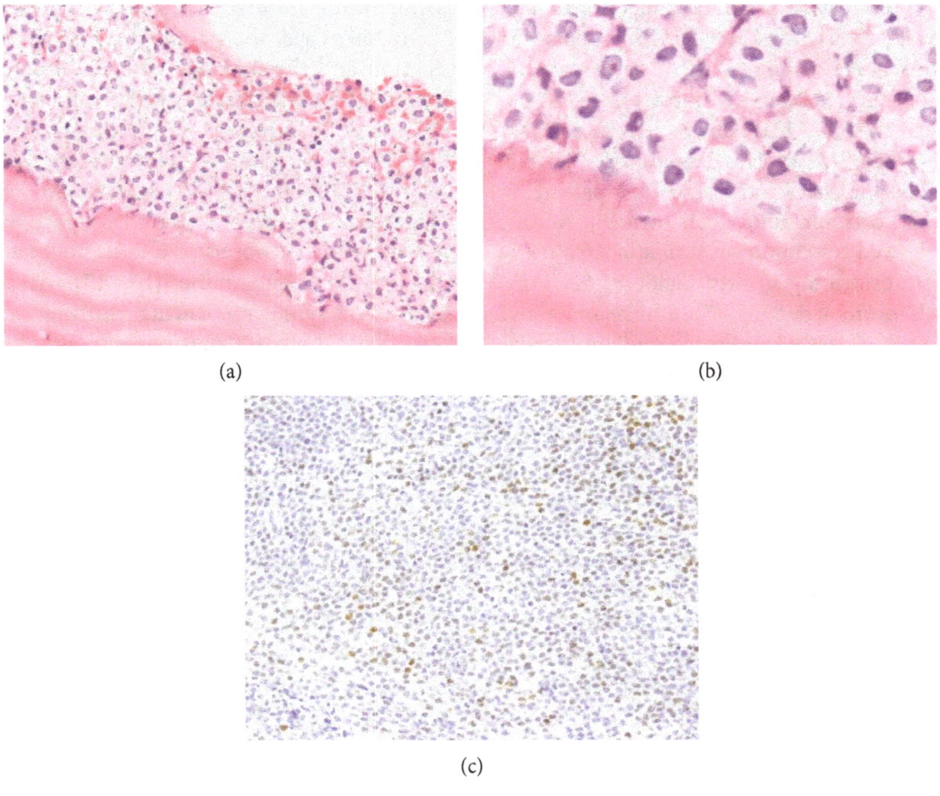

FIGURE 5: Histopathology of bone marrow biopsy at diagnosis. (a)-(b) Hematoxylin-Eosin stain showed that the bone trabecula border in contact with leukemic cells shows osteolysis-like appearance. (a) Magnification, 100x; (b) magnification, 400x; (c) parathyroid hormone-related protein stain. Positive cells were stained brown. Magnification, 100x.

and receptor activator of nuclear factor kappa-B ligand (RANKL), the molecules involved in bone remodeling, was performed. PTH-rP was positive in some of the leukemic cells (Figure 5(c)), while RANKL was negative (data not shown). Since these molecules activate osteoclasts, we performed TRAP staining to detect osteoclasts, which was negative (data not shown). In addition, immunostaining of osterix (Osx), an osteoblast-specific transcription factor, demonstrated multilayered osteoblasts along the trabecula in the bone marrow only after induction chemotherapy (Figure 6). Thus, prolonged myelosuppression was suspected to be caused by progressive BMF, although its exact mechanism was unclear.

3. Discussion

Bone marrow fibrosis (BMF) is characterized by an increased deposition of reticulin fibers, and in some cases collagen fibers, in the bone marrow [4]. BMF as a side effect of all-trans retinoic acid (ATRA) has been reported by

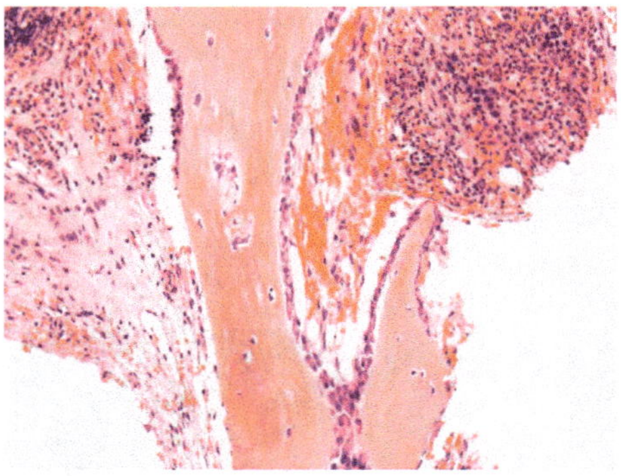

Figure 6: Multilayered osteoblasts in the bone marrow after induction chemotherapy. Osteoblasts multilayered along the trabecular bone. Magnification, 40x.

Hatake et al. [9]. Eleven of thirteen (84.6%) APL patients who received ATRA as induction therapy developed collagenous fibrosis after 1–8 weeks. Fibrosis resolved spontaneously or after consolidation therapy. Five of sixteen (31.3%) APL patients who received chemotherapy alone, without ATRA, developed collagenous fibrosis. However, collagenous fibrosis was not enhanced by anticancer drugs in AML patients [9]. In contrast, there are reports of marked BMF at APL diagnosis [5–7]. Abou Dalle et al. summarized the characteristics of nine patients in previously published reports, including their own [5]. Among them, four patients showed resolution of BMF after treatment. Mori et al. showed transforming growth factor-β_1 (TGF-β_1) secreted by APL cells promoted BMF [7]. Unlike the above reports, our case presented with irreversible and progressive BMF as treatment progressed (Figure 4). CR was achieved after induction therapy and was maintained until the third consolidation therapy, suggesting that ATRA treatment or APL cells did not cause BMF. In cases of MPN, BMF is associated with abnormal number or function of megakaryocytes and platelets, which secrete cytokines with fibrogenic potential (such as TGF-β and platelet-derived growth factor) [4, 10]. In our case, bone marrow biopsies after consolidation chemotherapies showed megakaryocytes were within the normal range without dysplasia. Splenomegaly was not observed in a CT scan just before death. Thus, it was unlikely that MPN developed during cytotoxic chemotherapy administration. *JAK2* or other mutations could not be tested due to lack of preserved specimens. BMF as a side effect of cytarabine or anthracyclines has not been reported in the literature.

In the bone marrow biopsy at the time of diagnosis, the border of bone trabecula in contact with APL cells was osteolytic (Figures 5(a) and 5(b)). Although the patient had coccygeal pain, magnetic resonance imaging of the pelvis during ATRA treatment demonstrated no apparent osteolytic lesions. Among hematological disorders, multiple myeloma and adult T-cell leukemia are the most frequent causes of hypercalcemia associated with bone resorption [11]. In these diseases, osteoclastic differentiation/activity is enhanced through PTH-rP and RANKL signaling pathways [11]. Despite this, hypercalcemia in AML is rare [11]. There were no previous reports of PTH-rP-positive AML cells from patients. Human cell line HL-60 cells, established from patient's APL cells, were able to secrete PTH-rP when stimulated with phorbol 12-myristate, 13-acetate (PMA), but not when unstimulated [12]. In our case, the serum calcium level on patient admission was not tested because she had no signs or symptoms of hypercalcemia. Although APL cells in our case were partially PTH-rP-positive (Figure 5(c)) and RANKL-negative (data not shown) by immunostaining, almost no osteoclasts were observed by TRAP staining (data not shown). Thus, the significance of PTH-rP-positive APL cells in our case was unknown.

Bone marrow biopsy after induction with ATRA showed multilayered osteoblasts along bone trabecula (Figure 6). There were also small pieces of trabeculae, which may have been regenerated. As it was only observed after induction with ATRA but not after two courses of consolidation chemotherapy, ATRA might be the cause of this phenomenon. ATRA acts on osteoblasts and osteoclasts and causes bone remodeling [13]. It would be worthwhile to examine the correlation between ATRA blood levels and osteoblast proliferation *in vivo* with a large sample size.

In our case, the patient had bone pain during the induction and the first two courses of consolidation chemotherapy. In the literature, bone pain was observed in 14 of 101 newly diagnosed APL patients during induction by ATRA with or without chemotherapy [14] and also seen in relapsed/refractory APL patients [15]. Bone pain due to cytarabine has been reported as part of "cytarabine syndrome" which is observed 6 to 12 hours after administration of high-dose cytarabine [16, 17]. There is a report of cytarabine syndrome during continuous injection of low-dose cytarabine (20 mg/m^2/day), but bone pain was not observed [18]. Primary and secondary myelofibrosis accompanies progressive bone pain in extremities due to extramedullary hematopoiesis [19]. In our case, bone pain occurred on day 18 of induction therapy with ATRA, on days 7–10 of the first consolidation therapy, and days 4–12 of the second consolidation therapy with a relatively small amount of cytarabine by continuous injection. Pain mainly occurred in the coccyx. However, no pain was recorded during the third consolidation therapy. Since the mechanism of bone pain caused by ATRA and cytarabine is unknown, it is unclear whether our patient was idiosyncratic or if bone pain was associated with the progression of BMF.

Phlegmonous gastritis (PG) is a rare but occasionally fatal stomach bacterial infection [20, 21]. Common symptoms include fever, epigastralgia, nausea, and vomiting, which resemble peritonitis and often present as acute abdomen. Hematemesis is also usually observed. Laboratory tests show elevation of white blood cell counts and CRP. Computed tomography demonstrates thickening of the stomach wall (localized or generalized) and the low-density area inside the wall. Gastroendoscopy shows thickened folds and extensive ulceration. The predisposing factors to PG are chronic gastritis, gastric trauma, alcoholism, debilitation, and achlorhydria caused by proton pump inhibitor use, infection, and immunosuppression. Treatment consists of antibiotics and surgical resection. There are only a few reports on PG in immunocompromised patients. In the literature, only four cases of PG were reported in blood disorders (multiple myeloma, gastric lymphoma, chronic myelomonocytic leukemia, and ALL) [21–24]. In our case, the patient suffered from pneumocystis pneumonia during prolonged myelosuppression, suggesting an extremely immunocompromised state. In addition, she was taking a proton pump inhibitor, another predisposing factor to PG. *Enterobacter cloacae*, *Enterococcus* species, and *Staphylococcus* species were detected in the gastric fluid culture, while the blood culture was negative. The clinical course was acute, and she died within two days. Physicians should keep in mind PG as a differential diagnosis of acute abdomen in patients with hematological diseases.

In AML patients, bone marrow biopsy might not be routinely performed for follow-up because minimal residual disease is mainly evaluated by karyotyping, FISH, and qPCR [2]. However, as our case illustrates, bone marrow biopsy can demonstrate progressive BMF, which predicts imminent myelosuppression and a resulting risk of severe infection.

4. Conclusion

Here, a rare case of APL with progressive BMF was reported. Evaluation of BMF by bone marrow biopsy after each treatment cycle may serve as a predictor of persistent myelosuppression leading to severe infection. Since there has been no report on PTH-rP-positive AML cells, association regarding stratification of osteoblasts, BMF, and bone pain during treatment for APL, further study is warranted.

References

[1] S. Swerdlow, E. Campo, N. Harris et al., *WHO Classification of Tumours of Haematopoietic and Lymphoid Tissues*, IARC, Lyon, France, 2017.

[2] M. A. Sanz, P. Fenaux, M. S. Tallman et al., "Management of acute promyelocytic leukemia: updated recommendations from an expert panel of the European LeukemiaNet," *Blood*, vol. 133, no. 15, pp. 1630–1643, 2019.

[3] M. Huang, Y. Ye, S. Chen et al., "Use of all-trans retinoic acid in the treatment of acute promyelocytic leukemia," *Blood*, vol. 72, no. 2, pp. 567–572, 1988.

[4] D. J. Kuter, B. Bain, G. Mufti, A. Bagg, and R. P. Hasserjian, "Bone marrow fibrosis: pathophysiology and clinical significance of increased bone marrow stromal fibres," *British Journal of Haematology*, vol. 139, no. 3, pp. 351–362, 2007.

[5] I. Abou Dalle, S. Nassif, and A. Bazarbachi, "Acute promyelocytic leukemia with increased bone marrow reticulin fibrosis: description of three cases and review of the literature," *Hematology/Oncology and Stem Cell Therapy*, vol. 11, no. 2, pp. 99–104, 2018.

[6] C. Shah and S. J. Grethlein, "Case report of rituximab-induced thrombocytopenia," *American Journal of Hematology*, vol. 75, no. 4, p. 263, 2004.

[7] A. Mori, H. Wada, M. Okada et al., "Acute promyelocytic leukemia with marrow fibrosis at initial presentation: possible involvement of transforming growth factor-beta(1)," *Acta Haematologica*, vol. 103, no. 4, pp. 220–223, 2000.

[8] K. Shinagawa, M. Yanada, T. Sakura et al., "Tamibarotene as maintenance therapy for acute promyelocytic leukemia: results from a randomized controlled trial," *Journal of Clinical Oncology*, vol. 32, no. 33, pp. 3729–3735, 2014.

[9] K. Hatake, T. Ohtsuki, M. Uwai et al., "Tretinoin induces bone marrow collagenous fibrosis in acute promyelocytic leukaemia: new adverse, but reversible effect," *British Journal of Haematology*, vol. 93, no. 3, pp. 646–649, 1996.

[10] A. Malara, V. Abbonante, M. Zingariello, A. R. Franco Migliaccio, and A. Balduini, "Megakaryocyte contribution to bone marrow fibrosis: many arrows in the quiver," *Mediterranean Journal of Hematology and Infectious Diseases*, vol. 10, no. 1, Article ID e2018068, 2018.

[11] J. T. Sargent and O. P. Smith, "Haematological emergencies managing hypercalcaemia in adults and children with haematological disorders," *British Journal of Haematology*, vol. 149, no. 4, pp. 465–477, 2010.

[12] J. Bolodeoku and R. Kusec, "Parathyroid hormone related protein (PTHrP) in acute myeloid leukaemia cells," *British Journal of Haematology*, vol. 98, no. 1, pp. 245-246, 1997.

[13] P. Henning, H. H. Conaway, and U. H. Lerner, "Retinoid receptors in bone and their role in bone remodeling," *Frontiers in Endocrinology*, vol. 6, p. 31, 2015.

[14] A. Kanamaru, Y. Takemoto, M. Tanimoto et al., "All-trans retinoic acid for the treatment of newly diagnosed acute promyelocytic leukemia. Japan Adult Leukemia Study Group (see comments)," *Blood*, vol. 85, no. 5, pp. 1202–1206, 1995.

[15] R. Ohno, H. Yoshida, H. Fukutani et al., "Multi-institutional study of all-trans-retinoic acid as a differentiation therapy of refractory acute promyelocytic leukemia. Leukaemia Study Group of the Ministry of Health and Welfare," *Leukemia*, vol. 7, no. 11, pp. 1722–1727, 1993.

[16] R. P. Castleberry, W. M. Crist, T. Holbrook, A. Malluh, and D. Gaddy, "The cytosine arabinoside (Ara-C) syndrome," *Medical and Pediatric Oncology*, vol. 9, no. 3, pp. 257–264, 1981.

[17] M. A. Jirasek and J. D. Herrington, "Cytarabine syndrome despite corticosteroid premedication in an adult undergoing induction treatment for acute myelogenous leukemia," *Journal of Oncology Pharmacy Practice*, vol. 22, no. 6, pp. 795–800, 2016.

[18] B. L. Powell, P. J. Zekan, H. B. Muss, F. Richards 2nd, E. S. Lyerly, and R. L. Capizzi, "Ara-C syndrome during low-dose continuous infusion therapy," *Medical and Pediatric Oncology*, vol. 14, no. 6, pp. 310–312, 1986.

[19] J. A. Cox, P. R. Sevak, L. L. Grumbles, T. A. Swanson, and S. S. Hatch, "Single-fraction radiotherapy for palliation of myelofibrosis-related extremity pain syndrome," *Journal of Pain and Symptom Management*, vol. 48, no. 2, pp. 299–304, 2014.

[20] M. Ishioka, N. Watanabe, M. Sawaguchi et al., "Phlegmonous gastritis: a report of three cases with clinical and imaging features," *Internal Medicine*, vol. 57, no. 15, pp. 2185–2188, 2018.

[21] M. Saito, M. Morioka, H. Kanno, and S. Tanaka, "Acute phlegmonous gastritis with neutropenia," *Internal Medicine*, vol. 51, no. 20, pp. 2987-2988, 2012.

[22] J. Guo, S. K. Young, C. R. Lorenzo et al., "Phlegmonous gastritis in a patient with myeloid sarcoma," *Applied Immunohistochemistry & Molecular Morphology*, vol. 17, no. 5, pp. 458–462, 2009.

[23] R. Harikumar, K. Pramod, M. Pushpa, K. Simi, and G. Arun, "Gastric lymphoma presenting as phlegmonous gastritis," *Journal of Gastrointestinal Cancer*, vol. 38, no. 1, pp. 24–27, 2007.

[24] A. Horsburgh, "Acute phlegmonous gastritis in a patient with myelomatosis," *The Lancet*, vol. 274, no. 7093, p. P89, 1959.

13

PD-1 Checkpoint Blockade in Patients for Acute Myeloid Leukemia after HSCT Relapse Resulted in Severe GVHD and sHLH

Zhi zhuo Du, Mi Zhou, Jing Ling, Lan Cao, Lingjun Kong, Shengqin Cheng, Peifang Xiao, and Shaoyan Hu

Children's Hospital of Suzhou University, Suzhou, China

Correspondence should be addressed to Shaoyan Hu; hsy139@126.com

Academic Editor: Håkon Reikvam

Treatment with immune checkpoint inhibitors (ICI) such as carrizumab leads to immune-mediated adverse effects including severe acute graft versus host disease (aGVHD) and secondary hemophagocytic syndrome (sHLH). Herein, we present two cases where aGVHD and sHLH developed after ICI administration, which was treated using methylprednisolone (MP). They developed high-grade fever complicated with liver dysfunction and diarrhea 1 day after ICI administration. Treatment with MP does not alleviate symptoms because of steroid resistance. Hyperbilirubinemia, rash with blisters, and watery diarrhea showed severe aGVHD. Hyperferritinemia, hypertriglyceridemia, and cytopenias suggested the diagnosis of HLH and met the criteria for sHLH diagnosis. They were thus administered intravenous high-dose MP, methotrexate (MTX), basiliximab, ruxolitinib, etc, which resolved these symptoms.

1. Introduction

With the progress of treatment, the therapeutic effect of acute myeloid leukemia (*AML*) has gradually increased from about 10% to about 70% [1], but allogeneic hematopoietic stem cell transplantation (*HSCT*) is the only treatment option for high-risk AML. AML recurrence after *HSCT* affects about 30–40% of *HSCT* recipients, and recurrence is still the primary cause of death in *AML* patients after *HSCT* [2]. The prognosis of *AML* recurrence after *HSCT* is poor. The 3-year survival rate is about 20–30% [3], and the treatment options are very limited. General management includes immunosuppressant withdrawal, chemotherapy, donor lymphocyte infusion (*DLI*), chimeric antigen receptor (CAR) T-cell therapy, and second transplantation, which are not very effective. At present, *ICI* is increasingly applied to solid tumors such as lymphoma, lung cancer, and melanoma, and has achieved encouraging therapeutic effects [4]. Therefore, increasing attention has been paid to the treatment of *ICI*. Some literature points out that highly expressed cells of programmed death 1 (*PD-1*) are closely related to leukemia relapse after *HSCT* [5–7], which provides a therapeutic target for leukemia recurrence after *HSCT*. However, *ICI*, including carrizumab, can activate T cells and induce serious autoimmune complications, such as immune-related adverse events (*irAE*), including *aGVHD*, secondary hemophagocytic lymphohistiocytosis (*sHLH*); *sHLH* is a potentially fatal disease, which can be manifested as fever, rash, cytopenia, coagulation dysfunction, liver dysfunction and hemophagocytic cells in the bone marrow. The occurrence of these two complications can endanger the lives of children.

Here, we report two *AML* patients who relapsed after HSCT treated with carrizumab, who developed *sHLH* and severe *aGVHD*, and were successfully treated with pulse therapy using high-dose *MP* and other immunosuppressants.

2. Case Report

2.1. Case 1. A 10-year-old girl was diagnosed with *AML (M4)*; chromosome: chromosome:46, *XX*; negative fusion gene; *Izkf1* negative; full exon sequencing: a frameshift mutation was detected in *WT1* gene; *RNA SEQ* detected after

TABLE 1: Frequency of acute treatment, emergent *GVHD*, and laboratory findings: pretreatment, day 14 after the administration of carrizumab.

	Case 1		Case 2	
	Pretreatment	Day 14	Pretreatment	Day 14
Stage of *aGVHD*				
Skin	Stage 0	Stage 4	Stage 1	Stage 4
GI	Stage 0	Stage 4	Stage 0	Stage 4
Liver	Stage 0	Stage 2	Stage 0	Stage 2
HLH				
Hemoglobin (g/L)	146	85	85	77
Platelet ($\times10^9$/L)	194	61	108	16
Neutrophil count ($\times10^9$/L)	1.64	1.58	1.64	0.03
Bilirubin (mg/dL)	0.88	4	0.22	4.11
Ferritin (ng/mL)	6253.6	20920	3796.7	10450
Fibrin (g/L)	2.81	0.71	2.85	4.94
Triglyceride (mmol/L)	1.76	4.94	2.56	5.35
sIL-2R (U/mL)	—	12365	—	76806
NK cell activity (<15.11%)	—	11.22	—	8.61

Acute GVHD stage/grade and responses were scored according to consensus and National Institutes of Health (NIH) criteria, GI = gastrointestinal.

the fusion gene: *PRDM16/SKI* positive. The patient received induction chemotherapy with daunorubicin, cytarabine, cytarabine, and etoposide (*DAE*) scheme in June 2020 and achieved a partial response (*PR*). Then, the patient received consolidation chemotherapy with idarubicin, cytarabine (*IA*) scheme, and 2 cycles of dicitabine, homoharringtonine, cytarabine, and recombinant human granulocyte colony-stimulating factor (*G-CSF*) (*DEC* + *HAG*) scheme and achieved a PR. After receiving dicitabine, cladribine, cytarabine, and *G-CSF (DEC* + *CLAG)* scheme, the patient achieved a complete response (*CR*); at this stage, the patient was positive for minimal residual disease (*MRD*), confirmed through flow cytometry (*FCM*). The patient underwent *allo-HSCT* from a *HLA*-mismatched related donor (5/10), after preconditioning with semustine, *CLAG*, cyclophosphamide, busulfan (*CCNU* + *CLAG* + *BuCy*), followed by cyclosporine A, mycophenolate mofetil, and short-term methotrexate for prophylaxis of *GVHD*. The patient achieved CR with *MRD* negativity (*CRMRD-*) 1 month after *allo-HSCT* and no *GVHD*. In May 2021, 4 months after *HSCT*, the disease progressed to relapse, and the evaluation of bone marrow (*BM*) showed that 16.5% of blasts, 84.6% of donor chimeric; 32.29% of *FCM–MRD*; and 7.57% of WT1. We performed the *HLA-loss* test, but no *HLA* gene loss was detected. So the patient was treated with azacytidine chemotherapy and *DLI*, but it was still not achieved *CR*. The second transplantation was performed 5 months after *HSCT1*. The patient underwent *allo-HSCT* from a HLA-mismatched unrelated donor (cord blood) (7/10), after preconditioning with total body irradiation (*TBI*), *CLAG*, mefallen, followed by cyclosporine A, mycophenolate mofetil, and short-term methotrexate for prophylaxis of *GVHD*. The patient achieved *CR MRD* 1-month after *allo-HSCT* and no *GVHD*. The patient was treated with azacytidine and interferon for preemptive therapy, but after that, the patient achieved *CR MRD*, but the copy number of *WT1* in the patient increased gradually. Three months after the *HSCT2*, the patient was treated with azacytidine and camrelizumab (3 mg/kg/d) injection. On that day, the child felt general pain and discomfort, low fever, gradually developed a skin rash, even blisters, diarrhea, dark green watery stool, jaundice, abnormal liver function, 4-degree *GVHD*, accompanied by repeated fever hyperferrinemia, hypofibrinogenemia, hypertriglyceridemia, cytopenias, and sIL-2R > 2500 pg/ml (Table 1), which was consistent with *sHLH*. The children were combined with four degrees of *GVHD* and *sHLH* and were gradually reduced and treated with methotrexate (*MTX*) and MP (5 mg/kg/d), and basiliximab. *GVHD* and *sHLH* were gradually controlled. The evaluation of bone marrow (*BM*) showed *CR*, no hemophagocyte was found, and the copy number of *WT1* decreased.

2.2. Case 2. A 2 years old girl was diagnosed with *AML (M7)*; frameshift mutation was detected in the *ETV6* gene of myeloid line 67, and *CBFA2T3-GLS2* was positive. The patient received induction chemotherapy with daunorubicin, cytarabine, cytarabine, and homoharringtonine (*DAH*) scheme in March 2021 and achieved a *CR* with *CR MRD+*. After receiving *HAG*, 2 cycle *HA*, cytarabine, and etoposide (*EA*) scheme, the patient still achieved a *CR* with *CR MRD*; The patient underwent *allo-HSCT* from a *HLA*-mismatched unrelated donor (cord blood) (8/10), after preconditioning with *CCNU* + *CLAG* + *BuCy*, followed by cyclosporine A, mycophenolate mofetil, and short-term methotrexate for prophylaxis of *GVHD*. The patient achieved *CR MRD- 1* month after *allo-HSCT* and with 1-degree skin *GVHD*. In November 2021, 3 months after *HSCT*, the disease progressed to relapse, and the evaluation of bone marrow (*BM*) showed that 34% of blasts, 97.6% of donor chimeric; 46.29% of *FCM–MRD*; and 87.91% of *CBFA2T3-GLS2*; considering the relapse of *AML*, and camrelizumab (3 mg/kg/d) targeted antitumor therapy was given. Fever occurred on the same day and then gradually appeared the same 4-degree *GVHD* symptoms as the first case, such as a rash (including blisters), diarrhea, abnormal liver function, and jaundice. At the same time, the child developed repeated fever, hyperferrinemia, hypertriglyceridemia, cytopenias, *sIL-2R* >2500 pg/ml, and decreased *NK* cell activity (Table 1), which was consistent with sHLH. The child was complicated with four degrees of *GVHD* and *sHLH*, which were gradually reduced after being treated with *MTX* and *MP* (10 mg/kg/d), basiliximab, ruxolitinib, etc. *GVHD* and *sHLH* were gradually controlled. The evaluation of *BM* showed that 88% of blast parents gave up treatment.

3. Discussion

At present, chemotherapy, *DLI*, cell therapy, *et, al* are still unsatisfactory for patients with AML relapse after *HSCT*. *PD-1* pathway can be used as a checkpoint to limit T-cell-mediated immune response. Blocking the *PD-1* receptor on T cells can lead to the activation and proliferation of T cells, and induce an effective antitumor effect of immunotherapy [8]. In recent years, it has achieved certain therapeutic effects for patients with AML relapse after transplantation. Blocking *PD-1* after *HSCT* can enhance the graft *versus* leukemia (*GVL*) effect, but at the same time, the activation and proliferation of T cells can also lead to fatal *aGVHD* [9, 10]. Bradley et al. reported that the application of PD-1 inhibitors can also induce severe *aGVHD* [11]. In this *GVHD* state, T cells are activated and promote the activation of secondary macrophages, IL-6, IL-1, and IFN-γ, It is reported that *PD-1* inhibitors may cause *sHLH*, mainly in lymphoma, lung cancer, and other solid tumors [12, 13]. However, *PD-1* leads to fewer reports of post-transplant *HLH*. At present, the overall mortality of post-transplant *sHLH* is high, which can reach 80% [14]. If large doses of glucocorticoids cannot be rapidly alleviated, immune activation will continue, leading to further progress of *sHLH* and a*GVHD*, which will endanger life.

After the application of *PD-1*, the incidence rate of *irAE* is high. Both *aGVHD* and *sHLH* are *irAE*, but rarely occur at the same time. High fever, rash, diarrhea, and liver dysfunction were initially considered as *aGVHD* until there were cytopenia, decreased natural killer (*NK*) cell activity, hepatosplenomegaly, and coagulation dysfunction, especially hyperferrinemia (serum ferritin >10000 μg/ml), which has important clinical significance for the diagnosis of *sHLH* [15], Will realize the occurrence of *sHLH*. For patients with these two complications at the same time, the treatment is often difficult. Single-use of glucocorticoids is considered effective for *irAE* [16, 17]. However, patients with *aGVHD* and *sHLH* may have glucocorticoid resistance, and other immunosuppressants such as basiliximab, *MTX*, and ruxolitinib need to be used to control the deterioration of *irAE*. Because of the high mortality rate of *sHLH* after transplantation, it is essential for early diagnosis and treatment of *sHLH*. For patients who have had *aGVHD*, if they have abnormal blood coagulation function, hyperferrinemia, splenomegaly, and other manifestations, they should be alert to the occurrence of *sHLH*.

Because the relapse of *AML* after *HSCT* is always a difficult point, the chemotherapy effect is poor and the overall survival rate is low. The treatment of *PD-1* inhibitors provides us with the possibility of treatment. In order to avoid the high incidence rate of *aGVHD* and *sHLH*, we may adopt the following methods: (1) whether to use *ICI* can be determined according to the values of *PD-1*, *PD-L1*, and *PD-L2*. Some studies point out that the proportion of *PD-1* or *PD-L1* is relatively high, which has a good therapeutic effect [18, 19]; (2) by reducing the therapeutic dose of *ICI*, the current conventional dose is 3 mg/kg, and the proportion of severe *aGVHD* or *sHLH* is relatively high, so the dose can be further reduced. Matthew et al. tried to reduce the dose to 1 mg/kg or even 0.5 mg/kg [20]. If children with *irAE* I or II can choose to receive *ICI* treatment again, or even increase the dose if it is level III or IV, it should be avoided; (3) at the same time as *ICI* treatment, we used glucocorticoid, cyclosporine, and other drugs to prevent *aGVHD* to reduce the incidence rate of *aGVHD* or *sHLH*. Once a*GVHD* occurs, we should be alert to *sHLH*. If *sHLH* occurs, the *HLH-94* regimen seems to achieve a better therapeutic effect.

4. Conclusion

In conclusion, these 2 cases represent a particularly early and aggressive form of *sHLH* with *PD-1* inhibitor therapy and report severe *aGVHD* caused by recurrent *PD-1* after *HSCT*. With the continuous exploration of new *PD-1* inhibitors in children with post-transplantation relapsed *AML*, it should be considered that the incidence rate of *sHLH* and *aGVHD* as possible severe *irAE* is increasing, and the methods and strategies for *ICI* treatment of post-transplantation relapsed *AML* can be improved, to achieve the best treatment effect and minimize toxic and side effects.

Consent

Written informed consent was obtained from the patient's relatives for the publication of this case report and any accompanying images.

Authors' Contributions

SH and PX were involved in the identification, selection, and management of the patient and manuscript review. ZD was involved in the management of the patient and manuscript drafting. SC and MZ were involved in the selection and management of the patient and manuscript review. LC, LL, and LK were involved in manuscript editing. All authors have read and approved the final manuscript.

Acknowledgments

This study was supported by research funding from National Natural Science Foundation of China (NSFC) (nos. 81970163 and 82170218).

References

[1] M. Lejman, I. Dziatkiewicz, and M. Jurek, "Straight to the point—the novel strategies to cure pediatric AML," *International Journal of Molecular Sciences*, vol. 23, no. 4, p. 1968, 2022.

[2] S. Leotta, A. Condorelli, R. Sciortino et al., "Prevention and treatment of acute myeloid leukemia relapse after hematopoietic stem cell transplantation: the state of the art and future perspectives," *Journal of Clinical Medicine*, vol. 11, no. 1, p. 253, 2022.

[3] A. Bazarbachi, C. Schmid, M. Labopin et al., "Evaluation of trends and prognosis over time in patients with AML relapsing after allogeneic hematopoietic cell transplant reveals improved survival for young patients in recent years," *Clinical Cancer Research*, vol. 26, no. 24, pp. 6475–6482, 2020.

[4] Q. Tang, Y. Chen, Xj Li et al., "The role of PD-1/PD-L1 and application of immunecheckpoint inhibitors in human cancers," *Frontiers in Immunology*, vol. 13, Article ID 964442, 2022.

[5] S. A. Minnie, R. D. Kuns, K. H. Gartlan et al., "Myeloma escape after stem cell transplantation is a consequence of T-cell exhaustion and is prevented by TIGIT blockade," *Blood*, vol. 132, no. 16, pp. 1675–1688, 2018.

[6] M. Noviello, F. Manfredi, E. Ruggiero et al., "Bone marrow central memory and memory stem T-cell exhaustion in AML patients relapsing after HSCT," *Nature Communications*, vol. 10, no. 1, p. 1065, 2019.

[7] T. Hutten, W. Norde, R. Woestenenk, R. C. Wang, F. Maas, and M. Kester, "Title: increased co-expression of PD-1, TIGIT and KLRG-1 on tumor-reactive CD8+ T cells during relapse after allo-SCT," *Biology of Blood and Marrow Transplantation*, vol. 24, 2017.

[8] R. A. Wilcox, A. L. Feldman, D. A. Wada et al., "B7-H1 (PD-L1, CD274) suppresses host immunity in T-cell lymphoproliferative disorders," *Blood*, vol. 114, no. 10, pp. 2149–2158, 2009.

[9] A. Saha, K. Aoyama, P. A. Taylor et al., "Host programmed death ligand 1 is dominant over programmed death ligand 2 expression in regulating graft-versus-host disease lethality," *Blood*, vol. 122, no. 17, pp. 3062–3073, 2013.

[10] H. Fujiwara, Y. Maeda, K. Kobayashi et al., "Programmed death-1 pathway in host tissues ameliorates Th17/Th1-mediated experimental chronic graft-versus-host disease," *The Journal of Immunology*, vol. 193, no. 5, pp. 2565–2573, 2014.

[11] Y. Tang, Z. Zhou, H. Yan, and Y. You, "Case report: preemptive treatment with low-dose PD-1 blockade and azacitidine for molecular relapsed acute myeloid leukemia with RUNX1-runx1t1 after allogeneic hematopoietic stem cell transplantation," *Frontiers in Immunology*, vol. 13, Article ID 810284, 2022.

[12] Q.-Y. Xu, H.-Y. Yang, M.-W. Li, Z.-D. He, H.-Y. Hong, and Z.-G. Peng, "Sintilimab combined with chidamide in the treatment of extranodal nature killer/T-cell lymphoma with secondary hemophagocytic lymphohistiocytosis Two case reports and literature review," *Medicine*, vol. 13, no. 2, pp. 49–52, 2022.

[13] R. Marar, S. Prathivadhi-Bhayankaram, and M. Krishnan, "Immune checkpoint inhibitor-induced hemophagocytic lymphohistiocytosis in a patient with squamous cell carcinoma," *Journal of Hematology*, vol. 11, no. 4, pp. 142–147, 2022.

[14] R. D. Sandler, R. S. Tattersall, H. Schoemans et al., "Diagnosis and management of secondary HLH/MAS following HSCT and CAR-T cell therapy in adults; A review of the literature and a survey of practice within ebmt centres on behalf of the autoimmune diseases working party (adwp) and transplant complications working party (tcwp)," *Frontiers in Immunology*, vol. 11, p. 524, 2020.

[15] M. Sadaat and S. Jang, "Hemophagocytic lymphohistiocytosis with immunotherapy: brief review and case report," *Journal for ImmunoTherapy of Cancer*, vol. 6, no. 1, p. 49, 2018.

[16] A. Hantel, B. Gabster, J. X. Cheng, H. Golomb, and T. F. Gajewski, "Severe hemophagocytic lymphohistiocytosis in a melanoma patient treated with ipilimumab + nivolumab," *Journal for ImmunoTherapy of Cancer*, vol. 6, no. 1, p. 73, 2018.

[17] P. A. Ascierto, M. Del Vecchio, M. Mandalá et al., "Adjuvant nivolumab versus ipilimumab in resected stage IIIB-C and stage IV melanoma (CheckMate 238): 4-year results from a multicentre, double-blind, randomised, controlled, phase 3 trial," *The Lancet Oncology*, vol. 21, no. 11, pp. 1465–1477, 2020.

[18] X. Yang, L. Ma, X. Zhang, L. Huang, and J. Wei, "Targeting PD-1/PD-L1 pathway in myelodysplastic syndromes and acute myeloid leukemia," *Experimental Hematology & Oncology*, vol. 11, no. 1, p. 11, 2022.

[19] J. R. Brahmer, H. Abu-Sbeih, P. A. Ascierto et al., "Society for Immunotherapy of Cancer (SITC) clinical practice guideline on immune checkpoint inhibitor-related adverse events," *Journal for ImmunoTherapy of Cancer*, vol. 9, no. 6, Article ID e002435, 2021.

[20] J. C. Albring, S. Inselmann, T. Sauer et al., "PD-1 checkpoint blockade in patients with relapsed AML after allogeneic stem cell transplantation," *Bone Marrow Transplantation*, vol. 52, no. 2, pp. 317–320, 2017.

14

Efficacy of Inotuzumab Ozogamicin plus Ponatinib Followed by Allogeneic Stem Cell Transplantation in a Patient with Relapsed Philadelphia Chromosome-Positive Acute Lymphoblastic Leukemia

Ilina Micheva, Vladimir Gerov, Stela Dimitrova, and Merlin Efraim

UMHAT "Sveta Marina" Medical University, Varna, Bulgaria

Correspondence should be addressed to Ilina Micheva; ilinamicheva@gmail.com

Academic Editor: Pier Paolo Piccaluga

Philadelphia chromosome-positive acute lymphoblastic leukemia (Ph + ALL) is an aggressive disease with poor outcomes. Despite the incorporation of tyrosine kinase inhibitors (TKIs) in the therapeutic strategies, patients who relapse after chemotherapy plus TKI have poor overall survival (OS) and less chance to proceed to hematopoietic stem cell transplantation (HSCT) which remains the only curative approach. Therefore, new drugs, such as antibody-targeted therapies alone or in combination with TKIs, offer new therapeutic options for those patients. However, the combination of inotuzumab plus ponatinib has limited application. We present a case of a patient affected by Ph + ALL with T315I mutation successfully treated after early relapse with inotuzumab plus ponatinib, followed by allogeneic HSCT and ponatinib maintenance.

1. Introduction

Philadelphia chromosome (Ph) is the most common cytogenetic abnormality in adult patients with acute lymphoblastic leukemia (ALL), found in about 20–30% of ALL cases [1]. The incidence of Ph + ALL increases with age, reaching 43.8% in patients older than 50 years of age [2]. Patients with Ph + ALL have poor prognosis with higher rates of relapse and worse overall survival.

In the era of tyrosine kinase inhibitors (TKIs), the outcome of those patients has dramatically improved, and currently, the standard of care in the frontline setting is TKI in combination with chemotherapy [3,4]. However, there is still high risk of relapse, especially among patients with resistant BCR-ABL1 mutations [5]. Allogeneic hematopoietic stem cell transplantation (HSCT) is considered in the first remission, especially for younger patients treated with imatinib combination therapy [6].

Novel drugs, such as potent later-generation TKIs, antibody-drug conjugates, bispecific monoclonal antibodies, and chimeric antigen receptor T-cell (CAR T) therapies, are being developed and investigated in patients with Ph + ALL [7].

Inotuzumab and Blinatumumab have shown promising results in relapse/refractory (R/R) Ph + ALL [8,9]. Ponatinib, a third-generation TKI, has proven to be the most potent TKI for patients with Ph + ALL and the only one capable of overcoming the T315I mutation [10].

Recently, the combination of monoclonal antibodies (MoAbs) and TKI has been evaluated in Ph + ALL in frontline or relapse/refractory settings [11,12]. However, the combination of inotuzumab plus ponatinib has limited application. There is only one report where these novel drugs have been used sequentially in a patient with relapsed Ph + ALL. Pirosa MC et al. describe a case of a young patient with Ph′+ALL, who relapsed after second HSCT, who reached long-term disease control with molecular remission by treatment with inotuzumab ozogamicin, donor lymphocyte infusion, and ponatinib [13].

2. Materials and Methods

We present a case of a patient affected by Ph + ALL with T315I mutation successfully treated after early relapse with inotuzumab plus ponatinib, followed by allogeneic HSCT and ponatinib maintenance.

3. Results

Our case represents a 54-year-old female who was was referred to our hospital in June 2019 with fatigue, petechiae on the lower limbs, splenomegaly, and abnormal complete blood count (CBC) with hemoglobin 8.7 g/dL, platelets 89×10^9/L, and white blood cell 72.01×10^9/L. The morphological exam of the peripheral blood and bone marrow showed about 90% lymphoid blast cells.

The flow cytometric analysis confirmed the diagnosis of precursor B-cell ALL with following phenotype: CD19++/+++, CD22++, CD10++/+++, HLA-DR++/+++, CD34++, CD38+/++, CD13+, CD33 low+, CD123+/++, CD71 low+, CD58++, CD20+, CD45 low+, cyCD79a+, and nTdT+. Conventional cytogenetic study of the bone marrow, using GTG banding, revealed the presence of the Ph chromosome in 80% of the metaphases (karyotype 46,XX,t(9;22) (q34; q11)) [14]. Additionally, a single metaphase with trisomy 8 and 9 was described (49,XX,+8,+9, t(9;22) (q34;q1), but considered insignificant. Molecular analysis by real-time PCR showed 0.0909% BCR-ABL Mbcr (b3a2, b2a2) transcripts.

Treatment with H-CVAD plus imatinib mesylate was initiated according to the protocol. After 2 courses of therapy, complete remission (CR) was achieved. Treatment continued with two more cycles, and the HSCT from HLA-identical sibling was planned for March 2020. A week before the planned admission to the transplant unit, the patient appeared for consultation asymptomatic with CBC, revealing extreme leukocytosis- 143.00 10^9/L, normal hemoglobin- 135 g/L, and platelets- 125 10^9/L. The morphology and immunophenotype were consistent with the initial diagnosis. The BCR-ABL/ABL transcript level was 40%. T315I mutation was detected.

In March 2020, inotuzumab therapy was initiated and administered according to the protocol: 0.8 mg/m^2 i.v. on day +1 and 0.5 mg/m^2 i.v. on days +8 and +15 as described by Kantarjian et al. [8]. Corticosteroids were given before the first infusion of inotuzumab in order to decrease the white blood cell count and decrease the risk of tumor lysis syndrome. Ponatinib in a dose of 30 mg daily was added with the first administration of inotuzumab. No serious toxicity grade 3 and 4 were registered. After the first cycle, the patient achieved complete CR with a deep molecular response (DMR) (BCR- ABL/ABL IS = 0.0023%, 4.5 log) and proceeded to HSCT.

In April 2020, HSCT was performed by a matched related donor using a myeloablative conditioning regimen (thiotepa 5 mg/kg for 2 days, fludarabine 30 mg/m^2 for 5 days, and busilvex 3.2 mg/kg for 3 days) and mobilized peripheral blood stem cells (CD34+ 2.14×10^6/kg). Revaluation on day +30 revealed DMR (BCR- ABL/ABL IS = 0.0047%, 4.3 log). Ponatinib maintenance was initiated at a dose of 30 mg/day. The patient was followed up monthly and maintained DMR. On month 6, an asymptomatic increase of the liver enzymes was registered with ALT-524.7 U/l (range 10–49 U/l), ASAT- 257.6 U/l (range 0–34 U/l), ALP- 358 U/l (range 45–129 U/l), GGT 208 U/l (range 0–38 U/l), and lactate dehydrogenase- 437 U/l (range 208–378 U/l). Infectious or autoimmune hepatitis was excluded, and there were no signs of graft versus host disease. Toxicity was suspected, and ponatinib was stopped. A month later, after treatment with ursodeoxycholic acid and silymarin, the liver indexes were normalized and Ponatinib was restarted at a dose of 15 mg/day.

At the time of reporting, the patient was asymptomatic, in sustained molecular response (BCR- ABL/ABL IS = 0.000097%, 6 log). Maintenance with ponatinib continues in a dose of 15 mg/day with excellent tolerability.

4. Discussion

Our case represents an early recurrence of ALL, with unfavourable T315 mutation, in which the possibility of using MoAb as a rescue therapy and bridge to HSCT was discussed. Both inotuzumab and blinatumomab have shown superiority over chemotherapy in terms of efficacy. The experience with inotuzumab in Ph + ALL patients comes from the clinical trials of inotuzumab. Among Ph + patients in the INO-VATE study, the rates of CR/CR incomplete, minimal residual disease (MRD) and subsequent HSCT were higher in the inotuzumab arm compared to standard chemotherapy [8].

Blinatumomab was tested in adults with R/R Ph + ALL in a phase 2 study ALCANTARA and showed a CR of 36%, including four of 10 patients with the T315I mutation, complete MRD response in 88% of CR responders, and a median OS of 7.1 months [9].

At the time of recurrence, blinatumomab was not approved for treatment of patients with Ph + ALL. Inotuzumab was applied based on the CD22 expression, the efficacy even in high tumour burden with >50% lymphoblasts in the bone marrow and taking into account the increased risk of veno-occlusive disease (VOD), reported as the major non-hematologic adverse event associated with inotuzumab [8].

It has been demonstrated that the presence of T315I mutation in Ph + ALL is associated with a highly aggressive disease phenotype and resistance to TKI therapy [5]. Analysis of 17 TKI-resistant Ph + leukemia patients who were found to have an ABL kinase domain mutation showed that combined use of different TKIs and complex chromosomal karyotypes may promote the development of the T315I mutation. Ratio of blast cells >50% and number of white blood cells $>20 \times 10^9$/L were related to poor survival prognosis [15].

Ponatinib is a third-generation TKI that is currently approved as per label when no other TKIs are indicated for the treatment of patients with CML and Ph + ALL after failing treatment with second-generation TKIs or if the presence of T315I mutation is discovered [14]. In the phase II PACE trial, among patients with Ph + ALL, 41% achieved a major hematologic response (MaHR) by 6 months with a median time to MaHR among responders 0.7 months (range, 0.4–5.5 months). The median duration of MaHR in responders with Ph^+ ALL was 3.2 months (range, 1.8–12.8 months). Major cytogenetic response (CyR) and complete CyR were achieved by 47% and 38% of patients, respectively. Median progression-free survival (PFS) was 3.0 months, and OS at 3 years was 12%. A multivariate analysis showed that the presence of T315I itself is not a predictor of response [16].

Recently, several studies have evaluated the efficacy of MoAb in combination with TKI.

A retrospective study showed high efficacy of the combination blinatumomab and TKI (ponatinib, dasatinib, or bosutinib) in R/R Ph + ALL and chronic myeloid leukemia (CML) in lymphoid blast phase with molecular responses of 75% and one-year OS rates of 73%. Two of the patients in the analysed group were with T315I mutation [17].

The combination blinatumomab-dasatinib was evaluated in front-line settings in a phase 2 single-group trial in adults with newly diagnosed Ph + ALL. CR was observed in 98%, and after two cycles of blinatumomab, 60% of the patients had molecular response. At a median follow-up of 18 months, overall survival was 95% and disease-free survival was 88% [11].

The combined use of inotuzumab and ponatinib, both drugs highly effective in Ph^+ ALL with T315I mutation, has been avoided due to high risk of hepatotoxicity. Efficacy of inotuzumab with less hepatotoxic TKI, particularly bosutinib, has been recently investigated. CR was detected in 50% of patients, with major molecular response (MMR) in 85%, and the OS was 0.7 months. Notably, patients with T315I mutation were excluded from this study [12].

Despite the limited experience and expected high liver toxicity, we used the combination inotuzumab plus ponatinib achieving CR and MRD negativity after one course of treatment, which allowed us to proceed to HSCT.

Maintenance with TKIs should be considered after transplant to reduce relapse rates in Ph + ALL. However, the choice of TKI and the duration of maintenance therapy remain uncertain. A systematic review, comparing survival outcomes of second-generation TKIs nilotinib and dasatinib with first-generation TKI imatinib after HSCT in Ph + ALL, showed that the use of all TKIs after allo-HSCT for patients in CR1 improved OS when given as a prophylactic or preemptive regimen. Limited data suggest that second-generation TKIs (i.e., dasatinib) have a better OS, especially in patients with MRD-positive status. Imatinib did not improve OS in patients who were >CR1 at the time of allo-HSCT [18].

In a recently published study, analyzing the impact of TKI maintenance after HSCT in Ph + ALL, 59% of patients received posttransplant TKI as prophylaxis or at the first MRD positivity (11 from 95 patients received ponatinib). Median time to TKI initiation after allo-HSCT was 2.4 months (range 19 days–35 months). The 2-year PFS for patients who initiated prophylaxis within 3 months after transplantation was 94.5% (95% CI: 74.3–99.0, med. PFS = 144 mo.) compared to 75% in patients who received TKI after 3 months of transplantation (95% CI: 46.8–82.0, med. PFS = 96 mo.) (P value = .041). In the TKI prophylactic group, the relapse rate was similar between patients receiving imatinib or newer-generation TKIs. In the MRD-triggered group, 75% of patients who received imatinib relapsed compared to 45% of patients who received newer-generation TKI. Newer-generation TKIs may overcome some of the unfavorable mutations and may lead to lower relapse rates in patients with more advanced disease [19].

During the course of ponatinib maintenance, we registered hepatotoxicity, requiring stopping of ponatinib and dose reduction.

Ponatinib was approved at the dose of 45 mg/day [16]. However, because of the close relationship between the dose of ponatinib and the risk of cardiovascular events, dose reduction was suggested. It has been demonstrated that each 15 mg reduction causes an approximate 33% reduction of the risk of arterial thrombosis with sustained antileukemic activity [20].

In the era of monoclonal antibodies and third-generation TKI, inotuzumab plus ponatinib appeared a potent combination inducing complete molecular response in an extremely high-risk Ph + ALL with T315I mutation. TKI maintenance after transplantation may play an important role decreasing the rate of hematological relapse and improving disease-free survival in such challenging and difficult-to-treat cases.

References

[1] T. Burmeister, S. Schwartz, C. R. Bartram et al., "Patients' age and BCR-ABL frequency in adult B-precursor ALL: a retrospective analysis from the GMALL study group," *Blood*, vol. 112, no. 3, pp. 918-919, 2008.

[2] L. M. Secker-Walker, J. M. Craig, J. M. Hawkins, and A. V. Hoffbrand, "Philadelphia positive acute lymphoblastic leukemia in adults: age distribution, BCR breakpoint and prognostic significance," *Leukemia*, vol. 5, no. 3, pp. 196–199, 1991.

[3] J.-M. Ribera, A. Oriol, M. González et al., "Concurrent intensive chemotherapy and imatinib before and after stem cell transplantation in newly diagnosed Philadelphia chromosome-positive acute lymphoblastic leukemia. Final results of the CSTIBES02 trial," *Haematologica*, vol. 95, no. 1, pp. 87–95, 2010.

[4] D. A. Thomas, S. Faderl, J. Cortes et al., "Treatment of Philadelphia chromosome-positive acute lymphocytic leukemia with hyper-CVAD and imatinib mesylate," *Blood*, vol. 103, no. 12, pp. 4396–4407, 2004.

[5] K. Watanabe, Y. Minami, Y. Ozawa, K. Miyamura, and T. Naoe, "T315I mutation in Ph-positive acute lymphoblastic leukemia is associated with a highly aggressive disease phenotype: three case reports," *Anticancer Research*, vol. 32, no. 5, pp. 1779–1783, 2012.

[6] I. Abou Dalle, E. Jabbour, N. J. Short, and F. Ravandi, "Treatment of philadelphia chromosome-positive acute lymphoblastic leukemia," *Current Treatment Options in Oncology*, vol. 20, no. 1, p. 4, 2019.

[7] V. A. Guerra, E. J. Jabbour, F. Ravandi, H. Kantarjian, and N. J. Short, "Novel monoclonal antibody-based treatment strategies in adults with acute lymphoblastic leukemia," *Therapeutic Advances in Hematology*, vol. 10, Article ID 2040620719849496, 2019.

[8] H. M. Kantarjian, D. J. DeAngelo, M. Stelljes et al., "Inotuzumab ozogamicin versus standard therapy for acute lymphoblastic leukemia," *New England Journal of Medicine*, vol. 375, no. 8, pp. 740–753, 2016.

[9] G. Martinelli, N. Boissel, P. Chevallier et al., "Complete hematologic and molecular response in adult patients with relapsed/refractory philadelphia chromosome-positive B-precursor acute lymphoblastic leukemia following treatment with blinatumomab: results from a phase II, single-arm, multicenter study," *Journal of Clinical Oncology*, vol. 35, no. 16, pp. 1795–1802, 2017.

[10] N. J. Short, H. Kantarjian, E. Jabbour, and F. Ravandi, "Which tyrosine kinase inhibitor should we use to treat Philadelphia chromosome-positive acute lymphoblastic leukemia?" *Best Practice & Research Clinical Haematology*, vol. 30, no. 3, pp. 193–200, 2017.

[11] R. Foà, R. Bassan, A. Vitale et al., "Dasatinib-blinatumomab for ph-positive acute lymphoblastic leukemia in adults," *New England Journal of Medicine*, vol. 383, no. 17, pp. 1613–1623, 2020.

[12] N. Jain, J. Cortes, F. Ravandi et al., "Inotuzumab ozogamicin in combination with bosutinib for patients with relapsed or refractory Ph+ ALL or CML in lymphoid blast phase," *Blood*, vol. 130, no. 1, p. 143, 2017.

[13] M. C. Pirosa, S. Leotta, A. Cupri et al., "Long-term molecular remission achieved by antibody anti-CD22 and ponatinib in a patient affected by Ph′+ acute lymphoblastic leukemia relapsed after second allogeneic hematopoietic stem cell transplantation: a case report," *Chemotherapy*, vol. 63, no. 4, pp. 220–224, 2018.

[14] C. Pavlovsky, O. Chan, C. Talati, and J. Pinilla-Ibarz, "Ponatinib in the treatment of chronic myeloid leukemia and philadelphia chromosome positive acute lymphoblastic leukemia," *Future Oncology*, vol. 15, no. 3, pp. 257–269, 2019.

[15] P. Xu, D. Guo, X. Shao, M. Peng, and B. Chen, "Characteristics and mutation analysis of Ph-positive leukemia patients with T315I mutation receiving tyrosine kinase inhibitors," *OncoTargets and Therapy*, vol. 10, pp. 4731–4738, 2017.

[16] J. E. Cortes, D.-W. Kim, J. Pinilla-Ibarz et al., "Ponatinib efficacy and safety in Philadelphia chromosome-positive leukemia: final 5-year results of the phase 2 PACE trial," *Blood*, vol. 132, no. 4, pp. 393–404, 2018.

[17] R. Assi, H. Kantarjian, N. J. Short et al., "Safety and efficacy of blinatumomab in combination with a tyrosine kinase inhibitor for the treatment of relapsed philadelphia chromosome-positive leukemia," *Clinical Lymphoma Myeloma and Leukemia*, vol. 17, no. 12, pp. 897–901, 2017.

[18] Z. Warraich, P. Tenneti, T. Thai et al., "Relapse prevention with tyrosine kinase inhibitors after allogeneic transplantation for philadelphia chromosome-positive acute lymphoblast leukemia: a systematic review," *Biology of Blood and Marrow Transplantation*, vol. 26, no. 3, pp. e55–e64, 2020.

[19] N. Saini, D. Marin, C. Ledesma et al., "Impact of TKIs post-allogeneic hematopoietic cell transplantation in Philadelphia chromosome-positive ALL," *Blood*, vol. 136, no. 15, pp. 1786–1789, 2020.

[20] M. Breccia, P. Pregno, P. Spallarossa et al., "Identification, prevention and management of cardiovascular risk in chronic myeloid leukaemia patients candidate to ponatinib: an expert opinion," *Annals of Hematology*, vol. 96, no. 4, pp. 549–558, 2017.

15

The First Autopsy Case of Fatal Acute Cardiac Failure after Administration of Carfilzomib in a Patient with Multiple Myeloma

Teruhito Takakuwa,[1] Ippei Otomaru,[1] Taku Araki,[1] Akiko Miura,[1] Yotaro Fujitani,[1] Yasuhide Mochizuki,[2] Yoshimi Miyagi,[3] Hideto Senzaki,[3] and Ryosuke Yamamura[1]

[1]*Department of Hematology, Osaka Saiseikai Nakatsu Hospital, Osaka, Japan*
[2]*Department of Cardiology, Osaka Saiseikai Nakatsu Hospital, Osaka, Japan*
[3]*Department of Pathology, Osaka Saiseikai Nakatsu Hospital, Osaka, Japan*

Correspondence should be addressed to Teruhito Takakuwa; t_takakuwa@med.osaka-cu.ac.jp

Academic Editor: Marie-Christine Kyrtsonis

Carfilzomib (CFZ) improves progression-free survival for patients with relapsed or refractory multiple myeloma (MM) but has shown higher frequency of cardiovascular adverse events (CVAEs) than other proteasome inhibitors. We report the first autopsy case of acute death from cardiac failure shortly after administration of carfilzomib. A 74-year-old female was diagnosed with IgA MM after a 2-year period of smoldering MM. She was refractory to both bortezomib plus dexamethasone and lenalidomide plus dexamethasone therapies, so she subsequently received CFZ in combination with lenalidomide and dexamethasone. The day after the start of the therapy, she complained of severe dyspnea with a significant decline in left ventricular ejection fraction. Her acute cardiac failure rapidly progressed, and she died on day 7 of the start of CFZ. The autopsy showed invasion of inflammatory cells between the myocardial cells and very little myocardial necrosis. There was no obvious thrombus in the coronary artery of the heart, and no infarction or amyloid deposition was observed in the myocardium. Pathological findings of hypersensitivity myocarditis, a drug-induced cardiomyopathy, appeared to agree with this case except for absence of an eosinophilic infiltration of the myocardium. A CFZ-induced CVAE is generally considered reversible. However, rapidly progressing fatal heart failure like in our case is rare. To characterize CFZ-associated CVAE, further case collection is needed.

1. Introduction

Over the past 10 years, new drugs have progressively become clinically applicable for the treatment of multiple myeloma (MM) [1]; thus, treatment strategies for MM have undergone a considerable change. Carfilzomib (CFZ) is a second-generation proteasome inhibitor (PI) that shows excellent outcomes for relapsed and/or refractory MM. In the ASPIRE study [2], using the lenalidomide (LEN) and dexamethasone (DEX) combination therapy in the control group, overall survival was significantly prolonged by adding CFZ to the therapy. Furthermore, in the ENDEAVOR study [3], the CFZ + DEX combination therapy significantly prolonged progression-free survival compared with the bortezomib (BOR) and DEX combination therapy. However, it has been found that CFZ increases the risk of cardiovascular events. In therapies containing CFZ, the abovementioned ASPIRE study showed heart failure in 6.4% of participants, whereas the ENDEAVOR study showed congestive heart failure in 10.8% of participants, both of which were higher than that in the control group. One of our patients died of severe cardiac hypofunction following CFZ administration, after which we performed pathological autopsy. To date, there has been no autopsy report of a patient who died of CFZ-induced cardiotoxicity; thus, in this report, we discuss the pathological findings of such a case.

2. Case Presentation

In 2016, a 74-year-old woman diagnosed with IgA κ-type smoldering MM was hospitalized after developing malaise and fatigability. Physical findings at admission included pale palpebral conjunctiva and edema of the bilateral lower limbs. Laboratory test results were as follows: calcium, 11.4 mg/dL; hemoglobin, 6.1 g/dL; creatinine, 1.54 mg/dL; total protein, 6.4 g/dL; albumin, 3.2 g/dL; IgA, 2923 mg/dL; IgM, 29 mg/dL; IgG, 2253 mg/dL; beta-2-microglobulin, 17.6 mg/L; free kappa light chain, 82.0 mg/L; and free lambda light chain, 18.7 mg/L. Computed tomography (CT) revealed extramedullary tumor in the mediastinum, bilateral axilla, and pulmonary hilum. On fluorescence in situ hybridization, t(14; 16), t(4; 14), t(11; 14), and deletion 17p results were all negative. Symptomatic myeloma (the International Staging System (ISS) stage III and revised ISS stage III) was diagnosed. After high-dose DEX therapy, BOR plus DEX therapy was administered. Although partial response was obtained with four courses, IgA levels had exacerbated by the end of eight courses, and progressive disease was determined. Treatment was switched to LEN (15 mg/day) plus DEX therapy; however, severe cytopenia developed, and treatment was discontinued after one course. CT revealed extramedullary tumor in the para-aortic region, which was thought to indicate disease progression, in addition to low uptake throughout the entire liver (Figure 1). Therefore, treatment was changed to CFZ (20 mg/m^2 on days 1 and 2; then 36 mg/m^2 on days 8, 9, 15, and 16) in combination with LEN (5 mg/day) and DEX (KRd) therapy. After administration of KRd therapy, peripheral oxygen saturation had been reduced to 88% early on the next day, and transnasal oxygen therapy was initiated. The brain natriuretic peptide level increased to 418 pg/mL; however, there was no increase in myocardial escape enzymes. Ejection fraction (EF) reduced from 59% to 28% (Figure 2), and radiography revealed pulmonary congestion with pleural effusions. Thus, CFZ-induced acute heart failure was diagnosed. On day 2 of the administration, CFZ was discontinued. Despite the use of norepinephrine, dobutamine, furosemide, and human atrial natriuretic peptide, diuresis was not improved. The patient's respiratory condition deteriorated, and on day 5 following the CFZ administration, noninvasive positive pressure ventilation was initiated. Oxygenation did not improve, and the patient died early morning on day 8 following the CFZ administration. Autopsy was performed following death with the consent of the patient's family.

Macroscopic findings on autopsy revealed multiple vertebral osteolysis, hepatosplenomegaly, renal enlargement, and innumerable lymph node lesions in the paratracheal, tracheal bifurcation, and para-aortic areas. Pathological findings of the bone marrow showed basophilic cells with an eccentric nucleus and proliferation of large cells, which were positive for IgA on immunostaining (Figure 3(a)). The spleen exhibited invasion of similar cells replacing the splenic white pulp, as well as invasion into the splenic red pulp. In the liver, tumor cell invasion was accompanied by destruction of the limiting plates, primarily in the portal region. With the tumor cell invasion, destruction or loss of interlobular ductules and dilation of bile canaliculus were observed. In the kidneys, tumor cell invasion of the interstitial tissue was observed, accompanied by glomerular and renal tubule destruction and loss. The distal convoluted and collecting tubules were filled with eosinophilic amorphous deposits, which was positive for κ light chain (Figures 3(b) and 3(c)). There was no obvious thrombus in the coronary artery of the heart, and no infarction was observed in the myocardium. Invasion of inflammatory cells, primarily CD3- (cluster of differentiation 3-) positive lymphocytes, was observed between the myocardial cells, and these myocardial cells showed basophilic degeneration. There was no clear tumor cell invasion or amyloid deposition, and very little myocardial cell necrosis was observed. Between the myocardial cells, fibrosis and disarray were observed (Figures 3(d)–3(f)).

3. Discussion

It is well known that CFZ is cardiotoxic, and its clinical use is often associated with cardiovascular events. A recent meta-analysis [4] reported that among 2,594 patients with MM, cardiovascular events of all grades were observed in 18.1% of the patients, whereas events with grade ≥3 in 8.2% of the patients. According to this report, cardiovascular events were divided into four types—heart failure, hypertension, arrhythmias, and ischemic events, with the incidence of the first two being high. While reports of reduced EF following CFZ administration are common, MM is generally considered reversible. In a report from the Mayo Clinic [5], 12 out of 136 patients developed reduced EF following CFZ administration; however, all patients recovered, and the median period until recovery was 2 months. In a different report [6] on 60 patients with MM, 12% experienced reduced EF, which was considered reversible in all of them. Alternatively, Lendvai et al. [7] reported that among 44 patients with MM who received CFZ, six patients developed severely reduced EF, which was irreversible in three of the six cases. Our patient was a rare case, in which reduced EF developed within 24 h of CFZ administration and did not improve but was followed by rapid progression until death. Furthermore, from our search, we found no autopsy reports of death from cardiac hypofunction caused by CFZ.

Several basic studies have addressed the underlying mechanism of CFZ-induced cardiotoxicity; however, the mechanism has not been entirely elucidated. An experiment with rats have reported that exposure to high concentrations of CFZ inhibited chymotrypsin-like proteasomal activity and induced myocardial cell apoptosis [8]. Furthermore, when CFZ is used in combination with doxorubicin, cardiac toxicity is thought to be further exacerbated. An experiment with rabbits has suggested that CFZ has an acetylcholine-mediated vasodilatory effect and increased coronary perfusion pressure by reducing nitroglycerin and nifedipine anticonvulsant activity [9]. It has long been known that high-dose PI downregulates the function of endothelial nitric oxide synthase, a nitric oxide synthesizing enzyme, and can cause vascular endothelial dysfunction [10]. CFZ irreversibly inhibits proteasomes. Compared with other PIs, it may be associated with a higher risk of severe vascular endothelial dysfunction. More recently, however, Efentakis et al. [11] demonstrated that the molecular mechanism of CFZ-induced cardiotoxicity is not related to the inhibition of the proteasome function but to the inhibition of AMPKα/

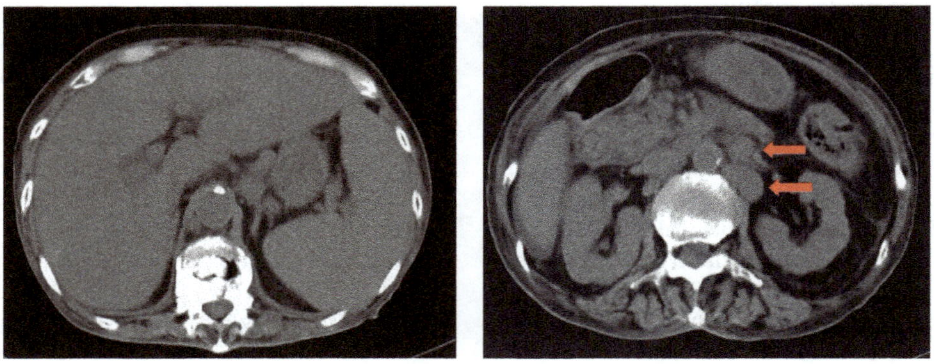

(a) (b)

Figure 1: CT image prior to carfilzomib administration. (a) Low uptake throughout the entire liver and splenomegaly could be observed. (b) Para-aortic lymph node swelling was observed (red arrow).

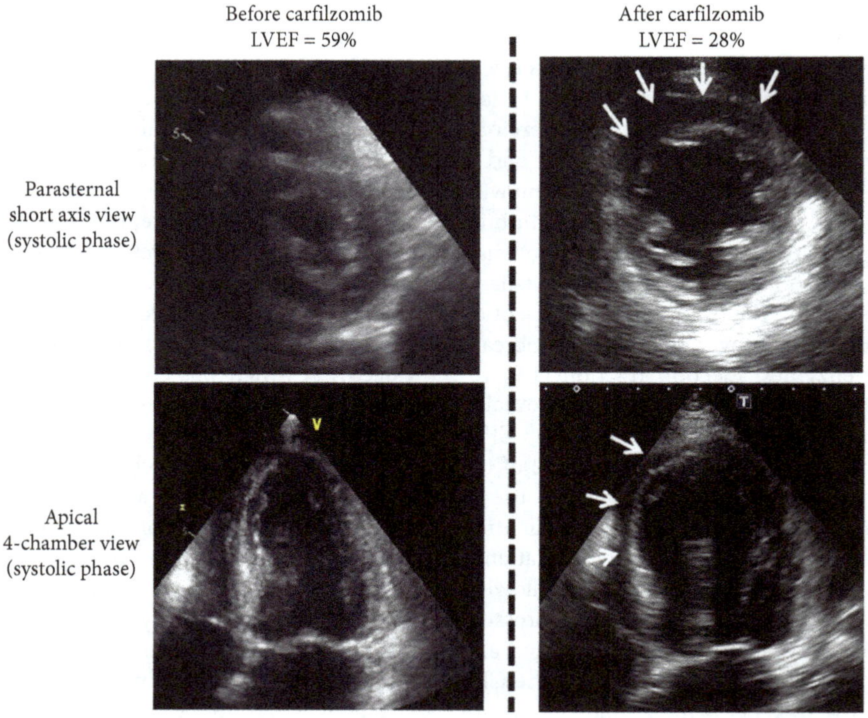

Figure 2: Transthoracic echocardiography beforeand after carfilzomib. After the administration of carfilzomib, the left ventricular ejection fraction decreased to 28% with diffuse wall motion abnormalities, particularly the anteroseptal segment.

mTORC1 pathways derived from increased PP2A activity, which is prevented by metformin.

Major pathological characteristics of the heart in our patient included CD3-positive lymphocyte invasion; however, myocardial cell necrosis was negligible. Myocardial cell disarray can occur in hypertrophic cardiomyopathy and dilated cardiomyopathy, which are the two major types of idiopathic cardiomyopathy. The thickened ventricular muscle and ventricular chamber enlargement, which are characteristics of cardiomyopathy [12], were not observed in our patient, and interstitial fibrosis in our patient was mild. Viral myocarditis is associated with lymphocyte invasion, as in the present case; however, had it been myocarditis, myocardial edematous changes and myocardial cell necrosis would have been remarkable [13], which was not the case in our patient. Sarcoidosis is characterized by epithelioid cell granuloma, which was not observed in our patient. Furthermore, no amyloid deposition was observed, which is a characteristic of cardiac amyloidosis, and no tumor infiltration was observed.

Alternatively, pathological findings of hypersensitivity myocarditis, a drug-induced cardiomyopathy, appeared to agree with this case. Doxorubicin is a drug that commonly causes myocardial impairment; however, the cumulative toxicity of doxorubicin often occurs during a median period of 3 months after administration. By contrast, in fulminant hypersensitivity myocarditis, severe heart failure has been reported to progress during the period from several days to one week following drug administration, and the progress is fatal in some cases [14, 15]. Characteristic histopathological

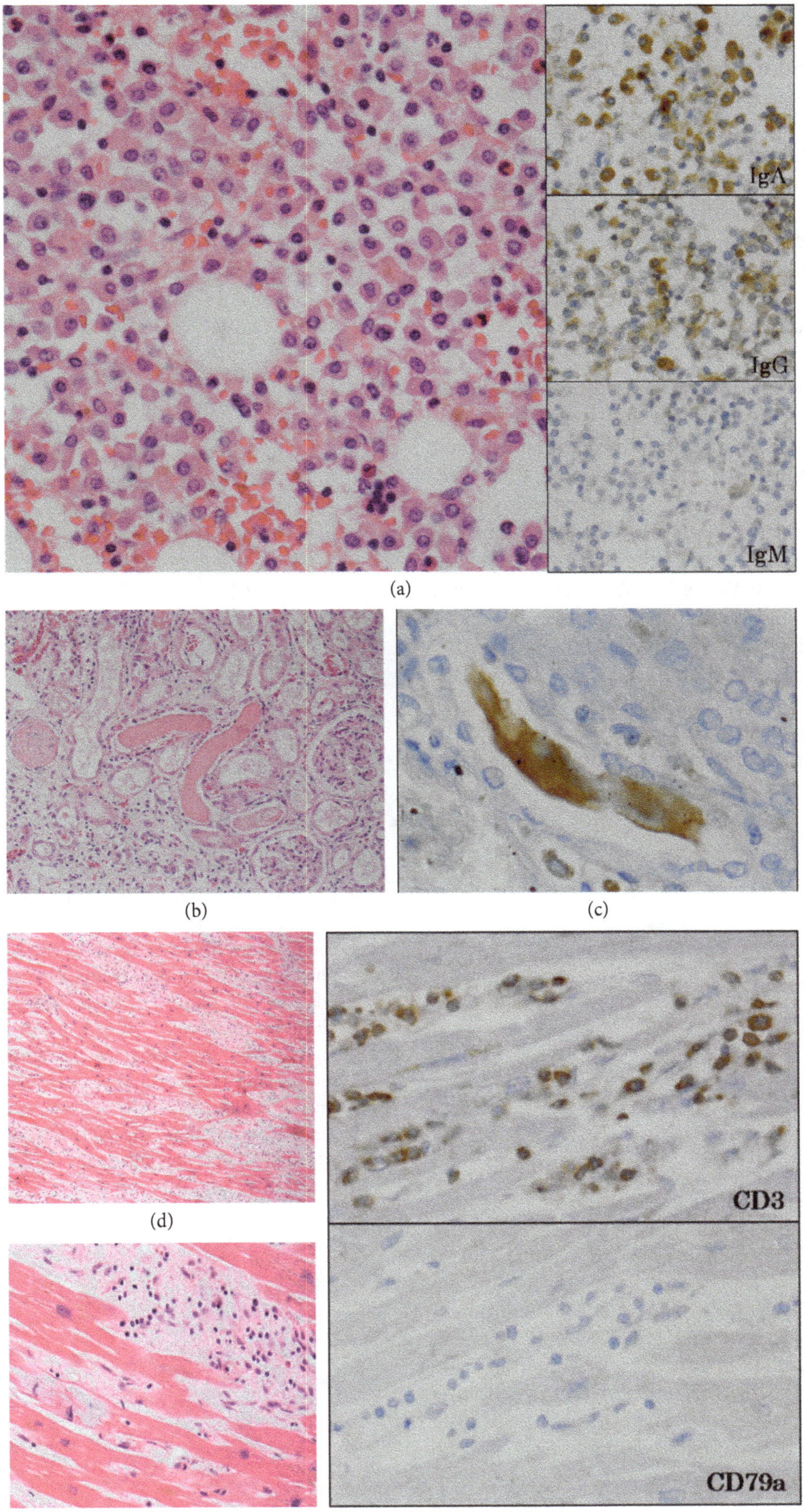

(a)

(b) (c)

(d)

(e) (f)

FIGURE 3: Pathological autopsy findings. (a) Bone marrow contained large basophilic cells with perinuclear halo and proliferation of large cells with distinct nucleoli, which were positive for IgA on immunostaining. (b, c) In the kidneys, the distal convoluted and collecting tubules were filled with eosinophilic amorphous deposits, which was positive for κ light chain. (d, e, f) Fibrosis and disarray were observed between the myocardial cells, and these myocardial cells showed basophilic degeneration. Invaded inflammatory cells were positive for CD3 but negative for CD79a.

findings of hypersensitivity myocarditis primarily include inflammatory cell invasion, such as lymphocytes in the myocardial stroma, and unremarkable myocardial necrosis [16]. Immunohistologically, cells are primarily CD3-positive lymphocytes, with few CD8-positive T lymphocytes [14]. Lesions have little myocardial cell necrosis; therefore, fibrosis is often unremarkable or mild. These pathological findings are consistent with our patient; however, eosinophilic infiltration, which is a characteristic finding of hypersensitivity myocarditis, was not observed in this case. Thus, it was difficult to make a definitive diagnosis from these pathological findings.

Although no clear relationship was found in a meta-analysis between the incidence of cardiovascular events and age prior to treatment, in the most recent treatment regimen [4], results from 3 phase I/II studies showed that CFZ-induced cardiovascular events are significantly higher in patients older than 75 and that the most important risk factor is hypertension [17]. Recently, the European Myeloma Network in collaboration with the Italian Society of Arterial Hypertension recommended accurate monitoring of blood pressure and early signs and symptoms of cardiac dysfunction in MM patients receiving CFZ [18]. The cardiac function may suddenly decrease as in the present case, although this is rare. Therefore, it is extremely important to carefully monitor the patient's condition for early detection of the onset of cardiovascular events.

References

[1] K. C. Anderson, "Progress and paradigms in multiple myeloma," *Clinical Cancer Research*, vol. 22, no. 22, pp. 5419–5427, 2016.

[2] A. K. Stewart, S. V. Rajkumar, M. A. Dimopoulos et al., "Carfilzomib, lenalidomide, and dexamethasone for relapsed multiple myeloma," *New England Journal of Medicine*, vol. 372, no. 2, pp. 142–152, 2015.

[3] M. A. Dimopoulos, P. Moreau, A. Palumbo et al., "Carfilzomib and dexamethasone versus bortezomib and dexamethasone for patients with relapsed or refractory multiple myeloma (ENDEAVOR): a randomised, phase 3, open-label, multicentre study," *The Lancet Oncology*, vol. 17, no. 1, pp. 27–38, 2016.

[4] A. J. Waxman, S. Clasen, W.-T. Hwang et al., "Carfilzomib-associated cardiovascular adverse events," *JAMA Oncology*, vol. 4, no. 3, article e174519, 2018.

[5] T. Jain, H. Narayanasamy, J. Mikhael et al., "Systolic dysfunction associated with carfilzomib use in patients with multiple myeloma," *Blood Cancer Journal*, vol. 7, no. 12, p. 642, 2017.

[6] M. A. Dimopoulos, M. Roussou, M. Gavriatopoulou et al., "Cardiac and renal complications of carfilzomib in patients with multiple myeloma," *Blood Advances*, vol. 1, no. 7, pp. 449–454, 2017.

[7] N. Lendvai, I. Tsakos, S. M. Devlin et al., "Predictive biomarkers and practical considerations in the management of carfilzomib-associated cardiotoxicity," *Leukemia & Lymphoma*, vol. 59, no. 8, pp. 1981–1985, 2018.

[8] B. B. Hasinoff, D. Patel, and X. Wu, "Molecular mechanisms of the cardiotoxicity of the proteasomal-targeted drugs bortezomib and carfilzomib," *Cardiovascular Toxicology*, vol. 17, no. 3, pp. 237–250, 2017.

[9] C. Chen-Scarabelli, G. Corsetti, E. Pasini et al., "Spasmogenic effects of the proteasome inhibitor carfilzomib on coronary resistance, vascular tone and reactivity," *EBioMedicine*, vol. 21, pp. 206–212, 2017.

[10] Q. Wei and Y. Xia, "Proteasome inhibition down-regulates endothelial nitric-oxide synthase phosphorylation and function," *Journal of Biological Chemistry*, vol. 281, no. 31, pp. 21652–21659, 2006.

[11] P. Efentakis, G. Kremastiotis, A. Varela et al., "Molecular mechanisms of carfilzomib-induced cardiotoxicity in mice and the emerging cardioprotective role of metformin," *Blood*, vol. 133, no. 7, pp. 710–723, 2019.

[12] S. Noda, "Histopathology of endomyocardial biopsies from patients with idiopathic cardiomyopathy; quantitative evaluation based on multivariate statistical analysis," *Japanese Circulation Journal*, vol. 44, no. 2, pp. 95–116, 1980.

[13] G. J. Berry and K. A. Atkins, *Pathology of Human Myocarditis*, pp. 325–370, Springer, Berlin, Germany, 2003.

[14] K. R. Chikwava, V. H. Savell Jr., and T. K. Boyd, "Fatal cephalosporin-induced acute hypersensitivity myocarditis," *Pediatric Cardiology*, vol. 27, no. 6, pp. 777–780, 2006.

[15] A. Frustaci, R. Verardo, P. Sale et al., "Hypersensitivity myocarditis induced by beta-blockers: an unexpected cause of abrupt deterioration in hypertrophic cardiomyopathy," *Intensive Care Medicine*, vol. 33, no. 10, pp. 1848-1849, 2007.

[16] J. J. Fenoglio Jr., H. A. McAllister Jr., and F. G. Mullick, "Drug related myocarditis," *Human Pathology*, vol. 12, no. 10, pp. 900–907, 1981.

[17] R. Mina, M. Teresa Petrucci, N. Giuliani et al., "Cardiovascular toxicity in newly diagnosed, transplant-ineligible multiple myeloma patients treated with carfilzomib, cyclophosphamide and dexamethasone: results from an integrated analysis of 3 phase I/II trials," *Clinical Lymphoma Myeloma and Leukemia*, vol. 17, no. 1, p. e7, 2017.

[18] S. Bringhen, A. Milan, M. D'Agostino et al., "Prevention, monitoring and treatment of cardiovascular adverse events in myeloma patients receiving carfilzomib A consensus paper by the European Myeloma Network and the Italian Society of Arterial Hypertension," *Journal of Internal Medicine*, Epub ahead of print, 2019.

16

Central Nervous System Involvement by Small Lymphocytic Lymphoma after a Myxoma-Related Embolic Event

Nicolas Gallastegui,[1] Daniel P. Cassidy,[2] Deborah O. Heros,[3] Francisco Vega,[2] and Jonathan H. Schatz[1]

[1]*Division of Hematology, Department of Medicine, University of Miami Leonard M. Miller School of Medicine/Sylvester Comprehensive Cancer Center, Miami, FL, USA*
[2]*Division of Hematopathology, Department of Pathology and Laboratory Medicine, University of Miami Leonard M. Miller School of Medicine/Sylvester Comprehensive Cancer Center, Miami, FL, USA*
[3]*Division of Neuro-Oncology, Department of Neurology, University of Miami Leonard M. Miller School of Medicine/Sylvester Comprehensive Cancer Center, Miami, FL, USA*

Correspondence should be addressed to Jonathan H. Schatz; jschatz@med.miami.edu

Academic Editor: Masayuki Nagasawa

Involvement of the central nervous system by chronic lymphocytic leukemia/small lymphocytic lymphoma is exceedingly rare, and currently no risk factors have been described. We report the case of a patient with concomitant chronic lymphocytic leukemia/small lymphocytic lymphoma and an embolic cerebrovascular accident related to a cardiac myxoma, who developed parenchymal central nervous system involvement of lymphoma on the ischemic bed. The patient was successfully treated with a high-dose fludarabine-based chemotherapy regimen, achieving a sustained remission. We propose that embolic breakage of the blood-brain barrier may be a major risk factor in producing central nervous system involvement. We also propose that a high-dose fludarabine-based chemotherapy regimen may be adequate to achieve a better CNS penetration and improved outcomes.

1. Introduction

Chronic lymphocytic leukemia (CLL) and small lymphocytic lymphoma (SLL) are considered the same entity under the spectrum of the B-cell non-Hodgkin lymphomas. Characterized by monoclonal accumulation of CD5/CD19/CD20+ B-cells, the disease is called CLL when presenting with peripheral blood counts exceeding 5.0×10^9/L and SLL when presenting with primarily lymphomatous involvement of spleen or lymph nodes [1].

Infiltration of CLL/SLL cells outside lymphoid tissues, called extramedullary CLL (EM-CLL), is rare. Though a common and potentially devastating complication of aggressive lymphomas like Burkitt lymphoma (BL), fewer than 200 cases of central nervous system (CNS) involvement by CLL/SLL are reported in the literature [2]. Most commonly, it is described in patients with high counts of malignant lymphocytes in peripheral blood [3]. A systematic review by Ratterman et al. found that up to 27% of EM-CLL was in the CNS [4], and Strati et al. reported it carried the worst prognosis of all EM-CLL, with an average survival of 12 months [5].

Cardiac myxomas are the most common type of rare cardiac tumors, constituting 50–85% of lesions in adults and localized to the left atrium in 60–80% of cases [6]. Among myxoma patients with neurologic manifestations, 89% are attributed to ischemic events. Between 30% and 50% of patients with cardiac myxomas manifest peripheral embolization as the initial sign of disease [7]. There is no known association in between myxomas and lymphomas. A prior case series described 12 cases of myxomas associated with non-Hodgkin lymphomas, primarily Epstein–Barr virus-positive nongerminal center diffuse large B-cell lymphomas, and only one was CLL/SLL. Embolic events occurred in two of these cases, and in one, lymphoma cells were found together with the embolic myxoma cells [8].

Here, we present a case of central nervous system involvement by CLL/SLL after an embolic event by a concomitant myxoma.

2. Case Description

A 62-year-old male with a history of hypertension and a remote in-situ melanoma treated with resection presented to our institution in May 2016 with acute left upper extremity weakness.

Initial magnetic resonance imaging (MRI) showed multiple mixed signal intensity mass lesions on the right posterior temporal and occipital lobes with areas of hemorrhage and restricted diffusion suggestive of blood products. (Figure 1(a)). Complete blood count (CBC) showed normal white blood cell count at $8.2 \times 10^3/\mu L$ (range: $4–10.5 \times 10^3/\mu L$) with normal differential and normal absolute lymphocyte count, as well as normal hemoglobin at 12.9 g/dl (range: 13–16 g/dl) and platelet count at $249 \times 10^3/\mu L$ (range: $140–400 \times 10^3/\mu L$).

Initial suspicion was for embolic cerebrovascular accident (CVA) or less likely CNS metastasis. Positron emission tomography-computed tomography (PET-CT) performed to assess for underlying neoplasm, showing a low-grade fluorodeoxyglucose (FDG) avid uptake (standardized uptake value 2.8) over left atrial mass and subcentimeter non-FDG avid axillary and mediastinal lymphadenopathy without additional suspicious lymphadenopathy in the abdomen or pelvis. Computed tomography (CT) scan of the chest, abdomen, and pelvis with intravenous contrast showed bilateral axillary nodules up to 1.9 cm and scattered nonsuspicious subcentimeter lymph nodes in the abdomen and pelvis.

Echocardiogram showed a 2.5 cm globular mass on the left atrium highly suspicious for myxoma. Cardiac MRI corroborated a polypoid mobile mass from the intra-atrial septum, measuring $2.5 \times 4.0 \times 2.8$ cm. The patient was managed conservatively as neurologic symptoms improved without intervention. An elective cardiac myxoma resection was recommended to remove the presumed source of emboli. One month later, the patient underwent cardiac mass resection, with pathology confirming cardiac myxoma.

Two months after the resection the patient was evaluated for progressive growth of tender subcutaneous nodules of 1-2 mm on the distal left fifth digit and distal right fourth digit. He underwent resection on November 2016. Pathology review reported myxoma from cardiac source. At this time, CBC showed normal white blood cell count at $4 \times 10^3/\mu L$ with normal differential and normal absolute lymphocyte count, as well as normal hemoglobin at 13.4 g/dl and platelet count at $158 \times 10^3/\mu L$. The new myxoma lesions were presumed metastases from the already resected primary tumor. No additional workup was performed.

The patient was stable and followed clinically until May of 2017 when he developed gradual onset of intermittent neurologic symptoms characterized by dysmetria, left upper extremity paresis, apraxia, mild amnesia, and prosopagnosia. The patient underwent evaluation by his primary care doctor who recommended a brain MRI, showing a right parieto-occipital mass (Figure 1(b)). On physical exam, he had palpable bilateral inguinal lymphadenopathy up to 2 cm. The patient reported noticing these nodes up to 2 months previously and reported intermittent cervical and inguinal lymphadenopathy for 2 years. CBC showed normal white blood cell count at $5.3 \times 10^3/\mu L$ with normal differential, as well as normal hemoglobin at 13.3 g/dl and platelet count at $170 \times 10^3/\mu L$.

The patient underwent craniotomy with resection in July 2017. The patient's neurologic symptoms improved progressively over a period of two weeks after surgery.

Unexpectedly, the biopsy showed SLL on an extensively hemorrhagic background. Lymphoma cells were small with a largely perivascular distribution but were also seen in small aggregates throughout the biopsy. No cardiac myxoma was present in the resected tissue. By immunohistochemistry, the lymphoma cells stained positive for CD5, PAX-5, and CD23 and negative for CD20, CD3, BCL6, and cyclin-D1. (Figure 2).

A bone marrow biopsy in October 2017 showed CLL/SLL characterized by small cell atypical infiltrates accounting for 90% of bone marrow cellularity and reduced trilineage hematopoiesis. By immunohistochemistry, atypical cells were positive for CD5, PAX-5, CD20 (dim), and CD23 and negative for CD3, BCL6, and cyclin-D1. Flow cytometry showed a monoclonal B-cell population positive for CD19, CD20 (dim), CD5, DC23, CD38, and dim kappa light chain restriction. Ki67 was positive in 3%. Karyotype was normal, but deletion 13q14 was detected by fluorescent in-situ hybridization, and a molecular profile was positive with IgVH mutation >2% and negative for TP53 mutation. Cerebrospinal fluid was negative for malignancy by cytology and flow cytometry.

Peripheral flow cytometry showed a monoclonal kappa light chain restricted (dim) B-cell population positive for CD19, CD20 (dim), CD5, CD38, and CD23 and negative for CD10. In sum, the picture was consistent with good-risk CLL/SLL.

Rereview of the pathology slides from the previously resected cardiac myxoma and its distal embolic complications did not reveal the presence of lymphoma cells.

The case was reviewed by the expert panel at our institution. Because monoclonal B-lymphocytes in the peripheral blood were less than $5.0 \times 10^9/L$, the disease was characterized as SLL Lugano stage IV with extralymphatic extension to the CNS. Although the patient did not meet standard criteria for treatment, the expert panel felt a local recurrence in the CNS could be catastrophic and recommended treatment with systemic therapy that penetrates CNS. The patient underwent treatment FCR chemoimmunotherapy (rituximab, cyclophosphamide, and fludarabine) every 28 days. We increased the dose of fludarabine to 30 mg/Kg from the standard 25 mg/Kg to increase penetration to the CNS. The patient completed three cycles by January of 2018 with complete resolution of palpable inguinal lymphadenopathy after the first cycle. The

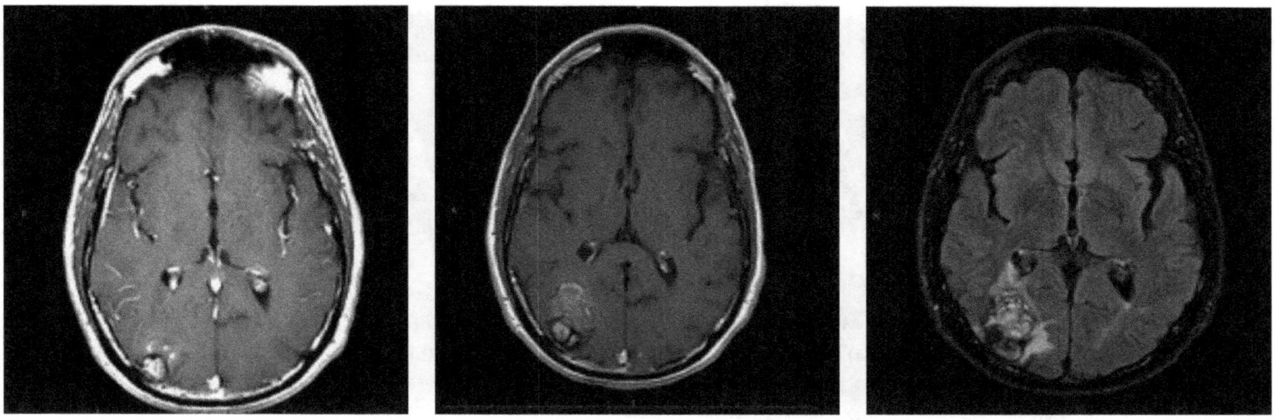

(a) (b) (c)

Figure 1: (a) Axial view T1 with Gadolinium at presentation, showing right posterior temporal lesion with a T1 hypointense rim suggestive of atypical stroke. Images of new findings at the previous area of stroke to evaluated new neurologic symptoms: (b) axial view T1 with Gadolinium showing an internal increase in size and (c) axial view FLAIR showing a heterogeneous lesion with hypointense foci within associated surrounding edema and enfacement of posterior horn or right lateral ventricle.

original plan was to complete four cycles, but the patient declined the fourth treatment.

Over time, the patient developed a focal tempor-ooccipital epilepsy and residual left homonymous hemianopia and presumed secondary to previous resection and remains under management by neurology. No paraneoplastic workup for seizures has been performed. Multiple CSF studies have been negative for malignancy by flow cytometry and cytology. Serial brain MRIs for surveillance have shown no evidence of recurrent tumors out to 12 months after completion of chemotherapy.

3. Discussion

Secondary involvement of the central nervous system (CNS) by non-Hodgkin Lymphoma (NHL) is a well-described phenomenon, estimated to happen in up to 5% of all subtypes [9]. The main risk factor overall is histology, with frequency as low as 2.8–5.3% for low-grade lymphomas [10–12] and as high as 30–50% for BL [13]. Other factors such as bone marrow involvement, retroperitoneal extension, and particular extranodal sites (breast, nasal/paranasal, testicular, gynecological, kidney, and adrenals) carry known increased CNS involvement risks for aggressive lymphomas [14]. CNS involvement by NHL is most commonly leptomeningeal, ~64% in the relapse setting, but up to 28% of cases are purely parenchymal (with some changes in this pattern emerging in the postrituximab area) [15].

In a large database analysis of low-grade lymphomas involving the CNS, CLL/SLL was found to be the third largest group with 8%, in comparison with follicular lymphoma with 38% [12]. The latter, despite being the most common leukemia diagnosed in the US with an annual incidence of 5 cases per 100,000 [16]. CNS involvement by CLL/SLL is, therefore, a rare phenomenon, and no specific risk factor has been established. The mean age of presentation is 64.5 and is more common in males than in females [2].

Overall, CNS infiltration by CLL/SLL has been estimated at 0.4%–2% [3, 5], but these numbers are discrepant with autopsy series in which involvement has ranged from 7–71% [17], suggesting most cases are not clinically significant.

Risk factors for CNS involvement by CLL/SLL are minimally studied [18]. Surprisingly, Moazzam et al. found involvement of CNS was more frequent in patients with a RAI staging of 0 compared with more advanced stages [17], but an autopsy series suggested increased frequency at later stagers and with increased number of organs involved [19]. Disease volume is therefore not strongly linked to CNS involvement, and additional unknown tumor- or host-specific factors may be at play.

Symptoms of CNS involvement by CLL/SLL are non-specific, with neurocognitive changes being the most common finding to prompt a workup [5]. Cranial nerve-related symptoms result commonly from CNS involvement, part of an overall constellation of headaches, cerebellar symptoms, altered mental status, and cognitive decline [2]. Workup for CNS involvement during initial evaluation of newly diagnosed CLL/SLL is not routine, as only 4% of patients prompted a workup to clarify neurologic symptoms in a large retrospective cohort analysis at a single institution, and from this group, only 10% were found to be positive [5].

Mechanisms by which CLL/SLL cells infiltrate the CNS remains undescribed clinically, though investigators have proposed transmigration through perforating cerebral vessels to the subarachnoid space and/or direct extension from seeded meninges or via perineural sheaths of cranial nerve roots [19]. The frequency of cranial nerve-related symptoms suggests perineural invasion of these nerves is important in many cases.

In this case, the patient had clinical presentation and MRI findings strongly consistent with embolic stroke, and workup revealed a cardiac myxoma, which was later known to have metastasized embolically to distal vascular beds in his fingertips. This history is, therefore, strongly consistent

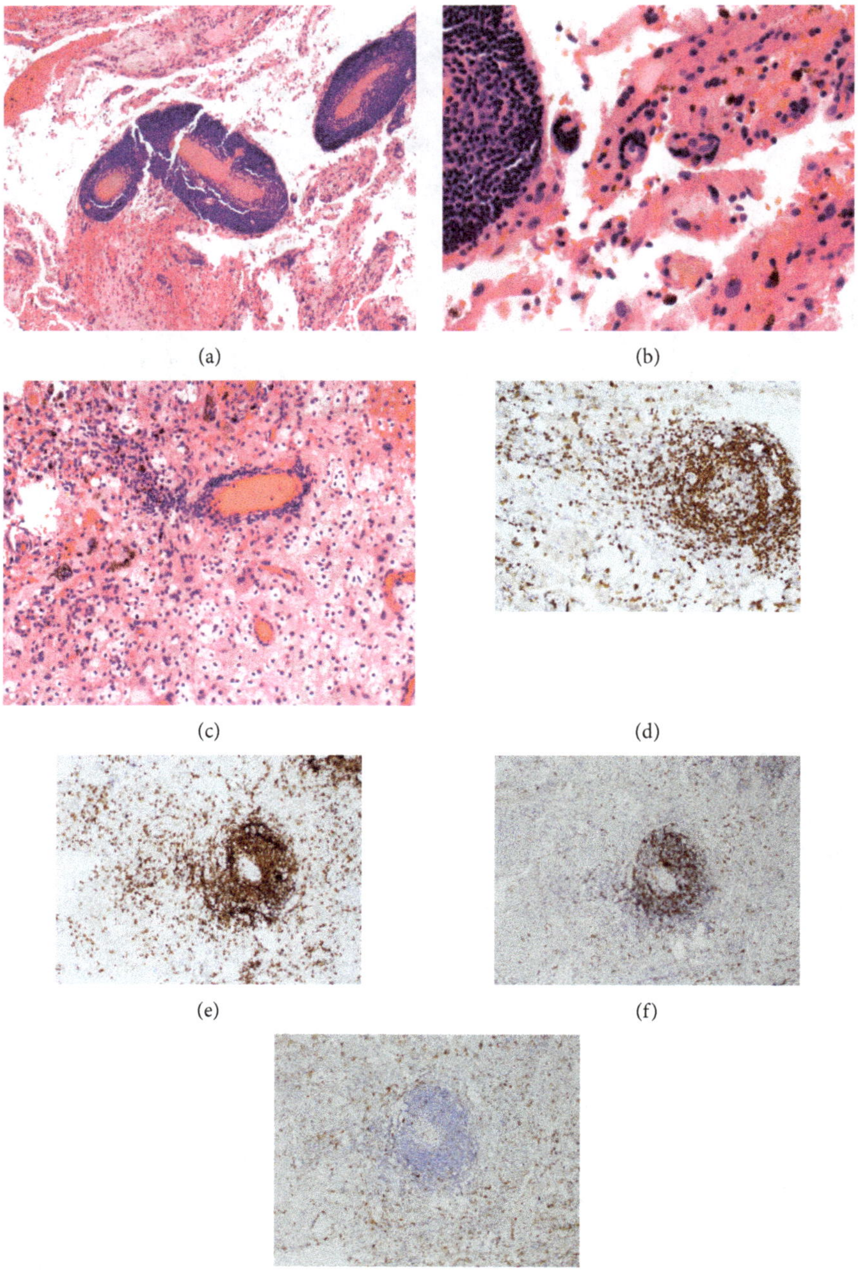

(a) (b) (c) (d) (e) (f) (g)

Figure 2: CNS biopsy: (a) lymphomatous infiltrate is predominantly perivascular that pushes into the surrounding brain parenchyma, which is hemorrhagic with numerous hemosiderin-laden macrophages. Intermediate and high-power photomicrographs of the perivascular lymphoid infiltrate: (b) the infiltrate is composed predominantly of lymphoid cells, which are small with mature nuclear chromatin and regular, rounded nuclear borders. (c) More invasive, rather than pushing, infiltrate involving the brain parenchyma. Immunohistochemistry: (d) PAX-5, (e) coexpression of CD5, (f) partial coexpression of CD23, and (g) cyclin-D1 is negative in the neoplastic lymphoid cells.

with embolic myxoma leading to his initial CVA and later CLL invastion to the same site, though we cannot definitively exclude the presence of CNS CLL upon initial presentation since CNS resection was not performed at that time.

To our knowledge, our report represents that first case of CNS involvement of CLL/SLL in the setting of a previous embolic event and the second report published of CLL/SLL co-occurring with a cardiac myxoma [20]. The parenchymal location restricted to the embolic bed is highly suggestive that the prior myxoma embolism was a key predisposing factor in this case, contrasting with clinical and autopsy reports that describe the leptomeningeal involvement as most frequent [21], though parenchymal disease is certainly also described [5].

Our report is also unusual in that the patient's presentation required emergent surgical intervention for an acute mass effect. Limb paralysis/paresis was found in only 12% of cases previously, with CNS involvement more commonly an asymptomatic incidental finding and generally arising 30 months or longer after initial CLL diagnosis [2].

No evidence of myxoma cells could be identified in the area of the brain embolism in this case, and no lymphoma cells were identified associated with the primary myxoma or its metasteses, supporting the idea that the prior emboli were enabling factors for lymphoma-cell entry to the CNS. Overall, we believe the interruption of the blood brain barrier was the major precipitating event, allowing the hematogenous spread of lymphoma cells.

We chose FCR treatment because high-dose fludarabine is known to penetrate CNS, based on neurotoxicity studies [22]. We decided to proceed with the standard FCR combination days 1 to 3, although with an increase of fludarabine from 25 mg/m^2 to 30 mg/m^2 to increase CNS penetration. Knop et al. [22] reported use of single-agent fludarabine 25 mg/m^2 (five days per cycle) in two patients with leptomeningeal CLL involvement, achieving remission for 11 months after 6 cycles and 25 months after 5 cycles, respectively. Elliot et al. [23] reported a six-month remission in a patient with extensive leptomeningeal CNS involvement using single-agent fludarabine 30 mg/m^2 from days one to five for six cycles. Wanquet et al. [24] also showed durable responses on CLL/SLL involving the CNS with fludarabine-based regimens. We also considered ibrutinib, which has adequate levels of brain distribution and has successfully been used as a single agent in the management of other types of lymphoma in the CNS [25] and specifically showed complete response as a second line therapy in a small retrospective cohort of CLL/SLL involving the CNS [24]. Our rationale was to save ibrutinib in case of later recurrence.

The patient here has sustained CNS remission so far as indicated by sequential imaging and clinical monitoring, providing anecdotal further support for fludarabine-containing chemotherapy for CLL cases in which CNS-directed therapy is indicated. Because CLL/SLL and CNS are most common in the elderly, we also suggest that in patients with CLL/SLL, CNS embolisms or other cerebrovascular accidents (CVAs) damaging the blood-brain barrier are potential risk factors for CNS invasion. CNS involvement by CLL/SLL should, therefore, be on the differential diagnosis for patients with CVA history and new neurologic signs or symptoms.

References

[1] E. Campo, S. H. Swerdlow, N. L. Harris, S. Pileri, H. Stein, and E. S. Jaffe, "The 2008 WHO classification of lymphoid neoplasms and beyond: evolving concepts and practical applications," *Blood*, vol. 117, no. 19, pp. 5019–5032, 2011.

[2] N. K. L. M. Timmers, J. S. de Maar, R. C. M. van Kruijsdijk, and S. K. Klein, "Central nervous system localisation of chronic lymphocytic leukaemia, description of two very distinct cases and a review of the literature," *Annals of Hematology*, vol. 97, no. 9, pp. 1627–1632, 2018.

[3] M. C. J. Hanse, M. B. Veer, K. Lom, and M. J. Bent, "Incidence of central nervous system involvement in chronic lymphocytic leukemia and outcome to treatment," *Journal of Neurology*, vol. 255, no. 6, pp. 828–830, 2008.

[4] M. Ratterman, K. Kruczek, S. Sulo, T. D. Shanafelt, N. E. Kay, and C. Nabhan, "Extramedullary chronic lymphocytic leukemia: systematic analysis of cases reported between 1975 and 2012," *Leukemia Research*, vol. 38, no. 3, pp. 299–303, 2014.

[5] P. Strati, J. H. Uhm, T. J. Kaufmann et al., "Prevalence and characteristics of central nervous system involvement by chronic lymphocytic leukemia," *Haematologica*, vol. 101, no. 4, pp. 458–465, 2016.

[6] I. Gosev, F. Paic, Z. Duric et al., "Cardiac myxoma the great imitators: comprehensive histopathological and molecular approach," *International Journal of Cardiology*, vol. 164, no. 1, pp. 7–20, 2013.

[7] V. H. Lee, H. M. Connolly, and R. D. Brown Jr., "Central nervous system manifestations of cardiac myxoma," *Archives of Neurology*, vol. 64, no. 8, pp. 1115–1120, 2007.

[8] C. K. Park, Y. A. Cho, M. Kim, and H. S. Shim, "Malignant lymphoma arising in cardiac myxoma, presenting with peripheral arterial emboli," *Cardiovascular Pathology*, vol. 32, pp. 26–29, 2018.

[9] N. Colocci, M. Glantz, and L. Recht, "Prevention and treatment of central nervous system involvement by non-Hodgkin's lymphoma: a review of the literature," *Seminars in Neurology*, vol. 24, no. 4, pp. 395–404, 2004.

[10] A. Hollender, S. Kvaloy, O. Nome, E. Skovlund, K. Lote, and H. Holte, "Central nervous system involvement following diagnosis of non-Hodgkin's lymphoma: a risk model," *Annals of Oncology*, vol. 13, no. 7, pp. 1099–1107, 2002.

[11] G. Spectre, A. Gural, G. Amir, A. Lossos, T. Siegal, and O. Paltiel, "Central nervous system involvement in indolent lymphomas," *Annals of Oncology*, vol. 16, no. 3, pp. 450–454, 2005.

[12] P. A. Pophali, G. Thanarajasingam, J. Pulido, P. B. Johnston, and R. S. Go, "Low grade b-cell non-Hodgkin lymphomas (NHL) involving the central nervous system (CNS): an analysis from the National Cancer Database (NCDB)," *Journal of Clinical Oncology*, vol. 35, no. 15, p. e13083, 2017.

[13] R. Buckstein, W. Lim, E. Franssen, and K. L. Imrie, "CNS prophylaxis and treatment in non-Hodgkin's lymphoma: variation in practice and lessons from the literature," *Leukemia & Lymphoma*, vol. 44, no. 6, pp. 955–962, 2003.

[14] E. Santambrogio, M. Nicolosi, F. Vassallo et al., "Aggressive non-Hodgkin lymphomas: risk factors and treatment of central nervous system recurrence," *Expert Review of Hematology*, vol. 12, no. 9, pp. 787–796, 2019.

[15] F.-J. Peñalver, J.-M. Sancho, A. de la Fuente et al., "Guidelines for diagnosis, prevention and management of central nervous system involvement in diffuse large B-cell lymphoma patients by the Spanish Lymphoma Group (GELTAMO)," *Haematologica*, vol. 102, no. 2, pp. 235–245, 2017.

[16] R. L. Siegel, K. D. Miller, and A. Jemal, "Cancer statistics, 2019," *CA: A Cancer Journal for Clinicians*, vol. 69, no. 1, pp. 7–34, 2019.

[17] A. A. Moazzam, J. Drappatz, R. Y. Kim, and S. Kesari, "Chronic lymphocytic leukemia with central nervous system involvement: report of two cases with a comprehensive literature review," *Journal of Neuro-Oncology*, vol. 106, no. 1, pp. 185–200, 2012.

[18] S. de Souza, F. Santiago, M. D. Ribeiro-Carvalho, A. Arnóbio, A. Soares, and M. Ornellas, "Leptomeningeal involvement in B-cell chronic lymphocytic leukemia: a case report and review of the literature," *BMC Research Notes*, vol. 7, no. 1, p. 645, 2014.

[19] S. C. Cramer, J. A. Glaspy, J. T. Efird, and D. N. Louis, "Chronic lymphocytic leukemia and the central nervous system: a clinical and pathological study," *Neurology*, vol. 46, no. 1, pp. 19–25, 1996.

[20] H. Laird-Fick, A. Tiwari, S. Narayanan, Y. Qin, D. Vodnala, and M. Bhutani, "A case of comorbid myxoma and chronic lymphocytic leukemia: not just a coincidence?," *Case Reports in Oncological Medicine*, vol. 2014, Article ID 142746, 4 pages, 2014.

[21] M. Barcos, W. Lane, G. A. Gomez et al., "An autopsy study of 1206 acute and chronic leukemias (1958 to 1982)," *Cancer*, vol. 60, no. 4, pp. 827–837, 1987.

[22] S. Knop, U. Herrlinger, U. Ernemann, L. Kanz, and H. Hebart, "Fludarabine may induce durable remission in patients with leptomeningeal involvement of chronic lymphocytic leukemia," *Leukemia & Lymphoma*, vol. 46, no. 11, pp. 1593–1598, 2005.

[23] M. A. Elliott, L. Letendre, C.-Y. Li, J. D. Hoyer, and J. E. Hammack, "Chronic lymphocytic leukaemia with symptomatic diffuse central nervous system infiltration responding to therapy with systemic fludarabine," *British Journal of Haematology*, vol. 104, no. 4, pp. 689–694, 1999.

[24] A. Wanquet, R. Birsen, C. Bonnet et al., "Management of central nervous system involvement in chronic lymphocytic leukaemia: a retrospective cohort of 30 patients," *British Journal of Haematology*, vol. 176, no. 1, pp. 37–49, 2017.

[25] L. Ysebaert, K. Beccaria, A. Ple, H. Sauvageon, and S. Mourah, "Ibrutinib brain distribution: a preclinical study," *Cancer Chemotherapy and Pharmacology*, vol. 81, no. 4, pp. 783–789, 2018.

17

Siltuximab-Related Favorable Clinical Outcome for a Patient Suffering from Idiopathic Multicentric Castleman Disease

Stamatios Chrysochoou,[1] Andreas Kreft,[2] and Eberhard Schneider[1,3]

[1]*GPR Gesundheits- und Pflegezentrum Rüsselsheim Gemeinnützige GmbH, August-Bebel-Straße 59, Rüsselsheim Am Main 65428, Germany*
[2]*Institute of Pathology, Johannes Gutenberg University, Langenbeckstraße 1, Mainz 55131, Germany*
[3]*Department of Biology, Julius Maximilians University, Am Hubland, Würzburg 97074, Germany*

Correspondence should be addressed to Eberhard Schneider; e.schneider@gp-ruesselsheim.de

Academic Editor: Pier Paolo Piccaluga

*Rational*Castleman disease is a rare lymphoproliferative disorder that can be subdivided into unicentric and multicentric forms, the latter of which causes a spectrum of serious medical conditions. Here, we present a case of idiopathic multicentric Castleman disease in the eighth decade of life. *Patient Concerns.* First hospitalized due to unexplained progressive anemia, the patient was readmitted to the hospital 18 months later with suspected lymphoma. Clinical examination revealed a progressive lymphadenopathy. *Diagnoses.* Histopathologic lymph node features, anemia, elevated CRP and IL6 levels, splenomegaly, and hypoalbuminemia indicated multicentric Castleman (MCD) disease. *Interventions.* The patient was treated intravenously with a dose of 11 mg/kg siltuximab every 3 weeks. *Outcomes.* Timely correct diagnosis through the stringent use of consensus diagnostic criteria and sufficient siltuximab therapy has considerably promoted favorable clinical outcomes in a patient suffering from MCD.

1. Introduction

Castleman disease (CD) is a rare lymphoproliferative disorder first reported by pathologist Benjamin Castleman in 1954 [1]. CD is subdivided into unicentric CD (UCD), involving just one enlarged lymph node, and multicentric CD (MCD), affecting multiple lymph nodes [2]. While UCD is considered a benign condition, MCD is characterized by a variety of clinical and laboratory abnormalities with a poor prognosis in otherwise untreated patients [3]. MCD can be caused by human herpesvirus-8 (HHV-8; HHV-8-associated MCD), with the majority of cases consisting of human immunodeficiency virus (HIV) infected or immunocompromised patients [4]. Little is known about the etiology of HHV-8-negative MCD, referred to as idiopathic MCD (iMCD). iMCD accounts for up to 50% of all MCD cases and can lead to cytokine storm-mediated multiple organ system dysfunction, apart from other severe clinical manifestations [4].

The diagnosis of iMCD can be challenging because it is both a rare disorder and a mimicker of other clinical conditions such as malignant lymphoma, cancer, or autoimmune diseases [5]. Recently, Fajgenbaum et al. established evidence-based consensus diagnostic criteria for HHV-8-negative/iMDC, which are subdivided in major, minor, and exclusion criteria [4]. Major criteria concise enlarged lymph nodes and histopathologic features consistent with the iMCD spectrum (i.e., regressed/atrophic/atretic/hyperplastic germinal centers (GC), follicular dendritic cell (FDC) prominence, and vascularity). Minor criteria consist of 6 laboratory and 5 clinical features (elevated ESR or CRP, anemia, thrombocytopenia/cytosis, renal dysfunction or proteinuria, polyclonal hypergammaglobulinemia, hypoalbuminemia and constitutional symptoms, large spleen and/or liver, fluid accumulation, eruptive cherry angiomata or violaceous papules, lymphocytic interstitial pneumonitis, respectively) of which at least 2 must match the patient's symptoms (with ≥1 laboratory criterion). iMCD can be further subclassified into iMCD-thrombocytopenia, ascites, reticulin fibrosis, renal dysfunction, organomegaly (iMCD-TAFRO), or iMCD, not otherwise specified (iMCD-NOS) [2]. Considering exclusion criteria, it is crucial to rule out malignant, infectious, and autoimmune conditions that can mimic iMCD [4].

While therapeutic strategies for UCD are more or less complete surgical removal, the multicentric form of the disease involves many more different approaches. Considering the guidance from van Rhee et al. [6], the consensus treatment algorithm for iMCD patients, regardless of clinical severity, starts with administering anti-IL6-directed treatment [6]. Up to now, siltuximab, an anti-IL6 chimeric monoclonal antibody, is the only approved drug for the treatment of HHV-8-negative iMDC in Europe and the USA (US Food and Drug Administration, 2014; European Medicines Agency, 2016) [7, 8]. For people who do not respond to siltuximab, a broad spectrum of other treatment options exist, like tocilizumab or rituximab-based therapeutic approaches, to name a few; however, it is currently difficult to clearly determine their effectiveness [3].

2. Report of a Case

We report on a 78-year-old female patient diagnosed with HIV-negative, HHV-8-negative iMCD in 2021, with a history of nicotine abuse and comorbidities such as hyperthyroidism, coronary sclerosis, and bilateral knee gonarthrosis, leading to right total knee replacement in November 2020. As permanent therapeutic intervention, the patient received Thyronajod (175 μg qd), pantroprazol (40 mg qd), Torasemid (5 mg qd), and Oxycodone (20 mg qd). During 2021, she received anti-SARS-CoV-2 vaccination (1st dose in April; 2nd dose in July).

As of November 2019, the patient was hospitalized due to progressive anemia (haemoglobin 10 g/dl, MCV 82 fl), persistent elevated levels of CRP (8–11 mg/dl), and weight loss (20 kg). Initially suspected as lymphoma, this diagnosis could not be clearly confirmed. CT scan of the thorax and abdomen revealed highly suspicious paraaortic and inter-aortocaval lymph nodes (largest paraaortic node: 3.3 × 2.6 × 1.1 cm). While subsequent examinations in March 2020 and March 2021 showed essentially steady lymph node progression (axillary lymph nodes from 6 to 8 mm; largest para-aortal node: 2.5 × 2.2 × .0 cm), these findings were considered not indicative for lymphoma.

The general condition of the patient appeared to be mainly stable since November 2019; Eastern Cooperative Oncology Group (ECOG) performance status has been assessed of 1 to 2.

However, as of June 2021, the patient was referred to our hospital by her general practitioner still with lymphoma as an initial tentative diagnosis. As well, she suffered from rheumatism-like musculoskeletal pain, mainly in the upper extremities.

Biopsy of a left-sided suprainguinal lymph node revealed atrophic germinal centers, positivity for CD21 in follicular dendritic cells, and a partial loss of proliferating B cells with abundant surrounding T-cells (Figure 1). Plasma cells were increased and appeared widely IgG-positive, exhibiting a polyclonal pattern for kappa and lambda light chains without enhanced expression of IgG4.

Both progressive lymphadenopathy in combination with histopathologic lymph node features are consistent with the iMCD spectrum (plasma cell subtype) and are referred to as major criteria.

Bone marrow aspirate studies including immunophenotyping of plasma cells showed a normal karyotype (46, XX) and could exclude myeloma due to low antigen expression (0.3%). Physical examination revealed splenomegaly, hypoalbuminemia (<35 g/l [32, 1 g/l]), pronounced increased soluble interleukin 2 receptor (sIL-2R) (1602 kU/l, normal 158–623), and highly elevated interleukin-6 (IL6) levels (64.1 pg/ml, normal <7.0 pg/ml). Further laboratory analyses were negative for HIV (serological testing), Epstein-Barr virus (EBV) (serological PCR and immunohistochemical testing), antinuclear antibodies (ANA), and HHV-8 infection (PCR testing). Vascular endothelial growth factor (VEGF) and interleukin-10 (IL) appeared in a normal range.

Since anemia, elevated CRP and IL6 levels, splenomegaly, and hypoalbuminemia meet 5 out of 11 minor consensus criteria, iMCD in the patient could be confirmed. The lack of thrombocytopenia, ascites, reticulin fibrosis, and renal dysfunction could clearly rule out iMCD-TAFRO, therefore we claimed the criteria are met for the existence of a less aggressive subtype iMCD-NOS.

Considering the consensus treatment algorithm for iMCD-NOS, the patient started therapy with siltuximab in August 2021 at a dose of 11 mg/kg intravenously every 3 weeks [6].

After 5 cycles of siltuximab, she presented in a general good condition with just a slight increase of lower limb edema. The therapy was well tolerated and no serious adverse side events could have been observed. Moreover, the patient experienced a remarkable decrease of rheumatism-like musculoskeletal pain. Haemoglobin as well as CRP and ferritin levels normalized (12.5 g/dl, normal 11.5–15.4 g/dl; 0.06 mg/dl, normal <0.50 mg/dl; 120.0 ng/ml, normal 13.0–150.0 ng/ml). TSH values decreased to 0.186 mU/l (normal <0.270–4.200 mU/l) while and FT4 values increased to 2.13 ng/dl (normal 0.90–1.70 ng/dl), both indicating hyperthyroidism which is an already known comorbidity in the patient.

CT scan of the thorax and abdomen revealed no essential changes in size of the spleen as well as of para-aortal and interaortocaval lymph nodes.

3. Discussion

More than half a century after Benjamin Castleman's initial description of a case, later termed as CD, a variety of lymphoproliferative disorders constitute the spectrum of CD. However, CD is a very rare and potentially serious lymphoproliferative disorder. International efforts have been made to define diagnostic criteria allowing to differentiate between particular forms of CD and to rule out mimickers of CD [4].

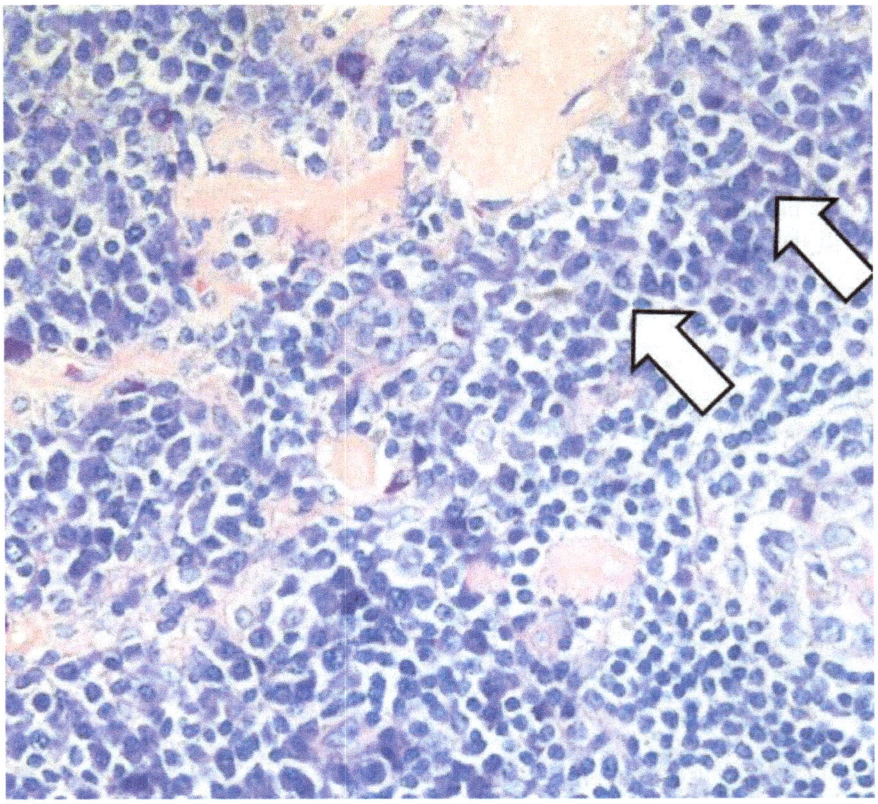

FIGURE 1: Histopathology. Involuted follicle (black arrow) with indistinct lymphocytic mantle and abundant perifollicular plasma cells (white arrows) (consistent with the plasma cell rich type of M Castleman).

The patient who attended our hospital was in her eighth decade of life and had a history of nicotine abuse and comorbidities. Her clinical presentation with features like progressive anemia and persistent elevated levels of CRP did not automatically trigger the suspicion of CD since CD is a rare condition with an estimated 10-year period prevalence of 2.5 cases per million in North America, which may also be applicable to Germany [9]. After ruling out lymphoma as an initial tentative diagnosis, we examined the possibility for CD. Because of the wide range of potential clinical outcomes, a correct diagnosis of not only CD but also the subtype is essential for treatment strategy [10]. Further, thorough differential diagnostic examination following the scheme of Fajgenbaum et al. [4] could reveal the MCD-subtype HHV-8-negative iMCD-NOS in our patient and rule out lymphoma as the initial tentative diagnosis.

Anti-IL6-directed therapy is recommended for the treatment of HHV-8-negative iMDC [7, 8]. Since siltuximab is an anti-IL6 chimeric monoclonal antibody, we decided to treat the patient with this therapeutic agent following established guidelines [6].

Therapeutic outcome after 5 cycles of siltuximab administration (3 weeks each cycle) can be considered very promising. The patient reported toleration of the treatment and decrease of rheumatism-like musculoskeletal pain. IL6 plays a role in rheumatoid arthritis and it is a common observation that inhibiting IL6 ameliorates the symptoms of both rheumatoid arthritis and iMCD [11, 12]. Therefore, a positive effect on rheumatism-like musculoskeletal pain of our patient was not unexpected.

Blood values improved generally, in particular haemoglobin as well as CRP and ferritin levels normalized. CT scan of the thorax and abdomen exhibited stable disease. However, a slight increase of lower limb edema could have been observed as well as a slight deterioration of indicators for hyperthyroidism. Overall, siltuximab appears to be a safe and effective treatment of HHV-8-negative iMDC in our patient.

4. Conclusions

Improving iMCD patient outcomes is essentially dependent on timely correct diagnosis and sufficient therapy of the disease. The consistent use of international, evidence-based consensus diagnostic criteria described by Fajgenbaum et al. [4] as well as consensus treatment strategies [3] helped us rule out lymphoma as an initial tentative diagnosis and to minimize unfavourable outcomes for an iMCD-NOS patient. The application of anti-IL6-directed therapy with siltuximab appeared as a safe and effective treatment strategy.

Abbreviations

ANA: Antinuclear antibodies
CD: Castleman disease
CT: Computed tomography

HHV-8: Human herpesvirus-8
HIV: Human immunodeficiency virus
IL: Interleukin
iMCD: idiopathic multicentric Castleman disease
TAFRO: Thrombocytopenia, ascites, reticulin fibrosis, renal dysfunction, organomegaly
UCD: Unicentric Castleman disease
VEGF: Vascular endothelial growth factor.

Consent

All procedures performed in studies involving human participants were in accordance with the ethical standards of the institutional and/or national research committee and with the 1964 Helsinki Declaration and its later amendments or comparable ethical standards.

Authors' Contributions

Eberhard Schneider conceptualized the study (e.schneider@gp-ruesselsheim.de). Andreas Kreft (andreas.kreft@unimedizin-mainz.de) and Eberhard Schneider curated the data. Stamatios Chrysochoou wrote the original draft (chrysochoou@gp-ruesselsheim.de). Eberhard Schneider reviewed and edited the manuscript.

Acknowledgments

The authors thank Heike Borchert for administrative and technical support. Publication fees are funded by EUSA Pharma(Germany) GmbH.

References

[1] B. Castleman and V. W. Towne, "Case records of the massachusetts general hospital: case no. 40231," *New England Journal of Medicine*, vol. 250, pp. 1001–1005, 1954.

[2] A. Dispenzieri and D. C. Fajgenbaum, "Overview of castleman disease," *Blood*, vol. 135, no. 16, pp. 1353–1364, 2020.

[3] A. Dispenzieri, J. O. Armitage, M. J. Loe et al., "The clinical spectrum of castleman's disease," *American Journal of Hematology*, vol. 87, no. 11, pp. 997–1002, 2012.

[4] D. C. Fajgenbaum, T. S. Uldrick, A. Bagg et al., "International, evidence-based consensus diagnostic criteria for HHV-8-negative/idiopathic multicentric Castleman disease," *Blood*, vol. 129, no. 12, pp. 1646–1657, 2017.

[5] Castleman disease collaborative network CDCN (2021), https://cdcn.org/castleman-disease/diagnosis-treatment/.

[6] F. van Rhee, P. Voorhees, A. Dispenzieri et al., "International, evidence-based consensus treatment guidelines for idiopathic multicentric Castleman disease," *Blood*, vol. 132, no. 20, pp. 2115–2124, 2018.

[7] European medicines agency (2021), https://www.ema.europa.eu/en/medicines/human/EPAR/sylvant.

[8] A. Deisseroth, C.-W. Ko, L. Nie et al., "FDA approval: siltuximab for the treatment of patients with multicentric castleman disease," *Clinical Cancer Research*, vol. 21, no. 5, pp. 950–954, 2015.

[9] D. Robinson Jr., M. Reynolds, C. Casper et al., "Clinical epidemiology and treatment patterns of patients with multicentric Castleman disease: results from two US treatment centres," *British Journal of Haematology*, vol. 165, no. 1, pp. 39–48, 2014.

[10] R. Riepl, T. Hoffmann, and J. Greve, "Morbus castleman-eine harmlose differenzialdiagnose einer lymphadenitis colli?—eine fallserie," *Laryngo-Rhino-Otologie*, vol. 21, no. 08, pp. 522–527, 2017.

[11] N. Nishimoto, K. Terao, T. Mima, H. Nakahara, N. Takagi, and T. Kakehi, "Mechanisms and pathologic significances in increase in serum interleukin-6 (IL-6) and soluble IL-6 receptor after administration of an anti-IL-6 receptor antibody, tocilizumab, in patients with rheumatoid arthritis and Castleman disease," *Blood*, vol. 112, no. 10, pp. 3959–3964, 2008.

[12] C. Garbers, S. Heink, T. Korn, and S. Rose-John, "Interleukin-6: designing specific therapeutics for a complex cytokine," *Nature Reviews Drug Discovery*, vol. 17, no. 6, pp. 395–412, 2018.

18

Successful Control of Hepatitis B Virus Reactivation following Restart of Ibrutinib in Chronic Lymphocytic Leukaemia

Sara Kristina Viberg Tjønnfjord[1,2] **Eirik Brekka Tjønnfjord,**[2] **Zbigniew Konopski,**[3] **and Geir Erland Tjønnfjord**[2,4]

[1]*Department of Nephrology, Odense University Hospital, Odense Kløverværnget 6, 5000 Odense C, Denmark*
[2]*Department of Haematology, Oslo University Hospital, P.O. Box 4950 Nydalen, No. 0424 Oslo, Norway*
[3]*Department of Gastroenterology, Oslo University Hospital, P.O. Box 4950 Nydalen, No. 0424 Oslo, Norway*
[4]*KG Jebsen Centre for B-Cell Malignancies, Institute of Clinical Medicine, University of Oslo, P.O. Box 4950 Nydalen, No. 0424 Oslo, Norway*

Correspondence should be addressed to Sara Kristina Viberg Tjønnfjord; sara.tjonnfjord@gmail.com

Academic Editor: Håkon Reikvam

Ibrutinib is a targeted therapy drug that blocks the activity of Bruton's tyrosine kinase, and it is an approved treatment for several mature B-cell malignancies including chronic lymphocytic leukaemia (CLL). Side effects include infections, cytopenia, nausea, and diarrhoea. In this report, we describe a case of hepatitis B reactivation in a female CLL patient undergoing treatment with ibrutinib. Diagnosis was confirmed with highly elevated hepatitis B virus DNA and a prior blood sample confirmed previous exposure. Ibrutinib was paused, and antiviral therapy was initiated with prompt clinical improvement. Ibrutinib was reinitiated shortly after clinical improvement. Thus, our case report demonstrates that systematic HBV screening is essential before starting treatment with ibrutinib. We suggest that antiviral prophylaxis is considered for patients at risk of reactivation, and ibrutinib may be continued following HBV reactivation with proper antiviral treatment.

1. Introduction

Ibrutinib is a small molecule drug that binds irreversibly to Bruton's tyrosine kinase (BTK), an important molecule in B-cell signalling. It is an orally administrated drug showing efficacy in mantle cell lymphoma (MCL), chronic lymphocytic leukaemia (CLL), and Waldenström's macroglobulinemia and compared to chemo-immunotherapy ibrutinib treatment has a lower risk of infections [1].

In preclinical studies using CLL cells, ibrutinib has been shown to promote apoptosis, inhibit proliferation, and prevent cells from responding to survival stimuli provided by the microenvironment resulting in a decreased expression of Mcl-1. In clinical studies, the activity of ibrutinib has been described to include a rapid reduction in lymphadenopathy accompanied by transient lymphocytosis, indicating that the drug has direct effects on cell homing and migration [2–5].

The efficacy of ibrutinib has been impressing progression free survival at 2 years >85% and 70% and overall survival at 2 years >95% and 65% in both treatment-naïve and relapsed or refractory CLL, respectively [3, 5, 6]. However, adverse effects have been documented. The most common are infections, cytopenias, diarrhoea, and muscle and joint pain (>10% frequency). Less common are nonmelanoma skin cancer, interstitial lung disease, tumour lysis syndrome, atrial fibrillation, and haemorrhage [7].

Reactivation of latent infections, particularly herpes and hepatitis B and C viridae, is well documented during treatment with anti-CD20 antibodies and purine analogues. However, only a few case reports describe tyrosine kinase inhibitor-induced HBV reactivation in patients with CLL,

Table 1: Time course of blood values obtained before, during, and after reactivation.

	February 16	April 16	May 16	June 16 (admission to hospital)	June 16 (ibrutinib paused, tenofovir prescribed)	June 16	August 16 (ibrutinib reinitiated with tenofovir)	October 16	January 17	January 18
P-AST (U/L)	30	↑40	↑62	↑714	↑618	↑133	28		23	16
P-ALT (U/L)	22	↑63	↑109	↑1553	↑843	↑304	27		18	24
P-ALP (U/L)		80	79	↑186	↑181	↑148	83		75	67
P-BILI (μmol/L)		9	7	↑182	↑232	↑186	12		7	13
P-INR		1.2		↑1.5	↑1.5	↑1.4	1.1			
HBV-DNA (IU/mL)					↑ 12 000 000	↑170 000		↑ 51	<20	<20

Reference ranges: AST (15–35 U/L), ALT (10–45 U/L), ALP (35–105 U/L), bilirubin (5–25 μmol/L), and INR (0,8–1,2).

and there are no guidelines on management of a reactivation.

2. Case Presentation

A 53-year-old female was diagnosed with CLL in 2009 [8]. She exhibited swelling of both parotic glands in 2002, but she was not diagnosed with Sjögren's syndrome until 2008 following clinical evaluation and biopsy of the parotic glands showing atrophy and chronic infection. Following a whole body CT scan disclosing generalized lymphadenopathy, she was referred for haematological evaluation. CLL was confirmed by flow cytometry, CLL score 5/5 [9]. Molecular analysis revealed that the CLL cells used the IGHV3-33 gene showing 100% homology to germ line.

First line treatment with six courses of fludarabine, cyclophosphamide, and rituximab (FCR) was initiated in 2011 due to progressive disease, Binet stage B. Complete remission with no residual disease detected by flow cytometry was accomplished. She had no medical history suggesting hepatitis, and she had been seen regularly at our hospital between 2002 and 2016 without any sign of liver enzymes being elevated. Serological screening for hepatitis was not performed.

Breast cancer was diagnosed in 2014 and treated by ablation and adjuvant radio-chemotherapy.

In January 2016, she suffered a CLL relapse, Binet stage C disease, and second-line treatment with FC without rituximab due to extreme lymphocytosis was initiated while waiting for the result of cytogenetic and molecular genetic assessment. She received one course of treatment with no effect, and as the genetic analysis showed homozygous deletion of 13*q*14 and heterozygous *TP*53-mutation (c.486del p.Tyr163ThrfsTer7), treatment was altered to ibrutinib 420 mg once daily from late February 2016.

In June 2016, she was admitted to the Department of Gastroenterology due to malaise, fever, jaundice, and elevated liver parameters (Table 1). Two months before the hospitalization, she had a kidney stone attack. Diclophenac had been administered for a couple of days due to epigastric and back pain. Obstructive uropathy with septicaemia or biliary obstruction was the initial diagnosis as a CT scan disclosed a kidney stone in the lower calyx of the right kidney with hydronephrosis, and empirical treatment with piperacillin and tazobactam was administered. Septicaemia was not confirmed, and hepatitis was then considered the proper diagnosis. A PCR test showed hepatitis B virus (HBV) DNA 12,000,000 IU/ml confirming HBV hepatitis. A serum sample from June 2009 was analysed which disclosed previous exposure to HBV (HBsAg positive, anti-HBc antibody positive, and anti-HBs antibody negative). No HBV-DNA was analysed at that time. She was unaware of any previous exposure to HBV.

When hepatitis B reactivation was diagnosed, ibrutinib was halted, and tenofovir 245 mg was administered once daily following which her condition rapidly improved (Table 1). Ibrutinib treatment was resumed in August 2016. Monotherapy with tenofovir was started as recommended by our infectious medicine consultant. Resistance rarely develops during monotherapy with tenofovir [10]. As of April 2019, she was doing very well on continuous treatment with ibrutinib and tenofovir, but two months later, she was diagnosed with a CLL relapse. Venetoclax monotherapy was initiated in October 2019, and tenofovir was continued. By May 2020, she experienced a complete haematological remission. However, three months later, there were signs of progression, and she succumbed from septicaemia in July 2021.

3. Discussion

Reactivation of viral infections is common in patients treated for haematological malignancies. The incidence and severity of viral reactivation relate to the severity of the immunosuppression. Antiviral prophylaxis has been shown to be effective. Guidelines generally recommend that any patient receiving immunosuppression or cytotoxic chemotherapy should be screened for HBsAg, anti-HBc, and HBV-DNA [10–12]. Hepatitis virus screening is recommended in lymphoproliferative disorders, in acute leukaemia, and in other patients treated with monoclonal anti-CD20 antibodies, anthracyclines, or corticosteroids, and in autologous stem cell transplantation [10].

Treatment can be either prophylactic or preemptive. Patients with positive HBsAg, where chemo-immunotherapy is planned, should be treated with antiviral prophylaxis for up to 12–18 months. HBV reactivation in patients with resolved hepatitis (positive anti-HBc and negative HBsAg) is an issue of relevance, particularly in cases of haematological malignancies. It is suggested that patients receiving high-risk treatment regimens are handled similarly to patients with chronic HBV. However, the best intervention strategy is not yet known for patients in the moderate risk group [10–12]. Ibrutinib is a relatively new drug targeting B-cell signalling approved for MCL and CLL. The Summary of Product Characteristics (SPC) states that HBV reactivation may occur during ibrutinib treatment and recommends serological testing for HBV and HCV to be done before treatment. Our patient's first line chemo-immunotherapy treatment, and later ibrutinib, was initiated years before national recommendations were introduced. The effect of ibrutinib on HBV reactivation has not been extensively addressed in the literature, and there are no guidelines on management of HBV reactivation during treatment with ibrutinib.

There are a few other case reports addressing handling of HBV reactivation. de Jésus Ngoma et al. observed an asymptomatic HBV reactivation with transaminitis and HBV-DNA elevation during ibrutinib treatment in an 80-year-old patient with CLL [13]. No antiviral prophylaxis was provided. It should be noted that slightly elevated HBV-DNA was measured before treatment, and ibrutinib was initiated only one month after chemo-immunotherapy was stopped without any universal prophylaxis. Herishanu et al. described reactivation of HBV in a patient with CLL previously treated with ibrutinib [14]. Ibrutinib was given as second-line treatment for twelve months, before it was unintentionally stopped. A rapid increase in ALT and AST occurred six weeks later together with a rapid elevation of HBV-DNA. Antiviral treatment was initiated, and ibrutinib was resumed together with antiviral therapy after full remission from HBV reactivation. A recent case report describes a CLL patient with occult HBV, who initially was treated with chemo-immunotherapy together with antiviral prophylaxis [15]. Ibrutinib was initiated three years later due to progression, and the patient developed HbeAg positivity and elevated HBV-DNA. Ibrutinib was paused, antiviral prophylaxis was prescribed, ibrutinib was reinitiated after fifteen days, and HBV-DNA became undetectable.

In contrast, Tedeschi et al. described a case series of 7 CLL patients with positive anti-HBc antibodies and undetectable HBV-DNA before ibrutinib treatment [16]. Patients were monitored every three months for reactivation. However, no reactivation events were detected during a follow-up period of 25 months.

More recently, Molica et al. reported on ibrutinib treatment in three patients with CLL and chronic active HBV infection [17]. The patients received antiviral therapy 2–10 months before initiation of treatment with ibrutinib. Ibrutinib could safely be administered for more than 2 years with continuous antiviral therapy. In our patient, like the patients reported by Molica et al., viral DNA could not be detected more than two years after the initiation of tenofovir while they are enjoying complete control of their CLL on continuous ibrutinib treatment. Whether antiviral therapy can be safely stopped in these patients when continuing ibrutinib therapy is elusive.

We chose to stop ibrutinib for eight weeks when HBV reactivation was diagnosed and tenofovir was initiated in our patient. Reactivation of HBV usually occurs after the second and third course of chemotherapy, and the median interval is 4 months [18]. Since the patient only received one course of chemotherapy, and HBV reactivation occurred more than 5 months later, ibrutinib is the possible cause of reactivation. Plasma HBV-DNA had started to decrease when ibrutinib was resumed. Whether the temporary discontinuation of ibrutinib was necessary remains unknown. At the time, the ECIL-5 guideline on management of viral hepatitis in patients with haematological malignancies had no specific recommendations on prophylaxis or treatment of HBV reactivation in patients treated with BTK inhibitors, but tenofovir or entecavir is recommended as first line treatment when indicated [19]. We, like Molica et al., chose tenofovir monotherapy which proved to be effective. To our knowledge, only one retrospective study has addressed the risk of HBV reactivation in this specific patient group. Hammond et al. found a cumulative incidence of 9.5% during ibrutinib treatment [20]. Thus, there is a relative high risk of reactivation, with possibly severe outcome. In patients with a history of HBV infection, prophylactic antiviral therapy is recommended by the German Society of Hematology and Medical Oncology to prevent reactivation during chemo-immunotherapy and should most likely be applied in patients treated with ibrutinib as well. However, we do not consider a history with HBV infection a contraindication for treating with ibrutinib or other signal inhibitors, if proper precautions are taken and antiviral prophylaxis provided in patients at risk of reactivation.

Additional Points

(i) All patients with CLL planning to start ibrutinib should be screened for HBV, and a double assurance of negative screening should be included in clinical practice before administration of chemotherapy in order to reduce the possibility of a reactivation. (ii) Previous HBV infection is not a contradiction for treatment with ibrutinib, if proper precautions are taken and antiviral prophylaxis provided in patients at risk of reactivation. (iii) There is a need for international guidelines on the management of viral hepatitis in CLL and related disorders specifically addressing treatment with signal pathway inhibitors.

References

[1] C. Sun, X. Tian, Y. S. Lee et al., "Partial reconstitution of humoral immunity and fewer infections in patients with chronic lymphocytic leukemia treated with ibrutinib," *Blood*, vol. 126, no. 19, pp. 2213–2219, 2015.

[2] N. Jain and S. O'Brien, "Ibrutinib (PCI-32765) in chronic lymphocytic leukemia," *Hematology-Oncology Clinics of North America*, vol. 27, no. 4, pp. 851-860, 2013.

[3] J. A. Burger, A. Tedeschi, P. M. Barr et al., "Ibrutinib as initial therapy for patients with chronic lymphocytic leukemia," *New England Journal of Medicine*, vol. 373, no. 25, pp. 2425–2437, 2015.

[4] J. C. Byrd, J. R. Brown, S. O'Brien et al., "Ibrutinib versus ofatumumab in previously treated chronic lymphoid leukemia," *New England Journal of Medicine*, vol. 371, no. 3, pp. 213–223, 2014.

[5] J. C. Byrd, R. R. Furman, S. E. Coutre et al., "Three-year follow-up of treatment-naïve and previously treated patients with CLL and SLL receiving single-agent ibrutinib," *Blood*, vol. 125, no. 16, pp. 2497–2506, 2015.

[6] J. A. Woyach, A. S. Ruppert, N. A. Heerema et al., "Ibrutinib regimens versus chemoimmunotherapy in older patients with untreated CLL," *New England Journal of Medicine*, vol. 379, no. 26, pp. 2517–2528, 2018.

[7] J. R. Brown, P. Hillmen, S. O'Brien et al., "Extended follow-up and impact of high-risk prognostic factors from the phase 3 RESONATE study in patients with previously treated CLL/SLL," *Leukemia*, vol. 32, no. 1, pp. 83–91, 2018.

[8] M. Hallek, B. D. Cheson, D. Catovsky et al., "iwCLL guidelines for diagnosis, indications for treatment, response assessment, and supportive management of CLL," *Blood*, vol. 131, no. 25, pp. 2745–2760, 2018.

[9] E. Matutes, K. Owusu-Ankomah, R. Morilla et al., "The immunological profile of B-cell disorders and proposal of a scoring system for the diagnosis of CLL," *Leukemia*, vol. 8, no. 10, pp. 1640–1645, 1994.

[10] European Association for the Study of the Liver, "EASL 2017 Clinical Practice Guidelines on the management of hepatitis B virus infection," *Journal of Hepatology*, vol. 67, no. 2, pp. 370–398, 2017.

[11] N. A. Terrault, A. S. F. Lok, B. J. McMahon et al., "Update on prevention, diagnosis, and treatment of chronic hepatitis B: AASLD 2018 hepatitis B guidance," *Clinical liver disease*, vol. 12, no. 1, pp. 33-34, 2018.

[12] M. Sandherr, M. Hentrich, M. von Lilienfeld-Toal et al., "Antiviral prophylaxis in patients with solid tumours and haematological malignancies-update of the guidelines of the infectious diseases working party (AGIHO) of the German society for Hematology and medical Oncology (DGHO)," *Annals of Hematology*, vol. 94, no. 9, pp. 1441–1450, 2015.

[13] P. de Jésus Ngoma, B. Kabamba, G. Dahlqvist et al., "Occult HBV reactivation induced by ibrutinib treatment: a case report," *Acta gastro-enterologica Belgica*, vol. 78, no. 4, pp. 424–426, 2015.

[14] Y. Herishanu, H. Katchman, and A. Polliack, "Severe hepatitis B virus reactivation related to ibrutinib monotherapy," *Annals of Hematology*, vol. 96, no. 4, pp. 689-690, 2017.

[15] I. Innocenti, F. Morelli, F. Autore et al., "HBV reactivation in CLL patients with occult HBV infection treated with ibrutinib without viral prophylaxis," *Leukemia and Lymphoma*, vol. 60, no. 5, pp. 1340–1342, 2019.

[16] A. Tedeschi, A. M. Frustaci, M. Mazzucchelli, R. Cairoli, and M. Montillo, "Is HBV prophylaxis required during CLL treatment with ibrutinib?" *Leukemia and Lymphoma*, vol. 58, no. 12, pp. 2966–2968, 2017.

[17] S. Molica, L. Levato, R. Mirabelli, A. Tedeschi, and M. Lentini, "Feasibility and safety of therapy with ibrutinib after antiviral control of hepatitis B virus (HBV) reactivation in chronic lymphocytic leukemia patients," *Leukemia and Lymphoma*, vol. 59, no. 11, pp. 2734–2736, 2018.

[18] H. I. Kawsar, J. Shahnewaz, K. V. Gopalakrishna, T. P. Spiro, and H. A. Daw, "Hepatitis B reactivation in cancer patients: role of prechemotherapy screening and antiviral prophylaxis," *Clinical Advances in Hematology & Oncology: Human Organization*, vol. 10, no. 6, pp. 370–378, 2012.

[19] V. Mallet, F. van Bömmel, C. Doerig et al., "Management of viral hepatitis in patients with haematological malignancy and in patients undergoing haemopoietic stem cell transplantation: recommendations of the 5th European Conference on Infections in Leukaemia (ECIL-5)," *The Lancet Infectious Diseases*, vol. 16, no. 5, pp. 606–617, 2016.

[20] S. P. Hammond, K. Chen, A. Pandit, M. S. Davids, N. C. Issa, and F. M. Marty, "Risk of hepatitis B virus reactivation in patients treated with ibrutinib," *Blood*, vol. 131, no. 17, pp. 1987–1989, 2018.

19

Aplastic Anemia and Good Syndrome in a Heavily Treated Stage IV Thymoma Patient: A Case Report and Review of the Literature

Sofia Chiatamone Ranieri,[1] Stefania Trasarti,[1] Maria Antonietta Arleo,[1] Luisa Bizzoni,[1] Livia Bonanni,[2] Valeria Di Battista,[3] Maria Assunta Limongiello,[1] Maria Grazia Nardacci,[1] Giuseppe Gentile,[1] and Robin Foà[1]

[1]*Department of Translational and Precision Medicine, University of Rome "Sapienza", Rome, Italy*
[2]*Department of Molecular Medicine, University of Rome "Sapienza", Rome, Italy*
[3]*Department of Medicine, Center of Hemato-Oncology Research (C.R.E.O.), University of Perugia, Perugia, Italy*

Correspondence should be addressed to Stefania Trasarti; trasarti@bce.uniroma1.it

Academic Editor: Sergio Storti

Thymoma is an uncommon slowly growing neoplasm. It usually presents with paraneoplastic syndromes including the immunodeficiency syndrome called Good syndrome and hematological disorders. Pure red cell aplasia is a well-recognized complication of thymoma, and aplastic anemia is very rare in association with GS. We report a case of GS in a heavily treated patient with stage IV thymoma associated with a pure red cell aplasia and an amegakaryocytic thrombocytopenia that evolved into an AA and provide an up-to-date review of the relevant literature. This is the first case of the association of GS and AA with the coexistence of a heavily treated stage IV thymoma. The fatal outcome was not related to the progression of the thymoma, but rather to the severe infectious complications. The combination of lymphopenia and hypogammaglobulinemia typical of GS, coupled to the neutropenia, caused by bone marrow failure, was the main predisposing factor for the unfavourable outcome.

1. Case Presentation

In October 2015, a 53-year-old man was admitted to our hospital due to an incidental finding of severe anemia. The patient had a long medical history of thymoma (B2/B3) started in 1981 with pleural and lymphatic metastatic repetitions and Masaoka stage IVb and received chemo-, immuno-, and radiotherapy following multiple recurrences. He underwent five surgical excisions and five traditional lines of chemotherapy associated with radiotherapy to the mediastinum and paravertebral tissue. Due to the progression of the disease, he was enrolled in different experimental protocols including receptor radionuclide therapy with somatostatin analogue, sorafenib, volasertib, nintedanib, and everolimus. From October 2013, he started a maintenance treatment with low-dose cyclophosphamide plus octeotride. Periodic CT/PET scans showed a stable disease with paracostal, paracardiac, paravertebral, and paramediastinic residual metastatic nodules.

When the patient was admitted to our institute (October 2015), the complete blood count was as follows: red blood cells 2.08×10^{12}/L, hemoglobin 6.9 g/dL, mean corpuscular volume 95 fL, mean hemoglobin concentration 34.1 g/dL, white blood cells 6.7×10^{9}/L (neutrophils 51% and lymphocytes 7%), platelets 447×10^{9}/L, and reticulocyte count 0.2%. Serologies and DNA tests were negative for viral infections (CMV, EBV, HIV, and Parvovirus). No immunological abnormalities were detected, except for positive antiacetylcholine receptor antibodies and reduced levels of immunoglobulin isotypes IgG, IgA, and IgM. A bone marrow aspirate and biopsy revealed a virtually absent erythropoiesis with a preserved granulocytic and megakaryocytic maturation without infiltration by thymocytes and CD1a + lymphocytes (Figure 1-2015). A myelodysplastic

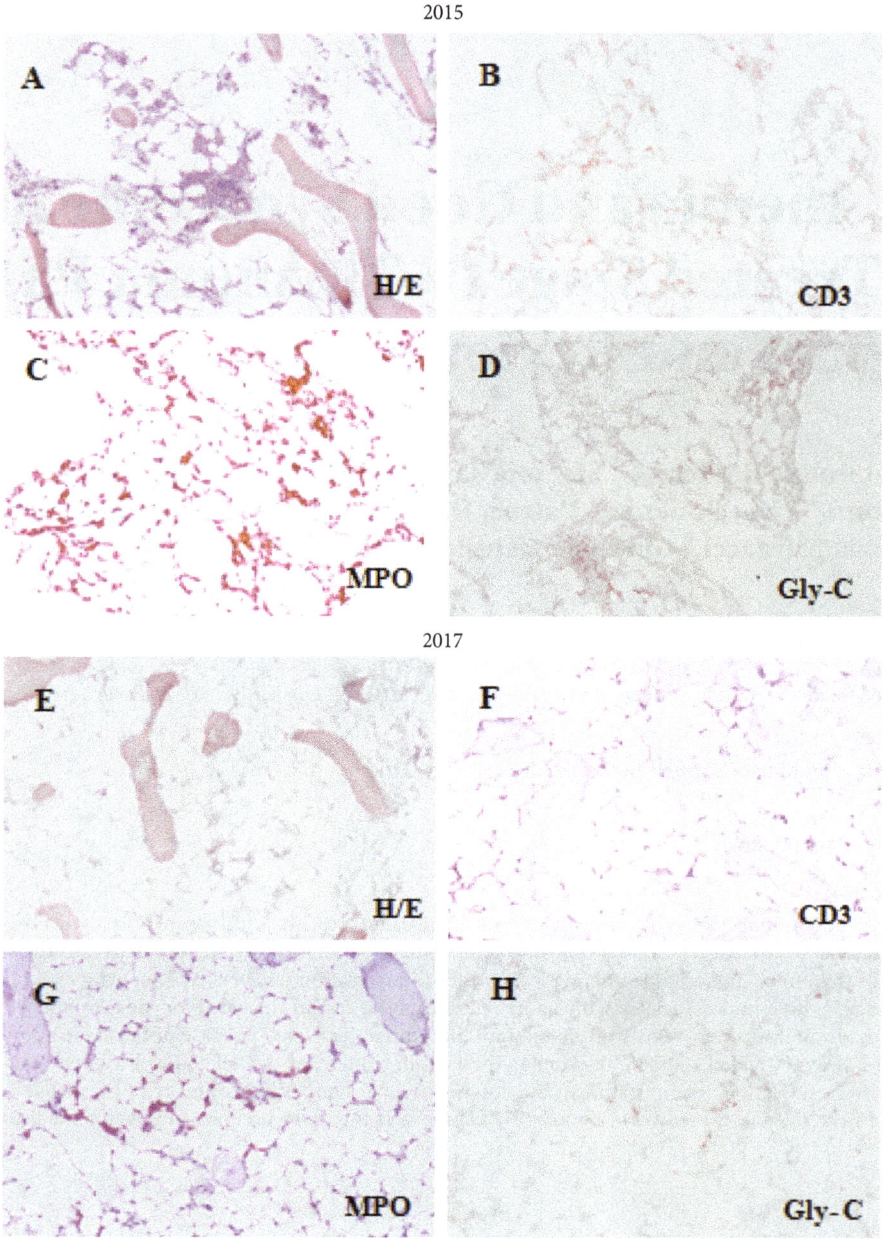

FIGURE 1: Histopathological images of the bone marrow (magnification 10x). (a) Biopsy section obtained on October 2015 showing a hypocellular bone marrow with preserved megakaryopoiesis (hematoxylin and eosin stain). (c) Myeloperoxidase staining revealed adequate numbers of myeloid cells. (d) Glycophorin C staining revealed a virtually absent erythropoiesis. (e) Biopsy section obtained on March 2017 revealed a severe hypocellular marrow (<5%) (hematoxylin and eosin stain). (g) Myeloperoxidase staining revealed a virtually absent myelopoiesis. (h) Glycophorin C staining revealed a virtually absent erythropoiesis. (b and f) In both biopsies, immunohistochemical stain for CD3 revealed a modest lymphoid component with interstitial distribution (CD3+).

syndrome was excluded by morphological evaluation, cytogenetic analysis, and mutational analysis, which revealed a normal karyotype and the absence of EZH2, GATA2, and TET2 mutations [1]. We also searched for rare mutations associated to sideroblastic anemia such as TRNT1. On this basis, we excluded the diagnosis of congenital sideroblastic anemia.

The study of the peripheral blood lymphocyte subpopulations showed the absence of B lymphocytes and an inversion of the CD4/CD8 ratio within the sCD3+ T lymphocytes, without a clonal restriction. Based on these findings, a diagnosis of PRCA associated to GS was made [2]. Cyclophosphamide was discontinued, and the patient remained on octeotride. The patient started supportive therapy with weekly blood transfusions, subcutaneous gammaglobulin (IG) infusions every three weeks, and erythropoietin and prednisone 75 mg daily. The last two drugs were suspended after 2 months due to lack of response. In May 2016, the patient developed a severe thrombocytopenia (platelets 15×10^9/L). A bone marrow aspirate revealed a new marked reduction in megakaryocytes, and data were compatible with a diagnosis of AATP

[3]. Treatment with high-dose ivIG (1gr/Kg) and steroids was started, which was followed by a slow and partial response that persisted for 9 months. Unfortunately, in February 2017, the patient showed again a severe thrombocytopenia (platelets 20×10^9/L), unresponsive to steroids and high-dose ivIG. After Institutional Ethical Committee approval, eltrombopag was started as compassionate therapy at 50 mg daily dose and thereafter increased to 100 mg daily. After 4 weeks, the patient presented a marked neutropenia, and a bone marrow biopsy showed a final evolution to AA (Figure 1-2017).

Treatment with growth factors was initiated without benefit. The patient was not considered eligible to transplant because of the persistent thymoma and severe immunodepression due to GS and previous multiple chemotherapic treatment, so antithymocyte globulin was proposed [4]. After the prephase treatment with high-dose steroids, the patient developed a digestive bleeding associated to an invasive aspergillosis with fever and a severe hemorrhagic cystitis. The patient finally died of infectious complications.

2. Discussion and Conclusions

To our knowledge, this is the first case of the association of GS and AA with the coexistence of a heavily treated stage IV thymoma. GS is a rare association of thymoma and immunodeficiency first described more than 50 years ago. It is defined by low or absent B-cells in the peripheral blood, hypogammaglobulinemia and (in some cases) defects in cell-mediated immunity (CD4 + T lymphopenia and an inverted CD4 + /CD8 + T-cell ratio), and susceptibility to infections [2]. PRCA, thought to be due to T-cell-mediated destruction of erythroid progenitor cells, is reported in 2% of patients with thymoma and is characterized by anemia, reticulocytopenia, and severe bone marrow erythroid hypoplasia [2]. AATP is a rare immune-mediated disorder characterized by thrombocytopenia resulting from an unexplained reduction in the number of bone marrow megakaryocytes in the presence of an otherwise normal hematopoiesis. The exact prevalence of amegakaryocytic thrombocytopenia is unknown. The available literature comprises case reports and small case series [5]. AA is an uncommon complication of thymic tumors (0–1.4%). It is characterized by bone marrow failure. Treatment of PRCA, AATP, and AA is based on immunosuppressive drugs; there is, however, no consensus on the optimal therapeutic strategy [2, 4, 5]. The association of GS, PRCA, and AATP evolving into an AA is extremely rare. There is a series of cases reported with a concomitant PRCA and GS [6], cases of thymoma with AA [7], and 7 cases of PRCA and AATP [3, 8–13], 3 of which progressed to AA [3, 8, 9], but never with evidence of a GS.

Very few cases of AA in GS have been described in the literature with many of them being associated with benign spindle cell tumors [14–16], different from our case (Table 1). In 3/6 cases, the diagnosis of GS and AA was simultaneous with the diagnosis of thymoma [14, 15, 18], and in 1 case, thymectomy was performed but without remission of the AA [14]. In 2 cases, the diagnosis of GS associated with a PRCA which then evolved into an AA was made years after the onset of the thymoma [16, 17]; in one of the 2 cases, surgery and local chemotherapy instillations were carried out after the onset of anemia, but they were ineffective for aplasia although there was no recurrence of thymoma [17]; and in the other case, there are insufficient data to define the state of the illness [16]. Five of the 6 cases died of infectious and hemorrhagic or thrombotic complications. In the more recently described case of pancytopenia, this appeared three years after thymectomy and without evidence of cancer recurrence, and the patient responded to eltrombopag [19].

In a recent review of AA and thymoma, cyclosporine therapy, both either alone or in combination with other agents such as ATG and G-CSF, was associated with a response rate of 66.6% [7]. Furthermore, there are 4 reports which have described patients who underwent an allogenic hematopoietic stem cell transplantation for aplastic anemia, 2 of which with metastatic thymoma, nobody with GS. All showed a good response [8, 20–22]. Considering the refractoriness of the tumor, in our case the administration of immunosuppressive agents to prevent tumor progression was excluded [23]; unfortunately, the response to corticosteroids and high-dose iv IG was ineffective for the PRCA and partially effective for the AATP and failed to contain the progression to AA.

ATG was proposed, but the patient died after the prephase treatment due to invasive aspergillosis. In view of the promising results obtained in AA [24] and in a case of GS with pancytopenia [19], we attempted to use eltrombopag, but could not assess its effectiveness due to the short time of administration. The prognosis of GS is considered worse than that of other primary immunodeficiencies, with an overall mortality rate of 46% [2].

The combination of lymphopenia and hypogammaglobulinemia typical of GS, coupled to the neutropenia, caused by bone marrow failure, was the main predisposing factor for the poor outcome of our patient [25].

In the literature, there have been 30 cases of AATP without significant comorbidities and autoimmune disease that have also shown a rapid progression to AA [26]. The rapid progression of AATP to AA in these cases suggests that thymoma-associated AATP may have a more aggressive disease course than thymoma-associated PRCA. In our case, the previous and prolonged chemo-, radio-, and immunotreatment could have caused a severe immunodepression with an acquired immunodeficiency syndrome (as observed, for example, in patients transplanted or subjected to long-term immunosuppressive treatments) associated with clonal/dysplastic changes responsible for the aplasia as observed in our patient. For this reason, our first goal was to exclude a myelodysplastic syndrome secondary to chemotherapy and radiotherapy treatments: no morphological changes suggestive of MDS were observed, the karyotype was normal, and also the mutations associated with myelodysplasia and rare forms of sideroblastic anemia associated with immunodeficiency such as TET2, GATA2, TRNT1, were negative.

On the other hand, the presence in the bone marrow of an expansion of T lymphocytes in the absence of clonality, the inversion of the CD4/CD8 ratio observed at the time of immunophenotyping, and the selective absence of B lymphocytes associated with the presence of selective red

Table 1: All reported cases of concomitant Good syndrome and aplastic anemia. The table is divided into seven horizontal rows illustrating reported cases including ours and twelve vertical columns illustrating literature, patient age and sex, disease progression, year of presentation of AA in relation to the diagnosis of thymoma, type of thymoma according to available WHO or traditional classification, bone marrow histology, information on serum immunoglobulins and lymphocyte subtypes, related manifestations, information on treatment received for thymoma, treatment for AA, and outcome and cause of death.

Report	Age (years) sex	Disease progression	Aplastic anemia and diagnosis of thymoma	Thymoma histology and stage	Bone marrow	Gammaglobulin and lymphocytes	Related features	Therapy for thymoma	Therapy for AA	Outcome	Cause of death
Chapin [16]	67 M	PRCA[1], GS[2], aplastic anemia	10 years after the onset of thymoma	Spindle cell thymoma	Aplasia with lymphoid infiltrate	Hypogamma	Na	None	Steroids	Death	Hemorrhage
Korn et al. [17]	75 M	GS[2]+ agenerative anemia, pancytopenia	7 years after the onset of thymoma	Mixed thymoma with plasmacytoid cells locally invasive	Aplasia + aggregates of mature lymphocytes	Hypogamma and severe impairment of cell immunity	Anti-AchR+[‡]	Surgery and nitrogen mustard instillation after the onset of anemia	Steroids and hormones	Death	Pulmonary embolus
Rogers et al. [14]	60 F	GS[2]+ aplastic anemia	Simultaneous	Spindle cell encapsulated thymoma	Marked hyopoplasia + few lymphocytes and plasma cells	Hypogamma	Ana+[†]	Surgery after the onset of anemia	Steroids and hormones	Death	Pneumonia and sepsis
Burrows and Carroll [15]	90 M	GS[2]+ aplastic anemia	Simultaneous	Spindle cell locally invasive	Marked hypoplasia + aggregates mature lymphocytes	Slightly hypogamma	None	None	Steroids	Death	Sepsis
Mir et al. [18]	68 M	GS[2]+ aplastic anemia	Simultaneous	Na	Hypoplasia	Hypogamma and lymphopenia	Na	None	Na	Death	Na
Kristiansen et al. [19]	61 M	GS[2], pancytopenia	3 years after the onset of thymoma	Na	Hypoplasia + *T* lymphocytosis	Hypogamma CD4/CD8 inverted	None	Surgery before the onset of aplastic anemia	ATG[α], steroids, CSA[β], CTX[γ], ivIG[δ], G-CSF[ε], eltrombopag	Response to eltrombopag + G-CSF#	
Our case	53 M	GS[2], PRCA[1], AATP[3], aplastic anemia	34 years after the onset of thymoma	Thymoma B2-B3 IV stage	Aplasia with modest lymphoid infiltrate	Hypogamma CD4/CD8 inverted absent B lymphocytes	Anti-AchR+[‡]	Surgery radiation and chemotherapy before the onset of aplastic anemia	Steroids, ivIG[δ], G CSF[ε], eltrombopag	Death	Sepsis

Na: not available; 1 PRCA: pure red cell aplasia; 2 GS: Good syndrome; 3 AATP: amegakaryocytic thrombocytopenia; [†]Ana+: antinuclear antibodies positive; [‡]AchR+: acetylcholine receptor *antibodies positive*; [α]ATG: antithymocyte globulin; [β]CSA: cyclosporine; [γ]CTX: cyclophosphamide; [δ]ivIG: intravenous gammaglobulin; [ε]G-CSF: granulocyte colony-stimulating factor.

series aplasia led us to believe that it was a paraneoplastic picture of altered maturation and disreactivity of autoimmune T lymphocytes. Before our clinical evaluation, we had no evidence of an immunoglobulin dosage, so we could not date the onset of Good syndrome. We only know that the patient has never had serious infections during previous treatments.

Every time a recurrence of the thymic disease occurred in our patient, therapy was immediately started (chemotherapy, radiotherapy, or immunotherapy) and complete remission was readily observed. Instead, at the time of our evaluation, the patient presented with a persistent although stable thymic-metastatic disease for at least 2 years, in maintenance with octeotride and cyclophosphamide. Therefore, it is assumed that the persistence of the thymic disease resulted in secondary pathologies such as PRCA, than evolved in AA and GS.

Our case highlights the challenging issue of treating a young fit patient with GS and AA, for whom, to date, we have no effective therapeutic tools. We describe this case not only for its rarity, but also for the complexity of the clinical management in an attempt to improve our understanding of this difficult-to-treat entity.

Abbreviations

Na: Not available
†Ana+: Antinuclear antibodies positive
‡AchR+: Acetylcholine receptor antibodies positive
$^{\alpha}$ATG: Antithymocyte globulin
$^{\beta}$CSA: Cyclosporine
$^{\gamma}$CTX: Cyclophosphamide
$^{\delta}$ivIG: Intravenous gammaglobulin
$^{\varepsilon}$G-CSF: Granulocyte colony-stimulating factor
AA: Aplastic anemia
GS: Good syndrome
AATP: Amegakaryocytic thrombocytopenia
PRCA: Pure red cell aplasia
CT/PET: Computed tomography/positron emission tomography
CMV: Cytomegalovirus
EBV: Epstein–barr virus
HIV: Human Immunodeficiency virus
ATG: Antithymocyte globulin.

Consent

Written informed consent was obtained from the patient's next-of-kin for publication of this case report and any accompanying images. A copy of the written consent is available for review by the editor-in-chief of this journal.

Authors' Contributions

Stefania Trasarti conceptualized the study. Stefania Trasarti and Sofia Chiatamone Ranieri designed the study. Stefania Trasarti, Sofia Chiatamone Ranieri, Maria Antonietta Arleo, Maria Assunta Limongiello, Maria Grazia Nardacci, and Valeria Di Battista acquired the data. Stefania Trasarti, Sofia Chiatamone Ranieri, and Giuseppe Gentile analyzed and interpreted the data. Stefania Trasarti and Sofia Chiatamone Ranieri prepared the manuscript. Stefania Trasarti and Giuseppe Gentile edited the manuscript. Giuseppe Gentile and Robin Foà reviewed the manuscript.

References

[1] M. Haider, E. J. Duncavage, K. F. Afaneh, R. Bejar, and A. F. List, "New insight into the biology, risk stratification, and targeted treatment of myelodysplastic syndromes," *American Society of Clinical Oncology Educational Book*, vol. 37, pp. 480–494, 2017.

[2] C. Bernard, H. Frih, F. Pasquet et al., "Thymoma associated with autoimmune diseases: 85 cases and literature review," *Autoimmunity Reviews*, vol. 15, no. 1, pp. 82–92, 2016.

[3] I. Maslovsky, D. Gefel, L. Uriev, D. Ben Dor, and G. Lugassy, "Malignant thymoma complicated by amegakaryocytic thrombocytopenic purpura," *European Journal of Internal Medicine*, vol. 16, no. 7, pp. 523-524, 2005.

[4] E. Di Bona, F. Rodeghiero, B. Bruno et al., "Rabbit antithymocyte globulin (r-ATG) plus cyclosporine and granulocyte colony stimulating factor is an effective treatment for aplastic anaemia patients unresponsive to a first course of intensive immunosuppressive therapy," *British Journal of Haematology*, vol. 107, no. 2, pp. 330–334, 1999.

[5] N. Agarwal, J. E. Spahr, T. L. Werner, D. L. Newton, and G. M. Rodgers, "Acquired amegakaryocytic thrombocytopenic purpura," *American Journal of Hematology*, vol. 81, no. 2, pp. 132–135, 2006.

[6] T. Kelesidis and O. Yang, "Good's syndrome remains a mystery after 55 years: a systematic review of the scientific evidence," *Clinical Immunology*, vol. 135, no. 3, pp. 347–363, 2010.

[7] A. V. Chintakuntlawar, S. A. Rizvi, S. D. Cassivi, and A. Pardanani, "Thymoma-associated pancytopenia: immunosuppressive therapy is the cornerstone for durable hematological remission," *Annals of Hematology*, vol. 94, no. 3, pp. 453–458, 2015.

[8] A. Simkins, A. Maiti, N. J. Short et al., "Acquired amegakaryocytic thrombocytopenia and red cell aplasia in a patient with thymoma progressing to aplastic anemia successfully treated with allogenic stem cell transplantation," *Hematology/Oncology and Stem Cell Therapy*, vol. 12, no. 2, pp. 115–118, 2019.

[9] S. Dahal, E. Sharma, S. Dahal, B. Shrestha, and B. Bhattarai, "Acquired amegakaryocytic thrombocytopenia and pure red cell aplasia in thymoma," *Case Reports in Hematology*, vol. 2018, Article ID 5034741, 3 pages, 2018.

[10] A. R. Cho, Y. J. Cha, H. R. Kim, E. K. Park, and E.-J. Cha, "Acquired amegakaryocytic thrombocytopenia after thymectomy in a case of pure red cell aplasia associated with thymoma," *The Korean Journal of Laboratory Medicine*, vol. 30, no. 3, pp. 244–248, 2010.

[11] C. M. Gay, W. N. William Jr., S. A. Wang, and T. H. Oo, "Thymoma complicated by acquired amegakaryocytic thrombocytopenia and pure red cell aplasia," *Journal of the National Comprehensive Cancer Network*, vol. 12, no. 11, pp. 1505–1509, 2014.

[12] A. Fujiwara, M. Inoue, H. Kusumoto, Y. Shintani, T. Maeda, and M. Okumura, "Myasthenic crisis caused by preoperative

chemotherapy with steroid for advanced thymoma," *The Annals of Thoracic Surgery*, vol. 99, no. 1, pp. e11–e13, 2015.
[13] T. Onuki, Y. Kiyoki, S. Ueda, M. Yamaoka, S. Shimizu, and M. Inagaki, "Invasive thymoma with pure red cell aplasia and amegakaryocytic Thrombocytopenia," *Hematology Reports*, vol. 8, no. 4, p. 6680, 2016.
[14] B. H. G. Rogers, J. R. Manaligod, and W. V. Blazer, "Thymoma associated with pancytopenia and hypogammaglobulinemia," *The American Journal of Medicine*, vol. 44, no. 1, pp. 154–164, 1968.
[15] S. Burrows and R. Carroll, "Thymoma associated with pancytopenia," *Archives of pathology*, vol. 92, no. 6, pp. 465–468, 1971.
[16] M. A. Chapin, "Benign thymoma, refractory anemia and hypogammaglobulinemia—case report," *The Journal of the Maine Medical Association*, vol. 56, pp. 83–87, 1965.
[17] D. Korn, A. Gelderman, G. Cage, D. Nathanson, and A. J. L. Strauss, "Immune deficiencies, aplastic anemia and abnormalities of lymphoid tissue in thymoma," *New England Journal of Medicine*, vol. 276, no. 24, pp. 1333–1339, 1967.
[18] M. A. Mir, C. G. Geary, and I. W. Delamore, "Hypoimmunoglobulinaemia and aplastic anaemia," *Scandinavian Journal of Haematology*, vol. 19, no. 3, pp. 225–229, 1977.
[19] H. A. Kristiansen, S. Fløisand, Y. Fløisand, and D. Heldal, "Eltrombopag in good's syndrome," *Case Reports in Hematology*, vol. 2014, Article ID 172139, 3 pages, 2014.
[20] V. Trisal, A. Nademanee, S. K. Lau, and F. W. Grannis Jr., "Thymoma-associated severe aplastic anemia treated with surgical resection followed by allogeneic stem-cell transplantation," *Journal of Clinical Oncology*, vol. 25, no. 22, pp. 3374-3375, 2007.
[21] A. Numata, K. Yasuda, T. Fukuda et al., "Non-myeloablative allogeneic haemopoietic stem-cell transplantation for treatment of metastatic invasive thymoma," *The Lancet Oncology*, vol. 6, no. 8, pp. 626–628, 2005.
[22] C. Lu, G.-S. He, S. Jin et al., "Haploidentical allogeneic hematopoietic stem cell transplantation for thymoma-associated severe aplastic anemia: a case report," *Chinese Medical Sciences Journal*, vol. 28, no. 3, pp. 189–191, 2013.
[23] A. Gaglia, A. Bobota, E. Pectasides, C. Kosmas, G. Papaxoinis, and D. Pectasides, "Successful treatment with cyclosporine of thymoma-related aplastic anemia," *Anticancer Research*, vol. 27, no. 4C, pp. 3025–3028, 2007.
[24] M. J. Olnes, P. Scheinberg, K. R. Calvo et al., "Eltrombopag and improved hematopoiesis in refractory aplastic anemia," *New England Journal of Medicine*, vol. 367, no. 1, pp. 11–19, 2012.
[25] C. Rivoisy, B. Besse, N. Girard et al., "Thymic epithelial tumor-associated cytopenia: a 10-year observational study in France," *Journal of Thoracic Oncology*, vol. 11, no. 3, pp. 391–399, 2016.
[26] J. P. Novotný, B. Köhler, R. Max, and G. Egerer, "Acquired amegakaryocytic thrombocytopenic purpura progressing into aplastic anemia," *Prague Medical Report*, vol. 118, no. 4, pp. 147–155, 2017.

20

Symptomatic Hypoalbuminemia as an Indication for Treatment of Waldenström Macroglobulinemia: A Case Report and Review of the Literature

Jeremy T. Larsen[1] **and Frederick D. Leonard**[2]

[1]*Division of Hematology and Medical Oncology, Mayo Clinic, Phoenix, Arizona, USA*
[2]*International Waldenstrom's Macroglobulinemia Foundation (IWMF), Sarasota, Florida, USA*

Correspondence should be addressed to Frederick D. Leonard; fdleonard@cableone.net

Academic Editor: Håkon Reikvam

Hypoalbuminemia has been reported as common in patients with symptomatic Waldenström macroglobulinemia (WM), but it is not typically mentioned as a manifestation of the disease in review articles or articles discussing indications for treatment. We present the case of a patient with WM for whom symptomatic hypoalbuminemia was the primary reason for initiating treatment. Except in rare cases of WM with renal or gastrointestinal involvement, hypoalbuminemia is thought to be due to the effects of elevated levels of inflammation-associated cytokines, and it has been associated with greater likelihood of progression of asymptomatic to symptomatic disease, greater disease severity, and poorer prognosis. Hypoalbuminemia in WM may become symptomatic, and it may be a reason to initiate treatment if symptoms affect quality of life.

1. Introduction

Waldenström macroglobulinemia (WM) is a B-cell lymphoproliferative disorder characterized by bone marrow infiltration with lymphoplasmacytic cells that secrete monoclonal immunoglobulin M (IgM). Its clinical manifestations can involve virtually any organ system since disease effects are due to both cellular infiltration and circulating IgM.

There is currently no cure for WM, so treatment is initiated when the disease becomes life-threatening or symptoms significantly affect quality of life. Suggested indications for treatment include symptomatic anemia with hemoglobin less than 10 g/dL; thrombocytopenia less than 100×10^9/L; symptomatic lymphadenopathy or hepatosplenomegaly; symptomatic hyperviscosity; symptomatic cryoglobulinemia, cold agglutinins, autoimmune-related events, or amyloidosis; moderate to severe peripheral neuropathy; constitutional symptoms (high fever, drenching sweats, significant weight loss, and severe fatigue); and symptomatic central nervous system involvement (Bing–Neel syndrome) [1, 2].

Not mentioned in the literature as an indication for treatment is symptomatic hypoalbuminemia. We present the case of a patient with WM for whom this was the primary reason for initiating treatment.

2. Case Presentation

A 66-year-old physician saw his internist for a routine annual visit. Over the previous six months, he had noted some decreased stamina while riding his mountain bike, but he was otherwise without symptoms. His exam was unremarkable, but initial laboratory studies showed a hemoglobin of 12.5 g/dL (reference value 13.2–16.6 g/dL) and an elevated total protein. Additional testing demonstrated an M spike of 2.4 g/dL. Albumin was low-normal at 3.5 g/dL (reference value 3.5–5.0 g/dL). A year prior, his hemoglobin and albumin had been within the normal range at 14.2 g/dL and 3.9 g/dL, respectively. In retrospect, these were both trending downward compared to previous results, and his hemoglobin had historically been significantly higher (15-16 g/dL) since he was quite physically fit and lived at 5,000 ft. elevation.

He was referred to our institution for further evaluation. A bone marrow biopsy, including cytogenetics, fluorescence in situ hybridization (FISH), and flow cytometry, was consistent with a diagnosis of WM with 70% bone marrow involvement by lymphoplasmacytic cells. Serum protein electrophoresis and immunofixation demonstrated an M spike of 2.1 g/dL with IgM kappa monoclonal protein. Quantitative IgM was 3,760 mg/dL (reference value 37–286 mg/dL), and hemoglobin was 12.7 g/dL. C-reactive protein (CRP) was 14.7 mg/L (reference range ≤8.0 mg/L). Lactate dehydrogenase and a comprehensive metabolic panel were normal with the exception of elevated total protein and slightly elevated alkaline phosphatase. Albumin was 3.7 g/dL. Twenty-four-hour urine protein was 269 mg (reference value <229 mg/24 h) of which 14% was albumin. Also present was an M spike of 111 mg/24 h. Follow-up a month later showed little change, and he was continued with evaluation and laboratory monitoring every three months. This included complete blood count, comprehensive metabolic panel, lactate dehydrogenase, serum viscosity, serum protein electrophoresis, quantitative serum immunoglobulins, serum free light chains, and erythrocyte sedimentation rate (later replaced with CRP).

At nine months after diagnosis his hemoglobin was 12.2 g/dL, IgM was 4,010 mg/dL, and albumin remained low-normal at 3.5 g/dL. He had seen his internist for evaluation of mild gynecomastia, and that evaluation showed a low free testosterone level. Based on a case report of a patient with WM who had improvement of both his anemia and IgM after being treated for low testosterone [3], he opted to start a trial of topical testosterone at a dose titrated to maintain his free and total testosterone within the normal range. His hemoglobin increased over the next six months to 13.4 g/dL though there was no significant change in his IgM or albumin levels.

By 2½ years after diagnosis, his hemoglobin and albumin had decreased to 12.1 g/dL and 3.1 g/dL, respectively. He had developed mild bilateral dependent edema that was noticeable toward the end of the day, mild inguinal adenopathy, and some intermittent myalgias and paresthesias/hyperesthesias. He had no fever, chills, or other constitutional symptoms, and he continued to exercise regularly. Iron studies had shown repeated low iron saturations that had failed to respond to oral iron. There was no evidence of blood loss, and a gastroenterology evaluation including colonoscopy was normal with the exception of four 2 mm adenomatous polyps that were resected. Because WM is associated with elevated hepcidin which interferes with iron absorption and utilization, and because parenteral iron has been reported to reverse both the low iron saturation and accompanying anemia [4], he was started on a trial of intravenous iron.

A month after his initial iron infusion, his hemoglobin had risen to 13.1 g/dL with an appropriate reticulocyte response. However, over the next six months despite stabilization of his anemia, he began to develop increasing lower extremity edema, nocturia, and more frequent and severe myalgias. All these symptoms significantly worsened in the month prior to initiating chemotherapy. The lower extremity edema was now accompanied by periorbital edema, and it was the symptom having the greatest impact on his quality of life and daily activities. By the time he started chemotherapy, his albumin had dropped to 2.4 g/dL, IgM had risen to 5,550 mg/dL, and hemoglobin remained stable at 12.9 g/dL.

The edema was generalized, bilateral, and symmetric. There was no venous insufficiency, venous congestion, or venous prominence to suggest proximal venous obstruction. His inguinal adenopathy did not change during the time his edema increased, and there was no hepatosplenomegaly or other adenopathy on exam. Imaging was not done to look for obstructing adenopathy since it was felt that the likelihood was low, it would not have explained his periorbital edema, and its presence would not have changed treatment. History, physical exam, and laboratory studies did not reveal any evidence of cardiac, gastrointestinal, or hepatic disease, and he had no gastrointestinal symptoms that might have suggested the possibility of a protein-losing enteropathy. His serum protein electrophoresis also did not suggest protein-losing enteropathy. Despite his increasing edema, his exercise tolerance remained well above average for age, and there were no symptoms of cardiopulmonary disease such as might be seen with amyloid involvement. There were also no other signs of amyloid on physical exam such as weight loss, ecchymosis, tongue enlargement, or shoulder pad sign. Other than his hypoalbuminemia and edema, he had no signs or symptoms to suggest nephrotic syndrome or other renal disease. His serum creatinine and estimated glomerular filtration rate had remained normal and stable since the time of his diagnosis, as had his blood pressure. His only medications were levothyroxine, which he had been on since the time of his WM diagnosis, and the topical testosterone previously described. His thyroid function studies were consistently within the normal range as were his testosterone levels on a relatively low dose of topical testosterone. He was on no over-the-counter medications or dietary supplements other than a daily multivitamin and calcium tablet.

He was treated with the combination of bendamustine and rituximab every four weeks, with the first cycle limited to bendamustine alone to avoid an IgM flare. During the week following his first treatment, he monitored his fluid status, recording daily weights and fluid intake and output. He diuresed over 5 liters of fluid; his weight decreased by 6 kilograms; and his peripheral edema resolved. A 24-hour urine protein study was collected prior to his second cycle of chemotherapy and showed a total protein of 132 mg/24 h of which 20% was albumin. The urine M spike was 39 mg/24 h. Serum albumin was 3.3 g/dL, IgM was 2,680 mg/dL, and hemoglobin was 13.3 g/dL. Three months after completing four cycles of chemotherapy, his albumin was 4.7 g/dL, hemoglobin was 16.8 g/dL, and IgM was 317 mg/dL. He was asymptomatic; he was on no medications except levothyroxine; his inguinal adenopathy had resolved; and his exercise capacity had returned to levels that exceeded those prior to his WM diagnosis. At two years after treatment, he remains asymptomatic with no evidence of gastrointestinal or renal disease and no progression of his WM. IgM is 254 mg/dL, CRP is <3.0 mg/L, and albumin and hemoglobin are stable at 4.6 g/dL and 16.5 g/dL, respectively.

3. Discussion

Albumin is the most abundant plasma protein in humans. It helps to maintain colloid osmotic pressure, it binds numerous endogenous and exogenous compounds, and it provides the bulk of plasma antioxidant activity. Measured albumin concentration is the net result of liver synthesis, tissue catabolism, renal and gastrointestinal losses, and any non-steady state albumin space shifts that may occur in acute conditions such as sepsis or trauma. Elevated levels of inflammation-associated cytokines are associated with both decreased synthesis and increased catabolism of albumin, and hypoalbuminemia is seen in a myriad of acute and chronic conditions. In these conditions, its presence has frequently been identified as a predictor of increased morbidity and mortality [5–9].

Peripheral edema is also seen in a wide variety of conditions. Anything that alters the delicate balance of intravascular and interstitial hydrostatic and osmotic pressures, or increases capillary permeability, can result in edema formation. Although albumin helps to maintain colloid osmotic pressure, low levels of albumin alone do not typically result in edema. However, when combined with alterations of hydrostatic pressure, as occurs with increased intravascular volume and altered venous or lymphatic return, or with increased capillary permeability, as occurs with local or systemic inflammation, edema results [7, 10].

In WM, hypoalbuminemia has been reported as associated with both more severe disease and poorer prognosis, and it has also been identified as frequently present in symptomatic WM patients and in patients requiring treatment for their disease [11–13]. In one report of a cohort of symptomatic WM patients, albumin <3.5 g/dL was found in 70% of patients identified as "poor risk" (patients who survived <2 years after the initiation of therapy) and in 45% of the remaining patients [14]. But unlike the more common malignant monoclonal gammopathy multiple myeloma, albumin level has not historically been used for prognostic scoring or staging in WM [1, 15]. However, a recent study identified an albumin of 3.5 g/dL or less as one of four independent predictors of progression of asymptomatic WM to symptomatic WM. The other three were IgM 4,500 mg/dL or greater, bone marrow lymphoplasmacytic infiltration 70% or greater, and $\beta 2$-microglobulin 4.0 mg/dL or greater. Using these four risk factors, the authors developed a validated risk model that categorizes patients as low, medium, or high risk based on median time to progression to symptomatic disease requiring treatment [16].

Despite these and other studies demonstrating a frequent association between hypoalbuminemia and WM, hypoalbuminemia is not typically identified as one of the manifestations of WM in review articles or in reference texts. It is also not identified as a factor to be considered in determining when to initiate treatment. This may be because gastrointestinal involvement, renal involvement, and nephrotic syndrome are rare in WM, and usually the result of amyloidosis, cryoglobulinemia, IgM or light chain deposition, or lymphoplasmacytic infiltration [17–20]. Yet most hypoalbuminemia seen in WM is not associated with these uncommon complications of WM, but is presumably due to the effects of elevated levels of inflammation-associated cytokines. This is consistent with what is seen in many other malignant and nonmalignant conditions in which acute and chronic inflammation are present [5–9].

This also appears to have been the case in our patient. The combination of his symptoms, physical findings, and laboratory results suggest that his WM resulted in a generalized inflammatory state that worsened as his disease progressed, and this inflammatory state did not resolve until his WM responded to treatment. This persistent inflammatory state likely resulted in a combination of hypoalbuminemia and increased capillary permeability that manifested as peripheral edema.

4. Conclusion

Hypoalbuminemia has been reported as common in patients with symptomatic WM, and it has recently been shown to be a risk factor for progression from asymptomatic to symptomatic disease requiring treatment. Despite this, it is not typically identified as a manifestation of WM in review articles or reference texts. As a result, clinicians seeing WM patients with hypoalbuminemia and edema might not attribute these findings to the disease but instead to other comorbid conditions commonly seen in the elderly population that is typical of WM. This case report and literature review illustrate that hypoalbuminemia is frequently associated with WM, it can improve when WM responds to treatment, and it should be included in lists of both the common and protean manifestations of the disease. Hypoalbuminemia may also become symptomatic, and it may be a reason to initiate treatment if symptoms affect quality of life.

References

[1] R. A. Kyle, S. M. Ansell, and P. Kapoor, "Prognostic factors and indications for treatment of Waldenström's macroglobulinemia," *Best Practice & Research Clinical Haematology*, vol. 29, no. 2, pp. 179–186, 2016.

[2] M. C. Minnema, E. Kimby, S. D'Sa et al., "Guideline for the diagnosis, treatment and response criteria for Bing-Neel syndrome," *Haematologica*, vol. 102, no. 1, pp. 43–51, 2017.

[3] L. F. Porrata and S. N. Markovic, "Androgenic therapy for Waldenstrom's macroglobulinemia," *American Journal of Hematology*, vol. 81, no. 11, pp. 892-893, 2006.

[4] S. P. Treon, C. K. Tripsas, B. T. Ciccarelli et al., "Patients with Waldenström macroglobulinemia commonly present with

iron deficiency and those with severely depressed transferrin saturation levels show response to parenteral iron administration," *Clinical Lymphoma Myeloma and Leukemia*, vol. 13, no. 2, pp. 241–243, 2013.
[5] C. Gabay and I. Kushner, "Acute-phase proteins and other systemic responses to inflammation," *New England Journal of Medicine*, vol. 340, no. 6, pp. 448–454, 1999.
[6] A. Gatta, A. Verardo, and M. Bolognesi, "Hypoalbuminemia," *Internal and Emergency Medicine*, vol. 7, no. S3, pp. 193–199, 2012.
[7] D. Levitt and M. Levitt, "Human serum albumin homeostasis: a new look at the roles of synthesis, catabolism, renal and gastrointestinal excretion, and the clinical value of serum albumin measurements," *International Journal of General Medicine*, vol. 9, pp. 229–255, 2016.
[8] D. Gupta and C. G. Lis, "Pretreatment serum albumin as a predictor of cancer survival: a systematic review of the epidemiological literature," *Nutrition Journal*, vol. 9, no. 1, p. 69, 2010.
[9] A. Akirov, H. Masri-Iraqi, A. Atamna, and I. Shimon, "Low albumin levels are associated with mortality risk in hospitalized patients," *The American Journal of Medicine*, vol. 130, no. 12, pp. 1465.e11–1465.e19, 2017.
[10] S. Cho and J. E. Atwood, "Peripheral edema," *The American Journal of Medicine*, vol. 113, no. 7, pp. 580–586, 2002.
[11] X. Cao, Q. Ye, R. Z. Orlowski et al., "Waldenström macroglobulinemia with extramedullary involvement at initial diagnosis portends a poorer prognosis," *Journal of Hematology & Oncology*, vol. 8, no. 1, p. 74, 2015.
[12] A. Anagnostopoulos, K. Zervas, M. C. Kyrtsonis et al., "Prognostic value of serum β2-microglobulin in patients with Waldenström's macroglobulinemia requiring treatment," *Clinical Lymphoma and Myeloma*, vol. 7, no. 3, pp. 205–209, 2006.
[13] M. A. Dimopoulos, A. Anagnostopoulos, M. C. Kyrtsonis et al., "Primary treatment of Waldenström macroglobulinemia with dexamethasone, rituximab, and cyclophosphamide," *Journal of Clinical Oncology*, vol. 25, no. 22, pp. 3344–3349, 2007.
[14] E. Kastritis, M. Gavriatopoulou, M. C. Kyrtsonis et al., "Prognostication of the high-risk WM patient," *Clinical Lymphoma Myeloma and Leukemia*, vol. 11, no. 1, pp. 127–129, 2011.
[15] A. Palumbo, H. Avet-Loiseau, S. Oliva et al., "Revised international staging system for multiple myeloma: a report from international myeloma working group," *Journal of Clinical Oncology*, vol. 33, no. 26, pp. 2863–2869, 2015.
[16] M. Bustoros, R. Sklavenitis-Pistofidis, P. Kapoor et al., "Progression risk stratification of asymptomatic Waldenström macroglobulinemia," *Journal of Clinical Oncology*, vol. 37, no. 16, pp. 1403–1411, 2019.
[17] K. W. Pratz, D. Dingli, T. C. Smyrk, and J. A. Lust, "Intestinal lymphangiectasia with protein-losing enteropathy in Waldenstrom macroglobulinemia," *Medicine*, vol. 86, no. 4, pp. 210–214, 2007.
[18] J. M. Vos, J. Gustine, H. G. Rennke et al., "Renal disease related to Waldenström macroglobulinaemia: incidence, pathology and clinical outcomes," *British Journal of Haematology*, vol. 175, no. 4, pp. 623–630, 2016.
[19] M. A. Gertz, G. Merlini, and S. P. Treon, "Amyloidosis and Waldenstrom's macroglobulinemia," *Hematology*, vol. 2004, no. 1, pp. 257–282, 2004.
[20] S. Zanwar, J. P. Abeykoon, S. M. Ansell et al., "Primary systemic amyloidosis in patients with Waldenström macroglobulinemia," *Leukemia*, vol. 33, no. 3, pp. 790–794, 2019.

Ibrutinib Plus R-ICE Induces Remission in Blastoid Variant Mantle Cell Lymphoma with CNS Relapse

Timothy S. Oh,[1] Madelyn Burkart,[2] Amir Behdad,[3] Hatice Savas,[4] and Reem Karmali[5]

[1]*Department of Medicine, Northwestern University Feinberg School of Medicine, Chicago, IL, USA*
[2]*Division of Hematology/Oncology, Robert H. Lurie Comprehensive Cancer Center of Northwestern University, Northwestern University Feinberg School of Medicine, Chicago, IL, USA*
[3]*Department of Pathology, Northwestern University Feinberg School of Medicine, Chicago, IL, USA*
[4]*Department of Radiology, Northwestern University Feinberg School of Medicine, Chicago, IL, USA*
[5]*Division of Hematology/Oncology, Robert H. Lurie Comprehensive Cancer Center of Northwestern University, Chicago, IL, USA*

Correspondence should be addressed to Reem Karmali; reem.karmali@northwestern.edu

Academic Editor: Pier Paolo Piccaluga

Mantle cell lymphoma (MCL) is an aggressive, difficult to treat subtype of lymphoma, resulting in relapses and poor outcomes. Novel agents such as Bruton tyrosine kinase (BTK) inhibitors have been studied in the treatment of relapsed/refractory (R/R) MCL. BTK inhibitor ibrutinib, in particular, has demonstrated improvement in survival outcomes of R/R MCL. Despite these advancements, many cases of MCL, including the more aggressive blastoid and pleomorphic variants, will undergo disease progression leading to poor survival outcomes. Blastoid variant MCL is associated with an increased risk of central nervous system (CNS) involvement, causing high mortality rates. In this case report, we discuss a patient with a diagnosis of blastoid MCL with CNS relapse who achieved a complete response (CR) after receiving standard rituximab plus ifosfamide-carboplatin-etoposide (R-ICE) salvage chemotherapy with the addition of ibrutinib. The patient subsequently underwent autologous stem cell transplantation (autoSCT) and maintained CR with ibrutinib maintenance.

1. Introduction

Mantle cell lymphoma (MCL) is an uncommon, aggressive subtype of non-Hodgkin lymphoma accounting for 3–10% of adult-onset lymphomas [1]. The common clinical course of MCL is characterized by recurrent relapses after initial therapy leading to poor survival outcomes, with a median survival of 4–5 years [2]. Current standard of care in fit patients broadly consists of three components: cytarabine-containing induction chemotherapy regimen followed by consolidation with autologous stem cell transplantation (autoSCT) and rituximab maintenance, while less fit patients receive less intensive therapy without autoSCT. There have been several novel agents studied for the treatment of relapsed/refractory (R/R) MCL including Bruton kinase (BTK) inhibitors. Ibrutinib, a first-generation BTK inhibitor, has shown notable improvement in survival outcomes in R/R MCL, with a 68% overall response rate when used as a single agent [3]. However, most patients will eventually progress, and survival remains poor for patients with high-risk disease features, including the aggressive morphologic variants (blastoid and pleomorphic variants), which comprise less than 20% of MCL cases [4].

Patients with blastoid variant MCL are at an increased risk for developing central nervous system (CNS) disease. CNS involvement in MCL is a rare, yet serious condition, and is known to have a high mortality rate with a median survival of 3.7 months [5]. It typically occurs later in the disease course during systemic relapse when treatment options are more limited. Prompt diagnosis and initiation of CNS-directed therapy is pertinent. We describe a case of blastoid MCL with CNS relapse demonstrating a complete response to treatment with the addition of ibrutinib to standard R-ICE salvage chemotherapy. Our patient was consolidated with an autoSCT and maintains response to ibrutinib maintenance therapy [6].

2. Case Presentation

Our patient is a 60-year-old male with no significant past medical history who presented with three weeks of worsening left-sided abdominal pain and a large, mobile right neck mass. He had no B-symptoms on presentation. Laboratory evaluation was significant for leukocytosis of 59.3 (cells/L) with a differential of largely atypical lymphocytes (Figure 1(a)) and LDH elevated to 1246 (IU/L). CT neck/chest/abdomen/pelvis showed diffuse lymphadenopathy (LAD) with marked splenomegaly, concerning lymphoma. A right cervical lymph node biopsy revealed a diagnosis of blastoid variant MCL, further characterized as cyclin-D1 negative, SOX-11 positive, and p53 negative with a Ki-67 index of approximately 90% (Figure 1(b)–1(f)). Bone marrow biopsy revealed MCL, blastoid variant, with 70–80% involvement. Mantel cell lymphoma international prognostic index (MIPI) score was 7.5, consistent with high-risk disease.

Staging PET/CT revealed diffuse hypermetabolic LAD above and below the diaphragm as well as known splenomegaly. The patient was treated with 6 cycles of rituximab plus cyclophosphamide, vincristine, doxorubicin, and dexamethasone (R-HyperCVAD) with intrathecal (IT) methotrexate (MTX). After 4 cycles, interim bone marrow biopsy showed no evidence of disease and interim PET/CT was consistent with complete response (CR). An autologous SCT after completion of induction chemotherapy was planned. However, 6 weeks after completion of therapy, the patient began experiencing double vision and facial paresthesias. A lumbar puncture was performed and showed elevated protein (>200 mg/dL) with negative cytometry and cytopathology for lymphoma. An MRI brain/orbits did not demonstrate signs of leptomeningeal disease or obvious abnormality to explain symptoms, but an MRI of the spine showed lumbar enhancement concerning disease involvement (Figure 2(a)). Two repeat cerebrospinal fluid (CSF) evaluations were similar to prior results, demonstrating elevated protein but negative cytometry and cytopathology. An autoimmune and infectious workup was negative. Given the CSF results and concerning MRI findings with known high-risk blastoid MCL, the patient was treated for presumed secondary CNS involvement with the addition of ibrutinib 560 mg daily to CNS-directed salvage chemotherapy with three cycles of R-ICE with IT MTX. The only complication of salvage therapy was IT MTX-induced myelopathy noted on the MRI spine. MTX was discontinued, and the patient completed a dexamethasone taper along with memantine with improvement in symptoms. No toxicities related to ibrutinib were noted. Repeat MRI spine after completion of therapy demonstrated CR (Figure 2(b)) with the resolution of symptoms and repeat PET/CT imaging showed CR2.

The patient underwent autoSCT with myeloablative busulfan and thiotepa conditioning after achieving a CR2. Ibrutinib was held during the peritransplant period. Post-transplant course was complicated by prolonged pancytopenia secondary to chemotherapy, for which the patient received granulocyte colony-stimulating factor (G-CSF) to assist with count recovery as well as intravenous immunoglobulin (IVIG).

Ibrutinib was resumed on day 46 post-transplant after count recovery. Reimaging on day 95 showed CR, and no enhancement was noted on MRI spine imaging. Currently, the patient continues ibrutinib 560 mg daily without any dose adjustments and has tolerated this well, with the only complication of ibrutinib being thrombocytopenia. The patient is now 31 months post-transplant and continues to be in CR.

3. Discussion

Management of relapsing CNS disease in MCL patients remains a challenging task. Currently, there is no consensus on standard treatment. Ibrutinib, however, has been a key focus in treatment and has been shown to be efficacious as a single-agent therapy. A 2013 phase 2 study, for example, demonstrated a response rate of 68%, estimated median response duration of 17.5 months, and estimated median progression-free survival (PFS) of 13.9 months in R/R MCL [3]. Of particular importance is the ability of ibrutinib to cross the blood-brain barrier to target CNS relapse, as demonstrated in prior pharmacokinetic studies [7].

Prior case reports have also shown promising outcomes by using ibrutinib in relapsing MCL patients with CNS involvement. A 2015 report of 3 patients with symptomatic CNS relapse showed rapid response after initiating ibrutinib as a single agent at a standard dose of 560 mg/d [8]. Clinical response times were noted after 3 days to 1 week after initiation of therapy. Two of the patients achieved CR at 9 months to 1 year while the third patient showed partial response (PR) at 2 months. A 2017 report of a patient with symptomatic CNS relapse also showed promising results with ibrutinib monotherapy (dose reduced to 280 mg/d in the setting of recurrent atrial fibrillation and concurrent treatment with amiodarone), sustaining CR 13 months after initiation of therapy [9].

More recently, a 2020 report of 84 patients compared outcomes between patients who received standard immune-chemotherapy (rituximab combined with either high-dose MTX, bendamustine, IT chemotherapy, or radiation therapy) versus ibrutinib alone for MCL with CNS relapse [10]. This is the first large cohort study of its kind examining the effectiveness of ibrutinib as a single agent in CNS relapse of MCL and showed improved overall response rate and CR rate (17% in the standard group vs 42% in the ibrutinib group) [10]. The ibrutinib group also showed improved 1-year overall survival (OS) compared to the standard cohort (61% vs 16%) [10]. It is evident that ibrutinib continues to act as a pivotal component of MCL with CNS relapse.

The outcome of the patient discussed in this case is particularly noteworthy given his multiple high-risk disease

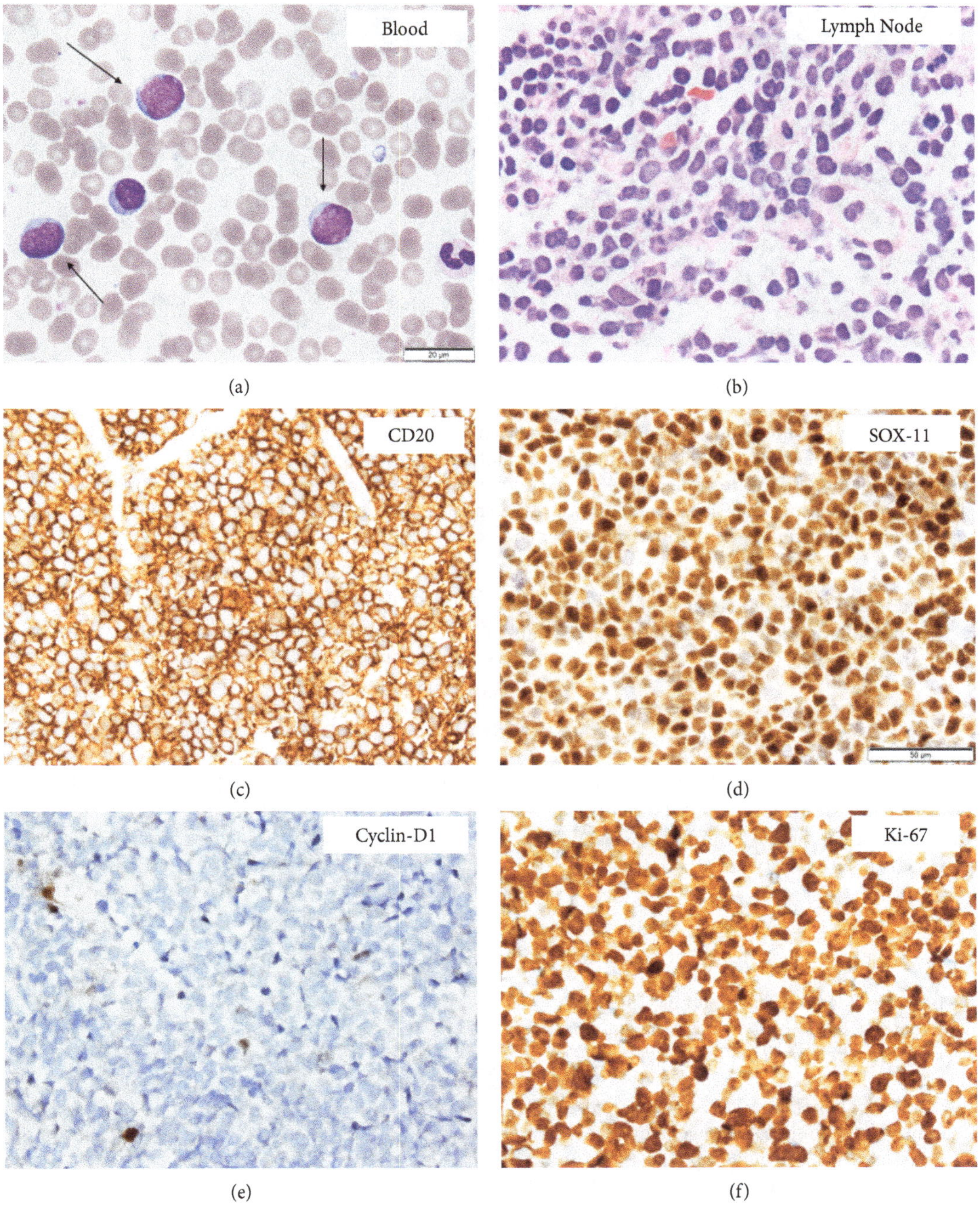

FIGURE 1: (a) Wright–Giemsa stain of peripheral blood smear shows circulating large atypical lymphoid cells, highlighted with arrows (1000×). (b) The hematoxylin and eosin section shows diffuse proliferation of large pleomorphic lymphoid cells in the cervical lymph node (600×). (c–f) Immunohistochemical stains (all 600×) demonstrate that the cervical lymph node neoplastic cells are positive for CD20 and SOX-11, while negative for cyclin-D1. Ki-67 highlights a very high proliferative index of ~90%.

characteristics, including blastoid variant, high Ki-67 index, and high MIPI score. Also, of particular interest is the fact that the patient has sustained a CR for over two years after completing salvage R-ICE combined with ibrutinib followed by an autologous SCT and ibrutinib maintenance, a combination which has not been reported elsewhere in the current literature specifically for R/R MCL. A phase I study demonstrated that ibrutinib combined with R-ICE for salvage therapy in R/R diffuse large B-cell lymphoma (DLBCL) had an overall response rate of 90% while being well-tolerated with low toxicity rates [6]. As seen in our patient, the translation of this approach with the addition of ibrutinib to R-ICE represents a promising new salvage chemotherapy regimen for relapsing MCL patients including those with CNS involvement. The addition of ibrutinib to R-ICE as salvage therapy and maintenance post autoSCT showed an impressive effectiveness in maintaining CR and preventing relapse in a patient with high-risk disease involving the CNS with an otherwise dismal prognosis. Our experience provides rationale for the evaluation of this

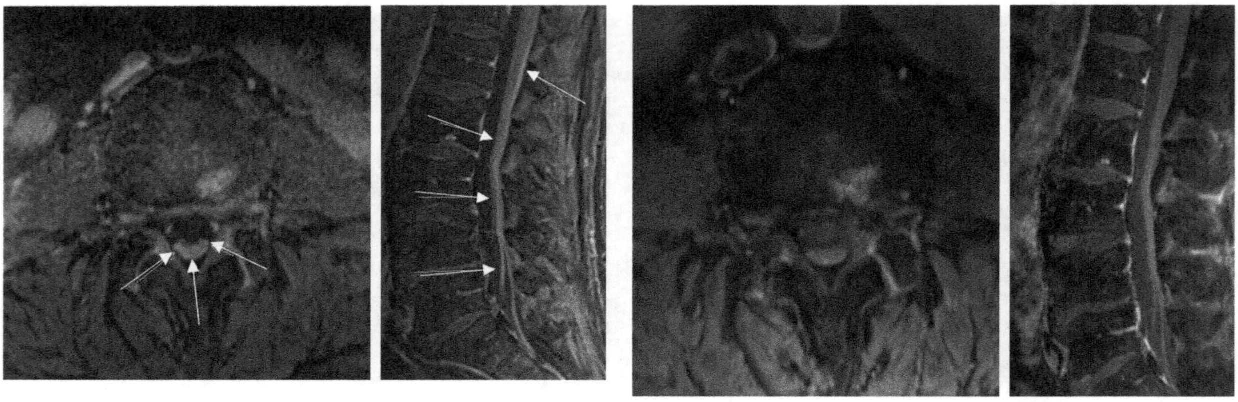

FIGURE 2: (a) Pretreatment axial and sagittal T1 weighted fat saturated postcontrast images show abnormal enhancement along the dorsal aspect of the spinal cord at the level of L1 and L2, with abnormal enhancement along the cauda equina nerve roots. Findings are highly suspicious for leptomeningeal disease with a differential of infectious and inflammatory etiologies. (b). Post-treatment axial and sagittal T1 weighted fat saturated postcontrast images show markedly improved enhancement at the level of L1 and L2 and of the conus medullaris and cauda equina nerve roots, with very subtle minimal enhancement.

approach on a larger scale in a clinical trial which may verify this approach as a promising new standard therapy in an otherwise challenging disease.

Disclosure

This research was performed as part of the employment of the authors under Northwestern University Feinberg School of Medicine and Robert H. Lurie Comprehensive Cancer Center of Northwestern University.

References

[1] P. Jain and M. Wang, "Mantle cell lymphoma: 2019 update on the diagnosis, pathogenesis, prognostication, and management," *American Journal of Hematology*, vol. 94, no. 6, pp. 710–725, 2019.

[2] J. M. Vose, "Mantle cell lymphoma: 2017 update on diagnosis, risk-stratification, and clinical management," *American Journal of Hematology*, vol. 92, no. 8, pp. 806–813, 2017.

[3] M. L. Wang, S. Rule, P. Martin et al., "Targeting BTK with ibrutinib in relapsed or refractory mantle-cell lymphoma," *New England Journal of Medicine*, vol. 369, no. 6, pp. 507–516, 2013.

[4] M. Schieber, L. I. Gordon, and R. Karmali, "Current overview and treatment of mantle cell lymphoma," *F1000Res*, vol. 7, Article ID F1000, 2018.

[5] C. Y. Cheah, A. George, E. Giné et al., "Central nervous system involvement in mantle cell lymphoma: clinical features, prognostic factors and outcomes from the European Mantle Cell Lymphoma Network," *Annals of Oncology*, vol. 24, no. 8, pp. 2119–2123, 2013.

[6] C. S. Sauter, M. J. Matasar, H. Schoder et al., "A phase 1 study of ibrutinib in combination with R-ICE in patients with relapsed or primary refractory DLBCL," *Blood*, vol. 131, no. 16, pp. 1805–1808, 2018.

[7] F. D. A. Clinical, *Pharmacology Reviews Ibrutinib 2055 52Orig1s000*, F. D. A, Silver Spring, MD, USA, 2013.

[8] S. Bernard, L. Goldwirt, S. Amorim et al., "Activity of ibrutinib in mantle cell lymphoma patients with central nervous system relapse," *Blood*, vol. 126, no. 14, pp. 1695–1698, 2015.

[9] D. Mannina and B. Loteta, "Ibrutinib treatment of mantle cell lymphoma relapse at central nervous system: a case report and literature review," *Case Rep Hematol*, vol. 2017, Article ID 9583257, 4 pages, 2017.

[10] C. Rusconi, C. Y. Cheah, D. Tucker et al., *Ibrutinib Compared to Immune-Chemotherapy for Central Nervous System Relapse of Mantle Cell Lymphoma: A Report from Fondazione Italiana Linfomi (FIL) and European Mantle Cell Lymphoma Network (EMCLN)*, EHA Library, The Hague, Netherlands, 2020.

22

Orbital Mucosa-Associated Lymphoid Tissue Lymphoma and Primary Cutaneous Classical Hodgkin Lymphoma: A Rare Case Report and Review of the Literature

Nicole Yun,[1] James Coggan,[2] Ira Miller,[3] and Parameswaran Venugopal[2]

[1]*Department of Internal Medicine, Rush University Medical Center, 1717 W. Congress Parkway, 1042 Kellogg, Chicago, IL 60612, USA*
[2]*Division of Hematology, Oncology and Cell Therapy, Rush University Medical Center, Chicago, IL, USA*
[3]*Department of Pathology, Rush University Medical Center, Chicago, IL, USA*

Correspondence should be addressed to Nicole Yun; nicole_k_yun@rush.edu

Academic Editor: Vincent Ribrag

A 60-year-old woman was diagnosed with isolated mucosa-associated lymphoid tissue (MALT) lymphoma of the ocular adnexa and treated with two years of weekly rituximab for eight doses followed by rituximab maintenance. After nearly two years of maintenance therapy, she developed a tender, indurated mass on the left neck. Biopsy results were consistent with primary cutaneous classical Hodgkin lymphoma (PCCHL).

1. Introduction

Classical Hodgkin lymphoma (HL) with cutaneous involvement is well described in the literature and usually occurs late in the course of the disease. The incidence has decreased in the recent decades, likely owing to improved chemotherapy and radiation therapy of patients with Hodgkin lymphoma, as well as the advent of stem cell transplantation [1]. PCCHL is extremely rare, with only 13 previous cases reported in the literature to date [2, 3]. It occurs when cutaneous Hodgkin lymphoma (CHL) arises in the skin as the primary tumor site, without evidence of systemic disease or of regional nodal involvement.

Non-Hodgkin lymphoma (NHL) and HL can present in the same host, either synchronously or metachronously and perhaps even in composite specimens. We describe the unique case of a patient initially treated for orbital MALT lymphoma who later presented with PCCHL. The combination of MALT lymphoma in the ocular adnexa followed by the appearance of PCCHL without any nodal or bone marrow involvement is exceedingly rare. To our knowledge, this is the first reported case of these two distinct entities occurring in the same host.

2. Case History

A 60-year-old woman presented with a 3-week history of left upper eyelid bruising and swelling without constitutional symptoms. Magnetic Resonance Imaging (MRI) revealed a 2.0 cm × 1.3 cm soft tissue mass in the medial extraconal compartment involving the oblique muscle. Biopsy was consistent with extranodal MALT-type marginal zone B-cell lymphoma. Staging workup with computed tomography (CT) and positron-emission tomography (PET) suggested possible cervical and inguinal lymph node involvement. Bone marrow biopsy did not show definitive evidence of involvement. The patient underwent treatment with weekly rituximab monotherapy for 8 weeks. Restaging PET of the orbital soft tissue mass demonstrated decrease in SUV from 11.2 to 4.7 in the orbital soft tissue mass and resolution of the hypermetabolic lymph nodes, indicating clinical and metabolic response to therapy. She was continued on maintenance rituximab every 2 months for 2 years.

The patient presented to clinic for her last dose of maintenance rituximab with a 3-4 cm tender, indurated, and slightly erythematous mass on the left side of her neck. She denied constitutional symptoms. CT of the neck

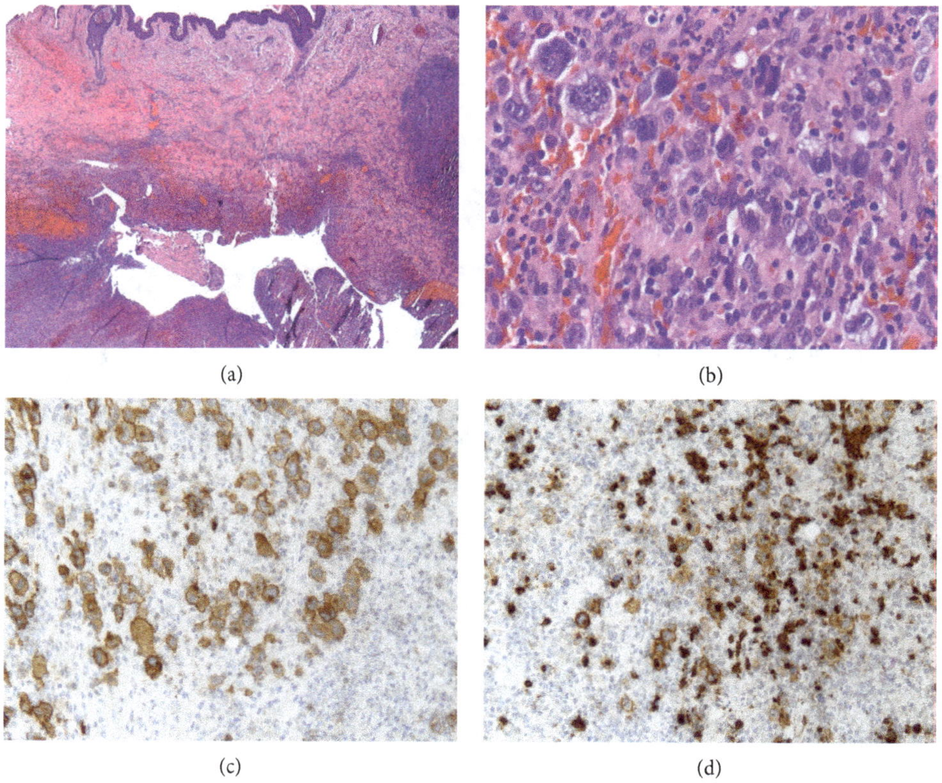

Figure 1: The specimen contained a cystic mass in the dermis, with overlying normal epidermis (a). The cystic areas were surrounded by neutrophils, histiocytes, and large binucleated and multinucleated malignant cells with Hodgkin and Reed–Sternberg morphology (b) that were positive for CD30 (c) and CD15 (d) on immunostains. CD15 also stains admixed neutrophils.

demonstrated a soft tissue mass on the left lateral aspect of her mid-neck extending into the overlying subcutaneous tissue and skin that was not seen on prior imaging. Excisional biopsy revealed tumor composed of large pleomorphic malignant cells and admixed inflammatory cells. The tumor was centered in the deep dermis, with satellite nodules (mainly microabscesses) in the superficial dermis. No evident lymph nodes were seen in the specimen. Immunohistochemical (IHC) staining showed that the malignant cells were strongly positive for CD30, CD15, PAX5, and CD79a and negative for CD45, diagnostic of classical Hodgkin lymphoma (Figure 1). Oct2 stained a minority of the malignant cells and BOB1 was completely negative, further supporting the diagnosis. Lack of CD20 and EBER excluded morphological variants of diffuse large B-cell lymphoma (DLBCL) and Epstein–Barr virus- (EBV-) positive mucocutaneous ulcer, and the absence of overlying skin ulceration also ruled out the latter. Interesting, the tumor cells expressed CD79a and partial CD2 which are unusual but not impossible findings in this entity. Staging PET-CT and bone marrow biopsy were negative for nodal or systemic involvement. She was treated with 2 cycles of ABVD followed by radiotherapy with no evidence of disease seen on restaging PET.

3. Discussion

Patients who have NHL have an increased incidence of developing HL years later. NHL has most commonly been associated with DLBCL, followed by follicular lymphoma. Proposed mechanisms include long-term effects of lymphoma treatment, immune defects, genetic susceptibilities, lifestyle or environmental factors, and likely interactions between these factors [4–6]. There is suspicion of a clonal link between HL and NHL with studies evaluating rare patients with both HL and DLCBL demonstrating that the Hodgkin/Reed–Sternberg cells and the DLBCL cells contain identical VDJ rearrangements of the Ig heavy chain (IGH) locus and contain shared somatic mutations within the VDJ region [7]. In 2016, Alvarez et al. described a woman who presented sequentially with splenic marginal zone lymphoma, Hodgkin lymphoma, and then DLBCL (also thought to be derived from MZL) [8]. Subsequent analysis of clonally rearranged IGH genes in the study revealed that the three histological types of lymphoma had the exact same clonal IGH rearrangement. We did not have enough evidence in our based-on-immunohistochemical staining to suggest that the PCCHL had involvement with prior diagnosis of MLZ/MALT-L. The specimens were never sent out for further molecular testing, and thus a definitive clonal relationship between the two processes could not be established.

13 cases of PCCHL have been reported to date (summarized in Table 1) with treatment and outcomes, if known. The cases have been described as idiopathic as well as iatrogenic. There are no clear guidelines on management and how much treatment is necessary. Previous cases of idiopathic PCCHL have been treated with topical corticosteroids, systemic combination chemotherapy, and/or radiotherapy with

Table 1: Current reported cases of primary cutaneous classical Hodgkin lymphoma, summarized from Koch et al. [3] and Kerstetter [2] with additions.

Reference	Age/ sex (M)	PMHx requiring IS	Disease site	Therapy	Outcome	EBV
Idiopathic						
[9]	50	None	Chest wall	MOPP-ABVD	Systemic disease after 2 months	N/A
	54	None	Left lower leg	RT	Systemic progression after 6 years	N/A
	45	None	Forearms and legs	Multiple chemotherapy	No progression at 5 years postchemo	N/A
	17	None	Right thigh	Topical CT	No progression at 9 years	N/A
	52	None	Right arm	None	No progression at 9 years	N/A
[10]	86	None	Left ankle	RT	Systemic disease discovered after 1 year	N/A
[11]	59	None	Left flank, inner thigh, and right foot	ABVD	No progression at 3 years	N/A
[12]	70	None	Right back	RT	No progression at 7 years	Negative
[3]	49	None	Right forearm	ABVD	Response to treatment but passed away from pulmonary tuberculosis	Negative
[13]	80	None	Left thigh	ABVD	No long-term follow-up data	N/A
Iatrogenic						
[14]	74	UC on infliximab	Scalp	Withholding immunosuppression, excision and chemo	Disease free at 10 months	Positive
[10]	25	DM, on MTX/ thalidomide/ steroids	Scalp	Withholding immunosuppression, chemo & radiation	Complete remission at 6 years	Positive
[2]	58	DM, on MTX/ CellCept/steroids	Elbow	Withholding immunosuppression, excision	Recurrence after 13 months	Positive

IS, immunosuppression; MOPP, mechlorethamine, vincristine, procarbazine, prednisone; ABVD, adriamycin, bleomycin, vinblastine, dacarbazine; RT, radiation therapy; CT, corticosteroids; UC, ulcerative colitis; DM, dermatomyositis; MTX, methotrexate; N/A, status not available.

varied responses. Iatrogenic PCCHL has been linked to EBV infection, and treatment consisted of withholding immunosuppression.

Our patient was treated with rituximab induction and nearly completed maintenance therapy at the time she was diagnosed with PCCHL. We considered the possibility of iatrogenic PCCHL, as rituximab induces a transient B-cell depletion and dose-dependent T-cell inactivation that could impair T-cell immunosurveillance. This could provoke development and progression of certain second primary malignancies (SPMs), including hematologic malignancies. However, there is no evidence that rituximab specifically contributes to later development of HL [15, 16], especially when EBV has been ruled out as a mediator. Furthermore, our patient was immunocompetent at the time of second lymphoma diagnosis. Complete blood count with differential showed WBC 7.74 K/μL, hemoglobin 13.4 g/dL, platelet count 185×10^9/L, absolute neutrophil count 5570/μL, and absolute lymphocyte count 1110/μL. Serum protein electrophoresis was not obtained. There were no clinically significant cytopenias and no infectious complications throughout the entire course of rituximab treatment and maintenance.

The only reported case of MALT with an extranodal HL was described in 2010. Oka et al. reported a patient with synchronous gastric MALT diagnosed at the same time as primary pulmonary Hodgkin lymphoma. Of note, this patient was infected with EBV, a known predisposing risk factor for Hodgkin lymphoma [17]. Both HRS-like and lacunar cells in the lung tumor and centrocyte-like cells in the MALT lymphoma expressed EBER, so it is likely that EBV was involved in the pathogenesis of both. EBV was excluded in our case.

In accordance with the Lugano Classification System, our patient is considered to have stage IE HL. Treatment rationale was based on National Comprehensive Cancer Network (NCCN) guidelines, which suggests treating early stage HL with extranodal involvement with two cycles of ABVD followed by either two additional cycles or radiation therapy. She tolerated and achieved complete remission with this treatment modality. We will continue to follow her progress.

4. Conclusion

In conclusion, PCCHL is an extremely unusual form of extranodal HL. As more reports begin to surface over the centuries, it becomes important to recognize potential risk factors that may be contributing to its pathogenesis, such as immunomodulating therapy, history of NHL, and viral infection/reactivation. Close longitudinal follow-up is recommended in order to identify systemic recurrence of disease, even after achieving remission. This will also lead to better understanding of treatment outcomes, prognostic factors in PCCHL, and primary extranodal HL as a whole and hopefully allow a more uniform consensus regarding therapy.

Authors' Contributions

Yun, Coggan, Miller, and Venugopal contributed to the manuscript of the project. Miller provided the images and description of Figure 1.

References

[1] C. E. Introcaso, J. Kantor, D. L. Porter, and J. M. Junkins-Hopkins, "Cutaneous Hodgkins disease," *Journal of the American Academy of Dermatology*, vol. 58, no. 2, pp. 295–298, 2008.

[2] J. Kerstetter, "Primary Coetaneous Hodgkin lymphoma: a revisit and case report," *International Clinical Pathology Journal*, vol. 3, no. 1, 2016.

[3] K. Koch, M. Patel, S. Pather, and D. Modi, "Primary Cutaneous Hodgkin lymphoma: a rare disease variant and review of the literature," *Journal of Case Reports and Studies*, vol. 4, no. 2, 2016.

[4] N. Baras, S. Dahm, J. Haberland et al., "Subsequent malignancies among long-term survivors of Hodgkin lymphoma and non-Hodgkin lymphoma: a pooled analysis of German cancer registry data (1990–2012)," *British Journal of Haematology*, vol. 177, pp. 226–242, 2017.

[5] L. B. Travis, C. S. Rabkin, L. M. Brown et al., "Cancer survivorship—genetic susceptibility and second primary cancers: research strategies and recommendations," *JNCI: Journal of the National Cancer Institute*, vol. 98, no. 1, pp. 15–25, 2006.

[6] L. B. Travis, W. D. Wahnefried, J. M. Allan, M. E. Wood, and A. K. Ng, "Aetiology, genetics and prevention of secondary neoplasms in adult cancer survivors," *Nature Reviews Clinical Oncology*, vol. 10, no. 5, pp. 289–301, 2013.

[7] A. Brauninger, M.-L. Hansmann, J. G. Strickler et al., "Identification of Common germinal- center B-cell precursors in two patients with both Hodgkins disease and non-Hodgkins lymphoma," *New England Journal of Medicine*, vol. 340, no. 16, pp. 1239–1247, 1999.

[8] S. Alonso-Alvarez, A. Redondo-Guijo, Ó. Blanco et al., "Lymphoma Heterogeneity: three different histological pictures and one unique clone," *Case Reports in Hematology*, vol. 2016, Article ID 3947510, 2016.

[9] N. Sioutos, H. Kerl, S. B. Murphy, and M. E. Kadin, "Primary Cutaneous Hodgkin's disease. Unique clinical, morphologic, and immunophenotypic findings," *The American Journal of Dermatopathology*, vol. 16, no. 1, pp. 2–8, 1994.

[10] J. Guitart and D. Fretzin, "Skin as the primary site of Hodgkins disease," *The American Journal of Dermatopathology*, vol. 20, no. 2, pp. 218–222, 1998.

[11] M. Mukesh, D. Shuttleworth, and P. Murray, "Primary Cutaneous Hodgkins lymphoma," *Clinical and Experimental Dermatology*, vol. 34, no. 8, 2009.

[12] G. Pranteda, M. F. Osti, M. C. Cox et al., "Primary Cutaneous Hodgkin lymphoma," *Journal of the American Academy of Dermatology*, vol. 63, no. 2, 2010.

[13] A. A. Ambekar and C. S. Soman, "Cutaneous Hodgkin's lymphoma," *South Asian Journal of Cancer*, vol. 6, no. 4, p. 170, 2017.

[14] S. Kumar, D. W. Kingma, W. B. Weiss, M. Raffeld, and E. S. Jaffe, "Primary Cutaneous Hodgkins disease with evolution to systemic disease," *The American Journal of Surgical Pathology*, vol. 20, no. 6, pp. 754–759, 1996.

[15] I. Fleury, S. Chevret, M. Pfreundschuh et al., "Rituximab and risk of second primary malignancies in patients with non-Hodgkin lymphoma: a systematic review and meta- analysis," *Annals of Oncology*, vol. 27, no. 3, pp. 390–397, 2016.

[16] L. Tao, C. A. Clarke, A. S. Rosenberg et al., "Subsequent primary malignancies after diffuse large B-cell lymphoma in the modern treatment era," *British Journal of Haematology*, vol. 178, no. 1, pp. 72–80, 2017.

[17] K. Oka, M. Shinonaga, R. Nagayama et al., "Coexistence of primary pulmonary Hodgkin lymphoma and gastric MALT lymphoma associated with Epstein-Barr virus infection: a case report," *Pathology International*, vol. 60, no. 7, pp. 520–523, 2010.

23

Successful Treatment of Concomitant Pleural Mucosa-Associated Lymphoid Tissue Lymphoma and Monoclonal Gammopathy of Undetermined Significance with Lenalidomide, Rituximab, and Dexamethasone

Yoshiki Uemura,[1] **Risa Maeda**,[2] **and Hiroyoshi Saegusa**[3]

[1]*Department of Hematology, Chikamori Hospital, 1-1-16, Okawasuzi, Kochi-shi, Kochi-ken 780-8522, Japan*
[2]*Department of Nephrology, Chikamori Hospital, 1-1-16, Okawasuzi, Kochi-shi, Kochi-ken 780-8522, Japan*
[3]*Department of General Medicine, Chikamori Hospital, 1-1-16, Okawasuzi, Kochi-shi, Kochi-ken 780-8522, Japan*

Correspondence should be addressed to Yoshiki Uemura; khs1040@chikamori.com

Academic Editor: Tatsuharu Ohno

Concomitant plasma cell and B cell neoplasms in a single patient have been infrequently reported. It is known that the prognosis of these patients is worse than that of patients with single-disease onset. Generally, the chemotherapy specific for each disease is provided sequentially. It has been suggested that the specific chemotherapy for lymphoma could lead to the occurrence of refractory multiple myeloma (MM). We present a case with the concomitant occurrence of mucosa-associated lymphoid tissue (MALT) lymphoma and monoclonal gammopathy of undetermined significance (MGUS). MGUS does not usually require aggressive treatment. However, the potential adverse effects of MGUS on the treatment course of the B cell lymphoma were concerning. Therefore, we explored a new therapeutic approach that is simultaneously effective against both diseases. Combination therapy of lenalidomide (LEN) and rituximab (RIT) gained indication for follicular lymphoma and MALT lymphoma recently. LEN is also a key drug in MM treatment. Both diseases in our patient were effectively treated with the combination of LEN, RIT, and dexamethasone. With this combination therapy, we expect a prognostic improvement in concomitant MM and B cell lymphoma cases.

1. Introduction

Rarely the simultaneous onset of B cell lymphoma and multiple myeloma (MM) has been reported. One study reported that six of 4165 patients with B cell lymphoma developed MM, and one of 804 patients with MM developed B cell lymphoma [1]. There is no standard therapeutic regimen for such patients. Despite both malignancies being derived from mature B cell, the characteristics of B cell lymphoma and MM are very different. The specific therapy for each malignant tumor is administered to the patients with two types of B cell malignancies. However, their prognosis is usually poor. There has been a previously reported case of a patient with the simultaneous onset of smoldering MM (SMM) and mucosa-associated lymphoid tissue (MALT) lymphoma [2]. SMM does not typically require treatment, as with monoclonal gammopathy of undetermined significance (MGUS). However, the patient's SMM deteriorated after complete remission of the MALT lymphoma was achieved by disease-specific treatment. In this case, the patient had the simultaneous onset of MALT lymphoma and MGUS. MGUS is also considered a preneoplastic condition of malignant lymphoma (ML). In fact, 1.2% of the patients with MGUS developed ML in a long-term follow-up study [3]. Environmental and genetic factors may modify a clonal, benign proliferation into a ML. We suspect that MGUS itself also has a possibility to worsen progress of

ML in the merger case of MGUS and ML, even if only a little.

The combination therapy of CD19- and B cell maturation antigen (BCMA)-chimeric antigen receptor (CAR) T cells was effective for the treatment of the patients with concomitant onset of B cell lymphoma and MM [4]. However, the CAR T therapy is costly and is not covered by insurance for MM yet in Japan. For resistant and refractory low-grade B cell lymphoma, the effectiveness of the combination of rituximab (RIT) and lenalidomide (LEN) has been recently shown [5]. It is well known that the combination of LEN and dexamethasone (DEX) is a standard regimen for MM [6]. In this case, RIT, LEN, and DEX were effective for both MALT lymphoma and MGUS.

2. Case Presentation

An 82-year-old male was hospitalized for fever and dyspnea (Figure 1). Chest radiography showed right pleural effusion. Chest drainage was carried out for the improvement of dyspnea. The pleural effusion cytopathology by Papanicolaou stain showed no malignancy. However, chromosomal karyotype analysis of the effusion demonstrated chromosome karyotype: −1, +der(?)t(?; 1)(?; p22)[5/20], XY[15/20]. Moreover, two-color flow cytometry (FCM) showed the expression of CD19, CD20, CD25, and λ chain, although their expression level was not high. CD25 expression is generally quite rare in MALT lymphoma. The lymphoma cells in bone marrow almost disappeared after R-THPCOP, and therapy. CD25+ cells almost disappeared after R-THPCOP; on the other hand, CD5+ cells did not decrease at all. Therefore, we thought that CD5+ cells might not be derived from lymphoma cells. We did not examine CD43 expression. FISH analyses showed no signal for IgH-CCND1 and BCL6. Computed tomography (CT) detected a pleural thickening (Figure 2(a)) in which gallium (Ga) scintigraphy showed an accumulation (Figure 2(b)). The serum soluble interleukin-2 receptor (sIL-2R) rises with the increase of the neoplastic cell in non-Hodgkin's lymphoma, reflecting the quantity of total tumor. The sIL-2R was high in our case (Table 1). We did not check the sIL-2R level just before R-THPCOP therapy. We deleted the sIL-2R level on May 21, 2021 to give an impression as if it rose after the R-THPCOP therapy (Figure 1). Primary pleural lymphoma was diagnosed because Ga scintigraphy and CT did not demonstrate any tumor lesions in other locations. Immunohistochemical staining of the pleural biopsy specimen demonstrated infiltration of λ-positive, monoclonal *B* cells presenting remarkable dysplasia (Figure 3(a)–3(d)). Based on morphological diagnosis and immunohistochemical staining, MALT lymphoma was strongly suspected. The expression of MIB-1 was around 30–40%. That is a little higher than that of usual MALT lymphoma. On admission, the bone marrow (BM) demonstrated that the lymphoma cells occupied about half of all nucleated cells (Figure 4(a), 4(b)). Two-color FCM of the BM expressed λ + CD19 + CD20 + CD25 + CD10-monoclonal malignant *B* cells, as did the pleural effusion (Figure 5). Chromosome analysis of the BM demonstrated a complex karyotype: −*Y*, del(20)(*q*11.2; *q*13.3), −1, +der(?)*t*(?; 1)(?; *p*22). Serum protein fractionation showed two *M*-peaks on admission. Immunoelectrophoresis detected the two clonal immunoglobulins of Ig*A*-κ and Ig*M*-λ. The BM smear specimen showed that the normal-sized, malignant plasma cells occupied 3%, and the large-sized, malignant plasma cell, like a foam cell, occupied 3% (Figure 4(a)). The immunostaining of the BM clot section showed that the large-sized plasma cells were IgA-positive (Figure 4(c)). However, it is not clear whether the normal-sized plasma cells express IgM because of high background level (Figure 4(d)). Both types of plasma cells were CD138-positive (Figure 4(e)). The immunostaining of the BM clot section could not clearly show the difference in the expression of the κ light chain and λ light chain because of a strong, nonspecific binding.

Our case was in an advanced stage because the pleural effusion contained lymphoma cells, and he complained of dyspnea. We thought that aggressive chemotherapy for MALT lymphoma would not cause a remarkable progression of gammopathy because serum IgA and IgM levels before the treatment were not so high, and the marrow plasma cells that mainly produce these immunoglobulins were few. We treated aggressively with R (RIT)-THPCOP (pirarubicin, cyclophosphamide, vincristine, and prednisolone). After R-THPCOP therapy, the thickened pleura became slightly thinner. However, the daily pleural fluid accumulation did not diminish. Therefore, pleurodesis was performed, and the pleural drain could be removed because the output gradually decreased. The BM smear showed that the lymphoma cells had mostly disappeared (Figure 6(a), 6(b)). FCM of the BM showed the disappearance of CD20, CD25, and the remarkable decrease in CD19 and λ light chain expression. Chromosome analysis of the BM before R-THPCOP therapy demonstrated a complex karyotype: 45, X, −Y [10/20]/46, XY, del(20)(q11.2q13.3) [2/20]/46, XY, −1, +der(?)t(?;1)(?;p22) [2/20]/46, XY [6/20], after R-THPCOP: 45, X, −Y [8/20]/46, XY, del(20) (q11.2q13.3) [1/20]/46, XY [11/20]. The chromosome aberration detected for pleural effusion before R-THPCOP: −1, +der(?)t(?;1)(?;p22) was lost from the BM after R-THPCOP. This indicates that the lymphoma cell has the chromosome karyotype: −1, +der(?) t(?;1) (?;p22), and the two MGUS clones have the chromosome karyotypes: −Y, del(20)(q11.2q13.3). However, we were not able to identify which chromosome karyotype each MGUS clone has.

Each drug of THPCOP had been used for MM treatment in the past. After R-THPCOP, the CD138-positive cells were slightly decreased (Figure 6(c)), and the serum levels of IgM and IgA as well as IgG decreased. In comparison with the large-sized plasma cells, the normal-sized plasma cells seemed to decrease in predominance. The chest tube was able to be removed after the pleurodesis. However, the right interlobar pleural effusion recurred (Figure 7(a)). Continuous treatment for MALT lymphoma was felt to be necessary. The combination therapy of LEN, RIT, and DEX was therefore initiated. This combination became indicated for MALT lymphoma recently. It is well known that LEN is also a key drug for MM. By adding DEX to this combination

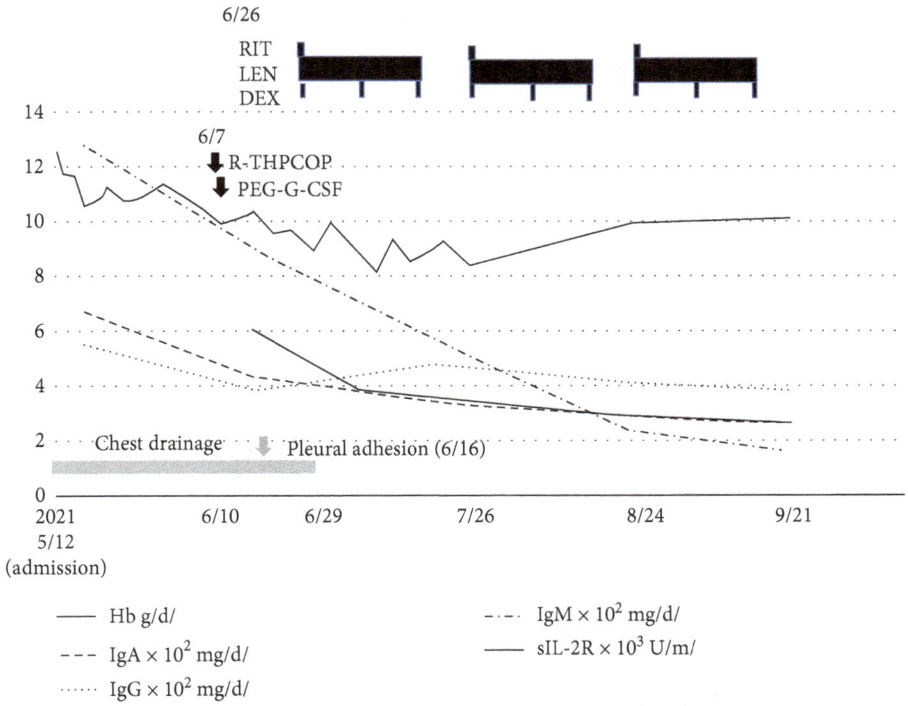

FIGURE 1: Clinical course. LEN, lenalidomide; RIT, rituximab; DEX, dexamethasone; sIL-2R, soluble interleukin-2 receptor; Hb, hemoglobin.

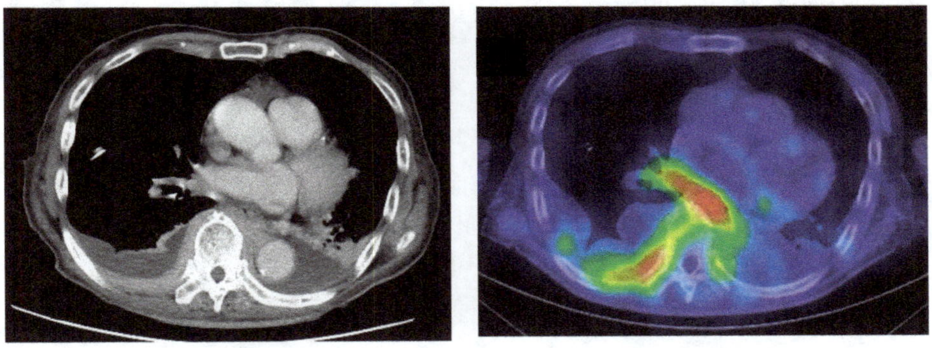

FIGURE 2: Image of pleural lymphoma. (a) Enhanced computed tomography. (b) Gallium scintigraphy.

therapy, we expected an improved prognosis for our patient. Specifically, LEN 10 mg/day orally for 21 days, RIT 375 mg/m^2 intravenously monthly, and DEX 20 mg/day orally weekly were given on a cycle of 28 days. After the third cycle of triple-drug therapy, we detected a significant decline in IgM concentration, a slow decline in the IgA and sIL-2R concentrations, and a slight residual of pleural effusion (Figure 7(b)).

3. Discussion

MALT lymphoma is thought to arise from postgerminal center memory *B* cells, which are able to differentiate into marginal zone *B* cells and plasma cells in germinal center [7]. MALT lymphomas most commonly express IgM. Differentiation to IgM-secreting plasma cells occurs in ca. 30% of MALT lymphoma [8]. It is likely that MALT lymphomas are malignancies of an IgM-only pathway of B cell development. Our case who merged MALT lymphoma and MGUS had two kinds of clonal globulins, IgM-λ and IgA-κ. We immunohistochemically detected the expression of IgM, and λ in MALT lymphoma. This suspected that IgM-λ type is derived from MALT lymphoma. The BM smear specimen showed that the normal-sized plasma cells and the large-sized plasma cell look like a foam cell. We showed that the large-sized plasma cells expressed IgA-κ type.

However, it is not clear whether the normal-sized plasma cells express IgM because of high background. We cannot deny that the normal-sized plasma cells might be inflammatory reactive cells. Li et al. reported the case who merged ML and three MM clones [4]. The germinal center is where somatic hypermutation of immunoglobulin and class-switch recombination occurs. MM was the neoplastic disease

Table 1: Laboratory data on admission.

Complete Blood Count		Biochemistry test		Serological test	
WBC	5,900/μl	TP	7.8 g/dl	C3	79 mg/dl
Banded neutrophil	1.0%	Alb	3.5 g/dl	C4	23 mg/dl
Segmented neutrophil	84.0%	AST	14 U/l	ANA	40 fold
Lymphocyte	4.0%	ALT	5 U/l	RF	6 IU/ml
Monocyte	3.0%	ALP	270 IU/ml	BNP	73 pg/ml
Eosinophil	8.0%	γ-GTP	16 IU/l	HCV Ab	(−)
RBC	$426 \times 10^4/\mu l$	CHE	186 U/L	HBs Ag	(−)
Hb	12.5 g/dl	LDH	208 U/l	IgG	546 mg/dl
Ht	37.5%	T-bil	0.6 mg/dl	IgA	662 mg/dl
MCV	88.0 fl	BUN	22.5 mg/dl	IgM	1272 mg/dl
Plt	$24.6 \times 10^4/\mu l$	Cr	1.66 mg/dl	sIL-2R	3190 U/ml
		UA	3.9 mg/dl		
Urinalysis		T-CHO	166 mg/dl	Coagulation	
Color	Yellow	TG	80 mg/dl	PT-INR	0.96
Protein	1(+)	Glu	109 mg/dl	APTT	33.4 sec
Glucose	(−)	HbA1c	5.3%	Fibrinogen	294.6 mg/dl
Occult blood	(+/−)	Na	137 mEq/l	FDP	6.5 μg/ml
		K	3.5 mEq/l	D-dimer	3.0 μg/ml
		Cl	102 mEq/l		
		CRP	0.17 mg/dl		

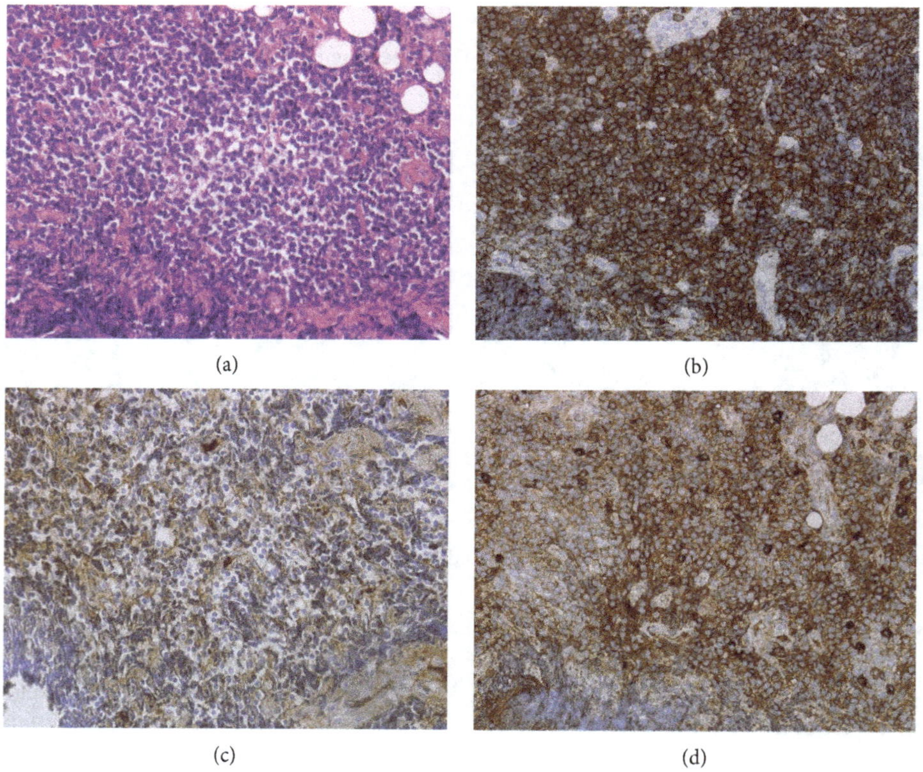

Figure 3: Pleural immunohistochemical staining. (a) Hematoxylin-eosin staining (×40). (b) CD20 (×40). (c) κ chain (×40). (d) λ chain (×40).

constructed from the cell already having received antigen stimulation in the germinal center [9]. We suppose that various genetic mutation, deletion, and amplification in MALT lymphoma might induce a mistargeting of somatic cell hypermutation and an abnormal class-switch, finally causing the multi-monoclonality of MGUS. However, it is unclear because we did not conduct a molecular analysis of our patient.

Generally, the merger cases of ML and MM were individually treated with a chemotherapy specific for each malignancy because of the lack of standard treatment guidelines. Li et al. reviewed 6 cases of coexistence of MM and ML, and 2 borderline cases with pathological and histological features of both tumors from the PubMed database [4]. Among the 6 cases, 2 patients could have clinical improvement; however, they were not followed after that.

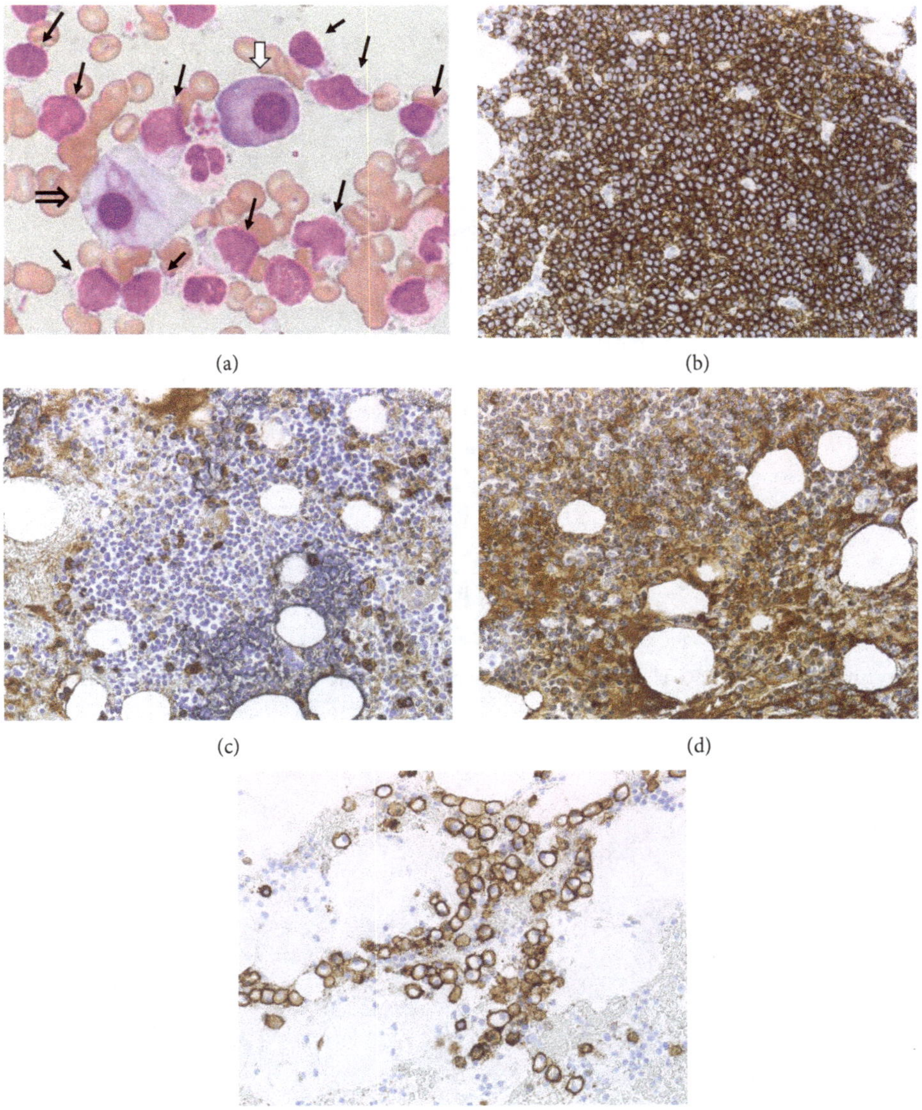

FIGURE 4: Immunohistochemical staining of bone marrow before R-THPCOP. (a) May Grunwald–Giemsa staining (×1000). (b) CD20 (×40). (c) IgA chain (×40). (d) IgM chain (×40). (e) CD138 (×40). Black arrow: lymphoma cell; white arrow: normal-sized plasma cell; double arrow: large-sized plasma cell.

Another 2 patient relapsed one or more times. One had no further report after the third complete remission. The other patient died of infection and disease development. The 2 borderline cases died because of disease development without effect of chemotherapy. These suggest that the conventional therapeutic approach might not be able to improve the prognosis of a merger case of MM and the ML. Our case merged MGUS with MALT lymphoma not MM. MGUS does not usually require aggressive treatment. The major indication of treatment is still against symptomatic MM and MM with clinical significance but not for MGUS. Such as MGUS and monoclonal B-cell lymphocytosis, in situ lymphomas have recently been described with minimal infiltrates of clonal B cells in morphologically reactive lymphoid tissues [10]. MGUS is known to predispose to B cell malignancies [3]. Environmental factors and genetic factors have a possibility to modify a clonal benign proliferation into a malignant lymphoma [11]. *H. pylori* could be also a crucial factor to develop gastric MALT lymphoma in patients with MGUS [12]. These things suggest that MGUS itself may worsen progress of ML in the merger case of MGUS and ML, even if only a little. Therefore, some treatment is likely necessary for not only ML but also MGUS to improve their prognosis. We searched for novel regimen to simultaneously treat these two diseases with acceptable toxicity and side effects. The recent study describes future directions for improving individual management of MGUS as well as the potential for developing early treatment strategies designed to delay and prevent the development of MM [13]. We have a report that B-cell lymphoma and MM led to remission by combination therapy of CD19- and BCMA-CAR T cell at the same time. However, the CAR

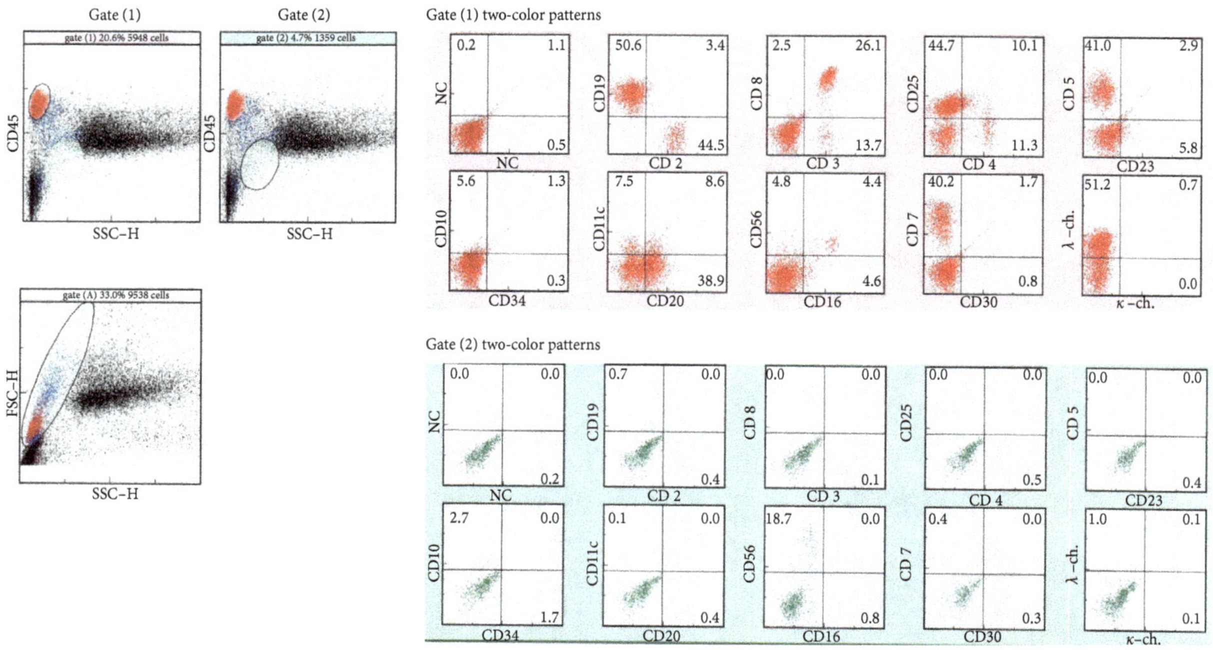

FIGURE 5: Flow cytometry analysis (CD45/SSC-H gating) of bone marrow before R-THPCOP. Two-color patterns in gate (1), and gate (2).

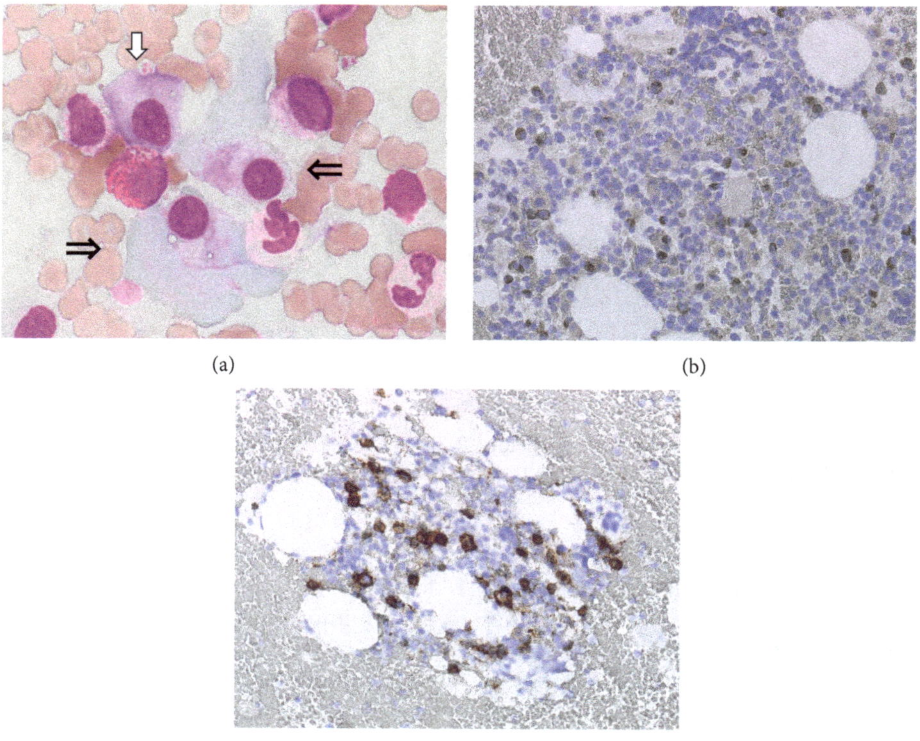

FIGURE 6: Immunohistochemical staining of bone marrow after R-THPCOP. (a) May Grunwald–Giemsa staining (×1000). (b) CD20 (×40). (c) CD138 (×40). White arrow: normal-sized plasma cell; double arrow: large-sized plasma cell.

T cell therapy carries a very high price, and it is not covered for elderly patients in our country. Thalidomide (THD) has an effect on standard therapy-failure MALT lymphoma through the significant downregulation of nuclear NF-κB expression [14]. LEN is a derivative of THD. It was revealed that single LEN administration also affected advanced MALT lymphoma [15]. The combination therapy of LEN and RIT recently gained indications for recurrent, refractory follicular lymphoma and MALT lymphoma. Furthermore, LEN is a key drug for MM treatment, and the combination of LEN and DEX is known as a standard MM regimen. Actually, in our case, the triple therapy with LEN, RIT, and

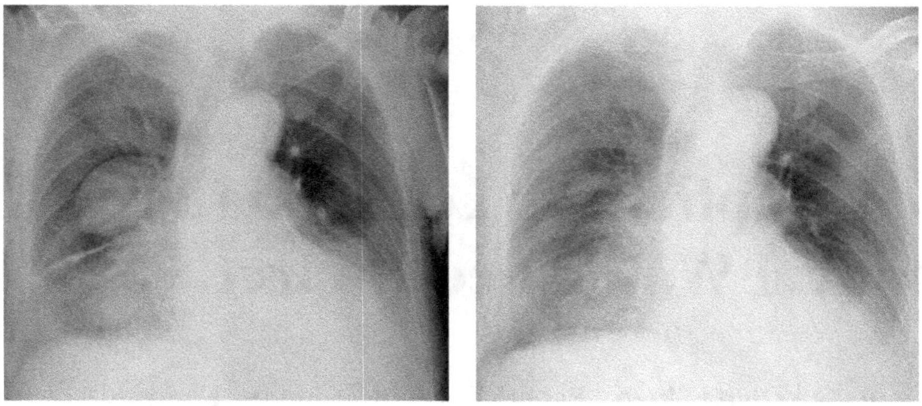

Figure 7: Chest radiograph. (a) Chest drainage removal date (June 28, 2021). (b) End date of 3 courses of triple therapy (September 9, 2021).

DEX persistently reduced the MALT lymphoma and the levels of IgA and IgM. It is necessary to evaluate more cases to clarify whether this triple therapy can improve the prognosis in merger cases of lymphoma and MM.

4. Conclusion

The patients with concomitant onset of plasma cell neoplasm and B cell lymphoma have been infrequently reported. The chemotherapy specific for each disease has typically been provided sequentially. The prognosis of these patients is usually poor. We thought that therapeutic approaches which could simultaneously treat both malignancies might be important. This is the first report where the combination of LEN, RIT, and DEX could effectively treat MALT lymphoma and MGUS simultaneously. We expect this combination therapy to improve the prognosis of the cases with concomitant onset of MM and B cell lymphoma.

Acknowledgments

The authors thank Editage for the English language editing.

References

[1] A. K. Mahindra, A. R. Sohani, C. E. Toomey et al., "B cell lymphoma in association with multiple myeloma: analysis of the biologic relationship," *Blood*, vol. 118, no. 21, p. 1590, 2011.

[2] S. Wöhrer, M. Raderer, B. Streubel, A. Chott, and J. Drach, "Concomitant occurrence of MALT lymphoma and multiple myeloma," *Annals of Hematology*, vol. 83, no. 9, pp. 600–603, 2004.

[3] P. Pasqualetti, V. Festuccia, A. Collacciani, and R. Casale, "The natural history of monoclonal gammopathy of undetermined significance," *Acta Haematologica*, vol. 97, no. 3, pp. 174–179, 1997.

[4] T. Li, J. Tan, L. Chen et al., "Case report: simultaneous occurrence of multiple myeloma and non-Hodgkin lymphoma treated by CAR T therapy," *Medicine*, vol. 99, no. 16, Article ID e19739, 2020.

[5] J. P. Leonard, M. Trneny, K. Izutsu et al., "AUGMENT: a phase III study of lenalidomide plus rituximab versus placebo plus rituximab in relapsed or refractory indolent lymphoma," *Journal of Clinical Oncology*, vol. 37, no. 14, pp. 1188–1199, 2019.

[6] S. V. Rajkumar, S. Jacobus, N. S. Callander et al., "Lenalidomide plus high-dose dexamethasone versus lenalidomide plus low-dose dexamethasone as initial therapy for newly diagnosed multiple myeloma: an open-label randomised controlled trial," *The Lancet Oncology*, vol. 11, no. 1, pp. 29–37, 2010.

[7] U. Novak, K. Basso, L. Pasqualucci, R. Dalla-Favera, and G. Bhagat, "Genomic analysis of Non-Splenic Marginal Zone Lymphomas (MZL) indicates similarities between nodal and extranodal MZL and supports their derivation from Memory B-cells," *British Journal of Haematology*, vol. 155, no. 3, pp. 362–365, 2011.

[8] P. G. Isaacson, J. Spencer, and T. Finn, "Primary B-cell gastric lymphoma," *Human Pathology*, vol. 17, no. 1, pp. 72–82, 1986.

[9] M. H. Bakkus, C. Heirman, I. Van Riet, B. Van Camp, and K. Thielemans, "Evidence that multiple myeloma Ig heavy chain VDJ genes contain somatic mutations but show no intraclonal variation," *Blood*, vol. 80, no. 9, pp. 2326–2335, 1992.

[10] L. Quintanilla-Martínez, P. Adam, and F. Fend, "In situ lymphoma and other early stage malignant non-Hodgkin lymphomas," *Pathologe, Der*, vol. 34, no. 3, pp. 244–253, 2013.

[11] D. Hurez, "Epidemiology of monoclonal gammopathies," *Revue du Praticien*, vol. 43, no. 3, pp. 271–274, 1993.

[12] A. Tursi and M. E. Modeo, "Monoclonal gammopathy of undetermined significance predisposing to Helicobacter pylori-related gastric mucosa-associated lymphoid tissue lymphoma," *Journal of Clinical Gastroenterology*, vol. 34, no. 2, pp. 147–149, 2002.

[13] N. Korde, S. Y. Kristinsson, and O. Landgren, "Monoclonal gammopathy of undetermined significance (MGUS) and smoldering multiple myeloma (SMM): novel biological insights and development of early treatment strategies," *Blood*, vol. 117, no. 21, pp. 5573–5581, 2011.

[14] S. H. Kuo, A. L. Cheng, C. W. Lin et al., "t(11;18)(q21;q21 translocation as predictive marker for non-responsiveness to salvage thalidomide therapy in patients with marginal zone B-cell lymphoma with gastric involvement," *Cancer Chemotherapy and Pharmacology*, vol. 68, no. 6, pp. 1387–1395, 2011.

24

Chronic Lymphocytic Leukemia Presenting as a Subcortical Watershed Infarct

Mridul Gupta,[1] **Divita Singh**,[2] **Patrick Lee**,[3] **and Sandhya Kadiyam**[1]

[1]*Internal Medicine, Monmouth Medical Center, Long Branch, New Jersey, USA*
[2]*Ambulatory Care Pharmacy Resident, University of Florida, Gainesville, Florida, USA*
[3]*Hematology and Oncology, Monmouth Medical Center, Long Branch, New Jersey, USA*

Correspondence should be addressed to Mridul Gupta; drmridulgupta90@gmail.com

Academic Editor: Kiyotaka Kawauchi

Internal watershed infarcts (WI) involve white matter between deep and superficial arterial systems of middle cerebral artery. These infarcts are considered to be either from low blood flow or microembolism. Anemia is an extremely rare cause of watershed infarcts. Very few cases of hemolytic anemia causing watershed cerebral infarcts have been reported. Chronic lymphocytic leukemia (CLL) is frequently complicated with secondary autoimmune cytopenia such as autoimmune hemolytic anemia (AIHA), immune thrombocytopenia (ITP), and pure red cell aplasia. AIHA is present in about 7–10% of patients with CLL. AIHA from CLL presenting as WI is an extremely rare phenomenon with no previously published case reports to the best of our knowledge.

1. Introduction

Chronic lymphocytic lymphoma (CLL) is a chronic lymphoproliferative disorder characterized by progressive monoclonal accumulation of functionally incompetent lymphocytes. It is the most common leukemia in the Western world and accounts for about 25–30% of all leukemia cases in the Unites States [1]. Autoimmune cytopenias are a relatively common hematologic complication and can be refractory to treatment often requiring prolonged steroid use in combination with second-line therapies and transfusion of blood products. Systemic hemodynamic compromise arising from autoimmune hemolytic anemia (AIHA) in CLL is a rare occurrence. We hereby present a case of cortical watershed infarct (WI) arising from AIHA which in turn was found to be the presenting manifestation of CLL.

2. Case Presentation

A 72-year-old man with a history of hypertension and cerebrovascular accident (CVA) 20 years ago without significant residual weakness presented to the emergency department with a 3-day history of right-sided facial droop, slurred speech, and clumsiness of the right hand. He had a 20 pack-year smoking history. His family history revealed a father who died suddenly at the age of 47 from an unknown cause, a brother with acute leukemia, and a sister with myocardial infarction at the age of 37 years.

On examination, he had mild right facial droop, mild dysarthria, right pronator drift, and 4/5 motor strength in the right upper and lower extremity. The remainder of the neurological examination was unremarkable. Other significant findings in physical examination were mild hepatosplenomegaly with axillary and cervical lymphadenopathy. Hematological investigations on admission showed severe anemia with a hemoglobin (Hb) level of 44 g/L, leukocytes 42.8×10^9/L, lymphocytes 35.95×10^9/L, neutrophils 4.28×10^9/L, and a platelet count of 120×10^9/L. Further investigations were most consistent with AIHA with an unconjugated hyperbilirubinemia (2.7 mg/dL), elevated LDH (444 IU/L), low haptoglobulin (<15 mg/dL), an elevated reticulocyte count 83.62×10^9/L (7.4%), and a positive direct antiglobulin test (DAT) with both IgG and anti-C3d.

Peripheral blood flow cytometry showed a monoclonal B-cell population with surface lambda-positive population and positive for CD 45, CD 19, CD 20 (weak), CD 22, CD 23, CD 5, and CD 38 (partial). This immunophenotype pattern was consistent with diagnosis of CLL. The clinical picture was consistent with modified Rai stage III CLL. The patient had multiple autoantibodies on cross match.

Computed tomography (CT) of the head was negative for acute bleed or mass effect but was suspicious for evolving stroke. It also showed an area of encephalomalacia in the left basal ganglia related to an old infarct or hemorrhage. The patient could not receive thrombolytic therapy due to severe anemia. Brain magnetic resonance imaging (MRI) showed multiple small areas of diffusion restriction with corresponding mild T2 hypersensitivity in the bilateral corona radiata and centrum semiovale. These findings were consistent with subcortical WI in a characteristic "string of pearls" pattern (Figure 1). Magnetic resonance angiogram (MRA) of the head and neck was negative for stenosis in any of the major vessels. Transthoracic echocardiogram showed normal left and right ventricle systolic function with normal ejection fraction. Subsequent transesophageal echocardiogram did not show any left atrial thrombus or atrial mass. Interatrial septum was also intact. No arrhythmias were noted on telemetry during the admission; however, on a subsequent admission the patient was noted to have paroxysmal atrial fibrillation.

The patient was transfused to a goal Hb of 8 g/dL with least incompatible packed red cell (PRBC) transfusions. A total of 7 units of PRBC were transfused during the hospital stay, which the patient tolerated without any significant reactions. AIHA was treated with intravenous immunoglobulin (IVIG) 1 g/kg body weight daily for five days followed by 1 mg/kg of prednisone daily. At the time of discharge, the patient's Hb was 8.8 g/dL and LDH had normalized. There was no significant change in the platelet count with steroids. At discharge, oral prednisone was continued for four months and gradually tapered off over the next two months.

His blood counts stabilized with steroids and IVIG. About 1 year after initial presentation, he was found to have worsening diffuse adenopathy in the posterior cervical and axillary areas. PET/CT done to evaluate the possibility of Richter's transformation showed extensive bulky hypermetabolic lymphadenopathy in the head and neck region, bilateral axilla, bilateral hila, mediastinum, and throughout the mesentery and retroperitoneal distribution of the abdomen and pelvis. Maximum standardized uptake value (SUV) of 4.64 was noted in the right posterior cervical region. At this time, the patient's LDH was 538 IU/L. Repeat flow cytometry showed a monoclonal surface lambda population which was positive for CD 20 (weak), CD 19, CD 5, CD 23, CD45, and CD 22. This pattern was again consistent with CLL.

The patient's clinical status declined rapidly. Plan for excision lymph node biopsy to rule out Richter's phenomenon had to be deferred due to severe debilitation and refractory AIHA. He was started on obinutuzumab with chlorambucil but had an anaphylactic reaction to obinutuzumab which led to discontinuation after 2 doses. His diffuse adenopathy did respond to the two doses of obinutuzumab with near-complete resolution over the next several days. The patient however remained very debilitated and confined to bed and further consideration of therapy was not appropriate and further staging of his lymphoma was deferred until his condition improved. His hospital course was complicated with recurrence of autoimmune hemolytic anemia, which was managed with blood product transfusions, steroids, and IVIG as before. He was eventually started on rituximab for refractory AIHA. He was in the middle of his second course of rituximab before his counts began to improve.

3. Discussion

CLL is the most common leukemia in the Western countries. In the United States, CLL accounts for approximately 25 to 30% of all leukemia cases [1]. It is more common in the elderly with a median age of 71 years at diagnosis [2]. There is also male predominance with a ratio of 1 : 6 : 1 approximately [1]. CLL is frequently complicated with secondary autoimmune cytopenias such as AIHA, immune thrombocytopenia (ITP), pure red cell aplasia (PRCA), and autoimmune agranulocytosis (AG). Incidence of these cytopenias is estimated to be approximately 4.3–9.7% in patients with CLL in most studies [3]. However, as these cytopenias often precede CLL diagnosis or occur at any time during the disease process, these numbers are likely to be an underestimation [4]. Systemic hemodynamic compromise arising from AIHA in CLL is an extremely rare occurrence. Our patient presented with a cortical WI arising from AIHA which in turn was found to be the presenting manifestation of CLL.

WI or border zone infarcts are ischemic lesions in the brain parenchyma located at the junction of territories supplied by 2 different non-anastomosing arterial systems. Two main types of WI described in literature are the cortical WI and the internal WI. The cortical WI occurs between cortical territories of anterior cerebral artery (ACA), middle cerebral artery (MCA), and posterior cerebral artery (PCA). The internal WI affects corona radiata between territories supplied by superficial and deep perforators of MCA and/or centrum semiovale between territories of superficial perforators of ACA and MCA [5].

WI represents about 10% of all brain infarcts in autopsy studies [6]. Actual incidence may be much higher since these infarcts are usually mild, asymptomatic, and nonfatal. In a study by Sorgun et al. to determine the etiologic subtypes of WI, out of 32 patients with a subcortical watershed infarct, 21 patients had large-artery atherosclerosis, 5 patients had cardio-embolism, and 3 had stroke due to causes such as aneurysm, hypercoagulability from chronic myeloid leukemia, and vasculitis [7]. Cortical WI are commonly related to microembolic phenomenon, while internal WI occur as a consequence of hemodynamic impairment [8].

Radiologically, internal WI can be either confluent or partial. Confluent infarcts are larger cigar shaped along the lateral ventricle. Partial internal WI can be either in the form of isolated single lesions or a chain-like "rosary" pattern.

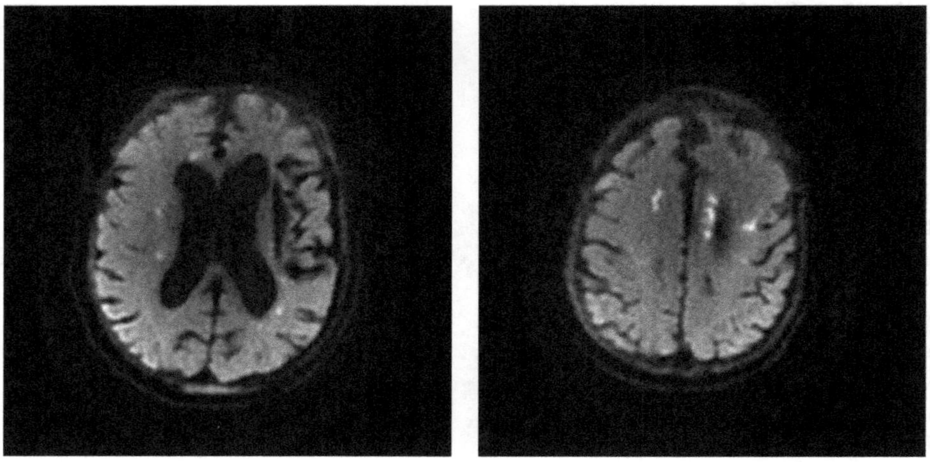

(a) (b)

Figure 1: Brain MRI showing small areas of diffusion restriction with T2 hyperintensity over (a) anterior horn of right lateral ventricle and (b) posterior horn of left lateral ventricle and left corona radiata, consistent with acute infarcts.

This rosary-like pattern in the centrum semiovale strongly supports the hemodynamic mechanism theory of causing WI [5]. Partial internal WI can sometimes be difficult to differentiate from leukoaraiosis and might even coexist in elderly patients.

Atrial fibrillation and atheromatous plaques are major offenders in causing microembolic diseases. Hemodynamic compromise leading to WI can arise from severe stenosis or occlusion of craniocervical arteries and/or systemic hypoperfusion in the setting of cardiac arrest or systemic hypotension. Hypoperfusion can further potentiate effects by affecting the clearance of microemboli [9]. Systemic hypotension and carotid disease are major etiologic causations of hemodynamic compromise leading to WI. Hemodynamic compromise from severe anemia leading to cerebral hypoperfusion and subsequent WI is an extremely rare phenomenon. Our patient presented with severe hemolytic anemia which was later found to be the presenting manifestation of CLL.

AIHA occurs in about 7% of patients with CLL and an additional 7–14% of patients may have a positive DAT without clinical evidence of hemolysis. [3] These numbers are variable based on the sample population and duration of follow-up. Moreno et al. [10] analyzed data from 960 Spanish CLL patients over 29 years and reported autoimmune cytopenias in 7.29% (70) patients out of which 5.1% (49) had AIHA, 2.08% (20) had ITP, and 0.10% (1) had Evan's syndrome. Out of these patients with CLL, 19 were found to have autoimmune cytopenias at diagnosis, 3 prior to diagnosis, and 48 during the course of the disease. In an observational study of 1750 CLL patients with a 10-year follow-up at Mayo Clinic, autoimmune cytopenias were diagnosed in 4.3% patients, with 2.3% patients developing AIHA and 2% developing ITP [11]. Data from 964 patients from an Israel CLL study group followed for 35 years revealed 11 (1.14%) cases with AIHA at diagnosis, 55 (5.70%) with DAT positivity without AIHA at diagnosis, and 43 (4.46%) developed AIHA during follow-up [12].

Various theories have been postulated to explain the pathophysiology behind these secondary cytopenias. Nonmalignant B cells in CLL can produce high affinity immunoglobulin G (IgG) directed against the antigens on erythrocytes and platelets, leading to AIHA and ITP [13]. CLL cells can also act as efficient antigen presenting cells, leading to T-cell response with subsequent autoimmunity [13]. Cytokines production from CLL cells can result in inhibition of normal erythropoiesis or megakaryopoiesis, leading to development of AIHA or ITP [14]. CLL cells can rarely act as effector cells, secreting a pathological monoclonal antibody [15]. CLL cells may also be stimulated through their polyreactive B-cell receptor (BCR) that recognizes autoantigens [15].

Although DAT is the most important diagnostic test, AIHA is also known to occur with a negative DAT. DAT-negative AIHA can arise from either lower affinity antibodies, antibodies in concentrations below threshold for the test, or autoantibodies of IgA class which are not detected with the current testing methods [14].

Warm AIHA is caused by warm agglutinins which are predominantly IgG antibodies that react with protein antigens on the red blood cell (RBC) surface at body temperature and cause extravascular hemolysis. Cold agglutinins cause cold AIHA and are predominantly IgM antibodies that generally react with polysaccharide antigens on the RBC surface only at temperatures below that of the core temperature of the body and commonly cause intravascular hemolysis. Differentiating between these two forms is important in terms of diagnosis and treatment.

Initial management of patients presenting with acute anemia consists of supportive care and may require transfusion of blood products based on local protocols that consider the blood count and patient symptoms. When treatment of CLL is not indicated, immunosuppression can be used alone. Immunosuppression with systemic glucocorticoids is used as a first-line treatment for AIHA from warm agglutinins. Prednisone 1 mg/kg is given for 4 weeks, which can be tapered over 1-2 months. Use of intravenous immunoglobulin (1 g/kg body weight daily for 5 days) in the beginning can also be considered. Chemotherapeutic agents are not to be used as first-line agents for CLL associated with AIHA or ITP [16]. Steroids are less effective for AIHA with cold agglutinins and are not considered as first-line treatment [14]. Instead rituximab is the preferred first-line agent for AIHA patients with cold antibodies [17].

If underlying CLL also needs to be treated, steroids can be used to manage AIHA while chemotherapeutic agents are being used. Rituximab also has some activity against CLL, so it can be used in monotherapy or in combination with other chemotherapy agents [18]. Rituximab has been used successfully in patients with warm AIHA in combination with or without steroids as first-line treatment or as a second-line agent following failure from first-line management. Recent consensus guidelines from an international workshop on CLL recommend against using targeted agents such as rituximab as first-line agents before steroids in the treatment of AIHA in CLL patients [16].

For patients who fail to respond to first-line therapy, cyclophosphamide, azathioprine, cyclosporine, and mycophenolate mofetil have been used as second-line agents in the treatment of DAT-positive AIHA [16]. The role of splenectomy in AIHA associated with CLL is not clearly defined. In a study by Akpek et al. in patients with AIHA in CLL, splenectomy resulted in partial response in half of the patients and no response in the other half [19]. More recently, Hill et al. concluded that laparoscopic splenectomy was safe and effective in treating AIHA associated with CLL in patients who had failed medical therapy [20]. Patient preference had often elevated use of rituximab prior to splenectomy.

Patients not responding to first- or second-line treatment within 4–6 weeks must be considered for alternate treatment options such as cyclophosphamide, mycophenolate mofetil, cyclosporine, or azathioprine [4]. Alternate causes of anemia should always be ruled out in refractory and relapsed cases prior to escalating treatment.

Rituximab has also been used in combination with other cytotoxic agents to provide more "CLL-directed treatment." Combination therapies with rituximab for autoimmune cytopenias include rituximab–cyclophosphamide–dexamethasone (RCD) [21, 22], rituximab–cyclophosphamide–vincristine–prednisone (R-CVP) [23], and rituximab–bendamustine [24]. Evidence for these combination modalities is limited to small case series.

Recently, newer monoclonal antibodies have been studied for their role in the treatment of refractory cases of AIHA with CLL. Nader et al. reported a case of rituximab-refractory AIHA associated with CLL which was successfully treated with ofatumumab [25]. Ibrutinib is a bruton tyrosine kinase inhibitor that has been approved for the initial treatment or in relapsed/refractory CLL cases. Furthermore, in patients with del(17p)/TP53 mutations, ibrutinib is the preferred choice for initial therapy. Although initial clinical trials of ibrutinib had excluded patients with uncontrolled hemolysis, recently there have been case reports of ibrutinib successfully being used for CLL-associated AIHA either as monotherapy or in combination with rituximab/steroids [26, 27].

In a randomized controlled trial from a German CLL study group, obinituzumab combined with chlorambucil was found to be superior to rituximab–chlorambucil combination or chlorambucil monotherapy in previously untreated patients [28]. Of note, in this trial, patients with AIHA were not considered suitable for enrollment.

Our patient was given a trial of obinituzumab–chlorambucil based on its superiority over the rituximab–chlorambucil combination. Despite favorable response in his lymph nodes after two treatments, it was not reinitiated due to severe reaction and near-complete remission of his adenopathy.

References

[1] R. L. Siegel, K. D. Miller, and A. Jemal, "Cancer statistics, 2018," *CA: A Cancer Journal for Clinicians*, vol. 68, no. 1, pp. 7–30, 2018.

[2] R. B. Rowswell-Turner and P. M. Barr, "Treatment of chronic lymphocytic leukemia in older adults," *Journal of Geriatric Oncology*, vol. 8, no. 5, pp. 315–319, 2017.

[3] K. Hodgson, G. Ferrer, A. Pereira, C. Moreno, and E. Montserrat, "Autoimmune cytopenia in chronic lymphocytic leukaemia: diagnosis and treatment," *British Journal of Haematology*, vol. 154, no. 1, pp. 14–22, 2011.

[4] M. Tsang and S. A. Parikh, "A concise review of autoimmune cytopenias in chronic lymphocytic leukemia," *Current Hematologic Malignancy Reports*, vol. 12, no. 1, pp. 29–38, 2017.

[5] I. Momjian-Mayor and J.-C. Baron, "The pathophysiology of watershed infarction in internal carotid artery disease," *Stroke*, vol. 36, no. 3, pp. 567–577, 2005.

[6] L. Jörgensen and A. Torvik, "Ischaemic cerebrovascular diseases in an autopsy series part 2. Prevalence, location, pathogenesis, and clinical course of cerebral infarcts," *Journal of the Neurological Sciences*, vol. 9, no. 2, pp. 285–320, 1969.

[7] M. H. Sorgun, S. Rzayev, V. Yilmaz, and C. T. Isıkay, "Etiologic subtypes of watershed infarcts," *Journal of Stroke and Cerebrovascular Diseases*, vol. 24, no. 11, pp. 2478–2483, 2015.

[8] C. Weill, L. Suissa, J. Darcourt, and M.-H. Mahagne, "The pathophysiology of watershed infarction: a three-dimensional time-of-flight magnetic resonance angiography study," *Journal of Stroke and Cerebrovascular Diseases*, vol. 26, no. 9, pp. 1966–1973, 2017.

[9] L. R. Caplan and M. Hennerici, "Impaired clearance of emboli (washout) is an important link between hypoperfusion, embolism, and ischemic stroke," *Archives of Neurology*, vol. 55, no. 11, pp. 1475–1482, 1998.

[10] C. Moreno, K. Hodgson, G. Ferrer et al., "Autoimmune cytopenia in chronic lymphocytic leukemia: prevalence, clinical associations, and prognostic significance," *Blood*, vol. 116, no. 23, pp. 4771–4776, 2010.

[11] C. S. Zent, W. Ding, M. S. Reinalda et al., "Autoimmune cytopenia in chronic lymphocytic leukemia/small

lymphocytic lymphoma: changes in clinical presentation and prognosis," *Leukemia and Lymphoma*, vol. 50, no. 8, pp. 1261–1268, 2009.

[12] A. Duek, L. Shvidel, A. Braester, and A. Berrebi, "Clinical and immunologic aspects of B chronic lymphocytic leukemia associated with autoimmune disorders," *Israel Medical Association Journal*, vol. 8, no. 12, pp. 828–831, 2006.

[13] A. M. Hall, M. A. Vickers, E. McLeod, and R. N. Barker, "Rh autoantigen presentation to helper T cells in chronic lymphocytic leukemia by malignant B cells," *Blood*, vol. 105, no. 5, pp. 2007–2015, 2005.

[14] C. Visco, W. Barcellini, F. Maura, A. Neri, A. Cortelezzi, and F. Rodeghiero, "Autoimmune cytopenias in chronic lymphocytic leukemia," *American Journal of Hematology*, vol. 89, no. 11, pp. 1055–1062, 2014.

[15] G. D'Arena, R. Guariglia, F. La Rocca et al., "Autoimmune cytopenias in chronic lymphocytic leukemia," *Clinical and Developmental Immunology*, vol. 2013, Article ID 730131, 8 pages, 2013.

[16] M. Hallek, B. D. Cheson, D. Catovsky et al., "iwCLL guidelines for diagnosis, indications for treatment, response assessment, and supportive management of CLL," *Blood*, vol. 131, no. 25, pp. 2745–2760, 2018.

[17] G. D'Arena, L. Laurenti, S. Capalbo et al., "Rituximab therapy for chronic lymphocytic leukemia-associated autoimmune hemolytic anemia," *American Journal of Hematology*, vol. 81, no. 8, pp. 598–602, 2006.

[18] K. A. Rogers and J. A. Woyach, "Secondary autoimmune cytopenias in chronic lymphocytic leukemia," *Seminars in Oncology*, vol. 43, no. 2, pp. 300–310, 2016.

[19] G. Akpek, D. McAneny, and L. Weintraub, "Comparative response to splenectomy in coombs-positive autoimmune hemolytic anemia with or without associated disease," *American Journal of Hematology*, vol. 61, no. 2, pp. 98–102, 1999.

[20] J. Hill, R. M. Walsh, S. McHam, F. Brody, and M. Kalaycio, "Laparoscopic splenectomy for autoimmune hemolytic anemia in patients with chronic lymphocytic leukemia: a case series and review of the literature," *American Journal of Hematology*, vol. 75, no. 3, pp. 134–138, 2004.

[21] N. Gupta, S. Kavuru, D. Patel et al., "Rituximab-based chemotherapy for steroid-refractory autoimmune hemolytic anemia of chronic lymphocytic leukemia," *Leukemia*, vol. 16, no. 10, pp. 2092–2095, 2002.

[22] J. Rossignol, A.-S. Michallet, L. Oberic et al., "Rituximab-cyclophosphamide-dexamethasone combination in the management of autoimmune cytopenias associated with chronic lymphocytic leukemia," *Leukemia*, vol. 25, no. 3, pp. 473–478, 2010.

[23] D. A. Bowen, T. G. Call, T. D. Shanafelt et al., "Treatment of autoimmune cytopenia complicating progressive chronic lymphocytic leukemia/small lymphocytic lymphoma with rituximab, cyclophosphamide, vincristine, and prednisone," *Leukemia and Lymphoma*, vol. 51, no. 4, pp. 620–627, 2010.

[24] A. Quinquenel, C. Willekens, J. Dupuis et al., "Bendamustine and rituximab combination in the management of chronic lymphocytic leukemia-associated autoimmune hemolytic anemia: a multicentric retrospective study of the French CLL intergroup (GCFLLC/MW and GOELAMS)," *American Journal of Hematology*, vol. 90, no. 3, pp. 204–207, 2015.

[25] K. Nader, M. Patel, and A. Ferber, "Ofatumumab in rituximab-refractory autoimmune hemolytic anemia associated with chronic lymphocytic leukemia: a case report and review of literature," *Clinical Lymphoma Myeloma and Leukemia*, vol. 13, no. 4, pp. 511–513, 2013.

[26] S. Manda, N. Dunbar, C. R. Marx-Wood, and A. V. Danilov, "Ibrutinib is an effective treatment of autoimmune haemolytic anaemia in chronic lymphocytic leukaemia," *British Journal of Haematology*, vol. 170, no. 5, pp. 734–736, 2015.

[27] C. Vitale, I. E. Ahn, M. Sivina et al., "Autoimmune cytopenias in patients with chronic lymphocytic leukemia treated with ibrutinib," *Haematologica*, vol. 101, no. 6, pp. e254–e258, 2016.

[28] V. Goede, K. Fischer, R. Busch et al., "Obinutuzumab plus chlorambucil in patients with CLL and coexisting conditions," *New England Journal of Medicine*, vol. 370, no. 12, pp. 1101–1110, 2014.

25

Combined Ruxolitinib and Venetoclax Treatment in a Patient with a *BCR-JAK2* Rearranged Myeloid Neoplasm

Coen J. Lap ,[1] Samah Nassereddine,[1] Min-Ling Liu,[2] Victor E. Nava,[2] and Anita Aggarwal[1,2]

[1] *The George Washington University Medical Faculty Associates, Washington, DC, USA*
[2] *Washington DC Veterans Affairs Medical Center, Washington, DC, USA*

Correspondence should be addressed to Coen J. Lap; clap@mfa.gwu.edu

Academic Editor: Håkon Reikvam

Hematological malignancies with a *BCR-JAK2* rearrangement have been described only sporadically in the literature over the last three decades. Although most patients suffer from a chronic myeloid neoplasm with marked eosinophilia, the clinical presentation varies significantly and can even manifest as a lymphoid malignancy. In this case report, we present a patient with a therapy-related *BCR-JAK2*$^+$ myeloid neoplasm with extensive extramedullary disease localizing in the lymph nodes. While treatment with a JAK2 inhibitor (ruxolitinib) was not able to stop disease progression, combination treatment with inhibitors of both JAK2 and BCL2 (venetoclax) resulted in disease control for over 1.5 years. Combining these two inhibitors might be strategic in these patients, not only because BCL2 is a downstream target of JAK/STAT signaling but also because BCL2 is crucial for JAK2 inhibitor resistance. The recent inclusion of *JAK2*-rearranged malignancies in major classification systems and guidelines emphasizes the importance of not only getting a better understanding of the clinical phenotype of these rare disorders but also of identifying alternative treatment options for patients ineligible for allogeneic stem cell transplantation. Considering the low toxicity of combination treatment with these two small molecule inhibitors, this regimen could be further explored in future studies.

1. Introduction

Activating mutations in Janus kinase 2 *(JAK2)*, which include *JAK2* V617F and mutations in exon 12, are found in a high proportion of patients diagnosed with chronic myeloproliferative neoplasms (MPN), including >95% of patients with polycythemia vera and approximately 55–65% of patients with essential thrombocytosis and primary myelofibrosis [1]. While these mutations are considered crucial molecular events in the pathogenesis of these disorders, rare chromosomal translocations involving *JAK2* have been described in patients suffering from both myeloid and lymphoid malignancies [2, 3]. The t(9; 22) (p24.1; q11.2) is a recurrent rearrangement that juxtaposes the *Breakpoint Cluster Region* gene (*BCR*; 22q11.2) to the *JAK2* gene (9p24.1), which leads to the formation of a *BCR-JAK2* fusion [4]. While this translocation has been identified in patients diagnosed with acute myeloid leukemia (AML) and B-cell acute lymphoblastic leukemia (B-ALL), most case reports have described it as the sole genetic abnormality observed in patients suffering from a clinical disease that resembles myeloid neoplasms, including MPN, myelodysplastic syndrome (MDS), or MPN/MDS overlap syndromes and is often associated with significant extramedullary hematopoiesis and/or bone marrow failure [2, 3, 5–8]. In most patients, the disease is highly therapy-resistant with rapid progression occurring within the first couple of months after diagnosis [9]. While JAK2 inhibitors have been suggested to be of some benefit in controlling disease, so far, long-term remissions have only been achieved after allogeneic stem cell transplantation (allo-SCT) [10, 11]. Here, we describe a case of a patient suffering from a therapy-related *BCR-JAK2*$^+$ myeloid neoplasm with significant disease localized in his lymph nodes. While monotherapy with a JAK2 inhibitor (ruxolitinib) was not able to control disease, combined treatment with inhibitors of JAK2 and BCL2 (venetoclax) resulted in disease control for over 1.5 years. A rationale for combining these two small molecule inhibitors is provided as an additional option, which could be further explored for patients with this rare hematological malignancy, especially when allo-SCT is not feasible.

2. Case Presentation

A 54-year-old male presented initially in February 2013 with left axillary lymphadenopathy. He was diagnosed with stage IIA nodular lymphocyte predominant Hodgkin lymphoma (NLPHL) and received two cycles of ABVD (adriamycin, bleomycin, vinblastine, and dacarbazine) before he became lost to follow-up. In March 2014, he presented again with biopsy-proven relapsing NLPHL. A bone marrow aspirate was performed at that time, revealing an unremarkable flow analysis and a normal karyotype (46XY [12]). He received three cycles of R-EPOCH (rituximab, etoposide, prednisone, vincristine, cyclophosphamide, and doxorubicin) with additional radiation therapy to the left axillary region for residual disease. He remained in complete remission until May 2018, when he presented with fatigue, a 25 kg weight loss over three months and was found to be anemic with a hemoglobin (Hgb) of 7.2 g/dL, platelet count (Plt) of $159 \times 10^3/\mu L$, and a white blood cell count (WBC) of $6.1 \times 10^{3/}\mu L$. Peripheral blood smear revealed a neutrophilic left-shift with 3% myelocytes, 2% metamyelocytes, and 6% eosinophils. Evaluation of the red blood cells (RBC) revealed marked anisopoikilocytosis, teardrop cells, and 2% nucleated RBC. No circulating blasts were seen. FDG-PET/CT displayed extensive FDG-avid lymphadenopathy (SUV_{max}~10) with splenomegaly measuring 18.4 cm. Bone marrow (BM) biopsy demonstrated a hypercellular BM with left-shifted myeloid hyperplasia but less than 1% blasts (Figure 1(a)), an increased myeloid to erythroid ratio (>5 : 1) and diffuse grade 3 reticulin fibrosis (Figure 1(b)). Cytogenetics revealed a 46XY, del(6) (p21.2p24), t(22; 9; 11) (q11.2, p24, p11.2) [11]/46XY, del(9) [9] karyotype with fluorescent in situ hybridization (FISH) analysis showing absence of a *BCR-ABL1* rearrangement, but three copies of *BCR* (Figure 2). The third copy of *BCR* was identified to be on the short arm terminus of chromosome 9 resulting in a *BCR-JAK2* fusion as suggested with an additional *JAK2* (9p24.1) probe (not shown). The rearrangement was confirmed with RNA sequencing, which revealed a break in exon 1 of *BCR* (nucleotide 1107 and codon 369) and a break in exon 17 of *JAK2* (nucleotide 2171 and codon 724) leading to an in-frame fusion. The resulting product included the coiled-coil oligodimerization domain of *BCR* as well as the area distal to the pseudokinase domain (JH2) of *JAK2*, thereby maintaining the active tyrosine kinase domain (JH1) in exon 19. Additional mutation analysis was negative for *JAK2* V617 F or alterations in *CALR*, *PDGFRA*, *PDGFRB*, or *FGFR1* but did reveal an alteration in *CD36* (c.157_158AA > G_p.N53 fs*24). Excisional biopsy of a lymph node ruled out lymphoma, but revealed extensive extramedullary involvement of the same myeloid malignancy with prominent erythroid precursors, atypical megakaryocytes, and left-shifted myeloid cells without increase of blasts (Figure 3). Importantly, the same *BCR-JAK2* translocation was identified in the biopsy and confirmed with RNA sequencing.

Pending the results of the molecular analysis, the patient was started on the *BCR-ABL1* tyrosine kinase inhibitor (TKI) imatinib mesylate 400 mg once daily due to an initial concern of CML. Because of limited response and upon identification of the *BCR-JAK2* translocation, treatment was switched to ruxolitinib and uptitrated to 20 mg twice daily. An early referral for allo-SCT was discussed, but the patient decided to postpone this. While initially an improvement in blood counts was observed (Hgb, 10.8 g/dL; Plt, $180 \times 10^3/\mu L$; WBC, $8.1 \times 10^{3/}\mu L$) with a reduced need for transfusions, he developed worsening anemia (Hgb, 7.8 g/dL), thrombocytopenia (Plt, $30 \times 10^3/\mu L$), and leukocytosis (WBC, $17.6 \times 10^{3/}\mu L$) with an elevated LDH (680 U/L) in January 2019. A peripheral smear revealed 6% promyelocytes, 3% metamyelocytes, 6% eosinophils, and 2% blasts, but repeated bone marrow evaluation only showed diffuse fibrosis and the previously identified *BCR-JAK2* translocation. The spleen remained enlarged at 19 cm on imaging. Ruxolitinib was continued, and because of disease progression, venetoclax was initiated and uptitrated to 400 mg daily. At that point, he was evaluated for allo-SCT but was found ineligible due to diminished pulmonary function. After several weeks, blood counts improved, and the patient became transfusion-independent and EPO support was discontinued. Over time, his blood counts normalized (Hgb, 12.4 g/dl; Plt, $167 \times 10^3/\mu L$; WBC, $5.7 \times 10^3/\mu L$ with 2% eosinophils) with repeat imaging, six months after the start of venetoclax, revealing a significant decrease in lymphadenopathy and a reduction in the spleen size to 13.1 cm. A new BM biopsy showed stable disease with extensive fibrosis, no increase in blasts, but persistence of the *BCR-JAK2* fusion and the *CD36* alteration, as well as a new *TET2* mutation (c.3782 G > A_p.R1261H). During this time, the patient tolerated the combination regimen well without development of infections, need for blood product support, or hospitalizations. Although no cytogenetic response was observed, the treatment significantly improved his quality of life. He remained stable under this combination treatment until May 2020, at which point he presented with abdominal complaints and renal failure as a result of bulky lymphadenopathy and splenomegaly due to disease progression. Ruxolitinib and venetoclax were discontinued. Blood counts revealed Hgb, 11 g/dL; Plt, $170 \times 10^3/\mu L$; and WBC, $12.1 \times 10^3/\mu L$ with a peripheral smear showing left-shifted hematopoiesis with 4% eosinophils and 1% blasts. Renewed bone marrow analysis only revealed fibrosis without a significant increase in blasts. The patient was started on azacytidine and re-evaluated for allo-SCT. However, allo-SCT was further postponed as a result of the patient contracting COVID-19. During that period, azacytidine was continued, and ruxolitinib was restarted. Unfortunately, the disease progressed with worsening bone marrow failure, without signs of transformation, and he passed away several months later.

3. Discussion

The 2017 revision of the World Health Organization (WHO) Classification of Myeloid Neoplasms and Acute Leukemia included a new provisional entity "*Myeloid Neoplasm with PCM1-JAK2 Rearrangement*" in the category of "*Myeloid/Lymphoid Neoplasms Associated with Eosinophilia and Rearrangement of PDGFRA, PDGFRB, or FGFR1,*

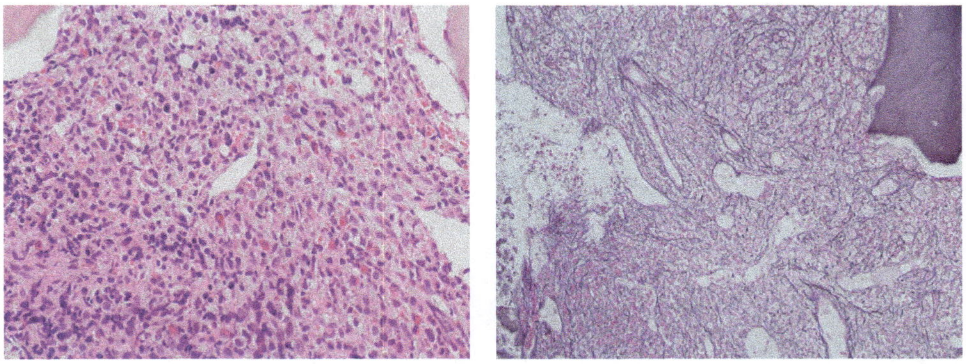

(a) (b)

FIGURE 1: Bone marrow biopsy showing a hypercellular marrow with marked myeloid hyperplasia with left shift ((a) hematoxylin and eosin stain, 400x) and grade 3 fibrosis ((b) reticulin stain, 200x).

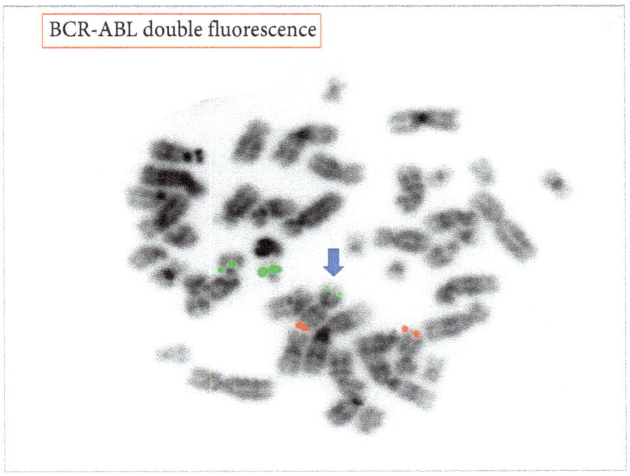

FIGURE 2: Fluorescent in situ hybridization with probes for *BCR* (22q11.2, green signal) and *ABL1* (9q34.1, red signal) was negative for a *BCR-ABL1* rearrangement. However, a third signal for the *BCR* probe (green signal, arrow) was observed, suggesting partial or complete gain of chromosome 22 or a translocation that involves *BCR* with a partner gene other than *ABL1*. Additional testing with a probe for *JAK2* (9p24.1, not shown) suggested the presence of a *BCR-JAK2* fusion, which was confirmed with RNA sequencing.

or with PCM1-JAK2" [12]. While the patient described here does not have a hematological malignancy with a *PCM1-JAK2* rearrangement, many experts in the field advocate to classify those rare cases with a *JAK2* rearrangement, including gene partners other than *PCM1*, in the same category because of similar clinical features [13]. This is also highlighted by the inclusion of patients with a *BCR-JAK2* rearrangement in the latest version of the U.S. National Comprehensive Cancer Network (NCCN) guidelines for "Myeloid/Lymphoid Neoplasms with Eosinophilia and Tyrosine Kinase Fusion Genes" (version 3.2021). Regardless of the classification, the presence of a *BCR-JAK2* translocation has not been linked to a specific clinical phenotype although most patients present as a chronic myeloid neoplasm with marked eosinophilia (~50–70%) (Table 1). However, eosinophilia can be notably absent and is not a requirement for the diagnosis. Additionally, *BCR-JAK2* rearrangements are sometimes identified in the new provisional entity of Philadelphia chromosome-like ALL, which are characterized by activated tyrosine kinase signaling as well as JAK/STAT signaling but lack the presence of a *BCR-ABL1* rearrangement [19]. The clinical heterogeneity may be the result of both disease factors (additional mutations and subclones) as well as existing host factors (germline allele diversity). Our patient presented with symptoms of a myeloid malignancy with a newly acquired *BCR-JAK2* rearrangement, four years after treatment for relapsing NLPHL. Considering that the patient had a normal bone marrow evaluation at the time of his relapsing NLHPL and was subsequently exposed to cytotoxic chemotherapy, including etoposide and cyclophosphamide, it supports a diagnosis of a therapy-related malignancy. It is likely that clonal evolution and expansion over time have resulted in a secondary myeloid neoplasm. Although the clinical significance of a *CD36* N53 fs*24 mutation is not clear at the moment, it is important to mention that it has been identified in patients with mixed phenotype acute leukemia's (MPAL) [20]. More importantly, the R1261H missense mutation in the epigenetic modifier *TET2* is a recurrent abnormality identified in (therapy-related) myeloid malignancies and is considered a driver of clonal hematopoiesis [21].

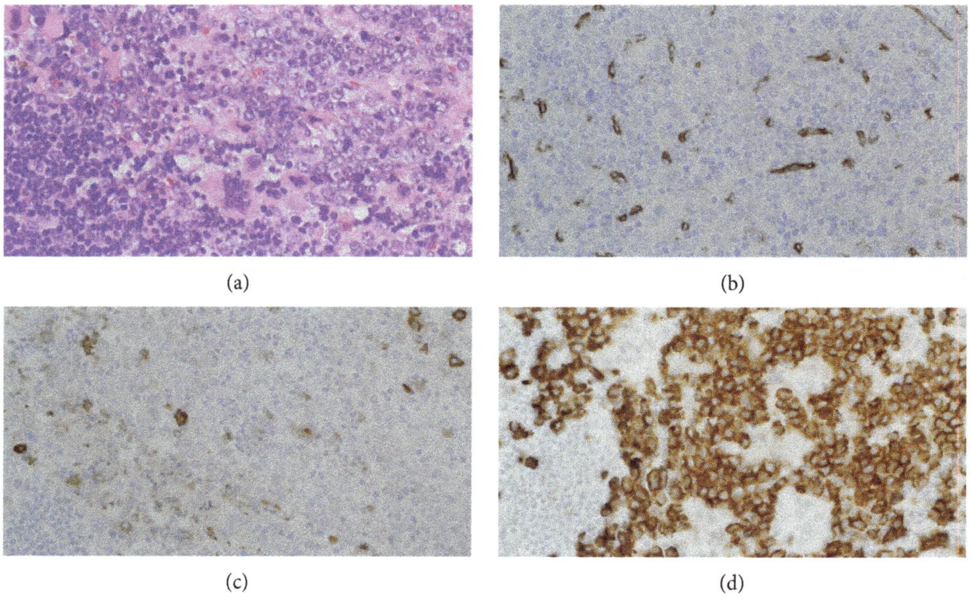

Figure 3: Lymph node showing extensive extramedullary involvement by a myeloproliferative neoplasm with numerous megakaryocytes ((a) hematoxylin and eosin stain, 400x), no increase in blasts ((b) CD34 immunostain, 400x), or significant myeloid cells ((c) MPO immunostain, 400x) but with prominent erythroid precursors ((d) CD71 immunostain, 400x).

Table 1: Summary of the literature regarding described phenotype, treatment, and response duration of patients with a *BCR-JAK2* fusion.

Reference	Age	Sex	Disease	Treatment	Follow-up
Griesinger et al. [2]	63	F	CML-like MPD, myeloid blast crisis	Imatinib, hydroxyurea, interferon-alpha	Complete hematological response. 20 months after diagnosis, she developed myeloid blast crisis and died.
Kantarcioglu et al. [3]	64	F	MDS	Not described	Died 3 months after diagnosis
Cuesta-Domínguez et al. [4]	58	M	B-ALL	Not described	Not described
Cirmena et al. [5]	67	F	AML	Not described	Not described
Tirado et al. [6]	14	M	B-ALL	Not described	Not described
Snider et al. [7]	59	M	MPN with eosinophilia, MPAL	Hydroxyurea, chemotherapy, allo-SCT	Transformation to MPAL 12 months after diagnosis. No evidence of disease 30 days after allo-SCT.
Elnaggar et al. [8]	84	M	CML-like MPD	Imatinib	Lost to follow-up
Schwaab et al. [10]	n/a	n/a	Myeloid neoplasm	Ruxolitinib 20 mg BID, allo-SCT	Complete hematological and cytogenetic remission on ruxolitinib. Relapsed after 18 months upon which referred for allo-SCT.
Schwaab et al. [11]	69	M	MDS/MPN	Ruxolitinib 20 mg BID, allo-SCT	Complete hematological, cytogenetic, and molecular response. AlloSCT while in remission
He et al. [14]	36	F	MPN with eosinophilia	Dasatinib, allo-SCT	No response of dasatinib. No evidence of disease 18 months after allo-SCT.
Bellesso et al. [15]	54	M	*BCR-ABL*$^-$ CML	Imatinib, dasatinib, allo-SCT	No response of imatinib or dasatinib. Died of aGvHD 53 days after allo-SCT
Impera et al. [16]	49	F	MPN-unclassifiable	Imatinib, dasatinib peg-interferon	No initial response with imatinib or dasatinib. Partial hematological response with peg-interferon
Lane et al. [17]	44	M	Atypical CML with leukemia cutis	Not described	Not described
Thakral et al. [18]	31	M	MPN with eosinophilia	Hydroxyurea, allo-SCT	No evidence of disease three months posttransplantation

CML, chronic myeloid leukemia; MPD, myeloproliferative disorder; MDS, myelodysplastic syndrome; B-ALL, B-cell acute lymphoblastic leukemia; AML, acute myeloid leukemia; MPN, myeloproliferative neoplasm; MPAL, mixed phenotype acute leukemia; allo-SCT, allogeneic stem cell transplantation; BID, twice a day; aGvHD, acute graft-versus-host disease; F, female; M, male.

As a result of the t(9; 22) (p24.1; q11.2), a fusion gene is formed in which the oligodimerization domain of *BCR* is juxtaposed to the *JAK2* tyrosine kinase domain resulting in constitutive activation of the JAK/STAT signaling pathway, which promotes cellular proliferation, differentiation, and growth [4, 22]. JAK inhibitors such as ruxolitinib (JAK1/2) have been used successfully in patients with *JAK2*-mutated MPN and, as such, have been proposed as a possible treatment for patients with a *BCR-JAK2*$^{+}$ myeloid malignancy [10, 11]. Unfortunately, responses seen in the handful of patients treated to date have been mixed with some progressing rapidly and others obtaining a complete cytogenetic response. However, even cytogenetic responses are usually short-lived due to the development of *JAK2* inhibitor resistance. Although our patient had an initial response after the start of ruxolitinib, he progressed five months later, prompting initiation of the BCL2 inhibitor venetoclax. Combining these two inhibitors may be strategic since downstream transcriptional targets of JAK/STAT signaling include antiapoptotic members of the BCL2 family, such as BCL2 and BCL-xl [23–25]. Several preclinical studies have suggested a beneficial synergistic effect of combining these two inhibitors in patients with *JAK2*-mutated hematological malignancies [25–27]. Moreover, resistance to JAK2 inhibitors has been attributed to overexpression of both BCL2 and BCL-xl. Although our patient did not develop a cytogenetic remission, the combination treatment stabilized the disease for over 1.5 years, achieving normal blood counts and significant reduction in splenomegaly and lymphadenopathy before final progression.

Even with combination treatment, our patient eventually developed progressive disease and succumbed before he was able to undergo allo-SCT. Although combined treatment might be able to control disease for a significant period of time, even when monotherapy with a JAK2 inhibitor fails, only allo-SCT results in long-term disease control, affirming the need for early referral. It needs to be emphasized that TKIs used for the treatment of *BCR-ABL1*$^{+}$ CML have not shown to be of any benefit and should be avoided in the treatment of these patients [11]. Considering the rarity of hematological malignancies with a *BCR-JAK2* translocation, it remains important to report cases to disseminate clinical experience, which may allow better characterization of the clinical phenotype and provide beneficial insights regarding targeted therapy regimens for patients who are not eligible for allo-SCT.

4. Conclusion

BCR-JAK2-rearranged hematological malignancies are rare disorders that can have a variable clinical presentation but should be classified as a "Myeloid/Lymphoid Neoplasms with Eosinophilia and Gene Rearrangement." Because eosinophilia can be discrete, or even absent, it highlights the importance of cytogenetic analysis in all patients that are presenting with a myeloid neoplasm. Combination treatment with inhibitors of JAK2 and BCL2 has minimal toxicity and can be beneficial in controlling disease.

Consent

Written informed consent was obtained from the patient for publication of this case report and any accompanying images.

Authors' Contributions

All authors contributed equally to this work.

References

[1] A. Tefferi, "Novel mutations and their functional and clinical relevance in myeloproliferative neoplasms: JAK2, MPL, TET2, ASXL1, CBL, IDH and IKZF1," *Leukemia*, vol. 24, no. 6, pp. 1128–1138, 2010.

[2] F. Griesinger, H. Hennig, F. Hillmer et al., "ABCR-JAK2 fusion gene as the result of a t(9;22)(p24;q11.2) translocation in a patient with a clinically typical chronic myeloid leukemia," *Genes, Chromosomes and Cancer*, vol. 44, no. 3, pp. 329–333, 2005.

[3] B. Kantarcioglu, I. Kaygusuz-Atagunduz, A. Uzay, T. Toptas, T. F. Tuglular, and M. Bayik, "Myelodysplastic syndrome with t(9;22)(p24;q11.2), a BCR-JAK2 fusion: case report and review of the literature," *International Journal of Hematology*, vol. 102, no. 3, pp. 383–387, 2015.

[4] Á. Cuesta-Domínguez, M. Ortega, C. Ormazábal et al., "Transforming and tumorigenic activity of JAK2 by fusion to BCR: molecular mechanisms of action of a novel BCR-JAK2 tyrosine-kinase," *PLoS One*, vol. 7, no. 2, Article ID e32451, 2012.

[5] G. Cirmena, S. Aliano, G. Fugazza et al., "A BCR-JAK2 fusion gene as the result of a t(9;22)(p24;q11) in a patient with acute myeloid leukemia," *Cancer Genetics and Cytogenetics*, vol. 183, no. 2, pp. 105–108, 2008.

[6] C. A. Tirado, W. Chen, L. J.-s. Huang et al., "Novel JAK2 rearrangement resulting from a t(9;22)(p24;q11.2) in B-acute lymphoblastic leukemia," *Leukemia Research*, vol. 34, no. 12, pp. 1674–1676, 2010.

[7] J. S. Snider, I. Znoyko, K. G. Lindsey et al., "Integrated genomic analysis using chromosomal microarray, fluorescence in situ hybridization and mate pair analyses: characterization of a cryptic t(9;22)(p24.1;q11.2)/BCR-JAK2 in myeloid/lymphoid neoplasm with eosinophilia," *Cancer Genetics*, vol. 247, pp. 44–47, 2020.

[8] M. M. Elnaggar, S. Agersborg, T. Sahoo et al., "BCR-JAK2 fusion as a result of a translocation (9;22)(p24;q11.2) in a patient with CML-like myeloproliferative disease," *Molecular Cytogenetics*, vol. 5, no. 1, p. 23, 2012.

[9] C. A. Smith and G. Fan, "The saga of JAK2 mutations and translocations in hematologic disorders: pathogenesis, diagnostic and therapeutic prospects, and revised World Health Organization diagnostic criteria for myeloproliferative neoplasms," *Human Pathology*, vol. 39, no. 6, pp. 795–810, 2008.

[10] J. Schwaab, M. Knut, C. Haferlach et al., "Limited duration of complete remission on ruxolitinib in myeloid neoplasms with PCM1-JAK2 and BCR-JAK2 fusion genes," *Annals of Hematology*, vol. 94, no. 2, pp. 233–238, 2015.

[11] J. Schwaab, N. Naumann, J. Luebke et al., "Response to tyrosine kinase inhibitors in myeloid neoplasms associated with

PCM1 - JAK2 , BCR-JAK2 and ETV6-ABL1 fusion genes," *American Journal of Hematology*, vol. 95, no. 7, pp. 824–833, 2020.

[12] S. Swerdlow, E. Campo, N Harris et al., *WHO Classification of Tumours of Haematopoietic and Lymphoid Tissues*, iARC Press, Lyon, France, 4th edition, 2017.

[13] A. Reiter and J. Gotlib, "Myeloid neoplasms with eosinophilia," *Blood*, vol. 129, no. 6, pp. 704–714, 2017.

[14] R. He, P. T. Greipp, A. Rangan et al., "BCR-JAK2 fusion in a myeloproliferative neoplasm with associated eosinophilia," *Cancer Genetics*, vol. 209, no. 5, pp. 223–228, 2016.

[15] M. Bellesso, R. Santucci, D. F. Dias, R. Centrone, and R. C. Elias, "Atypical chronic myeloid leukemia with t(9; 22)(p24, 11.2), a BCR-JAK2 fusion gene," *Revista Brasileira de Hematologia e Hemoterapia*, vol. 35, pp. 218-219, 2013.

[16] L. Impera, A. Lonoce, D. A. Fanfulla et al., "Two alternatively spliced 5′BCR/3′JAK2 fusion transcripts in a myeloproliferative neoplasm with a three-way t(9; 18; 22)(p23; p11.3; q11.2) translocation," *Cancer Genetics*, vol. 204, no. 9, pp. 512–515, 2011.

[17] S. W. Lane, D. J. Fairbairn, C. McCarthy, A. Nandini, J. Perry-Keene, and G. A. Kennedy, "Leukaemia cutis in atypical chronic myeloid leukaemia with a t(9; 22) (p24; q11.2) leading to BCR-JAK2 fusion," *British Journal of Haematology*, vol. 142, no. 4, p. 503, 2008.

[18] B. Thakral, T. Muzzafar, S. A. Wang, and L. J. Medeiros, "Myeloid neoplasm with eosinophilia and BCR-JAK2/t(9; 22)(p24; q11.2) morphologically mimicking chronic myeloid leukemia," *Annals of Diagnostic Pathology*, vol. 44, Article ID 151405, 2020.

[19] S. Jain and A. Abraham, "*BCR-ABL1*-like B-acute lymphoblastic leukemia/lymphoma: a comprehensive review," *Archives of Pathology & Laboratory Medicine*, vol. 144, no. 2, pp. 150–155, 2020.

[20] B. M. Getta, M. Roshal, J. Zheng et al., "Allogeneic hematopoietic stem cell transplantation with myeloablative conditioning is associated with favorable outcomes in mixed phenotype acute leukemia," *Biology of Blood and Marrow Transplantation*, vol. 23, no. 11, pp. 1879–1886, 2017.

[21] R. L. Bowman, L. Busque, and R. L. Levine, "Clonal hematopoiesis and evolution to hematopoietic malignancies," *Cell Stem Cell*, vol. 22, no. 2, pp. 157–170, 2018.

[22] E. Bousoik and H. Montazeri Aliabadi, "Do we know Jack" about JAK? A closer look at JAK/STAT signaling pathway," *Frontiers in Oncology*, vol. 8, p. 287, 2018.

[23] P. Sepúlveda, A. Encabo, F. Carbonell-Uberos, and M. D. Miñana, "BCL-2 expression is mainly regulated by JAK/STAT3 pathway in human CD34+ hematopoietic cells," *Cell Death & Differentiation*, vol. 14, no. 2, pp. 378–380, 2007.

[24] I. Sakai and A. S. Kraft, "The kinase domain of Jak2 mediates induction of bcl-2 and delays cell death in hematopoietic cells," *Journal of Biological Chemistry*, vol. 272, no. 19, pp. 12350–12358, 1997.

[25] A. Zeuner, F. Pedini, F. Francescangeli et al., "Activity of the BH3 mimetic ABT-737 on polycythemia vera erythroid precursor cells," *Blood*, vol. 113, no. 7, pp. 1522–1525, 2009.

[26] B. Will, T. Siddiqi, M. A. Jordà et al., "Apoptosis induced by JAK2 inhibition is mediated by Bim and enhanced by the BH3 mimetic ABT-737 in JAK2 mutant human erythroid cells," *Blood*, vol. 115, no. 14, pp. 2901–2909, 2010.

[27] M. Waibel, V. S. Solomon, D. A. Knight et al., "Combined targeting of JAK2 and BCL-2/BCL-XL to cure mutant JAK2-driven malignancies and overcome acquired resistance to JAK2 inhibitors," *Cell Reports*, vol. 5, no. 4, pp. 1047–1059, 2013.

26

Spontaneous Splenic Rupture and Rituximab-Induced Acute Thrombocytopenia in a Patient with High-Risk Mantle Cell Lymphoma

Jared Williams and Shingi Chiruka

Department of Haematology, Dunedin Hospital, 201 Great King Street, Dunedin 9016, New Zealand

Correspondence should be addressed to Jared Williams; jaredwilliams_@hotmail.com

Academic Editor: Sergio Storti

Mantle cell lymphoma is a relatively rare type of mature B-cell non-Hodgkin's lymphoma with an incidence of approximately 8 cases per million persons per year. In patients with mantle cell lymphoma, there are rare case reports of the potentially life-threatening consequences of splenic rupture and rituximab-induced acute thrombocytopenia (RIAT) occurring separately, but there are no reports of these occurring in the same patient. Whilst rare, they are important to be aware of as early detection may prevent fatal outcomes.

1. Introduction

Spontaneous splenic rupture secondary to malignancy and RIAT are both rare complications with only a limited number of case reports in the literature. Literature review revealed over 800 cases of spontaneous splenic rupture with only 8 cases in mantle cell lymphoma. The leading causes of spontaneous splenic rupture were malignancy (30%), infections (27%), inflammatory (20%), and drug/treatment related (9%) [1]. 22 cases of RIAT were identified with 13 of these occurring in patients with mantle cell lymphoma. We report a case of high-risk mantle cell lymphoma (Mantle Cell Lymphoma International Prognostic Index Score 7.9) who developed these 2 rare complications.

2. Case Summary

A 53-year-old Caucasian female presented to her general practitioner with a 2-month history of increasing lymphadenopathy in her groin and neck alongside drenching night sweats, fatigue, and left upper quadrant abdominal pain but no subjective weight loss. Her medical history was significant for depression and prior transient thyrotoxicosis due to thyroiditis (negative thyroid antibodies), and she was taking paroxetine 20 mg daily. Fine needle aspiration was performed on a cervical lymph node suggestive of mantle cell lymphoma, which was subsequently confirmed by excision biopsy (CD5+, CD20+, cyclin D1+, CD23−, CD10−, CD3−, and t(11; 14) on FISH with Ki-67 of 50%). She was initially referred for outpatient assessment but admitted for inpatient workup because a rapidly increasing peripheral lymphocyte count was noted. On admission, multiple small volume lymphadenopathy was present in her cervical, axillary, and inguinal areas, and she had hepatosplenomegaly, with the spleen palpable 8 cm below the costophrenic margin and liver palpable 12 cm below the costophrenic margin. Significant blood results were as follows: total white blood cell count 76.8×10^9/L, lymphocyte count 63.7×10^9/L, haemoglobin 128 g/L, platelets 156×10^9/L, neutrophils 10.5×10^9/L, B_2M 9.29 mg/L, LDH 704 U/L, uric acid 0.44 mmol/L, bilirubin 4 μmol/L, ALP 211 U/L, GGT 104 U/L, ALT 19 U/L, and albumin 27 g/L with normal calcium, phosphate, and renal function. Hepatitis B antigen, hepatitis B surface antibody, and hepatitis B core antibody were negative. Hepatitis C antibody was negative. The morphology of the lymphocytes on blood film was consistent with mantle cell lymphoma cells, pleomorphic variant. Staging CT revealed a maximal liver span of 25 cm and spleen 19.8 cm with low-volume lymphadenopathy, the largest being 32 × 26 mm in the right inguinal area. Bone marrow confirmed marrow involvement, and the morphology of the cells were consistent with the pleomorphic subtype. She was commenced on the Nordic protocol and had her first dose of R-Maxi-CHOP (rituximab, cyclophosphamide, doxorubicin, vincristine, and prednisone) as an inpatient over 2 days. She had fevers during rituximab but no other significant infusion reactions. The evening after receiving CHOP, she developed abdominal pain with the haemoglobin dropping from 106 to 78 g/L and CT scan showed a large splenic rupture, with a subcapsular splenic haematoma and blood extending around the liver and in the paracolic gutter. There was no active bleeding on angiography. Her platelets had dropped from 154 to 50×10^9/L. She remained haemodynamically stable. She was transfused 2 units of packed red blood cells and managed conservatively with no further decrease in haemoglobin. Routine pegfilgrastim (6 mg) had been previously charted and was given the following morning prior to medical review. She developed shortness of breath over the next 2 days, and chest X-ray revealed a significant left-sided pleural effusion which required thoracentesis. The effusion was an exudate with mantle lymphoma cells present. She was discharged from hospital a week later. Her 2nd cycle was rituximab and cytarabine, and during this, she developed multiple infusion reactions to the rituximab and was only able to finish 14% of the rituximab as a result. Her platelet count dropped from 591 to 136×10^9/L after the rituximab. Her lymphocyte count was normal after cycle 2 at 1.5×10^9/L. 3rd cycle of chemotherapy was delayed due to *Campylobacter* Gastroenteritis which was treated for 5 days with azithromycin. 11 days later following recovering from the infection, she presented for her 3rd cycle of chemotherapy but her lymphocyte count had risen to 20.7×10^9/L. Flow cytometry confirmed these were mantle cell lymphoma cells. Restaging CT showed stable disease compared with the original CT scan. Based on the increase in peripheral blood lymphocyte count, she was considered to have progressive disease. She was changed to salvage therapy with R-ICE (rituximab, ifosfamide, carboplatin, and etoposide). She again had recurrent infusion reactions with rituximab but this time developed significant acute thrombocytopenia following rituximab with platelet count falling from 197 to 22×10^9/L within 24 hours. Her coagulation studies remained normal, and no other cause for the thrombocytopenia was found. This was presumed to be an acute toxicity of rituximab. No further rituximab was subsequently given due to concerns regarding the progressive fall in the post-rituximab platelet count. Her platelet count recovered spontaneously without needing platelet transfusion. She tolerated the ICE well. Her lymphocytes fell to 2.5×10^9/L then rose again to 5×10^9/L. This was again thought to be progressive disease, and she was changed to DHAP (dexamethasone, cytarabine, and cisplatin). She tolerated this well, and lymphocytes decreased to 1.1×10^9/L before rising to 7.2×10^9/L 3 weeks later. DHAP was therefore ceased. At this stage, she had disease refractory to 3 lines of treatment and was considered for allogeneic stem cell transplantation. During workup for this, her disease was unable to be controlled and her management was changed to palliative and she passed away within 2 months.

3. Discussion

Splenic enlargement occurs in up to 40% of patients with mantle cell lymphoma but spontaneous splenic rupture is a rare phenomenon. Literature review has identified at least 800 cases of spontaneous splenic rupture, with 30% of these being related to malignancy [1]. There are 8 case reports of splenic rupture in mantle cell lymphoma [2–8]. In the majority of these, the mantle cell lymphoma was the blastoid variant and splenic rupture was the presenting complaint leading to the diagnosis, whereas in our patient, this occurred shortly after the 1st cycle of chemotherapy. Risk factors generated from case reports include degree of splenic enlargement, older age, male sex, aggressiveness of underlying disease, fungal infection, growth factor usage, particularly granulocyte colony-stimulating factor (G-CSF), and induction chemotherapy [5]. Our patient's splenic rupture occurred closely following induction chemotherapy. Induction chemotherapy, when the disease burden is at its highest, in theory may cause tumor lysis with release of enzymatic content from the cells, resulting in splenic damage and rupture [5]. Our patient was also taking paroxetine, which can impair platelet function. After the rituximab, she became acutely thrombocytopenic (platelet count 50×10^9/L); therefore, the paroxetine may have contributed to the bleeding. The pegylated G-CSF was given the day following the splenic rupture so was not contributory, but may have contributed to neutrophil activation exacerbating enzymatic digestion of the ruptured spleen. This had been charted alongside the chemotherapy and was routinely given the following morning prior to medical review. Management often involves splenectomy as the mortality in the case reports was high without surgical intervention. In the case reports of spontaneous splenic rupture in mantle Cell Lymphoma, 1 died at presentation and the majority of the others had some degree of haemodynamic instability and required urgent splenectomy. Our patient was haemodynamically stable, had no evidence of active bleeding, and therefore was managed conservatively without complication. Based on the limited number of mantle cell lymphoma case reports, it is hard to make recommendations for the management of spontaneous splenic rupture. However, splenectomy appears to be warranted, especially if there is any haemodynamic compromise.

Rituximab-induced acute thrombocytopenia (RIAT) is a rarely encountered side effect of rituximab. There are 22 case reports of this, and the majority of these have been in mantle cell lymphoma patients [9–25]. Omura et al. [9] listed the characteristics of these patients and noted the underlying diagnoses included mantle cell lymphoma (n = 13) [10–18], hairy cell Leukemia (n = 3) [11, 19, 20], follicular lymphoma (n = 2) [9, 21], prolymphocytic Leukemia (n = 1) [22], lymphoplasmacytic Lymphoma (n = 1) [23], pre-B cell acute lymphoblastic leukemia (n = 1) [24], and autoimmune haemolytic anaemia ($n = 1$) [25]. From the available characteristics given in these case reports, all had bone marrow infiltration and splenomegaly similar to our patient. Many, but not all of the cases, had recurrent infusion reactions during rituximab doses similar to our patient. Looking back at our patient, she had acute thrombocytopenia following rituximab shortly after the first dose, but this was overlooked due to other factors including the splenic rupture after cycle 1, and after cycle 2, her platelet count was 591×10^9 pre-rituximab masking the drop. The postrituximab percentage decrease in the platelet count was increasing with subsequent cycles (following cycle 1—68% decrease, cycle 2—77% decrease, and cycle 3—89% decrease). 5 of the 22 cases reports developed coagulopathy with the thrombocytopenia [9, 19–21, 24], suggesting consumption coagulopathy; however, our patient's coagulation studies remained normal. 12 cases attempted retrial of rituximab [9, 10, 12, 15–18, 23, 24] with 6 developing recurrence of thrombocytopenia [9, 10, 12, 15, 16, 24], making it difficult to decide clinically whether to continue it or not. It is likely that RIAT is underreported as it is not routine to monitor platelet counts after rituximab as most rituximab is given in the outpatient setting, and if the thrombocytopenia is mild-moderate, it may be overlooked.

The fact that these 2 seemingly rare events occurred in our patient may be a coincidence. From review of the literature, there are no case reports where these have occurred together. They are both rare events with limited case reports but both have a correlation with splenomegaly and mantle cell lymphoma.

4. Conclusion

This case report identified 2 rare events occurring in a patient with mantle cell lymphoma. As there are no other case reports of these occurring together, it is likely they are unrelated but highlight the importance of being aware of these potentially life-threatening complications.

References

[1] P. Renzuli, A. Hostettler, A. Schopfer, B. Gloor, and D. Candinas, "Systematic review of atraumatic splenic rupture," *British Journal of Surgery*, vol. 96, no. 10, pp. 1114–1121, 2009.

[2] J. Zieran, M. Paul, M. Scharfenberg, and J. Muller, "The Spontaneous Splenic rupture as first manifestation of Mantle Cell Lymphoma, a dangerous rarity," *American Journal of Emergency Medicine*, vol. 22, no. 7, pp. 629–631, 2004.

[3] K. D. Mason and S. K. Juneja, "Spontaneous rupture of the spleen as the presenting feature of the blastoid variant of mantle cell lymphoma," *Clinical and Laboratory Haematology*, vol. 25, no. 4, pp. 263–265, 2003.

[4] M. A. Lunning, M. Stetler-Stevenson, P. T. Silberstein, V. Zenger, and G. E. Marti, "Spontaneous (pathological) splenic rupture in a blastic variant of mantle cell lymphoma: a case report and literature review," *Clinical Lymphoma*, vol. 3, no. 2, pp. 117–120, 2002.

[5] C. Tan, D. Rajan, S. Majeed, S. Ahmed, L. Freedman, and P. Mustacchia, "Pathologic rupture of the spleen in mantle-cell-type non-hodgkin's lymphoma," *Case Reports in Medicine*, vol. 2012, Article ID 351275, 4 pages, 2012.

[6] Y. Maeda-Sakagami, Y. Tanaka, Y. Koba, I. Shinzato, and T. Ishikawa, "Mantle cell lymphoma presenting with spontaneous splenic rupture," *Rinsho Ketsueki-Japanese Journal of Clinical Hematology*, vol. 57, no. 8, pp. 1018–1025, 2016.

[7] A. Strickland, K. Marsden, J. McArdle, and R. Lowenthal, "Pathologic splenic rupture as the presentation of mantle cell lymphoma," *Leukemia & Lymphoma*, vol. 41, no. 1-2, pp. 197–201, 2001.

[8] R. Oinonen, K. Franssila, and E. Elonen, "Spontaneous splenic rupture in two patients with a blastoid variant of mantle cell lymphoma," *Annals of Hematology*, vol. 74, no. 1, pp. 33–35, 1997.

[9] Y. Omura, H. Shimazu, and T. Takahashi, "Rituximab-induced acute thrombocytopenia in a patient with follicular lymphoma: a case report and review of the literature," *Internal Medicine*, vol. 57, no. 8, pp. 1151–1154, 2018.

[10] C. Shah and S. J. Grethlein, "Case report of rituximab-induced thrombocytopenia," *American Journal of Hematology*, vol. 75, no. 4, p. 263, 2004.

[11] Z. Otrock, R. Mahfouz, G. Oghlakian, Z. Salem, and A. Bazarbachi, "Rituximab-induced acute thrombocytopenia: a report of two cases," *Haematologica*, vol. 90, article ECR23, 2005.

[12] M. Rosado, H. Chao, and M. Rose, "Severe acute thrombocytopenia following rituximab therapy," *Leukemia & Lymphoma*, vol. 48, no. 11, pp. 2239-2240, 2007.

[13] S. Dhand and H. Bahrain, "Rituximab-induced severe acute thrombocytopenia: a case report and review of literature," *Cancer Investigation*, vol. 26, no. 9, pp. 913–915, 2008.

[14] R. Ram, L. Bonstein, A. Gafter-Gvili, I. Ben-Bassat, O. Shpilberg, and P. Raanani, "Rituximab-associated acute thrombocytopenia: an under-diagnosed phenomenon," *American Journal of Hematology*, vol. 84, no. 4, pp. 247–250, 2009.

[15] J. H. Yi, S. J. Kim, H. K. Ahn, S. J. Lee, M. H. Chang, and W. S. Kim, "Rituximab-induced acute thrombocytopenia: a case report and review of the literature," *Medical Oncology*, vol. 26, no. 1, pp. 45–48, 2009.

[16] R. Parajui, E. Hire, and B. Shah, "Rituximab-induced acute severe thrombocytopenia," *British Journal of Haematology*, vol. 149, no. 6, p. 804, 2010.

[17] S. K. Sadashiv, R. Rao, S. Fazal, and J. Lister, "Rituximab-induced acute severe thrombocytopenia: a case series in patients with mantle cell lymphoma," *Clinical Lymphoma Myeloma and Leukemia*, vol. 13, no. 5, pp. 602–605, 2013.

[18] H. El-Osta and B. Nair, "Rituximab-induced acute thrombocytopenia: an underappreciated entity," *Leukemia & Lymphoma*, vol. 54, no. 12, pp. 2736-2737, 2013.

[19] J. Thachil, K. Mukherje, and B. Woodcock, "Rituximab-induced haemorrhagic thrombocytopenia in a patient with hairy cell leukaemia," *British Journal of Haematology*, vol. 135, no. 2, pp. 273-274, 2006.

[20] I. Kotsianidis, A. Goutzouvelidis, A. Anastasiades et al., "Severe thrombocytopenia and fibrinolysis mimicking disseminate intravascular coagulation after Rituximab infusion," *American Journal of Hematology*, vol. 85, no. 2, p. 146, 2010.

[21] H. Ureshino, A. Nishioka, K. Kojima et al., "Rituximab-induced acute thrombocytopenia in high tumor burden

follicular lymphoma," *Internal Medicine*, vol. 55, no. 15, pp. 2061–2064, 2016.

[22] G. E. Pamuk, S. Donmez, B. Turgut, M. Demir, and O. Vural, "Rituximab-induced acute thrombocytopenia in a patient with prolymphocytic leukemia," *American Journal of Hematology*, vol. 78, no. 1, p. 81, 2005.

[23] C. Rigamonti, C. Volta, S. Colombi et al., "Severe thrombocytopenia and clinical bleeding associated with rituximab infusion in a lymphoma patient with massive splenomegaly without leukemic invasion," *Leukemia*, vol. 15, no. 1, pp. 186-187, 2001.

[24] H. Rafei, S. Nassereddine, and I. Garcia, "Disseminated intravascular coagulation-like reaction following rituximab infusion," *BMJ Case Reports*, vol. 2017, Article ID bcr2016218443, 2017.

[25] S. Larrar, C. Guitton, M. Willems, and B. Bader-Meunier, "Severe hematological side effects following Rituximab therapy in children," *Haematologica*, vol. 91, no. 8, article ECR36, 2006.

27

Prolonged Remission of Cancer of Unknown Primary following Initiation of Eculizumab Therapy for Paroxysmal Nocturnal Hemoglobinuria

Ming Y. Lim[1], **Keith E. Volmar**[2] **and Nigel S. Key**[1]

[1]*Department of Medicine, Division of Hematology/Oncology, University of North Carolina, Chapel Hill, NC, USA*
[2]*Department of Pathology, UNC REX Healthcare, Raleigh, NC, USA*

Correspondence should be addressed to Nigel S. Key; nigel_key@med.unc.edu

Academic Editor: Kazunori Nakase

We report the case of a 64-year-old woman who presented with cancer of unknown primary treated with carboplatin and paclitaxel, followed by maintenance erlotinib. Her chemotherapy regimen was discontinued due to the development of profound hemolysis that was later identified to be due to paroxysmal nocturnal hemoglobinuria (PNH). She was started on a complement inhibitory antibody, eculizumab 900 mg every 2 weeks, with marked suppression of hemolysis. Eight years after diagnosis of cancer, the patient remains on eculizumab with no signs of cancer recurrence on regular imaging. Regardless of whether the co-occurrence of cancer and PNH was any more than coincidental in this patient, the uniqueness of the case is emphasized by the remarkable and sustained response of not only PNH but also possibly the associated cancer to eculizumab.

1. Introduction

Paroxysmal nocturnal hemoglobinuria (PNH) is an acquired clonal hemolytic anemia that is associated with other bone marrow failure syndromes including aplastic anemia and myelodysplastic syndrome [1]. Although PNH has recently been associated with $JAK2^{V617F}$ positive myeloproliferative neoplasms [2] and benign mesenchymal tumors [3], it has not been associated with solid tumor malignancies, to our knowledge. We report an unusual case of a patient who presented with an occult primary tumor which was followed shortly thereafter by the development of profound hemolysis due to PNH.

2. Case Presentation

A 64-year-old Caucasian woman presented at an outside hospital in March 2009 with shortness of breath two days after undergoing laparoscopic cholecystectomy for-choledocholithiasis. A chest radiograph demonstrated bibasilar and left upper lobe pulmonary opacities. Computed tomography (CT) of the chest revealed mediastinal and right supraclavicular lymphadenopathy, with right basilar and upper lobe consolidation, but no evidence of pulmonary embolism. She was diagnosed with postoperative pneumonia and discharged with oral antibiotics.

A follow-up CT chest in July 2009 demonstrated the continuing presence of right supraclavicular lymphadenopathy, now measuring 3 cm, and additional 1.5 cm lymph nodes in the pretracheal and subcarinal regions. The patient underwent an excisional lymph node biopsy on July 24, 2009, that revealed replacement of the lymph node by highly pleomorphic cells with prominent nucleoli and abundant cytoplasm, suggestive of high-grade metastatic carcinoma (Figure 1). Immunohistochemical evaluation showed that 100% of the cells were positive for cytokeratin (CK) (Figure 2) but negative for CK7, CK20, thyroid transcription factor-1 (TTF-1), melanoma antigen (Melan-A), CD30, and leukocyte common antigen. A few cells were positive for S100. There was no positive nuclear staining reaction for the estrogen or progesterone receptors in any of the tumor cells. In the absence of morphologic or histochemical features to identify a primary site, a positron emission tomography (PET)/CT was performed. This revealed right lower cervical and right

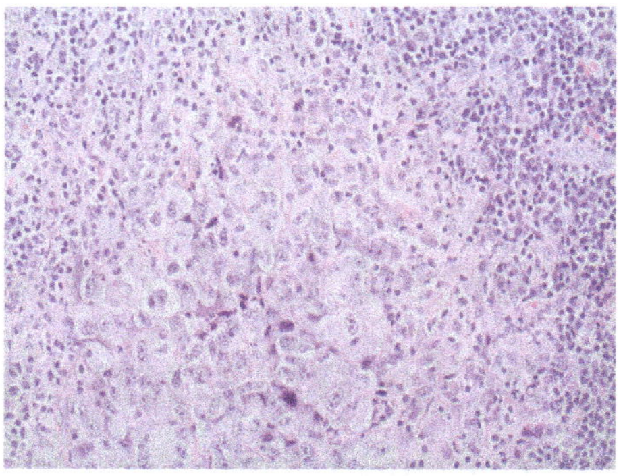

Figure 1: Lymph node biopsy. Sections show high-grade, pleomorphic malignant cells in a background of small lymphocytes (H&E, 200x).

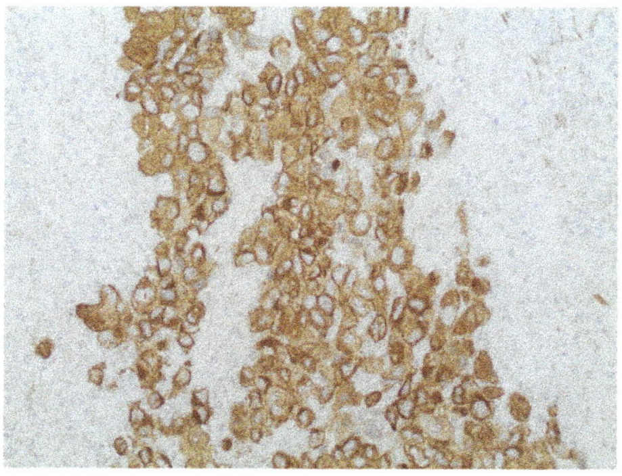

Figure 2: Lymph node biopsy. The malignant cells are strongly positive with antibodies to cytokeratin, indicating epithelial lineage and supporting the diagnosis of carcinoma (cytokeratin AE1/AE3, 200x).

supraclavicular lymphadenopathy with intense hypermetabolism and moderate hypermetabolic activity in the right peritracheal and precarinal lymph nodes. Increased fluorodeoxyglucose (FDG) uptake in the region of the left lateral oropharyngeal wall and base of the tongue without definite CT correlation was also noted. In addition, heterogenous uptake in the marrow of the axial and proximal appendicular skeleton without correlation on bone windows was noted. Clinically, the patient denied any localizing or systemic symptoms of malignancy. She was a nonsmoker with minimal alcohol intake. Endoscopic evaluation of her upper airways and breast magnetic resonance imaging (MRI) were unrevealing for a primary site.

The patient was diagnosed with carcinoma of unknown primary and was prescribed 4 cycles of carboplatin and paclitaxel, which was completed in February 2010. She was then switched to maintenance erlotinib in May 2010. Six days after initiation of erlotinib, the patient presented with jaundice and passage of dark red urine. Laboratory studies revealed hemoglobin (Hgb) of 7.1 g/dL (range: 12.0–16.0 g/dL), platelet count of $92 \times 10^3/\mu L$ (range: $150–450 \times 10^3/\mu L$), total bilirubin of 5.0 mg/dL (range: 0.2–1.0 mg/dL), and elevated liver enzymes and lactate dehydrogenase of 2,546 U/L (range: 81–234 U/L). The direct antiglobulin (Coomb's) test was negative. Urinalysis revealed a large amount of blood with zero RBC/hpf. The patient was started on prednisone 1 mg/kg for presumed erlotinib-induced hemolytic anemia. Bone marrow biopsy revealed a mildly hypercellular bone marrow with erythroid hyperplasia. The dose of erlotinib was reduced to 100 mg daily with waxing and waning of her hemolytic symptoms despite ongoing treatment with prednisone. Erlotinib was discontinued in July 2010, and the prednisone dose was tapered beginning in October 2010. In November 2010, the patient presented again with hemolytic anemia that failed to respond to high-dose prednisone. She was referred to our institution for further evaluation of her hemolysis.

She reported multiple episodes of intermittent coffee color urine in the preceding years, which resolved spontaneously. Urinalysis revealed 3+ hemosiderinuria. The highly sensitive flow cytometry assay (FLAER) revealed a PNH clone in 91% of granulocytes, 93% of monocytes, and 78% of red cells. With a confirmed diagnosis of PNH, prednisone was discontinued and eculizumab (900 mg every 2 weeks) was initiated. Treatment with eculizumab resulted in improvement of her laboratory values (Hgb 11.0 g/dL, white blood cells $4.6 \times 10^3/\mu L$ with a normal differential, and platelets $135 \times 10^3/\mu L$) with cessation of hemoglobinuria.

In early 2011, the patient developed acute thrombocytopenia to $<20 \times 10^3/\mu L$ with no significant change in other cell lines. With other possible causes excluded, a diagnosis of immune thrombocytopenic purpura (ITP) was made. She was treated with rituximab 375 mg/m^2 weekly for 4 weeks, with normalization of the platelet count. She has remained on eculizumab with no recurrence of hemolytic anemia.

With regards to the underlying malignancy, a staging CT in March 2011 showed minimal change in the previously noted right supraclavicular and mediastinal lymph nodes. Subsequent imaging in August 2011 demonstrated decreased prominence of the right supraclavicular and mediastinal lymphadenopathy with no other evidence of metastatic disease. As of April 2019, the patient remains on eculizumab 900 mg every 2 weeks, with no signs of cancer recurrence.

3. Discussion

Cancers of unknown primary (CUP), or occult primary tumors, are defined as histologically proven metastatic malignant tumors in which the primary site cannot be identified [4, 5]. These tumors confer a poor prognosis in most patients with a median survival of 8 to 12 months [6, 7]. As such, the fact that our patient with CUP remains disease-free more than 8 years after diagnosis is remarkable.

One possibility to explain this patient's long-term survival is the concomitant eculizumab for PNH management. Eculizumab is a humanized monoclonal antibody that binds to C5 and prevents its cleavage by C5 convertase, thereby inhibiting the generation of C5a and downstream formation of the membrane attack complex. In recent years, a substantial body of literature has linked complement factors C3a and C5a to various aspects of tumor biology. In addition to their recognized role in sustaining chronic inflammation, the anaphylatoxins C3a and C5a also promote a microenvironment that is immunosuppressive for tumor growth, is proangiogenic, and accelerates tumor growth through enhancement of tumor cell migration and subsequent tissue invasion and metastasis [8, 9]. Studies using animal models of lung cancer reported higher C5 deposition in lung cancer cell lines than in nonmalignant bronchial epithelial cells, thereby creating a favorable tumor microenvironment by inducing endothelial cell chemotaxis and blood vessel formation [10].

As such, the inhibition of C5 convertase by eculizumab could theoretically mediate an antitumor effect. Indeed, this has been demonstrated in several preclinical models of melanoma and lung cancer where pharmacologic inhibition of C5a potentiated blockade of the programmed cell death protein 1 (PD-1) pathway using immune checkpoint inhibitors [11, 12]. Animal models targeting complement pathways in cancer remain an area of active research. It would be of interest to determine if these findings could translate into clinical practice, given the favorable clinical outcomes seen using immunotherapy and checkpoint inhibitors in cancer therapy. In addition, given the traditional role of complement in enhancing the cytolytic effects of antibody-mediated immunotherapy, pharmacologic manipulation of complement will remain a challenge due to its uncertain benefit vs. harm in the cancer microenvironment [9].

In conclusion, our patient remains in prolonged remission for cancer of unknown primary following initiation of eculizumab therapy for PNH. Regardless of whether the co-occurrence of cancer and PNH was coincidental in this patient, the uniqueness of the case is emphasized by the remarkable and sustained response of not only the manifestations of PNH but also the underlying cancer, to eculizumab.

References

[1] T. Kinoshita and N. Inoue, "Relationship between aplastic anemia and paroxysmal nocturnal hemoglobinuria," *International Journal of Hematology*, vol. 75, no. 2, pp. 117–122, 2002.

[2] C. Sugimori, E. Padron, G. Caceres et al., "Paroxysmal nocturnal hemoglobinuria and concurrent JAK2V617F mutation," *Blood Cancer Journal*, vol. 2, no. 3, p. e63, 2012.

[3] N. Inoue, T. Izui-Sarumaru, Y. Murakami et al., "Molecular basis of clonal expansion of hematopoiesis in 2 patients with paroxysmal nocturnal hemoglobinuria (PNH)," *Blood*, vol. 108, no. 13, pp. 4232–4236, 2006.

[4] F. A. Greco and J. D. Hainsworth, "Cancer of unknown primary site," in *DeVita, Hellman, and Rosenberg's Cancer: Principles & Practice of Oncology*, V. T. DeVita, T. S. Lawrence, and S. A. Rosenburg, Eds., pp. 1720–1737, Lippincott Williams & Wilkins, Philadelphia, PA, USA, 10th edition, 2014.

[5] F. Losa, G. Soler, A. Casado et al., "SEOM clinical guideline on unknown primary cancer (2017)," *Clinical and Translational Oncology*, vol. 20, no. 1, pp. 89–96, 2018.

[6] N. Pavlidis and G. Pentheroudakis, "Cancer of unknown primary site," *The Lancet*, vol. 379, no. 9824, pp. 1428–1435, 2012.

[7] K. Hemminki, M. Bevier, A. Hemminki, and J. Sundquist, "Survival in cancer of unknown primary site: population-based analysis by site and histology," *Annals of Oncology*, vol. 23, no. 7, pp. 1854–1863, 2012.

[8] G. Hajishengallis, E. S. Reis, D. C. Mastellos, D. Ricklin, and J. D. Lambris, "Novel mechanisms and functions of complement," *Nature immunology*, vol. 18, no. 12, pp. 1288–1298, 2017.

[9] E. S. Reis, D. C. Mastellos, D. Ricklin, A. Mantovani, and J. D. Lambris, "Complement in cancer: untangling an intricate relationship," *Nature reviews Immunology*, vol. 18, no. 1, p. 518, 2018.

[10] L. Corrales, D. Ajona, S. Rafail et al., "Anaphylatoxin C5a creates a favorable microenvironment for lung cancer progression," *Journal of Immunology*, vol. 189, no. 9, pp. 4674–4683, 2012.

[11] D. Ajona, S. Ortiz-Espinosa, H. Moreno et al., "A combined PD-1/C5a blockade synergistically protects against lung cancer growth and metastasis," *Cancer Discovery*, vol. 7, no. 7, pp. 694–703, 2017.

[12] Y. Wang, S.-N. Sun, Q. Liu et al., "Autocrine complement inhibits IL10-dependent T-cell-mediated antitumor immunity to promote tumor progression," *Cancer Discovery*, vol. 6, no. 9, pp. 1022–1035, 2016.

28

Spontaneous Complete Remission of Acute Myeloid Leukemia in the Absence of Disease-Modifying Therapy following Severe Pulmonary Involvement by Coronavirus Infectious Disease-19

Maryam Barkhordar, Fatemeh Tajic Rostami, Marjan Yaghmaie, Mehrdad Abbaszadeh, Bahram Chahardouli, and Seied Asadollah Mousavi

Hematology Oncology and Stem Cell Transplantation Research Center, Tehran University of Medical Sciences, Tehran, Iran

Correspondence should be addressed to Seied Asadollah Mousavi; hsct2021@gmail.com

Academic Editor: Sudhir Tauro

Coronavirus infectious disease-19 (COVID-19) usually alters the innate and adaptive immune setting by excessive production of proinflammatory cytokines, leading to a deviation in the natural course of simultaneous malignant disease. In the absence of disease-modifying therapy, complete remission of acute myeloid leukemia (AML) is an extraordinary event caused mainly by an immune-related mechanism secondary to a severe infectious process. We present a 57-year-old woman with a new diagnosis of AML associated with a 11q23/KMT2A abnormality who had achieved temporary spontaneous remission in the absence of disease-modifying therapy following the severe pulmonary infection with coronavirus lasting for six months. We review the literature and explain the potential impact of stimulated immune responses by COVID-19 on induction of remission in a patient with AML that could provide an excellent opportunity for new immune-based therapies to evolve for the hematologic malignancies. Despite the high ability of the immune process to destroy the malignant cells, the remission of duration is usually short. Therefore, it seems that continuing treatment after SR of AML by a consolidation regimen or bone marrow transplantation, based on a risk-adapted treatment approach, may reduce the recurrence risk.

1. Introduction

During the coronavirus infectious disease-19 (COVID-19) pandemic, concurrent diagnosis of COVID-19 with various hematologic and nonhematologic malignancies has been reported. Acute myeloid leukemia (AML) is a life-threatening hematologic cancer characterized by the monoclonal proliferation of myeloblasts to more than 20% of bone marrow cellularity.

The co-occurrence of AML and COVID-19 as a considerable therapeutic challenge has been described in multiple reports with fatal outcomes in some patients [1, 2]. The panel of international experts recommended holding the induction therapy of AML until the improvement of COVID-19-related symptoms and obtained a negative polymerase chain reaction (PCR) test [3].

Spontaneous remission (SR) in a newly diagnosed AML without disease-modifying therapy is a rare event described infrequently. According to the previous reports, SR of AML was usually described following recovery of a severe infection process; furthermore, we believe that immune activation secondary to an infectious process could eradicate the leukemic cells and induce a complete or partial remission [4, 7].

Herein, we present a new case of AML with 11q23/KMT2A abnormality who achieved complete molecular cytogenetic remission in the absence of disease-modifying therapy following recovery from COVID-19. To our knowledge, this is the first report of SR in a patient with AML and concomitant COVID-19. Besides, we explain the potential impact of immune-mediated mechanisms on induction of SR in a patient with AML infected with coronavirus, contributing to the further development of new immune-based therapies for the hematologic malignancies.

2. Case Report

A 57-year-old woman without any past medical history had presented with the petechial skin rash and bruising on the trunk and lower extremities and fatigue for about two weeks. The initial workup revealed anemia (Hb, 9.0 g/dL), thrombocytopenia (15×10^9 platelets/L), and leukocytosis (13.4×10^9 white blood cells (WBC)/L) in the complete blood count (CBC), and circulating blasts on the peripheral blood smear (PBS).

Therefore, she was referred to our center, a tertiary referral center in Tehran, with the impression of AML and admitted to the hematology ward on September 3, 2020. On physical examination, the positive findings were conjunctival pallor, scattered bruises, and petechial hemorrhage over the body surface and lower extremities. Lungs were clear on auscultation. According to the panel of international experts, we performed the screening tests to rule out COVID-19 [3] that demonstrated the normal findings for the spiral chest CT scan and negative report for the PCR test.

After admission, BMA/B was performed and confirmed the initial diagnosis of AML M2 (Figure 1(a)). Pathologic evaluation revealed the 60% cellularity consisted of blast sheets occupying more than 65% of the bone marrow space with reduced megakaryocytes and scattered erythroid precursors. Immunophenotyping study by flow cytometry showed a predominant myeloblast population formed about 67% of the total cells with a positive expression of CD117, CD33, CD34, HLA-DR, and myeloperoxidase, aberrant expression of CD7, and negative for TdT, CD3, CD5, CD20, CD19, CD10, and CD14.

Chromosomal evaluation of 50 metaphase cells by G-banded cytogenetic revealed an abnormal female karyotype with abnormality of chromosome 11q23 and insertion in the long arm of chromosome 11 (11q22) accompanied with deletion of the long arm of chromosome 13 in the same abnormal clone. Fluorescence in situ hybridization (FISH) analysis was performed and showed the "nuc ish (KMT2A×1) (5′KMT2A con 3′KMT2A×1) [130/155]" by using the KMT2A break-apart probe in 83% of cells, illustrated in Figure 2 Molecular analyses of aspiration samples were negative for NPM1, FLT-3 ITD, and FLT-3 TKD mutations. Overall findings confirmed the diagnosis of AML M2 with 11q23/KMT2A abnormality.

During the first few days of hospitalization and before starting the induction chemotherapy, she developed fever (38 °C), shortness of breath, cough, and hypoxemia. Coarse crackles were heard on auscultation of the lungs, and arterial blood gas analysis indicated pH 7.43, $PaCO_2$ 42 mmHg, and PaO_2 46.7 mmHg on FiO_2 of 40%. She received empirical therapy with meropenem and azithromycin followed by vancomycin and voriconazole for neutropenic fever.

However, the pulmonary symptoms and hypoxemia became progressively worse, and blood culture samples were negative, which prompted us to rule out COVID-19 again. The second PCR for SARS-CoV-2 was performed, which turned positive, and a repeated CT scan showed bilateral and multifocal (dominantly peripheral) patchy ground-glass opacities suggestive COVID-19 (Figure 3(a)).

The patient was then transferred to the intensive care unit (ICU) on 13 September 2020 under the impression of COVID-19, received respiratory support by NIV (noninvasive ventilation), and was treated with remdesivir at 200 mg intravenously (IV) on the first day, followed by 100 mg daily for five days [8] and dexamethasone IV at 8 mg daily for ten days [9]. She was transfused by six units of packed red blood cells and ten units of platelets. Induction chemotherapy for AML was postponed to manage COVID-19 and achieve a negative PCR test [3].

After two weeks, she was returned to the hematology ward for starting the induction chemotherapy. However, she still required oxygen supplementation to maintain O_2 sat >90%, and her general condition was not suitable for starting chemotherapy. The chest CT scan was repeated on 29.09.2020 and showed notable progression in bilateral alveolar opacities with a coarse reticular pattern compared with the previous CT scan (Figure 3(b)). Therefore, pirfenidone, colchicine (0.6 mg twice daily), and oxygen therapy with a reserve bag mask were prescribed by our pulmonologist under the impression of COVID-19-related pulmonary fibrosis.

While waiting to improve her respiratory function to make an appropriate therapeutic decision based on her new condition, the blood cell counts improved and dramatically returned to normal. Therefore, we repeated bone marrow sampling to reevaluate leukemia on 2 November 2020, two months after the initial diagnosis. BMA revealed a normocellular marrow with 55% cellularity contained less than 5% blast and trilineage maturation (Figure 1(b)), and flow cytometry showed about 3% myeloblast having the expression of CD34 and CD117.

The findings interestingly showed spontaneous morphologic remission in the absence of disease-modifying therapy of acute leukemia. Given these normal results, she was discharged without induction chemotherapy and underwent follow-up in an outpatient clinic. However, due to pulmonary complications caused by COVID-19, oxygen therapy at 1-2 L/min via nasal prongs was administered at home.

After four weeks of discharge on November 30, 2020, while the blood cell count was normal, another BMA/B was performed to evaluate the remission status that illustrated the normal cellularity and maturation with no evidence of abnormal blasts. To assess the measurable residual disease (MRD), we repeated the FISH analysis on the BMA sample by baseline probe of KMT2A, which revealed a normal result and proved the molecular cytogenetic remission. During follow-up, the patient's respiratory function improved so that the need for oxygen therapy was eliminated, and antifibrotic drugs (pirfenidone and colchicine) were discontinued.

Six months after the initial presentation, on Feb 2021, the surveillance marrow with normal blood counts revealed the normal trilineage hematopoiesis with no evidence of the

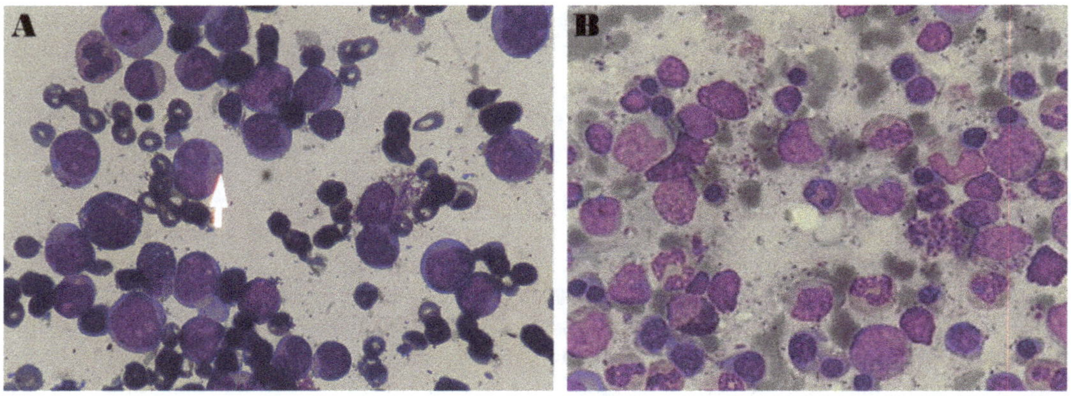

Figure 1: Bone marrow aspiration (BMA) morphology (1000 × Wright–Giemsa stain): (a) diagnostic BMA showing decreased trilineage hematopoiesis with a predominant medium-to-large-size myeloblast population with Auer rods in some blasts (arrow). (b) Follow-up BMA, after two months, showing maturing hematopoiesis with no abnormal myeloid blast population resembling complete remission.

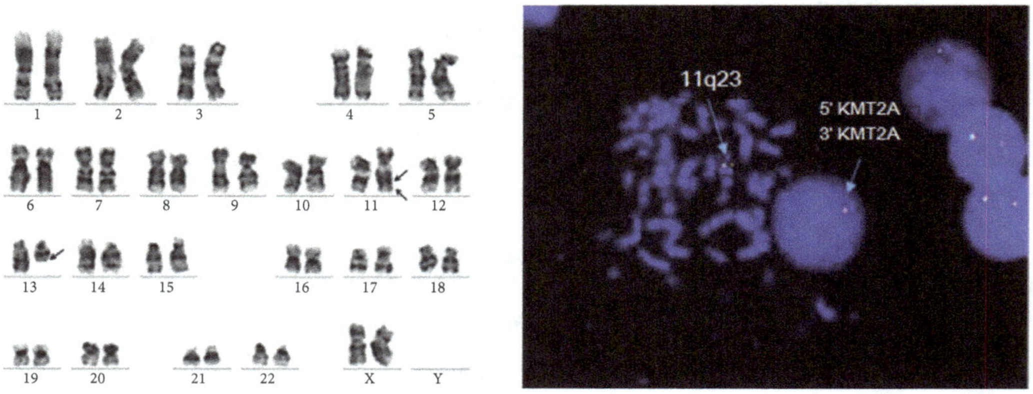

Figure 2: Karyotype: 46,XX,der (11) del (11) (q22 q23) ins (11; ?) (q22; ?), del(13) (q12q31) [50]. FISH (fluorescent in situ hybridization): nuc ish (KMT2A×1) (5′KMT2A con 3′KMT2A×1) [130/155], loss of 11q23.3 in 83% of cells.

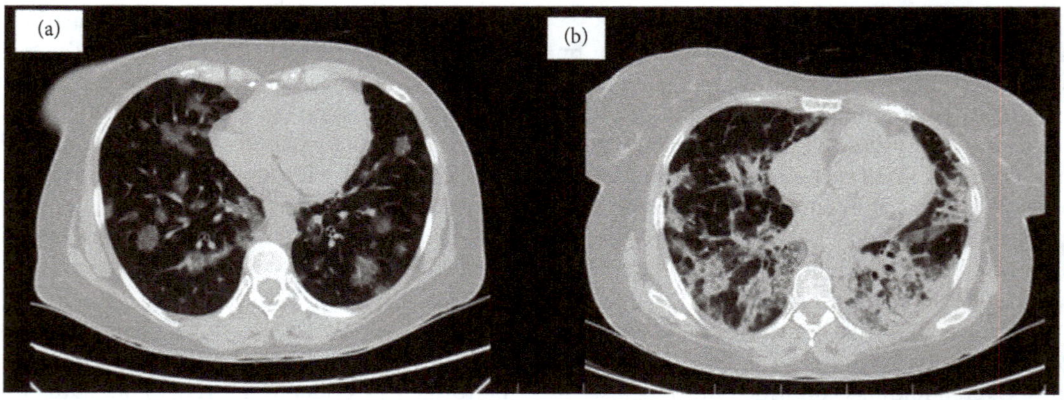

Figure 3: Spiral chest CT scans imaging: (a) diagnostic chest CT scan showing bilateral multifocal, dominantly peripheral, patchy ground-glass opacities suggestive of COVID-19 pneumonia. (b) Follow-up chest CT scan after 18 days showing notable progression in bilateral alveolar opacities with coarse reticular pattern (pulmonary fibrosis) in comparison with previous CT.

leukemia relapse by morphologic assessment. Although, according to the genetic evaluation, loss of 11q23/KMT2A reappeared in 50% of cells by karyotyping and 21% of cells by FISH, in favor of molecular relapse; however, she refused a recommended treatment to prevent overt hematologic relapse.

During the next two months, thrombocytopenia and anemia recurred (WBC, 9×10^9/L; Hb, 10 g/L; and PLT, 50×10^9/L), and a subsequent marrow test, undertaken on April 2021, demonstrated more than 30% blast cells and confirmed the hematological recurrence of the primary disease.

Therefore, the patient received the induction chemotherapy with cytarabine and daunorubicin (7 + 3) regimen and achieved a morphologic remission at BMA/B on day 28. In the second remission, she underwent allogeneic bone marrow transplantation from an HLA-matched sibling donor on 1 August 2021 using reduced-intensity conditioning with fludarabine and busulphan. Normal blood counts, morphologic remission, and full donor chimerism by short tandem repeat (STR) were achieved on day +28 after HSCT. At the last follow-up on day +90 after transplant, she was doing well, without any complication. The correlation between blood cells changes and the time point of COVID-19 diagnosis, spontaneous remission, and relapse are shown in Figure 4.

3. Discussion

We presented a new case of AML that the histologic diagnosis was confirmed by two subsequent examinations of the bone marrow. She achieved temporary SR in the absence of disease-modifying therapy after recovering from severe COVID-19, lasting six months. SR of AML is a relatively rare phenomenon in which the underlying mechanisms are not precisely known. Although based on existing published data, an immune-dependent mechanism secondary to the infectious process is considered the probable leading cause of SR [5–7], the other possible factors such as transfusion of blood products, corticosteroids, and colchicine that may contribute to the induction of remission in our case should be considered and discussed.

Colchicine is an alkaloid derivative of the plant (*Colchicum autumnale* L.), which has been known to possess a wide range of pharmacological activities, including antifibrotic, anti-inflammatory, and antiproliferative properties [10–12]. As an anti-inflammatory agent, colchicine is used to treat various inflammatory diseases such as gout, familial Mediterranean fever (FMF), and liver cirrhosis [11]. Colchicine has also been reported to exert an antiproliferative and anticancerous effect by mitotic arrest and cell death by inhibiting microtubules' formation, inducing oxidative stress, and increasing DNA damage [12].

Colchicine with pirfenidone was prescribed to our patient for the treatment of COVID-19-related pulmonary fibrosis [10] and was discontinued after two months. The first evidence of blood cell improvement appeared one month after starting colchicine. Therefore, the possible effect of colchicine in the induction of remission should be considered.

Blood product transfusion was discussed in some previous case reports as the possible cause of remission induction of acute leukemia in the absence of disease-modifying therapy and immunological mechanisms through the antileukemic effects of allogeneic lymphocytes, or inflammatory soluble cytokines are the probable underlying mechanism [13, 14]. Although our patient was transfused with low numbers of blood products before remission, the contribution of transfusion to the induction of remission could not be completely excluded.

In the current outbreak of COVID-19, corticosteroids have been widely used as anti-inflammatory agents that significantly reduce the complications among severe COVID-19 cases. Glucocorticoids are also an important part of the induction regimens for the lymphoid hematologic malignancies, but they have not a defined therapeutic role in myeloid leukemia. However, there is some evidence suggesting the possible efficacy of high-dose corticosteroids in inducing remission of AML in the absence of disease-modifying therapy [15, 16]. As our patient received low-dose dexamethasone for a short period, the impact of this agent to cause complete remission in our case seems unlikely but could not be excluded.

Rashidi et al. reported a case series study where 46 patients with SR of AML were reviewed. More than 70% of reported patients had confirmed pneumonia, soft-tissue infection, or bacteremia before SR [4]. According to the literature review, most patients did not receive any consolidation or maintenance therapy after achieving the SR, resulting in the experience of an early recurrence in most patients [4–7].

Theoretically, a standard immune system could potentially destroy the malignant cells by cellular and adaptive immune responses. Leukemia-derived dendritic cells (DCs) are the pivotal antigen-presenting cells (APCs) that initiate the antileukemic immune process by introducing the leukemia-associated antigens (LAAs) to the naïve T cells and stimulate the differentiation of naïve T cells into the CTLs [17]. DCs also stimulate the CTLs' and NK cells' activity to eradicate the leukemic cells by increasing the IFN-γ. A combination of cytokines including the granulocyte-macrophage colony-stimulating factor (GM-CSF), IL-4, TNF-α, IFN-α, IL-1β, IL-6, and PGE2 is necessary for converting the myeloid leukemia cells to the immature DCs and, subsequently, differentiation to the mature DCs [17–19].

However, the immune system is sometimes unable to destroy the abnormal cells, leading to various malignancies. Downregulation of MHC class II and costimulatory molecules on DCs can be responsible for antigen presentation impairment and antileukemic response failure [20]. The following possible mechanism is the immunosuppressive factors such as transforming growth factor-β (TGF-β), vascular endothelial growth factor (VEGF), and IL-10 that were secreted by leukemic cells [21].

On the other hand, some interfering events such as severe infection and excessive production of proinflammatory cytokines could alter the immune setting and overcome leukemia-induced immune suppression. The abovementioned process might lead to an antileukemia effect and even SR in the absence of disease-modifying therapy of acute leukemia described in some case reports [22].

COVID-19 usually affects both innate and adaptive immune responses. A large amount of chemokine is produced by DCs infected with the coronavirus [23]. Type 1 Interferon (IFN-α, β) and proinflammatory cytokines are secreted in the initial phases of the immune response. High plasma levels of G-CSF, IL-2, IL-7, TNF-α, and macrophage inflammatory protein 1 (MIP1) have been associated with severe lung damage in COVID-19 [24].

We introduced a case of AML with a 11q23/KMT2A abnormality that achieved SR in the absence of disease-modifying therapy lasting for six months following severe pulmonary involvement by COVID-19. Immune-dependent mechanisms secondary to COVID-19 can potentially

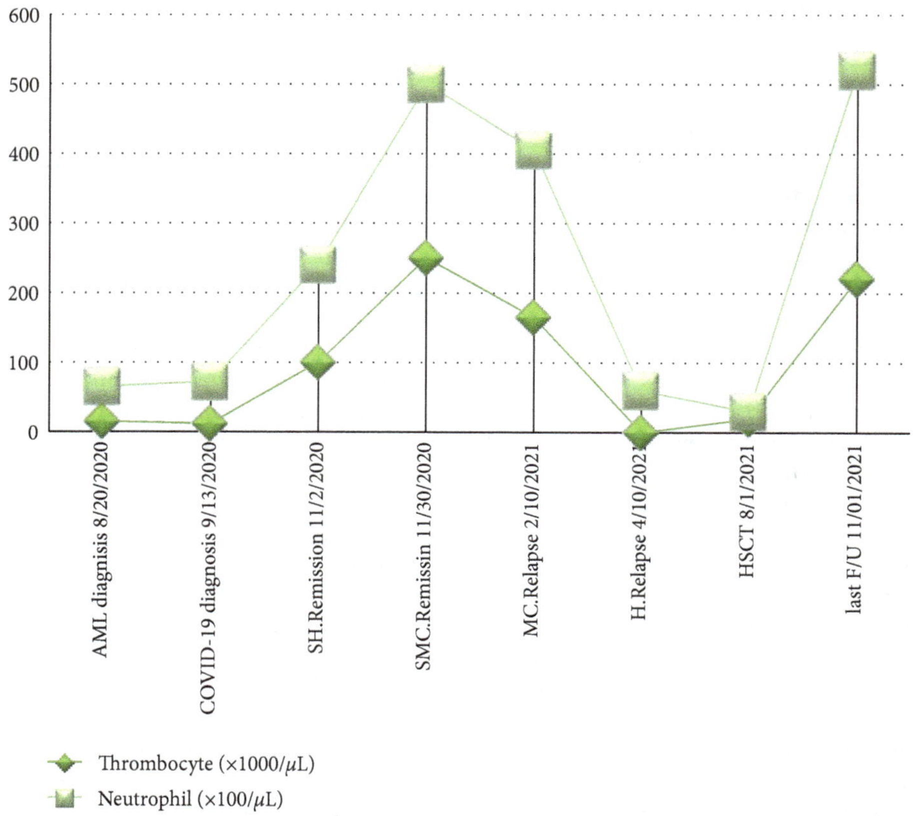

Figure 4: Blood cell changes and the time point of COVID-19 diagnosis, spontaneous remission, and relapse during the course of disease. SH.Remission, spontaneous hematologic remission; SMC.Remission, spontaneous molecular cytogenetic remission; H.Relapse, hematologic relapse; MC.Relapse, molecular cytogenetic relapse; HSCT, hematopoietic stem cell transplantation; and F/U, follow-up.

destroy leukemic cells in addition to virus-infected cells by excessive production of proinflammatory cytokines. Indeed, SR of AML offers supporting evidence for the crucial role of a patient's immune responses to kill the leukemic cells and induction of remission; it also provides an excellent opportunity to evolve new immune-based therapies for the hematologic malignancies. However, other less-likely causes of remission induction, such as transfusion of blood products, corticosteroids, and colchicine, should also be considered.

Despite the high capacity of the immune process to eliminate the malignant cells, the spontaneous immune-related remission in the absence of disease-modifying therapy, similar to what happens following the induction chemotherapy, is usually transient. Therefore, it seems that continuing treatment after SR of AML by a consolidation regimen or bone marrow transplantation, based on the risk-adapted treatment approach and according to ELN 2016 risk categorization, may improve the outcomes and reduce their recurrence risk. Additional work is needed to determine the pathogenesis of immune-related remission in acute leukemia to optimize therapeutic strategies to treat the disease and improve the durability of disease control.

Consent

The patient gave written informed consent for publication.

Authors' Contributions

All authors meet the ICMJE authorship criteria. Mehrdad Abbaszadeh and Fatemeh Tajic Rostami managed the patient and collected the data. Maryam Barkhordar wrote the manuscript. Marjan Yaghmaie performed the genetic analysis. Bahram Chahardouli performed the flow cytometric evaluation. Seied Asadollah Mousavi supervised the work.

References

[1] F. Ferrara, P. Zappasodi, E. Roncoroni, E. Borlenghi, and G. Rossi, "Impact of COVID-19 on the treatment of acute myeloid leukemia," *Leukemia*, vol. 34, no. 8, pp. 2254–2256, 2020.

[2] C. Núñez-Torrón, V. García-Gutiérrez, M. C. Tenorio-Núñez, G. Moreno-Jiménez, F. J. López-Jiménez, and P. Herrera-Puente, "Poor outcome in patients with acute leukemia on intensive chemotherapy and COVID-19," *Bone Marrow Transplantation*, vol. 56, no. 1, pp. 267–269, 2021.

[3] A. M. Zeidan, P. C. Boddu, M. M. Patnaik et al., "Special considerations in the management of adult patients with acute leukaemias and myeloid neoplasms in the COVID-19 era: recommendations from a panel of international experts," *The Lancet Haematology*, vol. 7, no. 8, pp. e601–e612, 2020.

[4] A. Rashidi and S. I. Fisher, "Spontaneous remission of acute myeloid leukemia," *Leukemia and Lymphoma*, vol. 56, no. 6, pp. 1727–1734, 2015.
[5] V. Camus, P. Etancelin, F. Jardin et al., "Spontaneous remission in three cases of AML M5 with NPM 1 mutation," *Clinical Case Reports*, vol. 3, no. 11, pp. 955–959, 2015.
[6] R. Mozafari, M. Moeinian, and A. Asadollahi-Amin, "Spontaneous complete remission in a patient with acute myeloid leukemia and severe sepsis," *Case Reports in Hematology*, vol. 2017, pp. 1-3, 2017.
[7] C. Rautenberg, J. Kaivers, U. Germing, R. Haas, T. Schroeder, and G. Kobbe, "Spontaneous remission in a patient with very late relapse of acute myeloid leukemia 17 years after allogeneic blood stem cell transplantation," *European Journal of Haematology*, vol. 103, no. 2, pp. 131–133, 2019.
[8] Y. Wang, D. Zhang, G. Du et al., "Remdesivir in adults with severe COVID-19: a randomised, double-blind, placebo-controlled, multicentre trial," *The Lancet*, vol. 395, no. 10236, pp. 1569–1578, 2020.
[9] J. A. C. Sterne, J. A. C. Sterne, S. Murthy et al., "Association between administration of systemic corticosteroids and mortality among critically ill patients with COVID-19amci: a meta-analysis," *JAMA*, vol. 324, no. 13, pp. 1330–1341, 2020.
[10] S. G. Peters, J. C. McDougall, W. W. Douglas, D. T. Coles, and R. A. DeRemee, "Colchicine in the treatment of pulmonary fibrosis," *Chest*, vol. 103, no. 1, pp. 101–104, 1993.
[11] G. Liantinioti, A. A. Argyris, A. D. Protogerou, and P. Vlachoyiannopoulos, "The role of colchicine in the treatment of autoinflammatory diseases," *Current Pharmaceutical Design*, vol. 24, no. 6, pp. 690–694, 2018.
[12] A. Kumar, P. R. Sharma, and D. M. Mondhe, "Potential anticancer role of colchicine-based derivatives," *Anti-Cancer Drugs*, vol. 28, no. 3, pp. 250–262, 2017.
[13] T. Maekawa, H. Fujii, S. Horiike et al., "Spontaneous remission of four months' duration in hypoplastic leukemia with tetraploid chromosome after blood transfusions and infection," *Nippon Ketsueki Gakkai Zasshi*, vol. 52, pp. 849–857, 1989.
[14] A. Tzankov, C. Ludescher, H.-C. Duba et al., "Spontaneous remission in a secondary acute myelogenous leukaemia following invasive pulmonary aspergillosis," *Annals of Hematology*, vol. 80, no. 7, pp. 423–425, 2001.
[15] Y. Shimohakamada, K. Shinohara, and N. Fukuda, "Remission of acute myeloblastic leukemia after severe pneumonia treated with high-dose methylprednisolone," *International Journal of Hematology*, vol. 74, no. 2, pp. 173–177, 2001.
[16] G. Hisconmez, S. Ozsoylu, and M. Tuncer, "Differentiation of myeloid leukemic cells induced by high-dose methylprednisolone in patients with acute myeloblastic leukemia and its therapeutic potential," *Leukemia Research*, vol. 15, pp. 537–541, 1991.
[17] A. Choudhury, J. L. Gajewski, J. C. Liang et al., "Use of leukemic dendritic cells for the generation of antileukemic cellular cytotoxicity against philadelphia chromosome-positive chronic myelogenous leukemia," *Blood*, vol. 89, no. 4, pp. 1133–1142, 1997.
[18] H. Cao, V. Vergé, C. Baron et al., "Cutting edge communication: in vitro generation of dendritic cells from human blood monocytes in experimental conditions compatible for in vivo cell therapy," *Journal of Hematotherapy and Stem Cell Research*, vol. 9, no. 2, pp. 183–194, 2000.
[19] T. M. Westers, I. Houtenbos, N. C. L. Snoijs, A. A. van de Loosdrecht, and G. J. Ossenkoppele, "Leukemia-derived dendritic cells in acute myeloid leukemia exhibit potent migratory capacity," *Leukemia*, vol. 19, no. 7, pp. 1270–1272, 2005.
[20] M. Vollmer, L. Li, A. Schmitt et al., "Expression of human leucocyte antigens and co-stimulatory molecules on blasts of patients with acute myeloid leukaemia," *British Journal of Haematology*, vol. 120, no. 6, pp. 1000–1008, 2003.
[21] H. Jonuleit, E. Schmitt, G. Schuler, J. Knop, and A. H. Enk, "Induction of interleukin 10-producing, nonproliferating Cd4+ T cells with regulatory properties by repetitive stimulation with allogeneic immature human dendritic cells," *Journal of Experimental Medicine*, vol. 192, no. 9, pp. 1213–1222, 2000.
[22] P. Musto, G. D'Arena, L. Meillo, N. Cascavilla, S. Ladogana, and M. Carotenuto, "Spontaneous remission in acute myeloid leukaemia: a role for endogenous productionof tumour necrosis factor and interleukin-2?" *British Journal of Haematology*, vol. 87, no. 4, pp. 879-880, 1994.
[23] H. K. W. Law, C. Y. Cheung, H. Y. Ng et al., "Chemokine up-regulation in SARS-coronavirus-infected, monocyte-derived human dendritic cells," *Blood*, vol. 106, no. 7, pp. 2366–2374, 2005.
[24] C. Huang, Y. Wang, X. Li et al., "Clinical features of patients infected with 2019 novel coronavirus in Wuhan, China," *The Lancet*, vol. 395, no. 10223, pp. 497–506, 2020.

Aggressive CD5-Positive Primary Bone Marrow Diffuse Large B-Cell Lymphoma with Leukemic Presentation

Mark G. Evans[1] **Sherif A. Rezk**[2] **Lauren C. Pinter-Brown**[3] **and Xiaohui Zhao**[2]

[1]*Department of Hematopathology, Division of Pathology and Laboratory Medicine, The University of Texas MD Anderson Cancer Center, Houston, TX, USA*
[2]*Department of Pathology and Laboratory Medicine, University of California Irvine (UCI) Medical Center, Orange, CA, USA*
[3]*Department of Medicine, Division of Hematology/Oncology, University of California Irvine (UCI) Medical Center, Orange, CA, USA*

Correspondence should be addressed to Mark G. Evans; markevans2011@gmail.com

Academic Editor: Pier Paolo Piccaluga

Primary bone marrow diffuse large B-cell lymphoma is an exceedingly rare form of non-Hodgkin lymphoma. It may demonstrate a leukemic presentation, and a proportion of cases have CD5 expression. The prognostic implications of this CD5-positivity remain unknown. Here, we present a 78-year-old man who presented with circulating peripheral blood lymphoma cells and a hypercellular marrow involved by diffuse large B-cell lymphoma, germinal center B-cell subtype. The patient responded favorably to six cycles of etoposide, prednisone, vincristine, cyclophosphamide, doxorubicin, and rituximab (EPOCH-R) and intrathecal methotrexate. He unfortunately relapsed in several enlarged inguinal lymph nodes and succumbed to the lymphoma approximately one year after diagnosis, demonstrating the particularly aggressive clinical course of his disease.

1. Introduction

Primary bone marrow lymphoma (PBML) accounts for only 1.16% of all lymphomas and most frequently presents as diffuse large B-cell lymphoma (DLBCL) [1]. PBML was initially described as bone marrow involvement at first presentation [1]. However, some authors have noted that initial bone marrow disease can also occur as a secondary manifestation of nodal lymphoma and that these cases should not be considered true PBML [2]. Alternatively, PBML has been defined as involving only the bone marrow [3] or without any lymphadenopathy [4]. Subsequently, additional PBML subtypes including small-cell B-cell lymphomas, and not DLBCL, have been observed [5].

Given the rarity of this disease, reliable epidemiologic information is not available. Only case reports and small case series have been published, which typically associate PBML with a poor prognosis [6]. Although one study described a cohort of patients who achieved potential cures [1], our case followed the aggressive course typically associated with such cases, where our patient quickly expired following relapsed disease and intensive chemotherapy.

2. Case Report

A 78-year-old man presented with a one-week history of anorexia and generalized weakness. His medical history was significant for metastatic papillary thyroid cancer, treated with radioactive iodine ablation, thyroidectomy, and axitinib. Computed tomography (CT) imaging demonstrated interval increase in splenic and hepatic size, but no concerning masses or lymphadenopathy. However, the patient's serum lactate dehydrogenase (LDH) was 4866 U/L, and his white blood cell count was $454 \times 10^3/\mu L$. His peripheral blood smear was notable for medium and large-sized lymphocytes with irregular nuclear contours accounting for 15% of circulating white blood cells (Figure 1(a)).

A subsequent bone marrow biopsy was hypercellular with 70–80% involvement by sheets of large cells demonstrating blast-like morphology with scant cytoplasm,

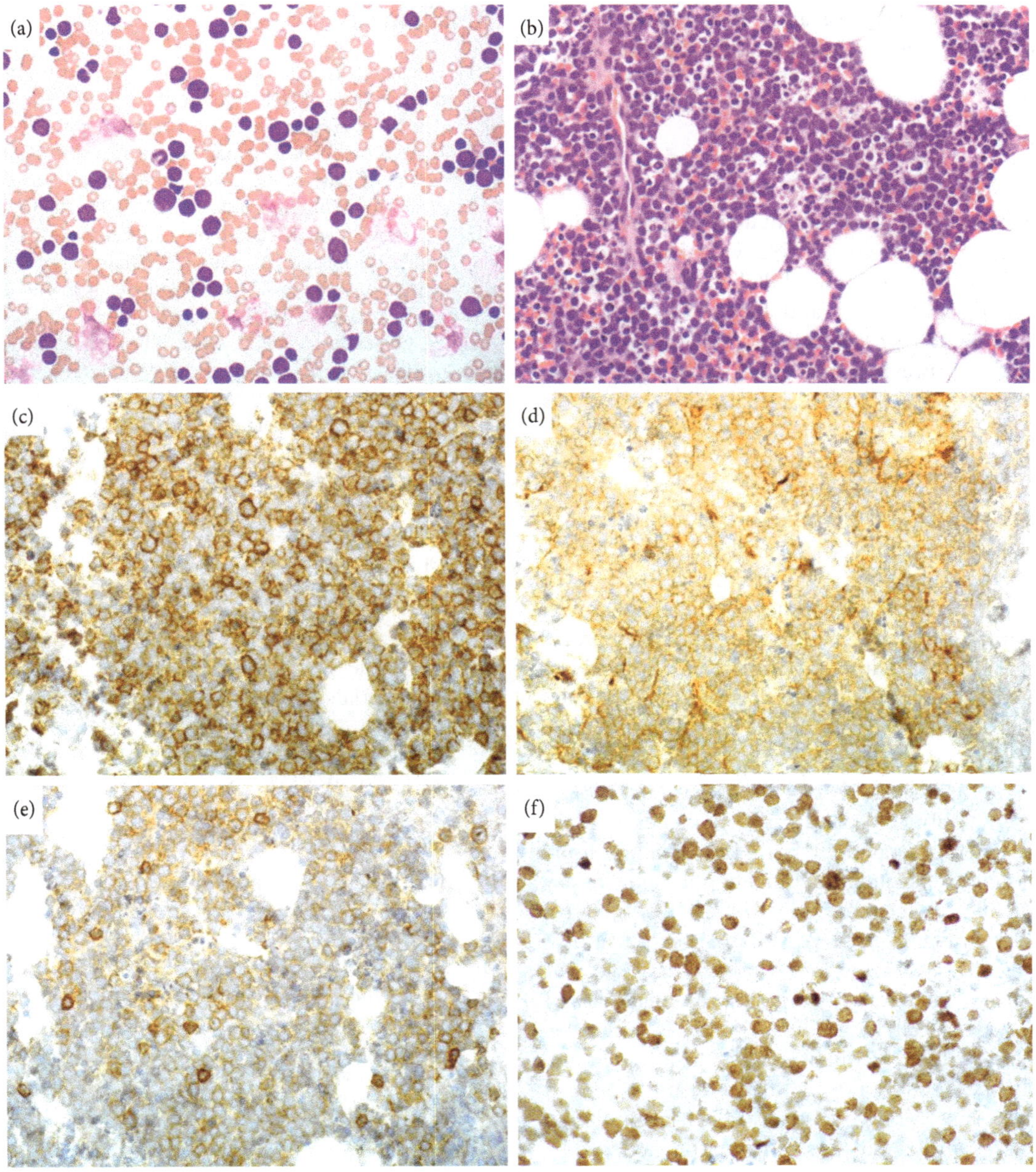

FIGURE 1: The patient's peripheral blood features medium and large-sized cells with scant cytoplasm and irregular nuclear contours (a; 400x magnification). Approximately 70–80% of the cellular elements within his hypercellular bone marrow biopsy show morphologic characteristics similar to those seen in the peripheral blood (b; 400x magnification). The cells are positive for CD20 (c), CD10 (d), and CD5 (e) by immunohistochemistry (400x magnification). Ki-67 demonstrates a high proliferation index of 80% (f; 400x magnification).

irregular nuclear contours, and prominent nucleoli. Numerous apoptotic bodies and mitotic figures were identified. By immunohistochemistry, the malignant cells were positive for CD20, PAX-5, CD5, CD10, MUM1, and BCL-2, while negative for EBV, CD30, BCL-6, cyclin D1, SOX-11, TdT, and MYC (Figures 1(b)–1(e)). A high Ki-67 proliferative index of 80–90% was observed. The bone marrow karyotype was reported as 47, XY, +7, del(13) (q12q22), add(14) (q32.3) (8)/46, and XY(12). Concurrent fluorescence in situ hybridization (FISH) was negative for BCR/ABL1, t(14; 18), IGH, BCL-6, and MYC rearrangements. Overall, these findings were consistent with CD5-positive diffuse large B-cell lymphoma, germinal center B-cell (GCB) subtype.

The patient received six cycles of etoposide, prednisone, vincristine, cyclophosphamide, doxorubicin, and rituximab (EPOCH-R), with intrathecal methotrexate and 50% dose reduction of doxorubicin and vincristine. Repeat bone marrow biopsy following the second cycle demonstrated a normocellular marrow with no lymphoma involvement, and follow-up imaging confirmed a complete response. Five months later, the patient developed relapse in several right inguinal lymph nodes, which demonstrated morphologic and immunohistochemical features identical to his initial bone marrow biopsy. He received six cycles of gemcitabine and oxaliplatin plus rituximab and intrathecal methotrexate, with radiologic evidence of a complete response after the third cycle. Unfortunately, the patient relapsed in the form of an enlarging abdominal mass and shortly thereafter expired, approximately one year after initial diagnosis.

3. Discussion

Primary bone marrow lymphoma is a rare lymphoma that usually presents as DLBCL. Our patient demonstrated relapse and an aggressive clinical course following leukemic presentation of primary bone marrow DLBCL. He was previously diagnosed with thyroid cancer and received axitinib. The published literature has yet to discuss a possible correlation between PBML and previous malignancies or their treatments. One case series has described a small cohort of patients with PBML, DLBCL subtype who demonstrated a better-than-expected prognosis [1], where each of the individuals presented with good performance status, favorable international prognostic index (IPI), and had received rituximab-based therapy. In most studies, the overall survival is dismal. While no recommended therapy exists for PBML, most studies document the use of rituximab, cyclophosphamide, doxorubicin, vincristine, and prednisone (R-CHOP) and a median survival of 9.6 months [7]. A review of 75 patients within the medical literature reported only 15 (20%) surviving, with follow-up times typically less than 24 months [1].

CD5-positivity is a relatively rare occurrence in DLBCL, observed in up to only 10% of cases [8]. Of interest, CD5 expression was demonstrated in both the patient's bone marrow biopsy and subsequent inguinal lymph node biopsy at relapse, with both specimens showing a CD10-positive GCB subtype. While the observed MUM1 expression is uncommon in GCB cases, it has been reported in 13% of 601 DLBCL patients in one study [9]. An alternate diagnosis of intravascular large B-cell lymphoma (IVLBCL) might be entertained, as it features frequent MUM1-positivity, bone marrow involvement, and CD5 expression in up to 38% of cases [10]. However, IVLBCL displays CD10-positivity in only 13% of cases and rarely occurs in lymph nodes [11]. Ultimately, the patient's findings favored the presence of a CD5-positive DLBCL, GCB subtype.

Yamaguchi et al. published a large series of 109 patients with DLBCL and CD5 expression [12]. The authors noted that these cases were more likely to present at the advanced stage, greater than 60 years of age, with elevated serum LDH and B symptoms compared to those without CD5-positivity. Overall, only 16 of the patients (14.7%) could be diagnosed as PBML. Nonetheless, the authors stated that bone marrow was the most common extranodal site of CD5-positive DLBCL. While CD5-positivity has been described in a large proportion of primary bone marrow DLBCL, CD5-negative cases have demonstrated similar features and outcomes [13, 14]. Whether CD5 expression influences outcome in PBML remains uncertain, although the devastating leukemic presentation and eventual relapse in our patient provide additional evidence for the poor prognostic significance of CD5.

References

[1] H. Chang, Y.-S. Hung, T.-L. Lin et al., "Primary bone marrow diffuse large B cell lymphoma: a case series and review," *Annals of Hematology*, vol. 90, no. 7, pp. 791–796, 2011.

[2] J. A. Strauchen, "Primary bone marrow B-cell lymphoma: report of four cases," *The Mount Sinai Journal of Medicine, New York*, vol. 70, no. 2, pp. 133–138, 2003.

[3] M. Hishizawa, K. Okamoto, K. Chonabayashi, H. Kaneko, M. Watanabe, and M. Tsudo, "Primary large B-cell lymphoma of the bone marrow," *British Journal of Haematology*, vol. 136, no. 3, p. 351, 2007.

[4] W. G. Staples and E. P. Gétaz, "Bone marrow involvement in malignant lymphoma without peripheral lymphadenopathy," *South African Medical Journal*, vol. 52, no. 5, pp. 60–63, 1977.

[5] K. Iwatani, K. Takata, Y. Sato et al., "Low-grade B-cell lymphoma presenting primarily in the bone marrow," *Human Pathology*, vol. 45, no. 7, pp. 1379–1387, 2014.

[6] C. L. Alvares, E. Matutes, M. A. Scully et al., "Isolated bone marrow involvement in diffuse large B cell lymphoma: a report of three cases with review of morphological, immunophenotypic and cytogenetic findings," *Leukemia and Lymphoma*, vol. 45, no. 4, pp. 769–775, 2003.

[7] G. Wang, Y. Chang, X. Wu et al., "Clinical features and prognostic factors of primary bone marrow lymphoma," *Cancer Management and Research*, vol. 11, pp. 2553–2563, 2019.

[8] X. Zhang, M. Sun, L. Zhang, and H. Shao, "Primary hepatosplenic CD5-positive diffuse large B-cell lymphoma: a case report with literature review," *International Journal of Clinical and Experimental Pathology*, vol. 6, no. 5, pp. 985–989, 2013.

[9] T.-X. Lu, Y. Miao, J.-Z. Wu et al., "The distinct clinical features and prognosis of the CD10+MUM1+ and CD10-Bcl6-MUM1- diffuse large B-cell lymphoma," *Scientific Reports*, vol. 6, no. 1, Article ID 20465, 2016.

[10] M. Ponzoni, E. Campo, and S. Nakamura, "Intravascular large B-cell lymphoma: a chameleon with multiple faces and many masks," *Blood*, vol. 132, no. 15, pp. 1561–1567, 2018.

[11] S. Nakamura, M. Ponzoni, and E. Campo, "Intravascular large B-cell lymphoma," in *WHO Classification of Tumors of Hematopoietic and Lymphoid Tissues*, S. H. Swerdlow, E. Campo, and N. L. Harris, Eds., pp. 317-318, IARC, Lyon, France, 4th edition, 2017.

[12] M. Yamaguchi, M. Seto, M. Okamoto et al., "De novo CD5+ diffuse large B-cell lymphoma: a clinicopathologic study of 109 patients," *Blood*, vol. 99, no. 3, pp. 815–821, 2002.

[13] S. Y. Kong, E. H. Cho, H. Y. Woo, Q. Park, Y. H. Ko, and S. H. Kim, "De novo CD5 positive diffuse large B-cell lymphomas with bone marrow involvement in Korea," *Journal of Korean Medical Science*, vol. 19, no. 6, pp. 815–819, 2004.

[14] K. Yoshida, H. Kayano, M. Akiba et al., "De novo CD-5 positive diffuse large B-cell lymphoma with leukemic dissemination diagnosed by immunohistochemical examinations of bone marrow clot sections," *Rinsho Ketsueki*, vol. 43, no. 10, pp. 943–948, 2002.

30

A Case of Myeloid Sarcoma following Allogeneic HSCT Presenting as Localized Hip Pain

Shannon Zhang, Casey Charlton, Akshay Amaraneni, and Keri Maher

University of Arizona, Tucson College of Medicine, Tucson, AZ, USA

Correspondence should be addressed to Keri Maher; krmaher@email.arizona.edu

Academic Editor: Pier P. Piccaluga

Myeloid sarcoma is a rare variant of acute myeloid leukemia (AML) which presents as an extramedullary soft tissue mass. Due to the rarity of this disease, along with nonspecific presenting symptoms, diagnosis can be delayed or missed without a high index of suspicion. In this case, we discuss a patient diagnosed with AML relapse in the form of myeloid sarcoma two years after allogeneic hematopoietic stem cell transplant (alloHSCT) for myelodysplastic syndrome (MDS) with the initial presentation for back pain misdiagnosed as spinal stenosis. This case report aims to help healthcare providers in recognizing the early signs and symptoms of this disorder as well as provide information in regards to treatment options and risk assessment.

1. Introduction

Myeloid sarcoma is a rare disease that can present as initial diagnosis or relapse of other hematologic disorders, most commonly acute myeloid leukemia (AML), as an extramedullary soft tissue tumor [1]. Due to the extremely low prevalence of this presentation, prospective knowledge on prognosis and optimal therapy is limited [1]. Presently, the literature consists of small retrospective studies or case reports. However, prognosis of myeloid sarcoma is thought to have a poorer prognosis than AML alone.

Myeloid sarcoma can precede, occur with, or occur after the diagnosis of AML, MDS, and other myeloproliferative neoplasms [2]. It can represent relapse after a hematopoietic cellular transplant and can occur in any organ. There has been a recent rise in reports of patients diagnosed with myeloid sarcoma after allogeneic stem cell transplant [1]. However, incidence is rare, occurring in less than 1% of transplanted patients. This form of relapse has been described up to five years after alloHSCT. Cases occurring after alloHSCT may represent failure of a graft-versus-leukemia effect with relapse of original disease or as a new therapy-related myeloid neoplasm [3].

In this case report, we discuss the findings of a 59-year-old Caucasian man presenting with back pain and leg weakness, who was ultimately diagnosed with myeloid sarcoma two years after receiving an allogeneic hematopoietic stem cell transplant for MDS.

2. Case Presentation

Our patient is a 59-year-old Caucasian male who was diagnosed in 2016 with MDS when he presented with thrombocytopenia (platelets 78,000) and neutropenia (ANC 800). Bone marrow biopsy showed trilineage dysplasia, and cytogenetics revealed a complex karyotype including −0, +3, 5q−, −7, +8, −9, and +22. He attained CR1 after 6 cycles of azacitidine, including normalization of cytogenetic studies. He underwent a reduced intensity matched unrelated donor peripheral blood stem cell transplant with fludarabine/melphalan + rabbit antithymocyte globulin conditioning in October 2016. His course was relatively uncomplicated, and one-year milestone visit revealed complete donor chimerisms and continued complete remission.

In March 2018, he began to complain of increasing pain in his lower back radiating down his right leg that ultimately resulted in decreased sensation and strength in his right leg.

He was seen by a chiropractor, and also an orthopedic surgeon, and was diagnosed with spinal stenosis. His orthopedic surgeon planned on operating to relieve this stenosis, and preop labs showed new-onset thrombocytopenia for which he was referred back to our transplant center. Workup at the transplant center showed parvovirus and EBV positivity as well as worsening cytopenias. He was started on IVIG for treatment of parvovirus; however, this was ineffective. Interestingly, peripheral blood chimerisms at this time showed continued complete engraftment, and bone marrow biopsy morphology showed no evidence of relapsed MDS or AML and was read as a hypocellular marrow consistent with parvovirus infection.

A repeat MRI was performed due to worsening pain that detected a large right-sided pelvic mass in the right iliac bone with acetabular and femoral head destruction measuring 14.2 × 13.6 × 18.3 cm (Figures 1 and 2). This mass was biopsied, and the final pathology report indicated myeloid sarcoma (CD45+, CD34+, CD1117+, and MPO+). Ultimately, bone marrow cytogenetics which resulted nine days after his biopsy revealed complex karyotype, albeit with different findings from his initial diagnostic marrow, likely indicating clonal evolution of his original disease. Repeat peripheral blood chimerisms were performed on the blood two weeks after the initial presentation to our center, revealed rapidly declining donor chimerisms at 23% donor DNA.

Given the patient's poor functional status, he was not an intensive therapy candidate. After discussion of therapy options including palliative radiation, hospice, and palliative chemotherapy, he opted for palliative radiation. However, he continued to decline clinically and was discharged to hospice.

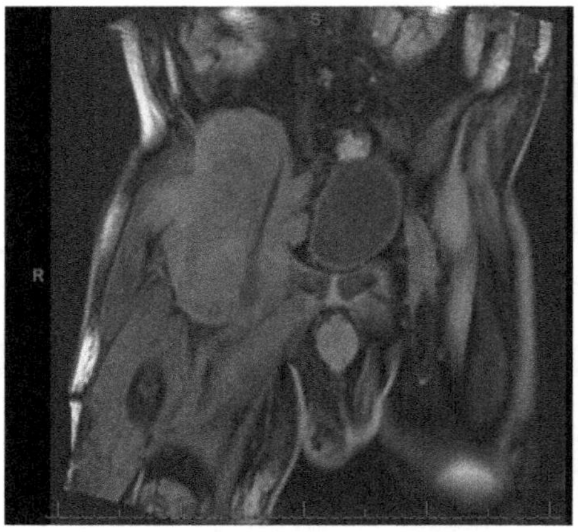

Figure 1: Large complex enhancing mass in the R iliac bone.

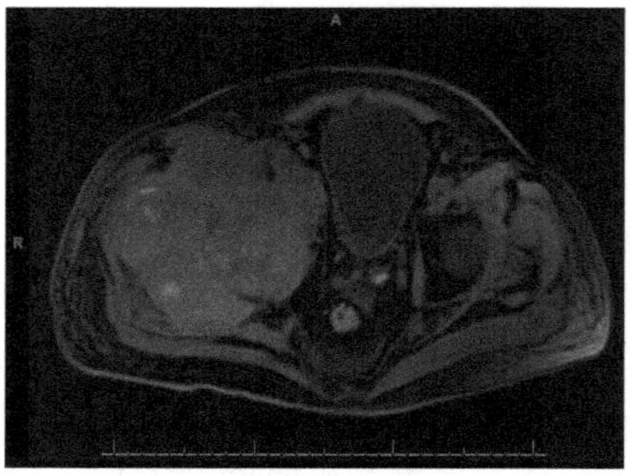

Figure 2: Large right iliac mass and associated destruction of surrounding osseous structures with involvement of right hip musculature.

3. Discussion

Extramedullary leukemia, including myeloid sarcoma, occurs when myeloid cells form tumors outside the bone marrow. This may indicate dysfunctional homing signals for leukemic blasts via chemokines, metalloproteinases, and leukocyte surface beta2 integrins [4]. The type of myeloid sarcoma is categorized according to the most abundant cell type and whether the cells present are immature or mature. The tumor can be further phenotyped immunologically which may guide therapy options [5].

A study published in 2007, analyzed the clinical, cytogenetic, and phenotypic factors of 92 adult patients with myeloid sarcoma. The average age of those affected was 55.8 years ranging from 16 to 87 years with a male to female ratio of 1.42 : 1. In 28.2% of cases, myeloid sarcoma was found localized to the skin. Other common sites included the lymph nodes (16.3%), testes (6.5%), bone (3.25%), and CNS (3.25%) [6]. Twenty-seven percent of cases presented as de novo myeloid sarcoma with approximately 40% of these originally misdiagnosed most commonly as diffuse large B-cell lymphoma. Approximately, 35% presented with simultaneous AML, MPN, or MDS. The remaining 38% of individuals in the study had a previous history of AML, MPN, and MDS. Of those with a previous history of AML (12 patients), 42% were found to have the M2 subtype. Of those with a previous history of MPN (13 patients), CML was the most common cause with 54% being affected. Other causes of MPN present before a diagnosis of myeloid sarcoma included polycythemia vera, essential thrombocytopenia, and mastocytosis. Histological studies of all 92 cases in this study concluded that the most prevalent histotype was blastic ($N = 42$), followed by monoblastic ($N = 20$) and myelomonocytic ($N = 20$). Of the 92 cases retrospectively presented in this study, only seven were still living, six of whom received an allogeneic HSCT as part of their therapy. There were no differences in survival between the group with de novo myeloid sarcoma, concomitant hematological disease and myeloid sarcoma, or previous history of hematological disease. The mean survival of those who underwent chemotherapy, imatinib mesylate (for CML patients in the blast type), surgery, and radiation therapy was 7.1 months, 5.6 months, 36 days, and 1 week, respectively [6].

In AML myeloid sarcoma, therapy mimics that for medullary AML and follows the paradigm of intensive induction and consolidation, followed by allogeneic hematopoietic stem cell transplant in individuals who are candidates based on disease characteristics as listed in ELN 2017 and performance status/medical comorbidities. If alloHSCT is used as part of the therapy paradigm, those with complete donor chimerisms have improved overall survival compared to those with mixed chimerisms, as expected [7]. Palliative therapy options include modest dose radiation (20–30 Gy), azacitidine, supportive care, and hospice.

4. Conclusion

In conclusion, the patient discussed initially developed an isolated myeloid sarcoma two years after alloHSCT for MDS. His diagnosis was delayed by several weeks due to non-specific presenting symptom of back pain and was only referred to hematology for further evaluation when he was incidentally noted to have thrombocytopenia on presurgical evaluation. At this time, the patient had declined significantly in functional status and was no longer a candidate for intensive therapy. While disease relapse after alloHSCT already portends a grim prognosis, this delay in diagnosis may have further worsened his overall prognosis. Vigilance for this diagnosis, especially in the post-transplant setting, is necessary due to its propensity for uncommon presentations.

References

[1] B. Avni and M. Koren-Michowitz, "Myeloid sarcoma: current approach and therapeutic options," *Therapeutic Advances in Hematology*, vol. 2, no. 5, pp. 309–316, 2011.

[2] W. Au, A. Chan, A. Lie, F. Chen, R. Liang, and Y. L. Kwong, "Recurrent isolated extramedullary relapses as granulocytic sarcomas following allogeneic bone marrow transplantation for acute myeloid leukemia," *Bone Marrow Transplantation*, vol. 21, no. 2, pp. 205–208, 1998.

[3] S. Johansen, H. K. Gjelberg, A. B. Ahmed, O. Bruserud, and H. Reikvam, "Myeloid sarcoma after allogeneic stem cell transplantation for acute myeloid leukemia: successful consolidation treatment approaches in two patients," *Case Reports in Oncological Medicine*, vol. 2018, Article ID 7697283, 5 pages, 2018.

[4] V. I. Broek, K. Vanderkerken, V. B. Camp, and V. I. Riet, "Extravasation and homing mechanisms in multiple myeloma," *Clinical & Experimental Metastasis*, vol. 25, no. 4, pp. 325–334, 2008.

[5] H.-Q. Wang and J. Li, "Clinicopathological features of myeloid sarcoma: report of 39 cases and literature review," *Pathology—Research and Practice*, vol. 212, no. 9, pp. 817–824, 2016.

[6] S. A. Pileri, S. Ascani, M. C. Cox et al., "Myeloid sarcoma: clinico-pathologic, phenotypic and cytogenetic analysis of 92 adult patients," *Leukemia*, vol. 21, no. 2, pp. 340–350, 2006.

[7] D. Antic, I. Elezovic, N. Milic et al., "Is there a "gold" standard treatment for patients with isolated myeloid sarcoma?," *Biomedicine & Pharmacotherapy*, vol. 67, no. 1, pp. 72–77, 2013.

31

Age-Adjusted Schedules of Venetoclax and Hypomethylating Agents to Treat Extremely Elderly Patients with Acute Myeloid Leukemia

Aaron M. Lee,[1] **Aaron M. Goodman**,[2] **and James K. Mangan**[2,3]

[1]*Department of Medicine, Internal Medicine Residency Program, University of California San Diego, La Jolla, CA, USA*
[2]*Department of Medicine, Division of Blood and Marrow Transplantation, Moores Cancer Center, University of California San Diego, La Jolla, CA, USA*
[3]*Moores Cancer Center, University of California, San Diego, 3855 Health Sciences Drive, Mail Code 0960, La Jolla, CA 92093, USA*

Correspondence should be addressed to James K. Mangan; jmangan@health.ucsd.edu

Academic Editor: Sudhir Tauro

Acute myeloid leukemia (AML) is associated with particularly poor outcomes in the elderly population, in whom the disease is most prevalent. BCL-2 has been identified as an antiapoptotic protein and promotes survival of leukemia stem cells. Recently, the United States FDA has approved venetoclax, a selective oral BCL-2 inhibitor, for use in conjunction with hypomethylating agents (azacitidine or decitabine) or low-dose cytarabine as a first-line treatment option for those AML patients ineligible for standard induction chemotherapy. However, there are nuances and challenges when using this regimen in the extremely elderly AML patients. Given the widespread adoption of this regimen and increasing prevalence of patients who are well into their 80 s, it is important to evaluate and understand how to safely use this regimen in this so-called "extremely elderly" population. We present here 3 case studies involving AML patients >85 years of age who were treated with venetoclax plus HMA and provide clinical knowledge on how this population should be appropriately managed.

1. Introduction

Acute myeloid leukemia (AML) commonly affects the elderly, with a median age at diagnosis of 67-68 years. Elderly patients (typically defined as >60 years old) often have poor responses to typical cytotoxic and intensive induction chemotherapy, given the propensity for adverse genomic features, drug-resistant phenotypes, and more comorbidities and compromised organ function than younger patients. Treating this population is a balancing act; low-intensity regimens often prove safe but ineffective, while intensive chemotherapy is associated with excess morbidity and mortality. For some time now, these elderly patients deemed unfit for induction chemotherapy have received low-intensity regimens typically consisting of monotherapy with a hypomethylating agent (HMA) or low-dose cytarabine, producing modest results and suboptimal outcomes.

In November 2018, venetoclax in combination with a hypomethylating agent (HMA) was granted accelerated approval by the FDA for AML patients ineligible for intensive chemotherapy or adults >75 years old. This has represented a major advancement in treatment of AML in the elderly. Several clinical trials studying venetoclax plus HMA showed tolerable safety profile as well as favorable response rates in patients with AML (Table 1). Dinardo et al. in a randomized phase III trial showed that in patients ineligible for standard induction therapy, use of venetoclax with decitabine or azacitidine led to overall survival advantage and higher incidence of remission compared to those who received azacitidine alone [1]. Venetoclax in conjunction with an HMA has now been widely used for those patients not fit for standard induction chemotherapy. While the median age in these trials ranged from 68 to 76

Table 1: Clinical trial outcomes in AML patients using venetoclax plus hypomethylating agents.

Study	Phase of study	Patient population	Number of patients	Treatment and dosing used	Median age, years (range)	# patients >75 years old	Response rate (CR + CRi)	CR	Median event-free survival	Median duration of CR + CRi	Median overall survival	Grade 3/4 adverse events
Dinardo et al., *Lancet Oncol*, 2018 [2]	1b	Age >65, treatment naïve, ineligible for standard induction	57	3 + 3 dose escalation; venetoclax-group A: target doses 400, 800, and 1200 mg/m^2; group B: target doses 400, 800, and 1200 mg/m^2; group C: target dose 400 mg/m^2; azacitidine-75 mg/m^2; decitabine-20 mg/m^2	Group A: 74 (71.5–79.0); group B: 75 (71.0–80.0); group C: 74 (69.0–79.5)	39	61.4% (35/57)	24.6% (14/57)	Not reported	Group A: 8.4 mos; group B: 12.3 mos; group C: 4.3 mos	12.3 months (all groups)	Thrombocytopenia; febrile neutropenia; neutropenia
Dinardo et al., *Blood*, 2019 [3]	1b	Age >65, treatment naïve, ineligible for standard induction	145	Venetoclax-ramp-up C1 from 20 (escalation phase) or 100 (expansion); target doses: 400, 800, and 1200 mg/m^2; in escalation expansion phase: 400 mg and 800 mg; azacitidine-42 mg/m^2, d1-7; decitabine-20 mg/m^2, d1-5	74 (65–86)	52	67%	37%	Not reported	11.3 months	17.5 months	Febrile neutropenia; anemia; thrombocytopenia; neutropenia; pneumonia
Dinardo et al., *NEJM*, 2020 [1]	3	Ineligible for intensive induction, age >75, all treatment naive	286 in variable group	Aza 75 mg/m^2, d1-7; VEN 400 mg daily, d1-28 w/3 day ramp-up C1	76 (49–91)	Not reported	66.4%	36.7%	9.8 months	17.5 months	14.7 months	Thrombocytopenia neutropenia; febrile neutropenia; anemia; leukopenia
Maiti et al., *Blood*, 2018 [4]	II	Age >69, ineligible for OR relapse/refractory AML	48	VEN days 1–28, cycle 1, D1-21; C2 and onwards VEN 200 mg PO daily in pts needing cyp3a4 decitabine-20 mg/m^2 IV daily D1–D10 until CR, followed by 5-day cycles	71 (22–82)	Not reported	71% (34/48)	CR alone not reported	Not reached	Not reached	Not reached	Infections; neutropenia; tumor lysis syndrome

Table 1: Continued.

Study	Phase of study	Patient population	Number of patients	Treatment and dosing used	Median age, years (range)	# patients >75 years old	Response rate (CR + CRi)	CR	Median event-free survival	Median duration of CR + CRi	Median overall survival	Grade 3/4 adverse events
Wei et al., *Journal of Clinical Oncology*, 2019 [5]	Ib/II	Age >60, treatment naïve, ineligible for intensive chemo	82	Venetoclax-initial 50 or 100 mg, titrated up to the target dose; phase II recommended dose: 600 mg; 800 mg in phase Ib w/ prolonged myelosuppression; low-dose cytarabine-20 mg/m^2 daily SC injection D1–10, 28-day cycles	74 (63–90)	40	54%	26%	Not reported	8.1 months	10.1 months	Cytopenia, febrile neutropenia; infections
Wei et al., *Blood*, 2020 [6]	3	Adults ≥18 y/o w/ ND AML ineligible for intensive chemo (38% had secondary AML, and 20% had received prior hypomethylating agent treatment)	210	Venetoclax + LDAC	76 (33–93)	82	48%	27%	4.7 months	Not reported	7.2 months	Febrile neutropenia; neutropenia; thrombocytopenia

years, additional information on using these regimens to manage older, "real-world" patients, particularly those over 85 years of age, would be helpful to clinicians in clinical practice. There remains a paucity of data on how to best manage these extremely elderly AML patients with venetoclax plus HMAs.

In this manuscript, we use three case studies to showcase how we treat AML in the extremely elderly. We will discuss our clinical experience and provide expert recommendations on treatment and management.

2. Case Reports

2.1. Patient 1. Patient 1 is an 87-year-old male who presented with fatigue and intermittent shortness of breath. The WBC count was 84,900 with a large number of circulating myeloblasts. Cytogenetic and molecular details are listed in Table 1.

The patient was admitted to the hospital and started on hydroxyurea for cytoreduction. Venetoclax and azacitidine were initiated when his WBC count dropped below 35,000. Due to high risk of tumor lysis, venetoclax was dose-escalated from 100 mg on day 1 to 400 mg by day 3 and was continued on 400 mg daily through day 21. Azacitidine was given intravenously at 75 mg/m^2 on days 1–7. His inpatient course was complicated by febrile neutropenia with a negative infectious workup and deep cytopenias requiring transfusion support.

Bone marrow biopsy on day 22 showed a hypocellular marrow with <5% blasts. His counts were allowed to recover, and he met criteria for complete remission after cycle 1. He subsequently received 10 additional cycles of therapy. He was maintained on venetoclax 400 mg daily on days 1–14 during the additional cycles with full-dose azacitidine, and cytopenias were managed with rare blood transfusions and occasional granulocyte colony stimulating factor (G-CSF). The patient's course was later complicated by Sweet's syndrome, believed to be secondary to G-CSF, at which time azacitidine and venetoclax were held. Repeat bone marrow showed his AML had relapsed, and he was restarted on azacitidine alone. He had a stable disease on azacitidine for 6 months before progressing with leukocytosis and circulating blasts. Next-generation sequencing revealed that the patient had acquired a FLT3 ITD mutation that was not previously present. He was switched to monotherapy with the FLT3 inhibitor gilteritinib and had a hematologic response before passing away from complications of AML 25 months after his original diagnosis.

2.2. Patient 2. Patient 2 is a 92-year-old male who presented with recurrent pneumonia and a biopsy-proven right lower lobe lung adenocarcinoma and was incidentally noted to be pancytopenic. A bone marrow biopsy was markedly hypocellular, with 43% myeloid blasts in scattered clusters. Cytogenetic and molecular data are displayed in Table 2.

The patient was referred to Thoracic Oncology and underwent successful radiation in 10 fractions of a stage I lung adenocarcinoma, and given his good performance status otherwise, he was admitted to the hospital and started on treatment with intravenous azacitidine (75 mg/m^2 on days 1–7) and venetoclax 400 mg daily on days 1–21. The patient tolerated induction well with minimal adverse effects, without neutropenic fever, and only mild weight loss and deconditioning. Repeat bone marrow biopsy on day 21 showed a markedly hypocellular marrow with a small myeloid blast population (3%), and he ultimately had good count recovery.

Following induction, the patient continued to tolerate the treatment well, with only symptoms of fatigue and occasional nausea. He did have persistent cytopenias, necessitating occasional transfusions and routine twice weekly G-CSF injections. The patient underwent 9 more cycles of therapy, including 5 cycles with azacitidine alone and 4 cycles with venetoclax given for only 14 days at the full dose of 400 mg daily. After 10 cycles of therapy, the patient showed evidence of relapsed disease and progression and passed away 17 months after the initial diagnosis.

2.3. Patient 3. Patient 3 is an 85-year-old male who had a transformation to acute myeloid leukemia after a yearlong history of MDS with multilineage dysplasia. He presented with leukocytosis and circulating blasts, and his bone marrow biopsy confirmed transformation to acute leukemia with both myeloid and T-lymphoid marker expressions. There was extensive marrow involvement. Cytogenetic and molecular details are displayed in Table 1.

The decision was made to start decitabine with venetoclax, and the patient was admitted for induction therapy. During induction, the patient received dose-reduced venetoclax 100 mg daily for 21 days due to concern for drug-drug interactions, given the concomitant use of posaconazole for fungal prophylaxis. A bone marrow biopsy following cycle 1 showed a cellular marrow with reduction of blasts from 80% down to 14%, with a normal absolute neutrophil count and stable thrombocytopenia (platelet counts stable around 20,000, compared to 25,000 on admission), and he was discharged without further complications.

On follow-up, the patient was continued on decitabine and venetoclax, receiving only 14 days of dose-reduced 100 mg venetoclax for each cycle, given persistent cytopenias. His course was complicated by anemia and fatigue, and the patient received G-CSF during periods of neutropenia between cycles and transfusions as needed. For cycles 2 and 3, the patient received a shorter dose of 14 days of venetoclax due to anemia. Bone marrow biopsy after cycle 3 showed ongoing reduction in the blast count (9% blasts). Cycle 4 was with decitabine alone, and the patient developed leukocytosis and a bacteremia, so after stabilization, cycle 5 was resumed with decitabine and venetoclax once again. Following cycle 5, the patient developed GI bleeding in the setting of thrombocytopenia. The patient was managed supportively on hydroxyurea and transfusion support, ultimately transitioning to hospice care, 6 months after his original diagnosis with AML.

Table 2: Clinical characteristics of three extremely elderly AML patients treated with venetoclax and azacitidine.

	Age at diagnosis	Medical comorbidities	Blood count at bone marrow diagnosis	Cytogenetics	Next-generation sequencing	Blast (%) in the marrow at diagnosis	Bridging therapy used prior to venetoclax plus HMA	Hospitalized for induction?	Complications from induction	Response to induction	Fungal prophylaxis during induction	Progression-free survival	Postinduction complications
1	87	Melanoma (*in situ*, resected); hyperlipidemia; hypertension	WBC: 84,900; Hgb: 9.3; platelet: 81; ANC: 5943	Karyotype: normal; FISH: normal	SF3B1 K666 N (VAF 47%), FLT3 D835Y (VAF 45%), and RUNX1 D93Afs * 31 (VAF 42%)	95	Hydroxyurea	Yes	Neutropenic fever; atrial fibrillation with rapid ventricular response; upper extremity phlebitis	CR	Micafungin	13 months, relapse following cycle 11	Sweet's syndrome following C11
2	92	Lung adenocarcinoma; prostate cancer (*localized*); hypertension	WBC: 0.4; Hgb: 8.6; platelet: 72; ANC: 136	Abnormal karyotype; deletion 6q; FISH: loss of 6q (33%) and 7q (29%)	Mutations in DNMT3A, SRSF2, RUNX1, BCOR, TET2, and BCR-ABL neg	43	None	Yes	None	CR	Micafungin	13 months	Neutropenic fever following C10; COVID-19 pneumonia
3	85	Prostate cancer (*localized*); minimal change disease; hypertension; hyperlipidemia	WBC: 38.3; Hgb: 7.6; platelet: 25; ANC: 5745	Karyotype: abnormal; deletion 20q; gain of *X* chromosome in two clones; FISH: diminished D20S108 (20q12) hybridization in 65% of cells	Mutations in RUNX1, SMC3, and TET2	80	Hydroxyurea	Yes	Tumor lysis syndrome	Partial response	Posaconazole	4 months on therapy, progression during cycle 4	GI bleeding and bacteremia following C5

Patient 1: C1 venetoclax 400mg 3 day ramp up to D21 + azacitidine 75 mg/m^2 D1-7. C2 venetoclax 400mg D1-21, azacitidine 75 mg/m2 D1-7. C3 venetoclax 400mg D1-14, azacitidine 75 mg/m^2 D1-7. C4-C5 azacitidine 75 mg/m^2 D1-7, venetoclax held due to cytopenia. C6-C11 Ven 400mg D1-14, azacitidine 75 mg/m2 D1-7. C12-17 azacitidine only. Gilteritinib thereafterPatient 2: C1 venetoclax 400mg (no escalation) D1-21, azacitidine 75 mg/m^2 d1-7. C2-3 venetoclax 400 D1-14 (avoid cytopenia), azacitidine 75 mg/m^2 D1-7. C4-5 azacitidine only secondary to cytopenias. C6-7 venetoclax 1-14d, with azacitidine. C8-10 azacitidine only. Patient 3: C1-3 venetoclax 100mg daily 1-21, Decitabine 20 mg/m^2 d1-5. C4 Decitabine 20 mg/m^2 d1-5. C5 venetoclax 100 mg daily, Decitabine 20 mg/m^2 d1-5.

3. Discussion

We present three cases of extremely elderly patients (>85 years old) with AML who have been treated with venetoclax and a hypomethylating agent (azacitidine or decitabine). There are several tools that have been used to assess fitness of elderly patients for AML therapy, some of which have been described by Min et al. [7]. We did not use a formal tool to select patients, but all patients selected were ambulatory, did not have any cognitive impairment, and had excellent family support and transportation to and from our center. The ECOG performance status was at least 2 at the time of treatment initiation. After receiving therapy, all three patients had bone marrow responses and two of the three patients completed over 10 cycles of therapy. All patients were treated with the full therapeutic dose of venetoclax when given in combination with HMA. After achieving initial response, we did modify subsequent cycles of VEN/HMA to use VEN only for 14 days instead of 21 and occasionally omitted venetoclax cycles and treated with HMA alone, all in an effort to manage cytopenias and avoid significant complications such as neutropenic fevers while the patients were on active treatment. Fungal prophylaxis and bacterial prophylaxis were used while the patients were neutropenic. Importantly, the patients were motivated for therapy, and two of three maintained a good quality of life while being treated. Patient 1 lived for 25 months after the initial diagnosis, and patient 2 survived for 17 months after the initial diagnosis. This case series illustrates that treatment with HMAs and venetoclax is feasible in the extremely elderly population and age alone should not rule out such patients from receiving active antileukemia therapy.

Disclosure

This research was performed as part of employment under UC San Diego Department of Medicine.

References

[1] C. D. DiNardo, B. A. Jonas, V. Pullarkat et al., "Azacitidine and venetoclax in previously untreated acute myeloid leukemia," *New England Journal of Medicine*, vol. 383, no. 7, pp. 617–629, 2020.

[2] C. D. DiNardo, K. W. Pratz, A. Letai et al., "Safety and preliminary efficacy of venetoclax with decitabine or azacitidine in elderly patients with previously untreated acute myeloid leukaemia: a non-randomised, open-label, phase 1b study," *The Lancet Oncology*, vol. 19, no. 2, pp. 216–228, 2018.

[3] C. D. DiNardo, K. Pratz, V. Pullarkat et al., "Venetoclax combined with decitabine or azacitidine in treatment-naive, elderly patients with acute myeloid leukemia," *Blood*, vol. 133, no. 1, pp. 7–17, 2019.

[4] Maiti, DiNardo, D. Courtney et al., "Interim analysis of phase II study of venetoclax with 10-day decitabine (DEC10-VEN) in acute myeloid leukemia and myelodysplastic syndrome," *Blood*, vol. 132, no. Supplement 1, p. 286, 2018.

[5] A. H. Wei, S. A. Strickland, J. Z. Hou et al., "Venetoclax combined with low-dose cytarabine for previously untreated patients with acute myeloid leukemia: results from a phase Ib/II study," *Journal of Clinical Oncology*, vol. 37, no. 15, pp. 1277–1284, 2019.

[6] A. H. Wei, P. Montesinos, V. Ivanov et al., "Venetoclax plus LDAC for newly diagnosed AML ineligible for intensive chemotherapy: a phase 3 randomized placebo-controlled trial," *Blood*, vol. 135, no. 24, pp. 2137–2145, 2020.

[7] G. J. Min, B. S. Cho, S. S. Park et al., "Geriatric assessment predicts nonfatal toxicities and survival for intensively treated older adults with AML," *Blood*, vol. 139, no. 11, pp. 1646–1658, 2022.

32

The Efficacy and Safety of Lenalidomide plus Rituximab in an Orbital Relapse of Diffuse Large B-Cell Lymphoma

R. Palmieri, F. Esposito, F. Meconi, V. M. Rapisarda, L. Anemona, G. Paterno, S. Vaccarini, D. Nasso, L. Pupo, and M. Cantonetti

Fondazione Policlinico Tor Vergata, Dipartimento di Biomedicina e Prevenzione, Rome, Italy

Correspondence should be addressed to R. Palmieri; raffaele.f.palmieri@gmail.com

Academic Editor: Vincent Ribrag

A 74-year-old male with diffuse large B-cell lymphoma, with an Ann Arbor stage IV-A, was submitted to immune-chemotherapy in 2014, with complete remission of the disease. Two years later, he presented with a left eye swelling leading to exophthalmos and blurred vision. A core biopsy was performed and revealed a local relapse of the disease. He was considered unfit for intensive salvage chemotherapy and was treated with a combination of rituximab and lenalidomide. After six courses of rituximab plus lenalidomide, the patient showed complete remission and was submitted to maintenance therapy with lenalidomide. After 24 months since the start of lenalidomide monotherapy, we did not observe any progression. In this experience, rituximab plus lenalidomide, without radiotherapy, was a safe and effective therapeutic combination in an elderly patient with a localized relapse of DLBCL who was unfit to receive more aggressive therapies.

1. Background

Diffuse large B-cell lymphoma (DLBCL), with an annual incidence of 7-8 cases per 100,000 people per year, is the most common subtype of aggressive non-Hodgkin's lymphoma [1], and notwithstanding recent chemotherapeutic advances, disease relapse occurs in up to half of all patients [2].

The extranodal presentation to the head at the onset of the disease is very uncommon [3]. However, orbital lymphomas represent about 5–15% of extranodal lymphomas and approximately 50% of all primary malignant tumors of the orbit. The incidence of an isolated recurrence at the orbit remains unknown [4]. It usually occurs in elderly patients. It is characterized by a poor prognosis, and until now, it lacks standard therapy [5].

Multiple therapies targeting the biological pathways of B-cell lymphomas are under clinical evaluation. Among them, lenalidomide, an immunomodulatory agent with both tumoricidal and immunomodulatory effects, appears particularly promising. Its tumoricidal effects include inhibition of vascular endothelial growth factor-mediated microvessels formation, leading to cancer cells' cycle arrest and apoptosis [6]. Immunomodulatory effects of lenalidomide include inhibition of proinflammatory cytokines such as tumor necrosis factor α, increased the cytotoxicity of natural killer (NK) cells, inhibition of regulatory T cells, and increased anti-inflammatory cytokines [7–9]. The association of lenalidomide with the anti-CD20 monoclonal antibody rituximab has been studied in several trials, showing encouraging results [10, 11].

2. Case Presentation

A 74-year-old male presented to our department with a red, ulcerated plaque on the left arm with three months of duration. Recently, the lesion was rapidly increasing in size and started bleeding. Excisional biopsy was performed, and the material was sent for histopathological examination. Microscopic examination revealed diffuse infiltrates of large noncleaved cells, with large nuclei and conspicuous nucleoli. Immunohistochemical evaluation revealed the abnormal cells to be CD20+ Bcl6+ MUM1+ CD10−c-Myc− and CD3−. The proliferative index (Ki 67) was 90%. A diagnosis of

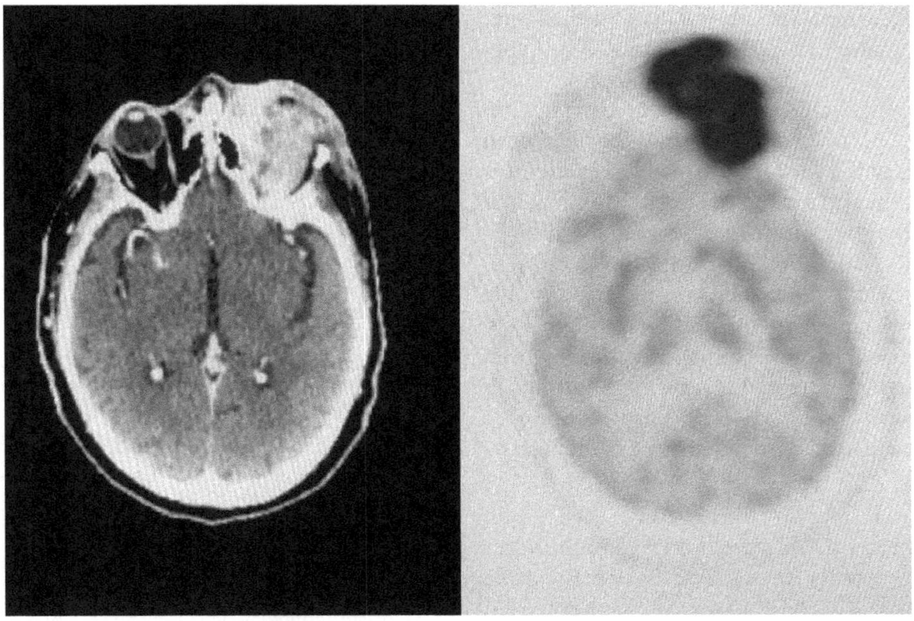

Figure 1: The FDG-PET/CT scan at relapse showed a huge tumor mass with high metabolic rate.

nongerminal center diffuse large B-cell non-Hodgkin's lymphoma (non-GCB DLBCL) was established. The bone marrow did not reveal any involvement of lymphoma. A fluorodeoxyglucose positron emission tomography (FDG-PET) was performed and it showed a diffuse involvement of mediastinal nodes.

The patient was subsequently started on systemic chemotherapy with rituximab combined with liposomal doxorubicin, cyclophosphamide, vincristine, and prednisone (R-COMP) for six cycles, followed by involved field radiotherapy on the arm. He well tolerated the therapy and obtained a complete remission.

Two years after the completion of therapy, the patient came to our observation with a left eye swelling leading to exophthalmos and blurred vision (Figure 1). A core biopsy was performed, and it revealed a disease with the same immunohistochemical panel of the diagnosis. Magnetic resonance imaging (MRI) showed a high-density process involving the left orbit and the surrounding soft tissues. An FDG-PET/Tc excluded any systemic involvement.

Bone marrow biopsy was not performed due to patient refusal.

At the time of the relapse, the patient was 76 years old and considered ineligible for high-dose second-line chemotherapy. Moreover, radiotherapy was not considered for the large extension of the disease because of the long-term side effects of rays on the patient's sight. In the absence of standardized therapy for these patients, we chose the combination of rituximab (375 mg/mq D1) plus lenalidomide (15 mg D1–21) every 28 days for 6 courses. At the end of the therapy, complete remission was confirmed by MRI and FDG-PET/CT scan evaluation (Figure 2).

After remission, lenalidomide (15 mg D1–21, every 28 days) monotherapy maintenance was started and planned to be continued until progression or unacceptable toxicity. After 24 months since the start of lenalidomide monotherapy, the patient is still in complete remission with an excellent quality of life.

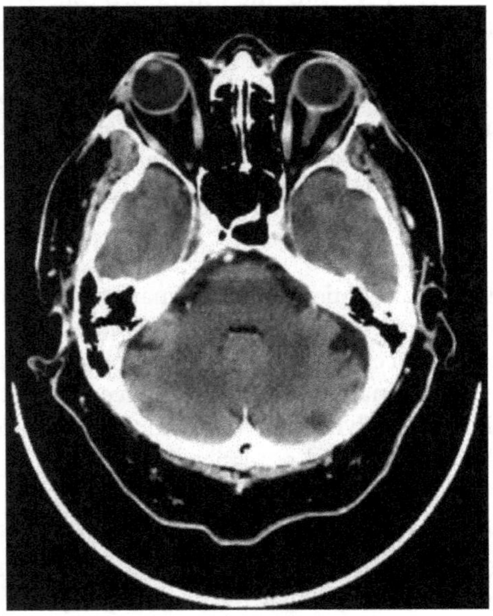

Figure 2: The CT scan performed after the end of the salvage therapy showed complete remission of the disease.

3. Discussion and Conclusions

Diffuse large B-cell lymphoma is the most common subtype of non-Hodgkin's lymphoma, accounting for approximately 30% of new cases. Despite the high rate of response to first-line standard chemotherapy R-CHOP, 30–40% of patients are refractory or relapse. High-dose chemotherapy followed by autologous stem cell transplant is considered a good option in relapsed/refractory young fit patients, with rates of overall survival at 4 years up to 60% [12]. Nevertheless, for patients not eligible for intensive salvage therapy, including most >70 years of age, front-line represents almost always the only chance for a cure, especially in non-GCB subtypes [13].

In our case, a 77-year-old patient presented with a relapsed non-GCB DLCBL involving the orbit. Long and even short-term prognosis of this localization in elderly patients is considered unfavorable, and we do not have a recommended therapy yet. Our patient was not eligible for standard high-dose chemotherapy, and radiotherapy was considered palliative. We decided to use the association of lenalidomide and rituximab as a manageable and well-tolerated therapy [14]. The efficacy of lenalidomide monotherapy has been investigated in heavily-pretreated DLBCL, resulting in higher overall response rate and longer progression-free survival as compared to standard intensive chemotherapy [15].

Furthermore, as recently observed in large multicenter randomized trials, a positive trend favoring lenalidomide plus R-CHOP versus R-CHOP alone was observed in previously untreated high-risk DLBCL [16]. Moreover, this drug association has also been tested in refractory/relapsed aggressive NHL involving the central nervous system and the ocular district, recording promising results [17]. Of note, the incidence of grade 3-4 toxicities was found remarkably higher among patients treated with standard chemotherapy as compared to those treated with lenalidomide plus rituximab [18], encouraging the use of this drug association for patients considered unsuitable for intensive treatment.

Finally, lenalidomide as maintenance therapy, meaningfully improved the outcome of patients with DLBCL if compared to placebo. Intriguing, the progression-free survival benefit of lenalidomide maintenance was equally important in patients who achieved complete remission as in those achieving a partial remission [19].

Therefore, our case report shows that the association of lenalidomide plus rituximab could be an option in the treatment of isolated orbital relapse of systemic non-GCB DLBCL. This strategy, improved by the following lenalidomide maintenance treatment, might be an attractive and well-tolerated therapeutic option in relapsed/refractory elderly patients who are unfit for intensive salvage chemotherapy.

Consent

Written informed consent was obtained from each patient for publication of this case report and accompanying images.

Acknowledgments

The authors thank Maria Stella Marchetti and L'Arcobaleno della Speranza Onlus.

References

[1] L. M. Morton, S. S. Wang, S. S. Devesa, P. Hartge, D. D. Weisenburger, and M. S. Linet, "Lymphoma incidence patterns by WHO subtype in the United States, 1992–2001," *Blood*, vol. 107, no. 1, pp. 265–276, 2006.

[2] P. Feugier, A. van Hoof, C. Sebban et al., "Long-term results of the R-CHOP study in the treatment of elderly patients with diffuse large B-cell lymphoma: a study by the groupe d'etude des lymphomes de l'adulte," *Journal of Clinical Oncology*, vol. 23, no. 18, pp. 4117–4126, 2005.

[3] R. Newton, J. Ferlay, V. Beral, and S. S. Devesa, "The epidemiology of non-Hodgkin's lymphoma: comparison of nodal and extra-nodal sites," *International Journal of Cancer*, vol. 72, no. 6, pp. 923–930, 1997.

[4] C. E. Margo and Z. D. Mulla, "Malignant tumors of the orbit," *Ophthalmology*, vol. 105, no. 1, pp. 185–190, 1998.

[5] R. C. Stacy, F. A. Jakobiec, M. C. Herwig, L. Schoenfield, A. Singh, and H. E. Grossniklaus, "Diffuse large B-cell lymphoma of the orbit: clinicopathologic, immunohistochemical, and prognostic features of 20 cases," *American Journal of Ophthalmology*, vol. 154, no. 1, pp. 87–98.e1, 2012.

[6] L. Lu, F. Payvandi, L. Wu et al., "The anti-cancer drug lenalidomide inhibits angiogenesis and metastasis via multiple inhibitory effects on endothelial cell function in normoxic and hypoxic conditions," *Microvascular Research*, vol. 77, no. 2, pp. 78–86, 2009.

[7] L. G. Corral, P. A. Haslett, G. W. Muller et al., "Differential cytokine modulation and T cell activation by two distinct classes of thalidomide analogues that are potent inhibitors of TNF-alpha," *Journal of Immunology*, vol. 163, no. 1, pp. 380–386, 1999.

[8] C. Galustian, B. Meyer, M.-C. Labarthe et al., "The anti-cancer agents lenalidomide and pomalidomide inhibit the proliferation and function of T regulatory cells," *Cancer Immunology, Immunotherapy*, vol. 58, no. 7, pp. 1033–1045, 2009.

[9] A. K. Hsu, H. Quach, T. Tai et al., "The immunostimulatory effect of lenalidomide on NK-cell function is profoundly inhibited by concurrent dexamethasone therapy," *Blood*, vol. 117, no. 5, pp. 1605–1613, 2011.

[10] A. Chiappella, A. Tucci, A. Castellino et al., "Lenalidomide plus cyclophosphamide, doxorubicin, vincristine, prednisone and rituximab is safe and effective in untreated, elderly patients with diffuse large B-cell lymphoma: a phase I study by the Fondazione Italiana Linfomi," *Haematologica*, vol. 98, no. 11, pp. 1732–1738, 2013.

[11] G. S. Nowakowski, B. LaPlant, W. R. Macon et al., "Lenalidomide combined with R-CHOP overcomes negative prognostic impact of non-germinal center B-cell phenotype in newly diagnosed diffuse large B-cell lymphoma: a phase II study," *Journal of Clinical Oncology*, vol. 33, no. 3, pp. 251–257, 2015.

[12] S. P. Robinson, A. Boumendil, H. Finel et al., "Autologous stem cell transplantation for relapsed/refractory diffuse large B-cell lymphoma: efficacy in the rituximab era and comparison to first allogeneic transplants. A report from the EBMT lymphoma working party," *Bone Marrow Transplantation*, vol. 51, no. 3, pp. 365–371, 2016.

[13] V. A. Morrison, P. Hamlin, P. Soubeyran et al., "Approach to therapy of diffuse large B-cell lymphoma in the elderly: the international society of geriatric oncology (SIOG) expert position commentary," *Annals of Oncology*, vol. 26, no. 6, pp. 1058–1068, 2015.

[14] P. L. Zinzani, C. Pellegrini, L. Gandolfi et al., "Combination of lenalidomide and rituximab in elderly patients with relapsed or refractory diffuse large B-cell lymphoma: a phase 2 trial," *Clinical Lymphoma Myeloma and Leukemia*, vol. 11, no. 6, pp. 462–466, 2011.

[15] M. S. Czuczman, M. Trněný, A. Davies et al., "A phase 2/3 multicenter, randomized, open-label study to compare the efficacy and safety of lenalidomide versus investigator's choice in patients with relapsed or refractory diffuse large B-cell lymphoma," *Clinical Cancer Research*, vol. 23, no. 15, pp. 4127–4137, 2017.

[16] U. Vitolo, T. E. Witzig, R. D. Gascoyne et al., "ROBUST: first report of phase III randomized study of lenalidomide/R-CHOP (R^2-CHOP) vs placebo/R-CHOP in previously untreated ABC-type diffuse large B-cell lymphoma," *Hematological Oncology*, vol. 37, no. 2, pp. 36-37, 2019.

[17] H. Ghesquieres, M. Chevrier, M. Laadhari et al., "Lenalidomide in combination with intravenous rituximab (REVRI) in relapsed/refractory primary CNS lymphoma or primary intraocular lymphoma: a multicenter prospective "proof of concept" phase II study of the French oculo-cerebral lymphoma (LOC) network and the lymphoma study association (LYSA)," *Annals of Oncology*, vol. 30, no. 4, pp. 621–628, 2019.

[18] F. Morschhauser, N. H. Fowler, P. Feugier et al., "Rituximab plus lenalidomide in advanced untreated follicular lymphoma," *New England Journal of Medicine*, vol. 379, no. 10, pp. 934–947, 2018.

[19] C. Thieblemont, H. Tilly, M. Gomes da Silva et al., "Lenalidomide maintenance compared with placebo in responding elderly patients with diffuse large B-cell lymphoma treated with first-line rituximab plus cyclophosphamide, doxorubicin, vincristine, and prednisone," *Journal of Clinical Oncology*, vol. 35, no. 22, pp. 2473–2481, 2017.

A Rare Presentation of HIV-Negative Plasmablastic Lymphoma: A Diagnostic Dilemma

Alaina J. Kessler,[1] Bridget K. Marcellino,[2] Scot A. Niglio,[2] Bruce E. Petersen,[3] and Adriana K. Malone[2]

[1]*Department of Medicine, Icahn School of Medicine at Mount Sinai, 1 Gustave L. Levy Place, New York, NY 10029, USA*
[2]*Tisch Cancer Institute, Icahn School of Medicine at Mount Sinai, New York, NY, USA*
[3]*Department of Pathology, Icahn School of Medicine at Mount Sinai, New York, NY, USA*

Correspondence should be addressed to Alaina J. Kessler; alaina.kessler@mountsinai.org

Academic Editor: Marie-Christine Kyrtsonis

Plasmablastic lymphoma (PBL) and plasmablastic plasma cell myeloma (PCM) have many overlapping characteristics. Clinical correlation can help make the distinction between the two entities. Human immunodeficiency virus- (HIV-) negative PBL is a rare disease, making the diagnosis more challenging. While there is no standard of care for PBL, current recommendations include dose-adjusted EPOCH (etoposide, vincristine, doxorubicin, cyclophosphamide, and prednisone), with or without bortezomib. We report an aggressive case of HIV-negative plasmablastic lymphoma and discuss the challenge in establishing a diagnosis. We review the literature regarding this disease and current recommendations for treatment.

1. Introduction

Plasmablastic lymphoma (PBL), a variant of diffuse large B-cell lymphoma (DLBCL), and plasmablastic plasma cell myeloma (PCM) have many overlapping features, often relying on clinical factors to make the distinction between the two entities. While the majority of cases of PBL are described in patients with human immunodeficiency virus (HIV), HIV-negative PBL is a rare disease associated with poor outcomes, making the diagnosis even more challenging [1]. The distinction between PBL and PCM is important to guide treatment. Although there is no current standard of care for PBL, the most recent literature recommends dose-adjusted EPOCH (etoposide, vincristine, doxorubicin, cyclophosphamide, and prednisone), with or without bortezomib, as first-line therapy [2]. Stem cell transplant (SCT) should be considered for chemosensitive patients [2]. This case highlights an aggressive presentation of a rare entity, HIV-negative PBL, and the challenges of diagnosis and treatment.

2. Case Presentation

An 81-year-old male with a history of heart failure with reduced ejection fraction, coronary artery disease with a history of coronary artery bypass grafting, atrial fibrillation (on warfarin), chronic obstructive lung disease, and diabetes mellitus presented to the emergency department with worsening shortness of breath. Two weeks prior to presentation, he had experienced sharp left-sided abdominal pain, which resolved without intervention. Approximately one week prior to presentation, he reported increased dyspnea and orthopnea, which remained present on admission. Additionally, he reported numerous episodes of spontaneous epistaxis for the past week.

On presentation to the emergency department, he was afebrile but tachycardic, tachypneic, and hypoxic to 83% on room air. No neurologic deficits were noted. Initial laboratory examination showed a white blood cell count of 21,500 cells/mm^3 (reference range 4,500–11,000 cells/mm^3) with 5% atypical lymphocytes, 22% band cells, 5%

metamyelocytes, 2% myelocytes, a hemoglobin of 12.1 g/dL (reference range 13.9–16.3 g/dL), and a platelet count of 42,000/μL (reference range 150,000–450,000/μL). The INR was 4.4, PT was 40.9 seconds (reference range 12.3–14.0 seconds), and APTT was 46.3 seconds (reference range 25.4–34.9 seconds). Chemistries were notable for a creatinine of 3.4 mg/dL (baseline 1.5 mg/dL), total protein 6.5 g/dL (reference range 6.0–8.3 g/dL), albumin 3.2 g/dL (reference range 3.5–4.9 g/dL), AST 310 U/L (reference range 1–35 U/L), ALT 22 U/L (reference range 1–45 U/L), uric acid > 30 mg/dL (reference range 4.0–9.0 mg/dL), and lactate dehydrogenase (LDH) 12,851 U/L (reference range 100–220 U/L). Calcium was within normal limits. Serum free light chain analysis demonstrated elevated free kappa 13,889 mg/L (reference range 3.3–19.4 mg/L) with a kappa/lambda ratio of 491.5 (reference range 0.26–1.65). M-spike was 0.00 g/dL. Testing for HIV was negative. Epstein–Barr virus (EBV) testing was consistent with prior exposure, with EBV IgM negative and IgG positive. Computerized tomography (CT) of the chest, abdomen, and pelvis without contrast showed extensive mediastinal and hilar lymphadenopathy (measuring up to 2 cm), which had increased in size and extent since imaging six months prior which was obtained as routine follow-up for a left lung nodule; no lytic lesions of the bone were identified. He was initiated on dialysis in the setting of worsening renal failure and subsequently intubated for hypoxemic respiratory failure. Bronchoscopy revealed diffuse alveolar hemorrhage.

Peripheral blood flow cytometry showed an aberrant kappa-restricted monotypic plasmacytoid population comprising 7-8% of total (CD138+, CD38 bright+, cytoplasmic kappa+, CD19−, CD56 dim+, CD45+, CD20−, and CD22−). Bone marrow biopsy (Figure 1) showed a hypercellular marrow (60–70%), with an infiltrate of markedly pleomorphic kappa-restricted monotypic plasmacytoid cells, many with immature features, comprising approximately 50% of overall cellularity (CD138+, kappa+, lambda−, CD117 focal+, CD56−, CD20−, and TdT−, by immunohistochemistry). *In situ* hybridization study for EBV-encoded RNA (EBER) was negative; however, sensitivity may have been limited due to decalcification. Flow cytometry showed an immunophenotype similar to that of the peripheral blood specimen.

Cytogenetic analysis demonstrated 100% of cells with a complex karyotype consisting of a jumping 1q translocation between *t*(1;3), *t*(1;11), and *t*(1;12) resulting in gains of 1q; a balanced translocation between the long arm of chromosomes 8 and 14, associated with MYC-IGH fusion; interstitial deletions of chromosomes 4*p* and 4*q*; gains/partial gains of chromosomes 7 and 12, and a derivative chromosome 21 as a result of an unbalanced translocation *t*(13; 21) resulting in three copies of 13q. FISH analysis showed 43% of cells with MYC-IGH [*t*(8;14)] fusion.

The differential diagnosis included plasmablastic lymphoma (PBL) and plasmablastic plasma cell myeloma (PCM). The favored diagnosis of PBL was largely based on clinical factors, including the highly aggressive presentation, lymphadenopathy both above and below the diaphragm, and absence of lytic lesions.

Due to advanced age, comorbidities, and impaired renal function, the decision was made to treat with dose-adjusted V-EPOCH (bortezomib, etoposide, dexamethasone, vincristine, cyclophosphamide, and doxorubicin) with the plan for 50% dose reduction of etoposide, doxorubicin, and vincristine and 25% dose reduction of cyclophosphamide on account of the patient being in acute renal failure. The patient received bortezomib (1.3 mg/m^2 on day 1), doxorubicin (5 mg/m^2 on days 1 and 2), etoposide (25 mg/m^2 on days 1 and 2), and vincristine (0.2 mg/m^2 on days 1 and 2). After two days of chemotherapy, he was noted to have unequal pupillary size. Magnetic resonance imaging (MRI) of the brain revealed watershed temporal lobe infarctions, and further chemotherapy was held. Based on his family's wishes, the patient was transitioned to comfort care measures and transferred to the palliative care unit. He was palliatively extubated and died 12 hours later.

3. Discussion

The case presented here exemplifies the difficulty of distinguishing between PBL, a variant of diffuse large B-cell lymphoma (DLBCL), and PCM with extramedullary involvement. Distinguishing between the two can be difficult as the two entities have many overlapping characteristics. It is imperative however to make this diagnostic distinction because the two entities are treated differently.

PBL and PCM have similar morphological and immunophenotypic features but subtle histological differences have been noted by Vega et al. [3]. PBL typically demonstrates a proliferation of plasmablasts and immunoblasts with rare cells showing mature plasmacytic differentiation. In contrast, cells with plasmacytic differentiation are typically more numerous in PCM. The two entities also have similar immunophenotypic profiles with both expressing plasma cell markers, such as CD38, CD138, and MUM1, without classic B-cell markers, such as CD19, CD20, and PAX-5 [3]. Monotypic light chain expression has been demonstrated in both PBL and PCM [3]. Complex karyotypes have also been shown to be associated with both entities [4]. Rearrangements in MYC, an oncogene originally described in Burkitt lymphoma, have been associated with both tumor progression in multiple myeloma as well as plasmablastic lymphoma [1, 4]. Despite these similar features, genomic profiling suggests PBL may be more closely related to DLBCL based on segmental gains such as 16p13.3 frequently seen in both diseases. [5].

Due to the overlapping pathologic features of PBL and PCM, clinical correlation is nearly always required to make the distinction between these two entities. PBL is highly associated with viral reactive lymphadenopathies such as HIV and EBV [3, 6, 7]. EBV positivity is detected more frequently in HIV-positive patients (75%) and posttransplant PBL (67%) compared to PBL in immunocompetent patients (50%) [1]. This patient was HIV-negative, and presence or absence of EBV could not be firmly established. While some criteria for multiple myeloma were present including anemia, renal insufficiency, and elevated free light-chain ratio, the patient lacked the presence of lytic lesions

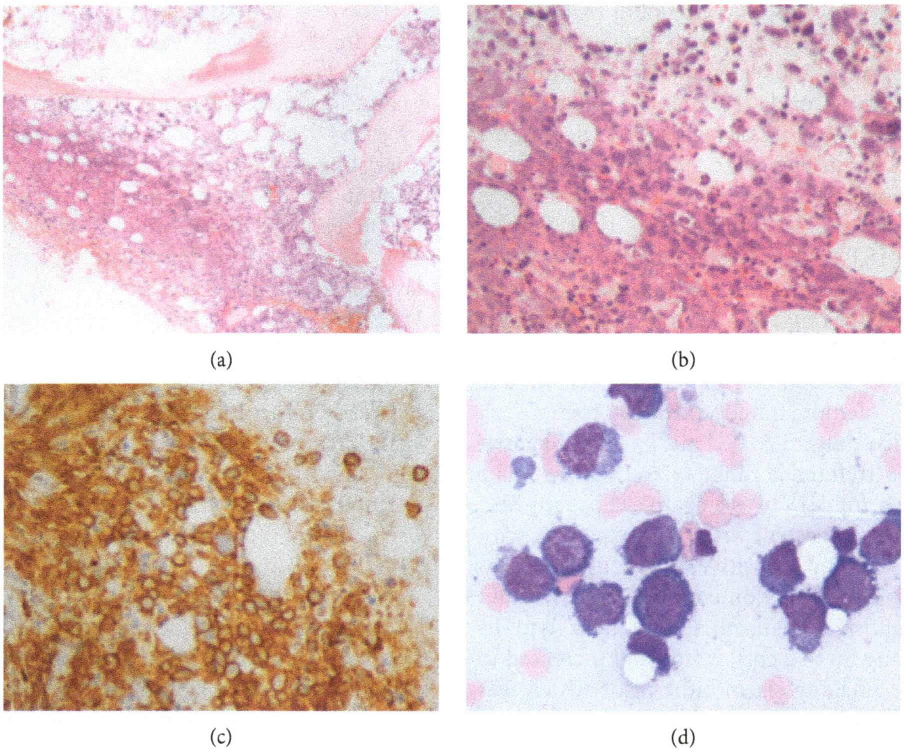

FIGURE 1: (a, b) Bone marrow biopsy with extensive infiltration by atypical plasmacytoid cells (original magnifications: ×100; ×400). (c) The cells are positive for CD138 by immunohistochemistry, indicative of plasma cell differentiation (original magnification: ×400). (d) Atypical plasmacytoid cells, including forms with plasmablastic morphology, as visualized on bone marrow aspirate smear (original magnification: ×1000).

and hypercalcemia that would have favored a diagnosis of multiple myeloma [8]. Ultimately, the diagnosis of PBL was favored over PCM due to the aggressive presentation associated with diffuse lymphadenopathy, elevated LDH, and hyperuricemia.

Although the actual incidence of HIV-negative PBL is unknown, the limited numbers of published cases suggest it is a rare entity. The largest case review from 1997 to 2014 revealed only 164 cases of HIV-negative PBL [2]. HIV-negative PBL is a male-predominant malignancy with a median age of 55 years [2]. The majority (75%) of patients with HIV-negative PBL are immunocompetent although PBL has been associated with lymphoproliferative and autoimmune disorders [9]. PBL has also been identified after solid organ transplantation [9]. A review of 76 patients with HIV-negative PBL showed the majority (89%) of patients presented with extranodal involvement, including disease in the oral cavity (21%), gastrointestinal tract (20%), soft tissue (17%), and bone marrow (15%) [9]. Poor prognostic factors include immunosuppression, Ann Arbor stage IV, EBV negativity, disease refractory to treatment, and C-MYC aberrations [1, 10]. Median overall survival of immunocompetent patients with PBL ranged from 11 to 19 months [1, 10].

While plasmablastic plasma cell myeloma is initially treated with VRd (bortezomib, lenalidomide, and dexamethasone), there is no standard of care for PBL [2, 11]. Given the poor outcomes and lack of response to commonly used chemotherapy such as CHOP (cyclophosphamide, doxorubicin, vincristine, and prednisone) and CHOP-like regimens, the National Comprehensive Cancer Network (NCCN) guidelines state that standard CHOP is not adequate treatment [12]. The NCCN recommends dose-adjusted EPOCH (etoposide, vincristine, doxorubicin, cyclophosphamide, and prednisone), CODOX-M/IVAC (cyclophosphamide, vincristine, doxorubicin, methotrexate alternating with ifosfamide, etoposide, and cytarabine), or Hyper-CVAD (hyperfractionated cyclophosphamide, vincristine, doxorubicin, and dexamethasone alternating with methotrexate and cytarabine).

Recent studies have focused on new therapeutic approaches, specifically the use of bortezomib, a proteasome inhibitor approved for the treatment of multiple myeloma and mantle cell lymphoma. There are limited case reports using bortezomib in patients with HIV-negative PBL. A recent review of the literature through March 2017 by Guerrero-Garcia et al. [13] identified 21 patients, ten of which (48%) were HIV-negative PBL. All had extranodal involvement. Of these ten patients, three (30%) patients achieved complete response and seven (70%) patients had partial response. Also of note in the frontline setting, the three patients (60%) who achieved complete response had received bortezomib as part of CYBORD (cyclophosphamide, bortezomib, and dexamethasone) or in combination with EPOCH. A recently published case report of PBL involving the right parotid gland in a HIV-negative patient showed continuous complete remission at 12 months using bortezomib plus lenalidomide upon relapse after CHOP [14]. Another case report of HIV-negative PBL utilizing a lenalidomide-based regimen with complete remission at 24 months suggests its usage as an alternative therapy for patients unable to tolerate intensive chemotherapy [8].

Stem cell transplant (SCT) should be considered for chemosensitive patients. A small case series of nine patients with HIV-negative PBL in which all were treated with CHOP or hyper-CVAD showed that seven patients achieved complete response and one patient achieved a partial response. [15] Three of the seven patients who achieved complete response and one patient who achieved partial response underwent consolidation with high-dose chemotherapy and autologous hematopoietic SCT. Of these four patients, two had no evidence of disease at 24 months. Although a small case series, these findings suggest that SCT can obtain durable and prolonged responses. The suggested treatment by Castillo et al. [2] is six cycles of infusional dose-adjusted EPOCH, with or without bortezomib, accompanied by intrathecal prophylaxis with each cycle of EPOCH as first-line therapy. For appropriate candidates, those authors also recommend consolidative high-dose chemotherapy followed by autologous SCT for patients in first remission. In patients who are chemorefractory in whom autologous SCT is not feasible, there is a single case report of an allogeneic SCT with cord blood transplantation achieving durable remission [16]. Recent data show SLAMF2 (CD319/CS1), targetable by elotuzumab, is expressed in PBL and has been proposed as a potential therapeutic target [17].

In conclusion, this case highlights an aggressive presentation of a rare entity, HIV-negative PBL, and discusses the clinical dilemma arriving at the diagnosis. As with this case, clinical correlation is frequently required to make the diagnosis. The distinction between these two entities is important for guiding treatment.

References

[1] J. Morscio, D. Dierickx, J. Nijs et al., "Clinicopathologic comparison of plasmablastic lymphoma in HIV-positive, immunocompetent, and posttransplant patients," *The American Journal of Surgical Pathology*, vol. 38, no. 7, pp. 875–886, 2014.

[2] J. J. Castillo, M. Bibas, and R. N. Miranda, "The biology and treatment of plasmablastic lymphoma," *Blood*, vol. 125, no. 15, pp. 2323–2330, 2015.

[3] F. Vega, C.-C. Chang, L. J. Medeiros et al., "Plasmablastic lymphomas and plasmablastic plasma cell myelomas have nearly identical immunophenotypic profiles," *Modern Pathology*, vol. 18, no. 6, pp. 806–815, 2004.

[4] L. Taddesse-Heath, A. Meloni-Ehrig, J. Scheerle, J. C. Kelly, and E. S. Jaffe, "Plasmablastic lymphoma with MYC translocation: evidence for a common pathway in the generation of plasmablastic features," *Modern Pathology*, vol. 23, no. 7, pp. 991–999, 2010.

[5] C.-C. Chang, X. Zhou, J. J. Taylor et al., "Genomic profiling of plasmablastic lymphoma using array comparative genomic hybridization (aCGH): revealing significant overlapping genomic lesions with diffuse large B-cell lymphoma," *Journal of Hematology and Oncology*, vol. 2, no. 1, p. 47, 2009.

[6] A. Carbone, E. Cesarman, M. Spina, A. Gloghini, and T. F. Schulz, "HIV-associated lymphomas and gamma-herpesviruses," *Blood*, vol. 113, no. 6, pp. 1213–1224, 2009.

[7] S. Montes-Moreno, C. Montalbán, and M. A. Piris, "Large B-cell lymphomas with plasmablastic differentiation: a biological and therapeutic challenge," *Leukemia & Lymphoma*, vol. 53, no. 2, pp. 185–194, 2011.

[8] J. M. Schmit, J. DeLaune, M. Norkin, and A. Grosbach, "A case of plasmablastic lymphoma achieving complete response and durable remission after lenalidomide-based therapy," *Oncology Research and Treatment*, vol. 40, no. 1-2, pp. 46–48, 2017.

[9] J. J. Castillo, E. S. Winer, D. Stachurski et al., "HIV-negative plasmablastic lymphoma: not in the mouth," *Clinical Lymphoma Myeloma and Leukemia*, vol. 11, no. 2, pp. 185–189, 2011.

[10] M. Liu, B. Liu, B. Liu et al., "Human immunodeficiency virus-negative plasmablastic lymphoma: a comprehensive analysis of 114 cases," *Oncology Reports*, vol. 33, no. 4, pp. 1615–1620, 2015.

[11] S. Yadav, R. Kumar, I. A. Jaiyesimi et al., "Aggressive plasmablastic multiple myeloma in a 42-year-old: is inflammatory bowel disease or infliximab treatment to be blamed?," *BMJ Case Reports*, December 2018.

[12] National Comprehensive Cancer Network, "Non- Hodgkin's lymphomas (version 4.2014). NCCN guidelines website," November 2017, https://www.nccn.org/about/nhl.pdf.

[13] T. A. Guerrero-Garcia, R. J. Mogollon, and J. J. Castillo, "Bortezomib in plasmablastic lymphoma: a glimpse of hope for a hard-to-treat disease," *Leukemia Research*, vol. 62, pp. 12–16, 2017.

[14] W. D. Marrero, A. Cruz-Chacón, C. Castillo, and F. Cabanillas, "Successful use of bortezomib-lenalidomide combination as treatment for a patient with plasmablastic lymphoma," *Clinical Lymphoma Myeloma and Leukemia*, vol. 18, no. 7, pp. e275–e277, 2018.

[15] J. J. Liu, L. Zhang, E. Ayala et al., "Human immunodeficiency virus (HIV)-negative plasmablastic lymphoma: a single institutional experience and literature review," *Leukemia Research*, vol. 35, no. 12, pp. 1571–1577, 2011.

[16] K. Nishi, S. Mitani, K. Hatanaka, and K. Imada, "Successful cord blood transplantation for an HIV-negative patient with refractory plasmablastic lymphoma," *Annals of Hematology*, vol. 96, no. 6, pp. 1057-1058, 2017.

[17] J. Shi, J. Bodo, X. Zhao et al., "SLAMF7 (CD319/CS1) is expressed in plasmablastic lymphoma and is a potential diagnostic marker and therapeutic target," *British Journal of Haematology*, 2018.

34

A Rare Case of BCL2-Positive Multiple Myeloma Complicated with Follicular Lymphoma

Yutaka Tsutsumi,[1] Shinich Ito,[1] Mirei Kobayashi,[1] and Takanori Teshima[2]

[1]*Department of Hematology, Hakodate Municipal Hospital, 1-10-1, Minato-cho, Hakodate 041-8680, Japan*
[2]*Department of Hematology, Hokkaido University Graduate School of Medicine, Sapporo, Japan*

Correspondence should be addressed to Yutaka Tsutsumi; yutsutsu@shore.ocn.ne.jp

Academic Editor: Kiyotaka Kawauchi

A 68-year-old woman presented with follicular lymphoma complicated by IgG kappa-positive multiple myeloma. In this case, both follicular lymphoma and plasma cells were positive for BCL2 by immunostaining. T-cell association in the FL and MM was also analyzed in this case. Some CD3-positive T-cells were found around the plasma cells. These cells were mainly CD8-positive T-cells and not CD4-positive T-cells. These results suggest that CD4-positive T-cells were not associated with the proliferation of the plasma cells in this case. Although the FL that developed was initially positive for BCL2 protein, this does not indicate that plasma cells were derived from FL cells because of the eventual complication that occurred in this case. Furthermore, in this case, rituximab and bendamustine were effective for FL. They were not effective for MM, however, demonstrating that additional treatment options are necessary for the simultaneous treatment of BCL2-positive MM with FL.

1. Introduction

Reports of multiple myeloma (MM) merged with malignant lymphoma (ML) are rare [1–3], and reports of MM merged with follicular lymphoma (FL) are even rarer [4].

Here, we report a 68-year-old woman with follicular lymphoma complicated by IgG kappa-positive myeloma. It was reported that marginal zone lymphoma (MALT) is differentiated into plasma cells by reactive CD4 T-cells in MALT patients [5, 6].

In the present case, both follicular lymphoma and plasma cells were positive for BCL2 by immunostaining. On the other hand, CD4-positive T-cells were not associated with the proliferation of the plasma cells. Although the MM that developed was initially positive for BCL2 protein, this does not indicate that plasma cells were derived from FL cells because of the eventual complication that occurred in this case. In the treatment, although rituximab and bendamustine were effective for the FL, they had no effect on the MM. Other treatment options may be necessary for the simultaneous treatment of BCL2-positive MM with FL.

2. Case Presentation

A 68-year-old woman with cervical lymphadenopathy visited our hospital in September 2016. She was diagnosed with follicular lymphoma grade 1 by biopsy of cervical lymphadenopathy (Figures 1(a) and 1(b)). The fusion gene IgH-BCL2 was detected by polymerase chain reaction (PCR) in a bone marrow examination. These suggested the bone marrow invasion by FL and we determined the clinical stage was IV, but the patient was followed closely without chemotherapy due to no symptoms. Plasma cells were 6.4% of this bone marrow specimen. In 2021, an increase in soluble interleukin 2 receptors (sIL2R: 834 U/mL) and β2 microglobulin (β2MG: 3.54 mg/L) was observed. An enlarging swelling of lymph nodes was also observed by computed tomography (CT). The patient had a white blood cell (WBC) count of $4\times10^3/\mu L$, a red blood cell (RBC) count of $3.99\times10^6/\mu L$, a hemoglobin (Hb) level of 12.2 g/dl, a platelet count (PLT) of $7.4\times10^4/\mu L$, and lactate dehydrogenase (LDH) of 181 U/L at the time of the treatment. A bone marrow examination and immunoelectrophoresis,

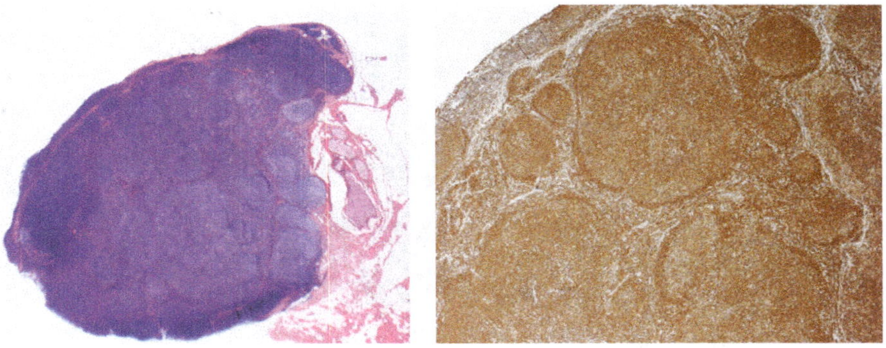

(a) (b)

Figure 1: (a) Lymph node specimen from this case; the nodular pattern was observed (×2). (b) Tumor cells were positive for BCL2 (×4).

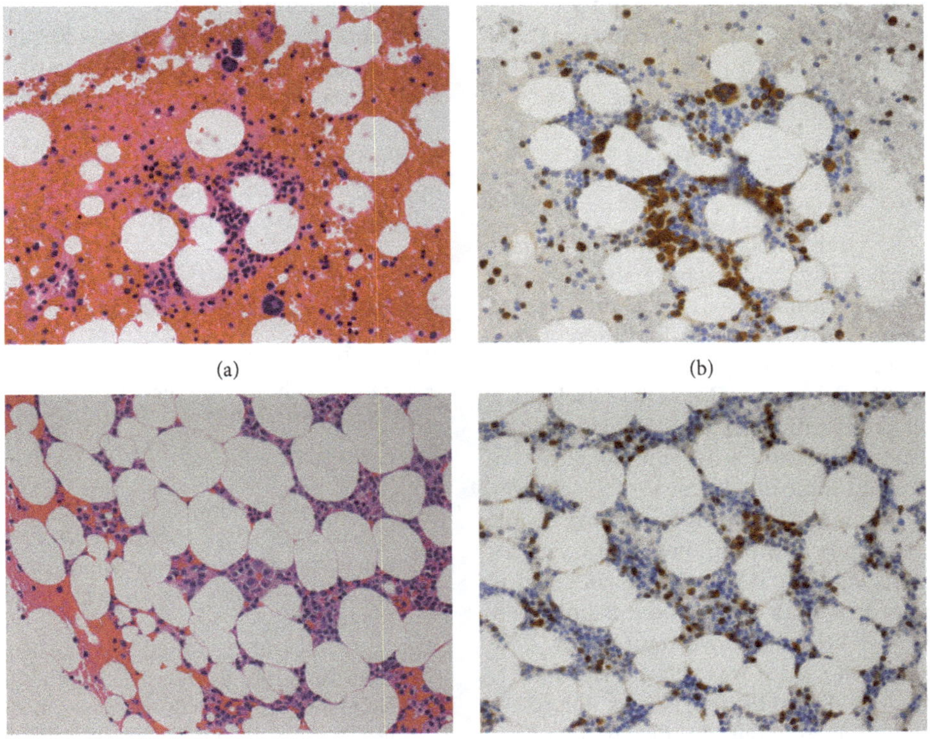

(a) (b)

(c) (d)

Figure 2: Bone marrow specimens in 2021: (a) atypical plasma cells with lymphocytes (×20). (b) Both lymphocytes and plasma cells are BCL2-positive (×20). Bone marrow specimens in 2016: (c) lymphocytes and plasma cells are observed (×20). (d) Plasma cells. Both cells and lymphocytes are BCL2-positive (×20).

therefore, were performed for reassessment. Immunoelectrophoresis was positive for immunoglobulin G-kappa (IgG-k), and the presence of neoplastic plasma cells was suspected. A bone marrow examination was performed to confirm IgH-BCL2 positivity. Furthermore, infiltration of B lymphocytes, nuclear enlargement, and 12.2% of multinucleated plasma cells were observed (Figure 2(a)). Serum calcium and creatine albumin levels were within normal limits, the osteolytic lesion was not visible in both CT and positron emission tomography (PET), and the free light chain (FLC) κ/λ ratio was 28.17 (501/17 mg/L). Although there were more dysplastic plasma cells, these results suggested the FL was complicated with smoldering MM (by IMWG criteria). These results showed that thrombocytopenia was due to FL in this case. Both lymphocytes and plasma cells were found to be BCL2-positive by immunostaining (Figure 2(b)). These observations indicated a follicular lymphoma complication with myeloma. The bone marrow specimen in 2016 was restained, and both lymphocytes and plasma cells were also found to be BCL2-positive (Figures 2(c) and 2(d)). In the bone marrow specimen from 2021, CD3-positive cells were observed around the plasma cells. These T-cells were mostly CD8-positive T-cells, wherein CD4-positive cells did not increase in number (Figures 3(a)–3(c)).

For the present case, rituximab at 375 mg/m^2 (day 1) and bendamustine at 90 mg/m^2 (days 2, 3) were administered in four courses for follicular lymphoma. After partial remission, rituximab maintenance therapy was performed once

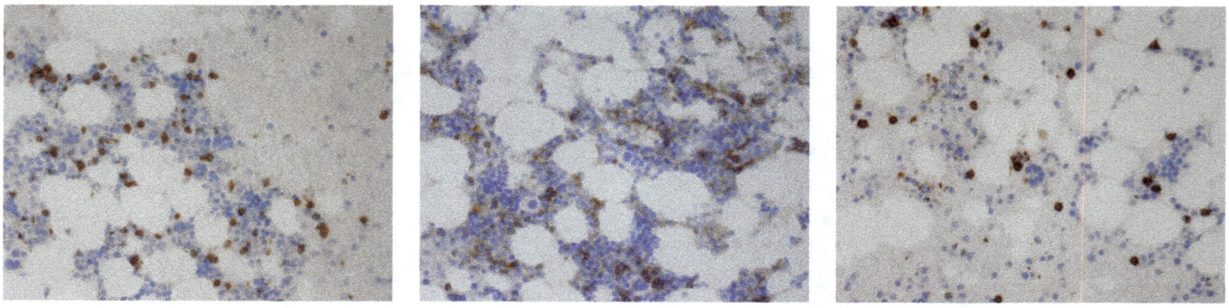

(a) (b) (c)

FIGURE 3: Bone marrow specimens in 2021: (a) CD3-positive T-cells around the myeloma cells (×40). (b) CD4-positive T-cells around the myeloma cells did not increase in number (×40). (c) CD8-positive T-cells around the myeloma cells (×40).

every 2-3 months. However, IgG remained around 3000 mg/dL, the FLC κ/λ ratio was 24.95 (297/11.9 mg/L), plasma cells were 16.0% after treatment, and no therapeutic effect of rituximab and bendamustine for smoldering MM was observed.

3. Discussion

Multiple myeloma is rarely associated with malignant lymphoma, and MALT, AITL, and FL have also been reported as associated with lymphoma [1–4]. Among these lymphomas, it has been reported that MALT is differentiated into plasma cells by reactive CD4 T-cells [5, 6]. In cases where AITL is complicated with MM, AITL itself may promote plasma cell proliferation [7–13]. In these reports [7–13], the proliferation of plasma cells with clonality was observed in five cases, and some involvement of T-cells was suspected, as in the case of MALT mentioned above [5, 6]. On the other hand, only one case of FL has been reported. The reason for the merging with MM is unknown; i.e., it is unknown whether it is derived from FL, and it is unknown whether activated CD4 T-cells were involved [4].

Likewise, in the present case, it was determined that FL was associated with MM from the beginning, but CD4 T-cells were not particularly abundant around plasma cells and B lymphocytes in the analysis of pathological specimens. Therefore, the involvement of CD4 T-cells in plasma cell proliferation and tumorigenesis is unknown.

On the other hand, both follicular lymphoma and plasma cells were positive for BCL2 by immunostaining. Puthier et al. reported high expression of BCL2 in slowly proliferating MM cells [14]. Zeng et al. reported that 43–75% of myeloma cells were BCL2-positive [15]. Thus, these reports show that although the FL that developed was initially positive for the BCL2 protein, the plasma cells were not derived from FL cells in this case.

As previously reported, rituximab and bendamustine were effective for FL. They were not effective for MM, however, demonstrating that MM requires a separate treatment. On basis of the positivity for the BCL2 protein, venetoclax could be one of the treatments options for this case. The effectiveness of venetoclax, however, was limited in the treatment of follicular lymphoma [16, 17]. In a report of FL complicated with MM, rituximab and bendamustine were administered for the treatment of FL, followed by lenalidomide and dexamethasone for the treatment of MM [4]. Although the BCL2 protein was not analyzed, lenalidomide was a useful treatment option for both FL and MM [17].

Further cases need to be examined to clarify treatment options for FL complicated with MM, where both tumor cells are positive for the BCL2 protein.

Authors' Contributions

Shinich Ito, Mirei Kobayashi, and Takanori Teshima contributed equally to this report.

References

[1] W. Caceres-Perkins, F. Cabanillas, G. San Vicente et al., "Gastric MALT lymphoma with biclonal gammopathy and bone marrow involvement mimicking multiple myeloma," *Puerto Rico Health Sciences Journal*, vol. 39, no. 3, pp. 275–277, 2020.

[2] G. E. Silva, R. S. Costa, F. Chahud et al., "Membranous glomerulonephritis associated with splenic marginal zone lymphoma mimicking multiple myeloma," *Clinical Nephrology*, vol. 79, no. 06, pp. 488–492, 2013.

[3] J. Xu, Y. Tang, S. Zhao et al., "Angioimmunoblastic T cell lymphoma with coexisting plasma cell myeloma: a case report and review of the literature," *Tohoku Journal of Experimental Medicine*, vol. 235, no. 4, pp. 283–288, 2015.

[4] M. Saito, K. Miyashita, Y. Miura et al., "Coexistence of primary colorectal follicular lymphoma and multiple myeloma: a case report," *International Journal of General Medicine*, vol. 11, pp. 363–367, 2018.

[5] C. E. Sever, J. R. Krause, and S. S. Kaplan, "Splenic lymphoma with circulating villous lymphocytes simulating plasma cell leukemia," *American Journal of Hematology*, vol. 42, no. 4, pp. 411-412, 1993.

[6] T. Bonnefoix, J. Q. Mi, P. Perron et al., "Terminal plasmocytoid differentiation of malignant B cells induced by autotumor-reactive CD4 (+) T cells in one case of splenic marginal zone B-cell lymphoma," *Blood*, vol. 99, no. 1, pp. 388–390, 2002.

[7] A. Yamane, N. Awaya, T. Shimizu, Y. Ikeda, and S. I. Okamoto, "Angioimmunoblastic T-cell lymphoma with

polyclonal proliferation of plasma cells in peripheral blood and marrow," *Acta Haematologica*, vol. 117, no. 2, pp. 74–77, 2007.

[8] H. Sakai, H. Tanaka, T. Katsurada, Y. Yoshida, E. Okamoto, and H. Ohno, "Angioimmunoblastic T-cell lymphoma initially presenting with replacement of bone marrow and peripheral plasmacytosis," *Internal Medicine*, vol. 46, no. 7, pp. 419–424, 2007.

[9] A. N. Ahsanuddin, R. K. Brynes, and S. Li, "Peripheral blood polyclonal plasmacytosis mimicking plasma cell leukemia in patients with angioimmunoblastic T-cell lymphoma: report of 3 cases and review of the literature," *International Journal of Clinical and Experimental Pathology*, vol. 4, pp. 416–420, 2011.

[10] H. Nagoshi, J. Kuroda, T. Kobayashi et al., "Clinical manifestation of angioimmunoblastic T-cell lymphoma with exuberant plasmacytosis," *International Journal of Hematology*, vol. 98, no. 3, pp. 366–374, 2013.

[11] O. Balagué, A. Martínez, L. Colomo et al., "Epstein-barr virus negative clonal plasma cell proliferations and lymphomas in peripheral T-cell lymphomas: a phenomenon with distinctive clinicopathologic features," *The American Journal of Surgical Pathology*, vol. 31, no. 9, pp. 1310–1322, 2007.

[12] A. R. Huppmann, M. R. Roullet, M. Raffeld, and E. S. Jaffe, "Angioimmunoblastic T-cell lymphoma partially obscured by an epstein-barr virus-negative clonal plasma cell proliferation," *Journal of Clinical Oncology*, vol. 31, no. 2, pp. e28–e30, 2013.

[13] A. Zettl, S. S. Lee, T. Rüdiger et al., "Epstein-barr virus–associated B-cell lymphoproliferative disorders in angioimmunoblastic T-cell lymphoma and peripheral T-cell lymphoma, unspecified," *American Journal of Clinical Pathology*, vol. 117, no. 3, pp. 368–379, 2002.

[14] D. Puthier, C. Pellat-Deceunynck, S. Barillé et al., "Differential expression of Bcl-2 in human plasma cell disorders according to proliferation status and malignancy," *Leukemia*, vol. 13, no. 2, pp. 289–294, 1999.

[15] W. Zeng, F. Meng, Z. Liu et al., "Bortezomib-based chemotherapy regimens can improve response in newly diagnosed multiple myeloma patients with bcl-2 and survivin overexpression," *International Journal of Clinical and Experimental Pathology*, vol. 7, no. 7, pp. 4239–4246, 2014.

[16] L. J. Costa, F. E. Davies, G. P. Monohan et al., "Phase 2 study of venetoclax plus carfilzomib and dexamethasone in patients with relapsed/refractory multiple myeloma," *Blood Advances*, vol. 5, no. 19, pp. 3748–3759, 2021.

[17] A. Freedman and E. Jacobsen, "Follicular lymphoma: 2020 update on diagnosis and management," *American Journal of Hematology*, vol. 95, no. 3, pp. 316–327, 2020.

35

Fatal Idiopathic Hyperammonemia after Induction Chemotherapy for Acute Myeloid Leukemia

Christophe Angelo,[1] Marie-Françoise Vincent,[2] Mina Komuta,[3] Philippe Hantson,[1,4] Nicole Straetmans,[5] and Edwige Boulet[5]

[1]*Department of Intensive Care, Cliniques St-Luc, Université Catholique de Louvain, 1200 Brussels, Belgium*
[2]*Department of Clinical Chemistry, Cliniques St-Luc, Université Catholique de Louvain, 1200 Brussels, Belgium*
[3]*Department of Pathology, Cliniques St-Luc, Université Catholique de Louvain, 1200 Brussels, Belgium*
[4]*Louvain Centre of Toxicology and Applied Pharmacology, Université Catholique de Louvain, 1200 Brussels, Belgium*
[5]*Department of Hematology, Cliniques St-Luc, Université Catholique de Louvain, 1200 Brussels, Belgium*

Correspondence should be addressed to Philippe Hantson; philippe.hantson@uclouvain.be

Academic Editor: Vincent Ribrag

Idiopathic hyperammonemia is a rare but potentially fatal complication occurring in patients with acute leukemia or bone marrow transplantation. The role of some specific anticancer drugs may be discussed, but the etiology of hyperammonemia is often multifactorial. We report the case of a 40-year-old woman who developed fatal idiopathic hyperammonemia two weeks after induction chemotherapy with idarubicin-aracytine for acute myeloid leukemia. Despite intensive care management and extrarenal epuration, the patient was declared brain dead two days after hyperammonemia onset.

1. Introduction

Idiopathic hyperammonemia (IHA) has been described for the first time in the 1980's after induction chemotherapy for acute leukemia [1]. It has also been occasionally reported in patients receiving bone marrow transplantation or suffering from multiple myeloma [2–4]. This complication occurs often with some delay after the start of chemotherapy, in the absence of underlying liver disease. Among the medications possibly associated with IHA, cytarabine has been frequently cited [1, 5]. As in the here reported observation, the role of other precipitating factors may also be debated. The possible involvement of parenteral nutrition or intestinal microbial proliferation is discussed.

2. Case Presentation

A 40-year-old woman without previous medical history was admitted to the Haematology Department for progressive fatigue and grade 2-3 dyspnoea which appeared one month before. The physical examination found a patient in a good general condition, but with extreme pallor. Laboratory investigations revealed hemoglobin 5.8 g/dl, white blood cell count 6040/mm^3 with 36% blasts, and platelet count 58,000/mm^3. Liver function tests were normal. The diagnosis of acute myeloid leukemia (AML) with inv(16)(p13.1q22), CBF-MYH11 (FISH analysis) was obtained. The induction chemotherapy included idarubicin 12 mg/m^2 (days 1–3) and aracytine 200 mg/m^2 (days 1–7). The diagnosis of acute myeloid leukemia (AML) with inv(16)(p13.1q22), CBF-MYH11 (FISH analysis) was obtained. On day 6, after the initiation of chemotherapy, the patient developed neutropenic fever and empiric treatment with piperacillin/tazobactam was started. She developed cytarabine-induced skin lesions and diffuse pancolitis with ascites. This was confirmed by the findings of the contrast-enhanced abdomen computed tomography (CT) that showed a major oedematous involvement of the caecal mucosa (22 mm) and of the right colonic mucosa; there was also a diffuse distension (3 cm diameter) of the small intestine with a thickening of the last loops (Figure 1). Due to this abdominal complication, parenteral nutrition (Aminomix Novum 3, Fresenius, 1500 ml/day, corresponding to 12 gN) was begun on day 10. The patient was transferred to the intensive care unit (ICU) on day 13 for tachycardia, hypotension, and respiratory distress. The abdomen was distended with absence of bowel sounds. The patient was conscious and oriented, and neurological testing was normal. Chest-X-ray examination did not reveal pneumonia. Arterial blood gas analysis showed pH 7.30, pCO_2 32 mmHg, and bicarbonate 20 mmol/l. Serological testing for HBV and HCV antibodies was negative; CMV IgG were >500 U/l. Antimicrobial therapy was switched for ceftazidime and vancomycin after the identification of *Enterococcus faecium* in bronchoalveolar lavage and blood culture. Hemodynamics remained stable, without need of vasopressors, and repeated blood culture was sterile. Stool culture revealed Gram-positive flora, but no *Clostridium difficile* nor other pathogens, with the limitation that stool culture was not repeated. On day 16, there was an unexpected impairment of consciousness leading to intubation for coma progression. The plasma ammonia level was 688 μmol/l, with the other relevant laboratory investigations displayed in Table 1. Abdomen ultrasound examination excluded the presence of a portal-systemic shunt. The brain computed tomography did not demonstrate cerebral edema. The electroencephalogram confirmed severe slowing of electrical activity (delta waves, 4 Hz), but without triphasic waves. Analysis of serum amino acids revealed high levels of glutamine, low levels of citrulline, and normal levels of ornithine. There was an extremely high glutamine concentration (7976 μmol/l) into the cerebrospinal fluid (CSF). Parenteral nutrition was interrupted, without any possibility of enteral feeding. Continuous venovenous hemofiltration (CVVH) was started and completed by intermittent hemodialysis, without significant efficacy on ammonia clearance. The patient received also intravenous carnitine supplementation (100 mg/kg/d), lactulose intrarectally, and two doses of rifaximin 550 mg via the nasogastric tube. Coma persisted, with a Glasgow Coma Scale score at 3/15 and delta-wave coma but no seizure activity at repeat EEG. Other causes of encephalopathy were excluded (uremic or sepsis-associated encephalopathy, infectious encephalitis, etc.). According to clinical and electrophysiological criteria, the patient was declared brain dead on day 18 after the start of chemotherapy. At postmortem examination, the liver architecture appeared relatively well preserved with about 10–20% of the hepatocytes presenting ballooning and nuclear loss in the pericentrolobular area. There was no evidence of intestinal necrosis.

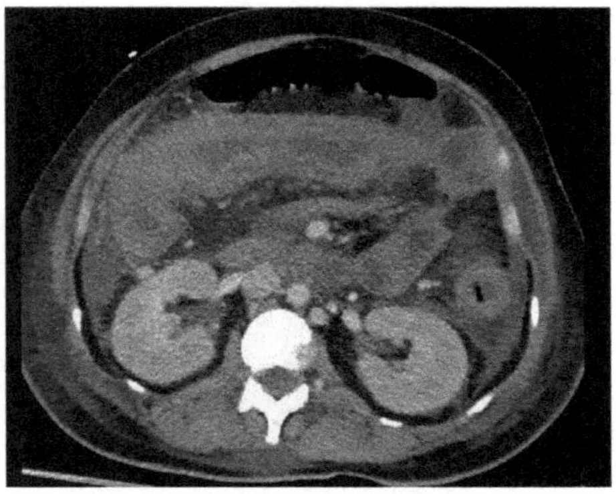

Figure 1: Contrast-enhanced abdomen computed tomography with oedematous thickening of the caecal and colonic mucosa.

3. Discussion

This patient developed fatal hyperammonemic encephalopathy less than 3 weeks after the start of induction chemotherapy based on the combination cytarabine-idarubicin to treat a recently diagnosed AML. This delay is consistent with a previous case who developed a similar clinical course on day 21 after having received high-dose cytarabine and mitoxantrone for AML and with other literature cases, even if a shorter delay (a few hours) was occasionally observed [6, 7]. The true incidence of IHA in patients receiving chemotherapy for acute leukemia is not known, as ammonia levels are usually not measured in asymptomatic patients, but reached 2.4% in the largest literature series [8]. Most of these cases occurred in the absence of severe hepatic dysfunction and other causes of hyperammonemia could also be ruled out. Therefore, this hyperammonemia is often classified as idiopathic [1, 2]. We can however assume that most of the systemic ammonia pool is originally generated in the gastrointestinal tract and this was likely the case in the present observation. The clinical presentation is usually characterized by rapidly progressive signs of central nervous system dysfunction including coma and seizures [9]. The prognosis is usually extremely poor, with a mortality rate around 80% [1, 2]. At postmortem examination, brain swelling and herniation are commonly observed. Our observation confirmed the presence of high glutamine levels in the CSF; as a metabolite of ammonia, the intracellular accumulation of glutamine may be responsible for an osmotic effect with astrocyte swelling [1]. The liver is usually free from preexisting disease. Ultrastructural liver changes differ from those observed in Reyes syndrome and usually reveal congestion, fatty infiltration, and cholestasis.

The origin of hyperammonemia is likely multifactorial. Cytarabine itself contributes very slightly to ammonia formation through a metabolic process of deamination [4]. Among other chemotherapy agents, 5-fluorouracil (5-FU) has also been associated in some cases with hyperammonemia [6]. However, ammonia is a product of 5-FU metabolism, and the clinical course of hyperammonemia is usually transient and benign. L-asparaginase is also often related to IHA with a mechanism that is also not fully understood [10]. There is insufficient evidence to prove that a congenital metabolic disorder is responsible for hyperammonemia. For the patients explored by plasma amino acid determinations, no specific profile could be identified. In our case, a urea cycle defect was unlikely based on slightly low plasma levels of citrulline, but normal plasma levels of ornithine and arginine, absence of argininosuccinate, and normal urinary levels of orotic acid [11]. Our patient had also no evidence of a preexisting congenital liver disease (Wilson's disease, for example). The role of some additional

Table 1: Laboratory data before and after hyperammonemic coma.

	Normal range	Day 1 (start of chemotherapy)	Day 7 (end of chemotherapy)	Day 13 (ICU admission)	Day 16 (coma onset)	Day 17	Day 18 (death)
Maximal daily temperature (°C)		36.6	38.4	38.8	37.3	37.2	35.8
CRP (mg/l)	<5	2.6	236.4	463.8	313.6	292.1	340.5
Ammonia (μmol/l)	<64	n.d.	n.d.	n.d.	688	1989	992
Total bilirubin (mg/dl)	<1.2	0.5	0.8	5.8	6.5	5.7	6.4
Alkaline phosphatase (IU/l)	35–105	40	28	21	35	37	42
Gamma-glutamyl transpeptidase (IU/l)	<40	16	46	28	32	36	41
Aspartate aminotransferase (IU/l)	15–35	12	12	45	28	37	42
Alanine aminotransferase (IU/l)	7–35	12	9	31	22	21	23
International normalized ratio	0.80–1.20	1.15	1.53	1.64	1.39	1.42	1.46
Arterial lactate (mmol/l)	0.5–2.2	n.d.	n.d.	2.8	2.1	2.9	2.7
Triglycerides (mg/dl)	<150	n.d.	n.d.	n.d.	n.d.	513	390

n.d., not done.

Table 2: Common therapeutic options for hyperammonemia.

Intervention	Mechanism
Lactulose	Acceleration of intestinal transit time
Intestinal antibiotics (digestive decontamination)	Reduction of intestinal microbial proliferation
Administration of probiotics	Changes in intestinal microbiota
Sodium benzoate/phenylacetate	Conjugation with glycine to form hippuric acid and promote urea excretion
Carnitine	Regulation of fatty acids metabolism
Reduction in protein intake, avoidance of catabolism	Decreased activity of urea cycle and ammonia production
Epuration techniques (HD, CVVH, MARS)	Increased ammonia elimination

precipitating factors may also be discussed. Among them, sepsis, dehydration, and nitrogen load by parenteral nutrition are commonly found and were present in our patient [1, 9, 12]. The ammonia production could also have been increased by the ileus-related microbial proliferation [13]. Reports of hyperammonemia due to urease-producing bacteria such as *Klebsiella spp.*, *Proteus spp.*, *Corynebacterium spp.*, and *Staphylococcus spp.* are commonly found, while *Enterococcus faecium* is not frequently cited [14].

Several strategies have been proposed to control hyperammonemia (Table 2) [15]. Some pharmacological agents (sodium benzoate and sodium phenylacetate) have been proposed to promote the elimination of ammonia, with variable outcomes [16]. In addition to ammonia-trapping agents, hemodialysis should be initiated early to promote ammonia elimination [17]. It has been suggested to continue hemodialysis until the blood ammonia concentration has dropped below 200 μmol/l for a period of at least 24 hours. Continuous venovenous hemofiltration (CVVH) is a possible alternative to hemodialysis. Even if it appears less effective than hemodialysis, CVVH is a continuous method that could be maintain for a longer period and could clear newly produced nitrogen [18]. However, these techniques may be limited by ammonia overproduction. The molecular adsorbent recirculating system (MARS) is an epuration technique based upon albumin dialysis. It could promote the elimination of bilirubin, bile acid, ammonia, and cytokines. It has been used with some efficacy in a case of L-asparaginase-related hyperammonemia [19]. Adequate nutritional support is essential to avoid protein catabolism or excessive protein intake by parenteral nutrition. Any medication impairing intestinal motility should be avoided. Finally, the long-term oral administration of a strain (SF68) of *Enterococcus faecium* was able to reduce the production of ammonia and the severity of encephalopathy in a single study of patients with cirrhosis and a normal dietary nitrogen intake [20]. Other strains (*Lactobacillus*, *Bifidobacterium*, etc.) have been tested using the same probiotic approach [15].

Consent

Informed consent was obtained from the relatives.

Authors' Contributions

Christophe Angelo and Edwige Boulet wrote the paper. Marie-Françoise Vincent performed the specialized laboratory investigations. Mina Komuta performed the post-mortem analysis. Philippe Hantson and Nicole Straetmans supervised the patient's management and revised the paper.

References

[1] A. J. Watson, J. E. Karp, W. Gordon Walker, T. Chambers, V. R. Risch, and S. W. Brusilow, "Transient idiopathic hyperammonaemia in adults," *The Lancet*, vol. 326, no. 8467, pp. 1271–1274, 1985.

[2] S. M. Davies, E. Szabo, J. E. Wagner, N. K. Ramsay, and D. J. Weisdorf, "Idiopathic hyperammonemia: a frequently lethal complication of bone marrow transplantation," *Bone Marrow Transplantation*, vol. 17, no. 6, pp. 1119–1125, 1996.

[3] L. Kwan, C. Wang, and L. Levitt, "Hyperammonemic encephalopathy in multiple myeloma," *New England Journal of Medicine*, vol. 346, no. 21, pp. 1674-1675, 2002.

[4] P. Fine, K. Adler, and D. Gerstenfeld, "Idiopathic hyperammonemia after high-dose chemotherapy," *The American Journal of Medicine*, vol. 86, no. 5, p. 629, 1989.

[5] Y.-H. Chen, T.-J. Chiou, Y.-N. Hsu, and C.-Y. Liu, "Idiopathic hyperammonemia after chemotherapy with vinorelbine, topotecan, and cisplatin in a patient with acute lymphocytic leukemia," *Hematology/Oncology and Stem Cell Therapy*, vol. 3, no. 4, pp. 199–202, 2010.

[6] K. H. Metzeler, S. Boeck, B. Christ et al., "Idiopathic hyperammonemia (IHA) after dose-dense induction chemotherapy for acute myeloid leukemia: case report and review of the literature," *Leukemia Research*, vol. 33, no. 7, pp. e69–e72, 2009.

[7] C. C. Liaw, H. M. Wang, C. H. Wang et al., "Risk of transient hyperammonemic encephalopathy in cancer patients who received continuous infusion of 5-fluorouracil with the complication of dehydration and infection," *Anticancer Drugs*, vol. 10, no. 3, pp. 275–281, 1999.

[8] R. B. Mitchell, J. E. Wagner, J. E. Karp et al., "Syndrome of idiopathic hyperammonemia after high-dose chemotherapy: review of nine cases," *The American Journal of Medicine*, vol. 85, no. 5, pp. 662–667, 1988.

[9] L. Nott, T. J. Price, K. Pittman, K. Patterson, and J. Fletcher, "Hyperammonemia encephalopathy: an important cause of neurological deterioration following chemotherapy," *Leukemia & Lymphoma*, vol. 48, no. 9, pp. 1702–1711, 2007.

[10] J. V. Leonard and J. D. S. Kay, "Acute encephalopathy and hyperammonaemia complicating treatment of acute lymphoblastic leukaemia with asparaginase," *The Lancet*, vol. 327, no. 8473, pp. 162-163, 1986.

[11] A. Laemmle, D. Hahn, L. Hu et al., "Fatal hyperammonemia and carbamoyl phosphate synthetase 1 (CPS1) deficiency following high-dose chemotherapy and autologous hematopoietic stem cell transplantation," *Molecular Genetics and Metabolism*, vol. 114, no. 3, pp. 438–444, 2015.

[12] S. Kobayashi, M. Ito, H. Sano et al., "Idiopathic hyperammonemia that developed during initial treatment with steroid in a patient with newly diagnosed leukemia," *Journal of Pediatric Hematology/Oncology*, vol. 37, no. 6, pp. e361–e363, 2015.

[13] E. A. Jones, A. Craigie, A. S. Tavill, G. Franglen, and V. M. Rosenoer, "Protein metabolism in the intestinal stagnant loop syndrome," *Gut*, vol. 9, no. 4, pp. 466–469, 1968.

[14] K. Otsuji, S. Simizu, T. Endo et al., "A case of infectious enterocolitis with hyperammonemia," *Journal of UOEH*, vol. 39, no. 4, pp. 271–276, 2017.

[15] S. Matoori and J.-C. Leroux, "Recent advances in the treatment of hyperammonemia," *Advanced Drug Delivery Reviews*, vol. 90, pp. 55–68, 2015.

[16] M. del Rosario, S. L. Werlin, and S. J. Lauer, "Hyperammonemic encephalopathy after chemotherapy," *Journal of Clinical Gastroenterology*, vol. 25, no. 4, pp. 682–684, 1997.

[17] G. T. Berry, N. D. Bridges, K. L. Nathanson et al., "Successful use of alternate waste nitrogen agents and hemodialysis in a patient with hyperammonemic coma after heart-lung transplantation," *Archives of Neurology*, vol. 56, no. 4, pp. 481–484, 1999.

[18] K. Y. Wong, S. N. Wong, S. Y. Lam, S. Tam, and N. S. Tsoi, "Ammonia clearance by peritoneal dialysis and continuous arteriovenous hemodiafiltration," *Pediatric Nephrology*, vol. 12, no. 7, pp. 589–591, 1998.

[19] G. Beziat, S. Tavitian, M. Picard, S. Faguer, C. Recher, and F. Huguet, "Multiple severe toxicities of L-asparaginase and their innovative management during induction therapy of acute lymphoblastic leukemia in an adult patient," *Case Reports in Hematology*, vol. 2019, Article ID 9086570, 6 pages, 2019.

[20] C. Loguerci, R. Abbiati, M. Rinaldi, A. Romano, C. D. V. Blanco, and M. Coltorti, "Long-term effects of Enterococcus faecium SF68 versus lactulose in the treatment of patients with cirrhosis and grade 1-2 hepatic encephalopathy," *Journal of Hepatology*, vol. 23, no. 1, pp. 39–46, 1995.

36

Hairy Cell Leukemia Masquerading as Pancytopenia in Pregnancy

Louisa Shackleton,[1] Stephen E. Langabeer,[2] David O'Brien,[1] Sarah L. McCarron,[2] Bridgette Byrne,[3] Rupert Barry,[4] Richard Flavin,[5] C. Larry Bacon,[1] and Catherine M. Flynn[1]

[1]*Department of Haematology, St. James's Hospital, Dublin 8, Ireland*
[2]*Cancer Molecular Diagnostics, St. James's Hospital, Dublin 8, Ireland*
[3]*Maternal Medicine Service, Coombe Women and Infants University Hospital, Dublin 8, Ireland*
[4]*Department of Dermatology, St. James's Hospital, Dublin 8, Ireland*
[5]*Department of Histopathology, St. James's Hospital, Dublin 8, Ireland*

Correspondence should be addressed to Stephen E. Langabeer; slangabeer@stjames.ie

Academic Editor: Tomás J. González-López

Thrombocytopenia is one of the most common hematological abnormalities observed during pregnancy, and in rare cases, this may be the first indicator of an underlying hematological malignancy. Hairy cell leukemia (HCL) is an uncommon B-cell lymphoproliferative disorder of which thrombocytopenia is a recurrent presenting feature. A case of pancytopenia presenting in pregnancy is described in which the thrombocytopenia persisted postpartum coincidental with a vesicular, pustular rash characterised as Sweet's syndrome. Hematological, histological, immunophenotypic, and molecular investigations confirmed the presence of HCL. The patient was treated with cladribine resulting in resolution of Sweet's syndrome, hematological remission from HCL, and achievement of a normal platelet count. This case highlights the need to maintain a wide differential diagnosis for presentations of pancytopenia or thrombocytopenia in pregnancy and the requirement for follow-up investigation of unusual cases with a lack of response to steroids or immunoglobulin.

1. Introduction

Thrombocytopenia develops in up to 10% of women during pregnancy or in the immediate postpartum period with approximately three quarters of cases attributed to gestational thrombocytopenia where the thrombocytopenia is mild and does not necessitate active management [1, 2]. Immune thrombocytopenia (ITP) is the most common cause in the first trimester but only accounts for approximately 4% of cases. Recent evidence suggest that in those patients with a platelet count less than 100×10^9/L, a cause other than pregnancy or its complications should be considered [3]. In rare cases, the thrombocytopenia may be the first presenting feature of a hematological malignancy with this incidence ranging from one in one thousand to one in ten thousand pregnancies; subsequent management remains a challenging endeavour [4]. Of those hematological malignancies reported during pregnancy, hairy cell leukemia (HCL) is exceedingly rare [5, 6].

HCL is an uncommon B-cell lymphoproliferative neoplasm usually presenting in the sixth decade with pancytopenia and splenomegaly and which is five times more common in men than women [7]. Morphologically, hairy cells possess distinct cytoplasmic projections and by immnophenotyping characteristically express CD11c, CD25, and CD103 in addition to pan-B cell antigens. The discovery of the *BRAF* V600E mutation in nearly all cases of classical HCL has led to the introduction of targeted agents in those cases refractory to standard therapies of purine nucleoside analogues [8, 9]. An unusual case of thrombocytopenia in pregnancy leading to a subsequent postpartum diagnosis of HCL is presented.

2. Case Report

A 37-year-old woman was noted to have pancytopenia on routine blood screening during the first trimester of pregnancy. Complete blood count demonstrated a platelet count of 85×10^9/L, white cell count of 2.3×10^9/L (of which neutrophils were 1.3×10^9/L and monocytes were 0.2×10^9/L), and hemoglobin 10.6 g/dL. She reported occasional easy bruising in the last two months with no other bleeding issues, lymphadenopathy, or splenomegaly. The patient had one previous uncomplicated pregnancy delivered thirteen months previously with normal platelet counts throughout and had been in good health prior to this pregnancy. She had a personal history of equivocal hypothyroidism, had a family history of hypothyroidism and systemic lupus erythematosus, was on no regular medications, and had not commenced any new medications in pregnancy. Thyroid function tests, immunoglobulins, and folate and vitamin B_{12} levels were within normal range with a negative antinuclear antibody test. As a low serum ferritin level was noted, she commenced on iron supplementation. The patient was given a presumptive diagnosis of immune thrombocytopenia in pregnancy. During pregnancy, fatigue was her only symptom and she had no bleeding complications with her platelet count remaining static. There were no clinical findings to suggest preeclampsia or HELLP (hemolysis, elevated liver enzymes, and low platelet count) syndrome. Blood film examination was performed routinely throughout pregnancy with no morphological abnormalities observed. At 38-week gestation (platelets 61×10^9/L), she was commenced on prednisolone 20 mg oral daily, but the platelet count showed no response (platelets 65×10^9/L) prompting immunoglobulin therapy at 1 g/Kg of booking weight (70 g once-only dose), but this again had no effect on the platelet count (platelets 52×10^9/L). Soon after, she presented to a maternity hospital in spontaneous labor and had a normal vaginal delivery at full term with minor bleeding and no postpartum hemorrhage. The platelet count was 52×10^9/L at the time of delivery, and no therapy was given. Her male infant had a normal platelet count at birth.

At review five weeks postpartum, the patient had developed a pustular skin rash on her left upper arm, lower abdomen, and lower back. A skin biopsy demonstrated dermal neutrophils producing upper dermal edema and a subepidermal blister consistent with bullous Sweet's syndrome (acute febrile neutrophilic dermatosis) (Figure 1(a)). Her hematological indices displayed persistent cytopenias with a hemoglobin of 13.0 g/dL, a white cell count of 1.7×10^9/L (of which neutrophils were 0.5×10^9/L and monocytes were 0.1×10^9/L), and a platelet count of 49×10^9/L. Occasional hairy cells were noted for the first time on blood film examination. Immunophenotyping demonstrated a population of B lymphocytes that represented 5% of non-erythroid cells. These B cells were kappa-restricted and positive for CD10, CD11c, CD19, CD20, CD25, and CD103. The bone marrow aspirate was normocellular for age and showed 23% lymphocytes with 10% having hairy projections. Trephine biopsy demonstrated an infiltration of hairy cells with typical morphology (Figure 1(b)) with immunohistochemistry of these hairy cells demonstrating positivity for CD10, CD20, CD25, CD72, and *BCL2* (Figure 1(c)). The *BRAF* c.1799T > *A*; p.(Val600Glu) mutation was detected in genomic DNA from the bone marrow by a next-generation sequencing approach; all of which were consistent with a diagnosis of HCL.

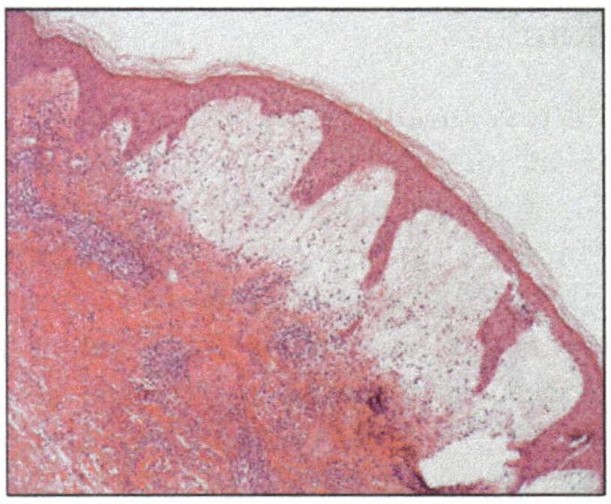

(a)

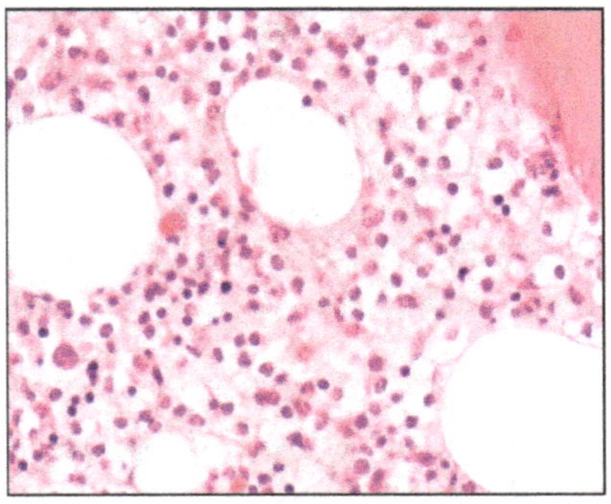

(b)

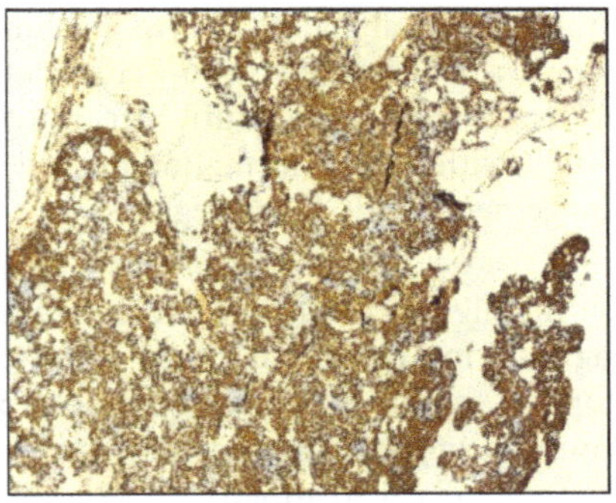

(c)

Figure 1: (a) Dermal infiltration of neutrophils of Sweet's syndrome, (b) bone marrow trephine demonstrating hairy cell leukemia infiltration, and (c) bone marrow trephine immunohistochemistry for CD20.

Following this diagnosis of HCL, the patient received a single five-day course of cladribine at a dose of 0.1 mg/kg/day by continuous intravenous infusion at nine weeks postpartum. This was complicated by an episode of febrile neutropenia and a diffuse erythematous rash secondary to allopurinol and co-trimoxazole which resolved following cessation of these medications. At the last follow-up seven months after cladribine treatment, the patient is well with hemoglobin of 13.1 g/dL, a white cell count of 4.2×10^9/L (of which neutrophils were 2.9×10^9/L and monocytes were 0.3×10^9/L), and platelet count of 207×10^9/L with resolution of Sweet's syndrome. At this center, in such a case of favorable dermatological and hematological response, repeat bone marrow analysis to assess immunophenotypic or molecular residual disease is not routinely performed unless clinically indicated.

3. Discussion

The family history of autoimmune disease for this patient suggested a diagnosis of ITP that can occur in the first or early second trimester of pregnancy and in which the platelet count does not necessarily improve postpartum, unlike gestational thrombocytopenia. However, the absence of thrombocytopenia in a previous pregnancy and, more tellingly, the lack of response to steroids and immunoglobulins were the atypical, discordant clinical features suggestive of an alternative etiology.

This patient's presentation is unusual in its association of a vesicular eruption consistent with bullous Sweet's syndrome with HCL. Sweet's syndrome is a neutrophilic dermatosis with a known association with hematological malignancies particularly acute myeloid leukemia [10] but rarely associated with HCL [11–13]. Consistent with another case, the patient's rash in this case resolved following chemotherapy [13].

HCL is uncommon in women of reproductive age and has only been sporadically reported during pregnancy [14]. In such instances, successful treatment has been documented with interferon-alpha, rituximab, purine analogues, and laparoscopic splenectomy [14–16]. However, given the rarity of this presentation, no definitive treatment guideline has been possible with more information needed to establish the best management of HCL in pregnancy.

This case highlights the need to maintain a wide differential diagnosis for presentations of pancytopenia and thrombocytopenia in pregnancy and for reevaluation of persistent thrombocytopenia postpartum particularly when unresponsive to standard treatments.

References

[1] D. B. Cines and L. D. Levine, "Thrombocytopenia in pregnancy," *Blood*, vol. 130, no. 21, pp. 2271–2277, 2017.

[2] A. E. Fogerty, "Thrombocytopenia in pregnancy: mechanisms and management," *Transfusion Medicine Reviews*, vol. 32, no. 4, pp. 225–229, 2018.

[3] J. A. Reese, J. D. Peck, D. R. Deschamps et al., "Platelet counts during pregnancy," *New England Journal of Medicine*, vol. 379, no. 1, pp. 32–43, 2018.

[4] T. Rizack, A. Mega, R. Legare, and J. Castillo, "Management of hematological malignancies during pregnancy," *American Journal of Hematology*, vol. 84, no. 12, pp. 830–841, 2009.

[5] J. K. Williams, "Hairy cell leukemia in pregnancy: a case report," *American Journal of Obstetrics and Gynecology*, vol. 156, no. 1, pp. 210-211, 1987.

[6] B. Pastner, R. W. Penney, and C. M. Walsh, "Recurrent hairy cell leukemia during pregnancy: a case report," *American Journal of Obstetrics and Gynecology*, vol. 170, no. 5, pp. 1380-1381, 1994.

[7] R. J. Kreitman and E. Arons, "Update on hairy cell leukemia," *Clinical Advances in Hematology & Oncology*, vol. 16, no. 3, pp. 205–215, 2018.

[8] B. Falini, M. P. Martelli, and E. Tiacci, "*BRAF*V600E mutation in hairy cell leukemia: from bench to bedside," *Blood*, vol. 128, no. 15, pp. 1918–1927, 2016.

[9] M. R. Grever, O. Abdel-Wahab, L. A. Andritsos et al., "Consensus guidelines for the diagnosis and management of patients with classic hairy cell leukemia," *Blood*, vol. 129, no. 5, pp. 553–560, 2017.

[10] S. M. Kazmi, N. Pemmaraju, K. P. Patel et al., "Characteristics of sweet syndrome in patients with acute myeloid leukemia," *Clinical Lymphoma Myeloma and Leukemia*, vol. 15, no. 6, pp. 358–363, 2015.

[11] C. Kramers, J. M. M. Raemaekers, H. M. J. van Baar, B. E. de Pauw, and A. M. Horrevorts, "Sweet's syndrome as the presenting symptom of hairy cell leukemia with concomitant infection by mycobacterium kansasii," *Annals of Hematology*, vol. 65, no. 1, pp. 55–58, 1992.

[12] F. Ventura, J. Rocha, T. Pereira, M. Herlander, P. Fernando, and B. Celeste, "Sweet syndrome as the presenting symptom of hairy cell leukaemia," *Dermatology Online Journal*, vol. 15, no. 2, p. 12, 2009.

[13] M. Alkayen and W. Cheng, "A case report of hairy cell leukemia presenting concomitantly with sweet syndrome," *Case Reports in Medicine*, vol. 2014, Article ID 823286, 3 pages, 2014.

[14] N. Daver, A. Nazha, H. M. Kantarjian, R. Haltom, and F. Ravandi, "Treatment of hairy cell leukemia during pregnancy: are purine analogues and rituximab viable therapeutic options," *Clinical Lymphoma Myeloma and Leukemia*, vol. 13, no. 1, pp. 86–89, 2013.

[15] M. R. Baer, H. Ozer, and K. A. Foon, "Interferon-α therapy during pregnancy in chronic myelogenous leukaemia and hairy cell leukaemia," *British Journal of Haematology*, vol. 81, no. 2, pp. 167–169, 1992.

[16] B. A. Adeniji, M. Fallas, M. Incerpi, S. Hamburg, R. Katz, and D. Ogunyemi, "Laparoscopic splenectomy for hairy cell leukemia in pregnancy," *Case Reports in Medicine*, vol. 2010, Article ID 136823, 2 pages, 2010.

Subdural Hygroma: A Morbid Complication of Intrathecal Chemotherapy in a Patient with B-Cell Acute Lymphocytic Leukemia

Mina Shenouda,[1] Madhulika Urella,[2] Jennifer Dotson,[1] Hassaan Yasin,[1] and Yehuda Lebowicz[1]

[1]*Marshall University, Department of Hematology and Oncology, 1400 Hal Greer Blvd, Huntington, WV 25701, USA*
[2]*Marshall University, Department of Internal Medicine, 1249 15th St., Suite 2000, Huntington, WV 25701, USA*

Correspondence should be addressed to Jennifer Dotson; rose67@marshall.edu

Academic Editor: Sergio Storti

A subdural hygroma is an accumulation of cerebrospinal fluid in the subdural space that may occur secondary to trauma and surgery, or for iatrogenic reasons, such as a lumbar puncture. Lumbar puncture is a procedure used commonly for intrathecal chemotherapy for patients with B-cell acute lymphocytic leukemia (B-ALL) though subdural hygroma is a very rare complication. We present a case of a fatal, refractory subdural hygroma in a patient with B-ALL.

1. Introduction

Subdural hygroma is an uncommon complication after lumbar puncture. A subdural hygroma is the accumulation of cerebrospinal fluid (CSF) in the subdural space that may occur for a number of reasons. Subdural hygromas are encountered in all age groups. Subdural hygroma affects the critical age groups of less than 5 years and more than 60 years, when the dural space is large enough for the fluid to accumulate [1]. The demographics vary based on the underlying etiology: it may occur from trauma and iatrogenic causes related to spontaneous intracranial hypotension or idiopathic. Patients vary in clinical presentation, ranging from asymptomatic to symptomatic with headache, changes in mental status, nausea and vomiting, focal neurological deficits, and seizures [2]. The pathogenesis of subdural hygromas is not entirely understood. The most commonly encountered explanation is a tear in the arachnoid layer forming a ball valve opening allowing CSF a one-way passage into the subdural space. It has been proposed that subdural hygromas represent prominent subdural effusions in which there is a separation of the dural border cell layer with an accumulation of the fluid [1, 3]. Intrathecal chemotherapy (IT) is administered by performing a lumbar puncture and is widely used in hematological and systemic malignancies for either prophylactic or therapeutic intentions. We present a case of bilateral subdural hygroma as a rare complication of intrathecal methotrexate administration.

2. Case Presentation

A 69-year-old male with a past medical history of recently diagnosed Philadelphia-positive B-cell acute lymphoblastic leukemia (B-ALL), coronary artery disease, diabetes mellitus, and hypertension was admitted to the hospital with severe nausea and vomiting, generalized weakness, and a headache for one-day duration. The patient had been discharged from the hospital three days prior after undergoing induction treatment for a new diagnosis of B-ALL with dasatinib, vincristine, dexamethasone, and prophylactic intrathecal methotrexate. The patient completed 4 cycles of dexamethasone 40 mg daily (given as 10 mg intravenously every 6 hours) for two days each weekly cycle. The diagnosis of B-ALL was made a month prior to this hospital admission when the patient had presented with severe pancytopenia. A peripheral blood flow cytometry sent at the time of initial presentation showed positive for CD10, CD79a, CD34, and terminal deoxynucleotidyl transferase (TdT) and was negative for myeloperoxidase (MPO), CD117, and CD33. Fluorescence in situ hybridization from the bone marrow biopsy sample showed BCR-ABL translocation and gain of RUNX1T1/8q, RUNX1/21q, MYC/8q, and chromosome 5. These findings were consistent with a diagnosis of B-ALL. Due to his age and comorbidities, his treatment consisted of dasatinib 140 milligrams (mg) orally daily along with two cycles of vincristine, four cycles of dexamethasone 40 mg daily, and three cycles of prophylactic intrathecal methotrexate. Additional cycles of vincristine were not given due to cytopenias. CSF cytology samples obtained during administration of intrathecal methotrexate were negative for any involvement of ALL. The patient obtained a complete hematologic and molecular remission after his first course of treatment. He was due for his next course of intrathecal methotrexate on the day of admission but was admitted to the hospital due to the above complaints. Over the prior few weeks, he had been complaining of generalized weakness throughout his arms and his legs and gait instability associated with balance issues. He also reported intermittent left-sided headaches. On physical examination, he was afebrile with 4/5 strength in all extremities but with no cranial nerve deficits. Laboratory evaluation demonstrated the white cell count was 3.300 k/cmm, hemoglobin was 7.3 g/dL, and platelet count was 92,000 along with hypokalemia. He was initially treated supportively with intravenous fluids and antiemetics. Subsequent magnetic resonance imaging (MRI) of the brain revealed development of large bilateral extra-axial fluid collections which appeared to be subdural in location, most suggestive of subdural hygromas. There was also an associated mass effect with sulcal effacement and approximately 3 mm rightward midline shift (Figure 1). The patient denied any recent falls or trauma. His most recent lumbar puncture was performed six days prior to his current presentation. Lumbar puncture was performed under aseptic precautions following the optimized technique to avoid CSF leakage. Neurosurgery then performed a burr hole procedure with evacuation of subdural fluid with subsequent CT head showing improvement in the subdural fluid collections (Figure 2). Postoperatively, the patient's neurological status wavered. A repeat CT of the brain was obtained on postoperative day four due to new onset slurring of speech and increased lethargy but was unchanged when compared to the recent MRI of the brain. Neurosurgery placed an epidural blood patch due to suspicion of a low-pressure cerebrospinal fluid leak. He was also instructed to place his bed in the Trendelenburg position as tolerated. Repeat MRI of the brain revealed an increase in the bilateral fluid collection (Figure 3). The patient's mentation and motor function improved, and subsequent CT head showed mild improvement in the fluid collection. The patient was discharged home and presented to the oncology clinic within a week with worsening altered mental status, confusion, agitation, weakness in the lower extremities, and balance

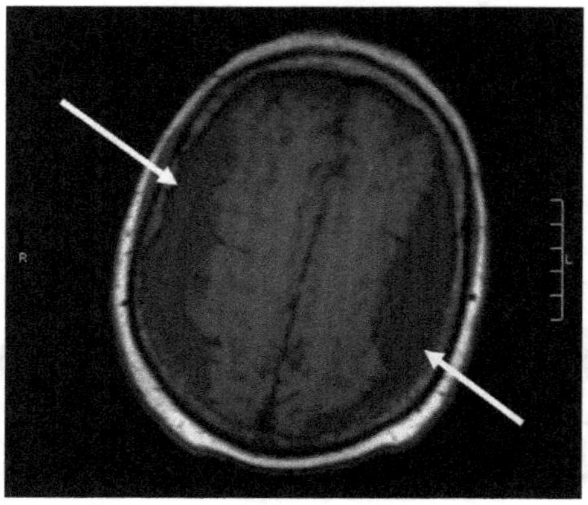

FIGURE 1: Axial T1 sequence from magnetic resonance imaging (MRI) of the brain.

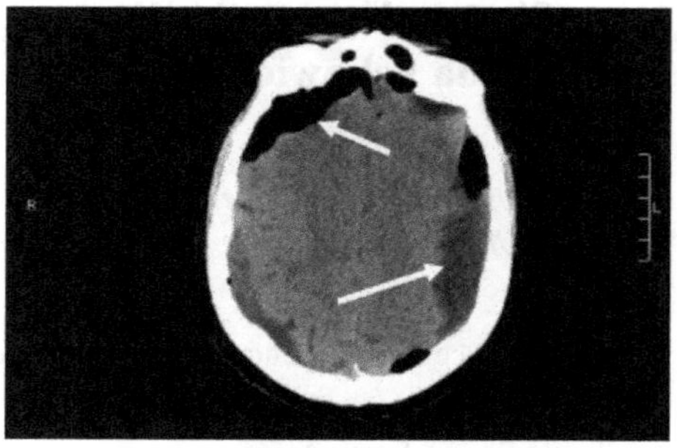

FIGURE 2: Computed tomography (CT) imaging of the brain after the bilateral burr hole procedure.

issues. Repeat CT of the head showed recurrent enlarged fluid collections (Figure 4). He had burr holes placed by neurosurgery bilaterally with subdural evacuating port systems. The fluid collections would resolve and recur over the hospital course. Repeat scans continued to show persistent mass effect, and his neurologic status continued to decline. The patient's family decided that he should be discharged with hospice, and he subsequently died a few days later.

3. Discussion

Acute lymphoblastic leukemia is responsible for 20% of adult leukemia cases and carries a significantly poorer prognosis than in children with overall five-year survival rates of 30–40% [4]. Among adults older than 55–60 years, the probability of survival decreases to 20% at three years [5]. With standard intensive induction chemotherapy, however, approximately 85–90% of adult patients will achieve a complete remission [6]. Patients with acute lymphoblastic leukemia (ALL) have substantial risk for developing leptomeningeal disease. In the absence of central nervous system (CNS) prophylaxis, as many as 50–75% of patients may develop CNS disease; thus, intrathecal (IT) methotrexate with or without cytarabine via lumbar puncture or Ommaya reservoir is a well-established component of induction therapy [7].

The mechanism for subdural hygroma via lumbar puncture (LP) is not well established but is presumed to

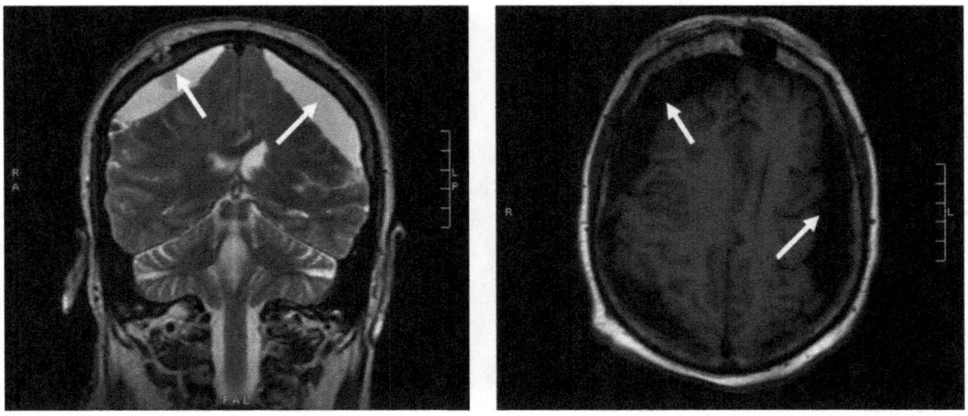

(a) (b)

FIGURE 3: (a) T2-weighted coronal sequence from an MRI of the brain. (b) An axial T1 flair image.

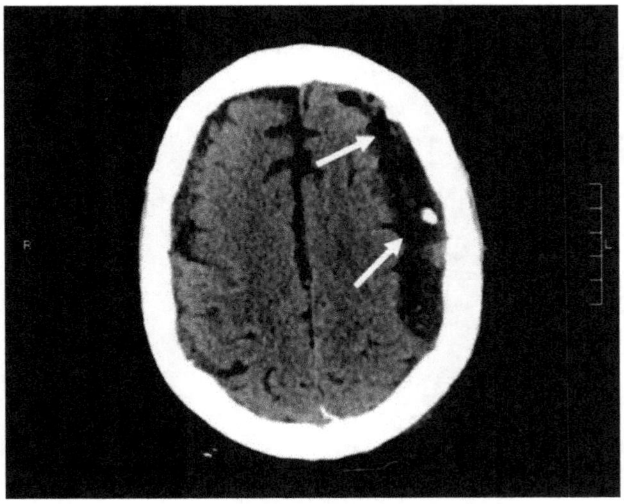

FIGURE 4: Computed tomography of the head.

involve a lumbar CSF leak with a reduction in CSF pressure, resulting in downward displacement of the brain with CSF accumulation in the inner dural layers of the cerebral convexities [8]. Bilateral subdural hygromas following prophylactic IT methotrexate is a very rare complication that has only been sporadically reported in the literature [8, 9]. A study of patients with subdural hygromas after haemopoietic stem cell transplant concluded that patients were at increased risk of developing subdural collections if they had an LP, with or without IT chemotherapy [10]. The risk of symptomatic subdural hygroma after LP is estimated to be only 1-2% [10]. In our patient, since there was no evidence for a prior structural or traumatic etiology for reduced CSF pressure, the IT administration of chemotherapy in this patient was most likely the causative mechanism of hygroma formation. In the DASISION trial, myelosuppression was commonly reported with tyrosine kinase inhibitor (TKI) therapy. Dasatinib has been known to cause serious and fatal bleeding due to platelet dysfunction, and the incidence of serious hemorrhage has been reported in a few patients, mostly associated with severe thrombocytopenia [11].

Patel et al. report an increased risk of CNS bleeding in association with tyrosine kinase inhibitor (TKI) therapy due to its effect on platelet function [12]. Though hygromas and hemorrhage are different clinical entities, subtle prohemorrhagic changes may favor the continuous meningeal leakage of CSF.

Initial management of subdural hygromas involves conservative measures, including bed rest combined with fluid supplementation, analgesic agents, and even caffeine. The epidural blood patch (EBP) is indicated if the conservative treatment is ineffective, as in our patient [13]. Other management options include an increase in platelet transfusion parameters above 50,000–75,000 per μl, continuous epidural saline infusion, or epidural injection of dextran or fibrin glue. However, even with optimal management, the size of the subdural hygroma may increase [14, 15]. Subdural hygromas may become membrane-bound and may produce mass effect on the cerebral hemispheres requiring surgical decompression, as in our patient (Figure 1). Lumbar puncture for intrathecal therapy in these patients with cerebral mass effect may lead to fatal brain herniation.

In this report, we describe a rare but potentially fatal complication of IT chemotherapy that oncologists should be aware of. Unfortunately, our patient appeared to be a complete hematologic and molecular remission, and his death was iatrogenic, a complication from the treatment. It should be noted that IT chemotherapy is not without risk. Intrathecal chemotherapy should be deferred if any neurologic symptoms become apparent or if there are any concerning findings during the lumbar puncture, such as low opening pressures or a traumatic tap which may occur because the spinal needle is advanced beyond the collapsed subarachnoid space. Headache after lumbar puncture is a potential warning sign that has been reported by few patients prior to the diagnosis of hygroma, and if this occurs, the patient should be promptly evaluated with the consideration of imaging to rule out hygroma or hemorrhage.

References

[1] K.-S. Lee, "History of chronic subdural hematoma," *Korean Journal of Neurotrauma*, vol. 11, no. 2, pp. 27–34, 2015.

[2] K. S. Lee, "The pathogenesis and clinical significance of traumatic subdural hygroma," *Brain Injury*, vol. 12, no. 7, pp. 595–603, 1998.

[3] K.-S. Lee, "Review natural history of chronic subdural haematoma," *Brain Injury*, vol. 18, no. 4, pp. 351–358, 2004.

[4] A. Kansagra, S. Dahiya, and M. Litzow, "Continuing challenges and current issues in acute lymphoblastic leukemia," *Leukemia & Lymphoma*, vol. 59, no. 3, pp. 526–541, 2018.

[5] R. Bassan and D. Hoelzer, "Modern therapy of acute lymphoblastic leukemia," *Journal of Clinical Oncology*, vol. 29, no. 5, pp. 532–543, 2011.

[6] N. Gokbuget, M. Kneba, T. Raff et al., "Adult patients with acute lymphoblastic leukemia and molecular failure display a poor prognosis and are candidates for stem cell transplantation and targeted therapies," *Blood*, vol. 120, no. 9, pp. 1868–1876, 2012.

[7] U. R. Surapaneni, J. E. Cortes, D. Thomas et al., "Central nervous system relapse in adults with acute lymphoblastic leukemia," *Cancer*, vol. 94, no. 3, pp. 773–779, 2002.

[8] H. Lewis, A. J. Mahdi, and C. Rowntree, "Bilateral subdural hygromas following administration of intrathecal methotrexate chemotherapy," *BMJ Case Reports*, vol. 2015, 2015.

[9] P. Lokireddy and M. J. S. Dyer, "Bilateral subdural hygromas following intrathecal methotrexate," *British Journal of Haematology*, vol. 155, no. 5, p. 536, 2011.

[10] H. Openshaw, J. A. Ressler, and D. S. Snyder, "Lumbar puncture and subdural hygroma and hematomas in hematopoietic cell transplant patients," *Bone Marrow Transplantation*, vol. 41, no. 9, pp. 791–795, 2008.

[11] H. Kantarjian, N. P. Shah, A. Hochhaus et al., "Dasatinib versus imatinib in newly diagnosed chronic-phase chronic myeloid leukemia," *The New England Journal of Medicine*, vol. 362, no. 24, pp. 2260–2270, 2010.

[12] S. B. Patel, I. Gojo, M. L. Tidwell, E. A. Sausville, and M. R. Baer, "Subdural hematomas in patients with Philadelphia chromosome-positive acute lymphoblastic leukemia receiving imatinib mesylate in conjunction with systemic and intrathecal chemotherapy," *Leukemia & Lymphoma*, vol. 52, no. 7, pp. 1211–1214, 2011.

[13] E. C. Williams, B. R. Buchbinder, S. Ahmed, T. A. Alston, J. P. Rathmell, and J. Wang, "Spontaneous intracranial hypotension: presentation, diagnosis, and treatment," *Anesthesiology*, vol. 121, no. 6, pp. 1327–1333, 2014.

[14] J. A. Aldrete, "Persistent post-dural-puncture headache treated with epidural infuson of dextran," *Headache: The Journal of Head and Face Pain*, vol. 34, no. 5, pp. 265–267, 1994.

[15] B. J. P. Crul, B. M. Gerritse, R. T. M. van Dongen, and H. C. Schoonderwaldt, "Epidural fibrin glue injection stops persistent postdural puncture headache," *Anesthesiology*, vol. 91, no. 2, pp. 576-577, 1999.

Primary Cutaneous T-Cell Lymphoblastic Lymphoma: Case Report and Literature Review

Sharad Khurana, Manuel Beltran, Liuyan Jiang, Ernesto Ayala, and Vivek Roy

Mayo Clinic, Jacksonville, FL, USA

Correspondence should be addressed to Sharad Khurana; khurana.sharad@mayo.edu

Academic Editor: Chihaya Imai

Cutaneous involvement by precursor T-cell lymphoblastic leukemia/lymphoma (T-ALL/LBL) is rare, and almost all cases are seen in association with bone marrow, blood, and/or lymph node involvement. Presentation with isolated skin involvement is very rare. Literature review revealed only one case report of primary cutaneous T-cell LBL. We discuss here another patient diagnosed with primary cutaneous T-cell LBL at our institute. This patient was initially misdiagnosed as having peripheral T-cell lymphoma NOS. Cytogenetic analysis showed the CDKN2A deletion (−9p21×2) in addition to three intact copies of ABL1 (+9q34). Although she failed multiple lines of intensive chemotherapy, her disease remained confined to the skin. We believe that this presentation of T-LBL is underreported, and many patients are likely misdiagnosed as having high-grade cutaneous T-cell lymphomas. With this case and literature review, we would like to highlight the importance of keeping lymphoblastic lymphoma on the differential diagnosis of cutaneous T-cell lymphoma-like lesions to avoid delay in diagnosis and inappropriate treatment of this aggressive disease.

1. Introduction

T-cell ALL/LBL accounts for ~20% of all cases of ALL and is more commonly seen in adults than children [1]. Cutaneous involvement by T-cell leukemia/lymphoma is a rare occurrence with a reported frequency of around 4.3% [2–4]. We present a patient diagnosed with primary cutaneous T-cell LBL at our institute. This patient was initially misdiagnosed as having peripheral T-cell lymphoma NOS as immunohistochemical staining for immature T-cell markers was not performed at presentation. The patient had an aggressive course with disease relapse and progression after multiple lines of intensive chemotherapy. However, her disease remained confined to the skin. Literature review revealed primary cutaneous T-LBL to be a very rare entity with only one previously reported case [5].

2. Case Description

A 52-year-old woman with past medical history of diabetes mellitus type 2, atrial fibrillation, and hypertension presented with multiple, small, and reddish papular lesions on both lower extremities. She described these lesions as "bug bites" which rapidly progressed in size and number, involving most of her body in a matter of eight weeks. She had no other symptoms at this time. The patient underwent excisional biopsy of one of the lesions which showed diffuse infiltrate by atypical lymphoid cells. Flow cytometry and immunohistochemical studies showed these atypical cells as CD4+ T cells that expressed CD2, CD3, CD5, partial CD57, partial CD52, partial CD26, and alpha/beta receptors (Figure 1). CD7, CD8, and CD30 were not expressed. These atypical lymphocytes had weak and focal expression for BCL2 but negative CD20 and BCL-6 expression. Myeloperoxidase (MPO), CD34, and CD117 were not expressed ruling out myeloid lineage malignancy. The proliferative rate by Ki-67 was moderate at 70%. Polymerase chain reaction (PCR) study for T-cell receptor gamma gene rearrangement was positive and for T-cell receptor, beta gene was oligoclonal. Terminal deoxynucleotidyl transferase (TdT) immunostaining was not performed. No metaphases were available for karyotyping. A final diagnosis of peripheral T-cell lymphoma NOS was made after evaluation by two different pathology centers. The lymphoma was limited to

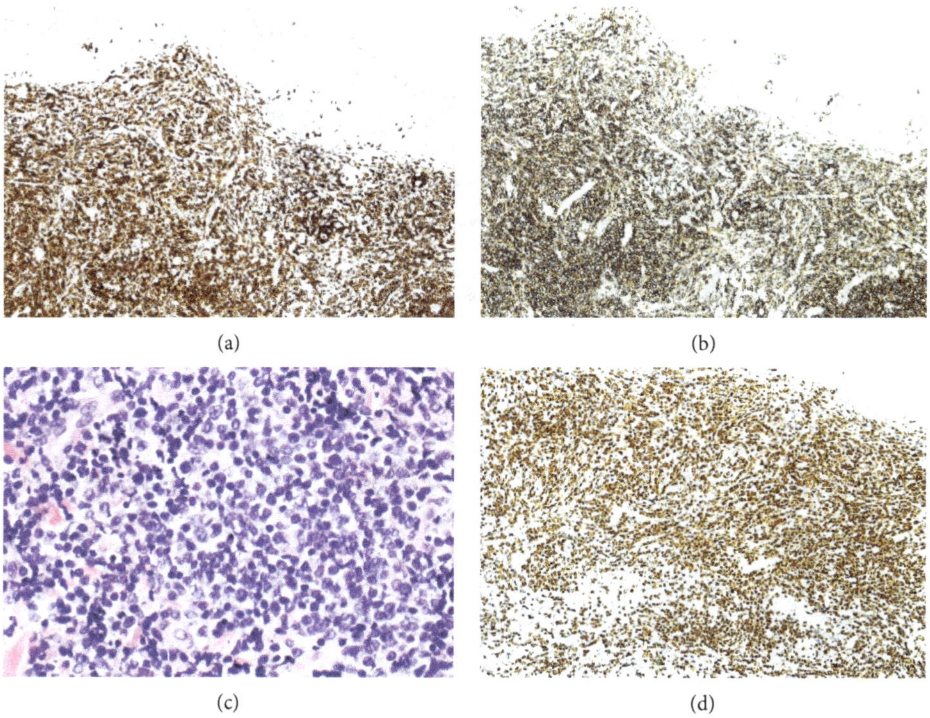

Figure 1: (a) Positive CD3 immunostaining. (b) Positive CD4 immunostaining. (c) H&E stain with blastic appearing lymphocytes. (d) Positive immunostaining with terminal deoxynucleotidyl transferase (TdT) of the lymphocytes.

the skin with no involvement of bone marrow and lymph nodes or any extranodal organ/tissue as confirmed by a positron emission tomography (PET-CT). HTLV-1 and HIV blood testing were negative. The patient was treated with six cycles of CHOEP (cyclophosphamide, doxorubicin, vincristine, etoposide, and prednisone) and went into complete clinical remission. Posttreatment PET scan showed resolution of all the metabolically active skin lesions. She was then referred to our institution for consideration of autologous stem-cell transplant as consolidation.

Three months after completion of chemotherapy while undergoing pretransplant evaluation, the patient noticed a slightly raised, erythematous 2×1 cm lesion on the right lower quadrant of her abdominal wall (Figure 2). Biopsy of this lesion showed neoplastic lymphocytes, demonstrating a similar immunophenotype as that was seen on the initial skin biopsy. However, both the dermatopathologist and hematopathologist noticed that the morphology of the lymphocytes appear to be blastic in appearance; therefore, immunostain for terminal deoxynucleotidyl transferase (TdT) was performed, which showed diffuse nuclear positivity in the lymphocytes, confirming lymphoblastic nature of these cells (Figure 1). As such, a final diagnosis of T-cell lymphoblastic lymphoma was made. Fluorescence in situ hybridization (FISH) study revealed homozygous CDKN2A deletion ($-9p21 \times 2$) and three intact copies of ABL1 (+9q34) (Figure 2), which aided in confirming the final diagnosis. Subsequent bone marrow biopsy was negative for involvement by T-cell lymphoblastic lymphoma/leukemia. No suspicious foci of increased FDG uptake were noted on the PET-CT of the whole body. We also reviewed the original skin biopsy and performed immunostain of TdT, which was again diffusely positive in the neoplastic lymphocytes. Further, we repeated and compared the PCR studies for TCR gene rearrangement between these two skin biopsies using multiple master mixes target conserved regions within the variable (V) and the joining (J) regions for T-cell receptor gamma gene and conserved regions within the variable (V), diversity (D), and the joining (J) regions for T-cell receptor beta gene. In each biopsy, a clone (amplicon at 264 dp) in the V-J region of beta gene and another clone (amplicons at 201 dp and 220 dp) at the V-J region of gamma gene were identified; and the results appeared to be identical. Therefore, the diagnosis of cutaneous T-cell lymphoblastic lymphoma at initial presentation and at relapse was confirmed.

She was treated with high-dose methotrexate and cytarabine along with prophylactic intrathecal chemotherapy with cytarabine and methotrexate, with the plan of proceeding with allogeneic hematopoietic stem cell transplantation. Unfortunately, her disease progressed after 2 cycles of chemotherapy as evidenced by enlarging right lower abdominal wall lesion, now almost 15 cm wide and 11.5 cm in length with ulceration (Figure 2). PET-CT showed hypermetabolic right lower abdominal wall subcutaneous lesion with associated reactive inguinal and external iliac lymphadenopathy. Repeat skin biopsy confirmed T-LBL, and chromosomal microarray (CMA) analysis performed using molecular inversion probes on a whole genome array showed multiple complex genomic alterations. Therapy was now switched to second-line nelarabine to obtain disease control before proceeding with allogeneic stem cell transplantation. The patient however had no response to

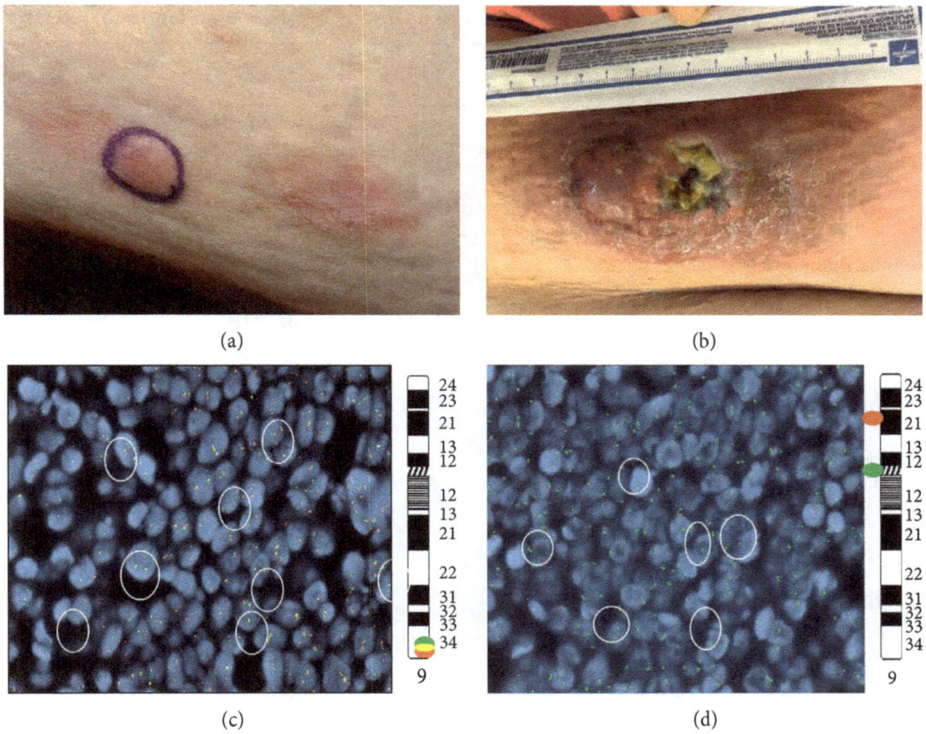

FIGURE 2: (a) 2 × 1 cm lesion on the right lower quadrant of the abdominal wall at first relapse. (b) Enlarging right lower abdominal wall lesion now almost 15 cm × 11.5 cm with ulceration. (c) Break-apart ABL1 fluorescence in situ hybridization (FISH) circles indicate 3 intact ABL1 signals (5′ABL1 (green)/3′ABL1 (red) {9q34}). (d) Enumeration for 9p-circles indicates homozygous loss of CDKN2A (CDKN2A(9p16) red/D9Z19(CEN) green).

nelarabine and her skin lesion kept progressing, for which she was referred to radiation oncology for palliative radiation to the ulcerated enlarging tumor.

3. Discussion

Approximately 5,960 new cases and 1,470 deaths attributable to acute lymphoblastic leukemia/acute lymphoblastic lymphoma (ALL/LBL) are estimated in 2018 in the United States of America [6]. T-cell ALL/LBL accounts for ~20% of all cases of ALL and is more common in adults than children [1]. It accounts for 20% of all cases of leukemia in adults [7] with a 2 : 1 male predominance. Lymphoblastic neoplasms can present as either leukemia or lymphoma forms depending on the extent of the bone marrow (BM) infiltration by the neoplastic cells. Lymphoblastic presentation is more often of T-cell lineage than B cell, with an approximate ratio of 9 : 1 [4].

Lymphoblastic lymphomas comprise around 3.5% to 7% of all skin lymphomas [8]. Cutaneous involvement by T-cell leukemia/lymphoma is a rare occurrence with a frequency of around 4.3% as compared to 16–33% patients with B-LBL/ALL [2–4]. T-LBL usually presents as multiple skin lesions throughout the body as compared to B-LBL which can present as a solitary skin lesion [2, 3, 9]. Almost all cutaneous T-LBL cases reported in the literature are seen in association with bone marrow (T-ALL) and/or mediastinal (most common T-LBL site), lymph node, or extranodal involvement (Table 1). Cutaneous LBLs present as diffuse monomorphous infiltrate located in the entire dermis and subcutis without epidermotropism. Immunophenotyping studies are required to distinguish ALL/LBL from other high-grade cutaneous lymphomas like peripheral T-cell NOS. T-LBL is distinguished from peripheral T-cell lymphoma by the presence of immature T-cell phenotypes such as TdT, CD7, and cytoplasmic CD3.

While great progress has been made in recent years in understanding the biology and genetic makeup/mutations associated with T-cell ALL [10], cytogenetic and molecular abnormalities are not well defined in T-LBL and more so in cutaneous T-LBL due to rarity of the disease. A linkage between abnormal expressions of genes located at 9q34 and 17q22–23 has been described [11]. ZNF79, ABL1, or THRAP1 have been noted in the "lymphoma phenotype" such as in bulky masses in the mediastinum with minimal BM involvement [11]. Schraders et al. described a cohort of 12 cases of T-LBL, showing recurrent genomic aberrations affecting gene loci with known roles in cell cycle regulation. The most frequent genomic abnormality in this cohort, observed in 11 cases (92%), was the deletions of the CDKN2A locus, which encodes two tumor suppressor genes, p16INK4a and p14ARF. Deletions of RB1 (16%), a tumor suppressor gene, duplications of MYB (16%), an oncogene locus, and an amplification of ABL1 were also reported [12]. Vezolli et al. reported trisomy 4 and gain of 1p36.33-p22.1 on microarray-comparative genomic hybridization in early-stage disease and multiple chromosomal alterations in the late-stage of primary cutaneous T-LBL [5].

Table 1: T-cell lymphoblastic lymphomas with cutaneous involvement reported in the literature.

Source	Sex/ age	Cutaneous location	Extracutaneous involvement	Immunohistochemical profile	Treatment	Disease status at last follow-up
Nascimbeni et al. [13]	M/66y	Scalp and trunk	BM and retroperitoneal LN	CD2, CD7, CD3, CD99, TdT, C-kit	Four cycles of CHOP with intrathecal MTX	Complete remission
Ginoux et al. [14]	M/75y	Right arm and occipital area	Bilateral LN on axillary, cervical, and inguinal areas, BM	CD3, CD5, CD4, Ki67, TdT	CHOP	Died 8 Mo after diagnosis
Lee et al. [2]	M/16y	Subcutaneous nodule on the neck	BM, LN	CD99, CD3, CD45RO, TdT	Unspecified chemotherapy	Died 2 y after diagnosis
Lee et al. [2]	M/20y	Multiple scalp nodules	Prostate	CD3, CD4, CD8, CD10, CD99, CD45RO, TdT	Unspecified chemotherapy	Died 5 Mo after diagnosis
Lee et al. [2]	M/25y	Multiple subcutaneous nodules on face, scalp, chest wall	BM, LN, scrotal involvement	CD3, CD10, CD99, CD45RO, TdT	Unspecified chemotherapy	Complete remission 8 y after diagnosis
Lee et al. [2]	M/17y	Subcutaneous nodules on neck and abdomen.	Mediastinal mass, BM, LN	CD3, CD99, CD45RO, TdT.	Unspecified chemotherapy	Complete remission 9 y after diagnosis
Lee et al. [2]	F/25y	Multiple subcutaneous nodules on right breast, neck, chest wall, legs	BM, LN	CD3, CD4, CD8, CD33, CD99, TdT	Unspecified chemotherapy	Relapse
Lee et al. [2]	M/39y	Multiple nodules on scalp	Mediastinal mass, LN, BM, left kidney, pleura	CD3, CD4, CD8, CD10, CD1a, TdT	Unspecified chemotherapy	Complete remission 3 y after diagnosis
Lee et al. [2]	M/22y	Multiple subcutaneous nodules on back	Mediastinal mass, LN, tonsil, nasopharynx	CD3, CD8, CD10, CD45RO, TdT	Unspecified chemotherapy	Partial remission
Vezzoli et al. [5]	F/29y	Multiple nodules on face, breast, thoracomammary region, abdomen, thighs	Primary cutaneous with axillary LN, 23 Mo after diagnosis	CD3, CD5, CD7, CD99, CD45RA, CD79a, KI67, TdT	DHAP + pro MACE cytaBOM + ABSCT	Died after 28 Mo diagnosis
Yaar et al. [15]	M/27y	Cutaneous nodule right cheek and forehead	Mediastinal mass, BM	CD3, CD5, CD7, CD45, CD34, Ki-67	Not described	Not described
Prasad et al. [16]	M/5y	Noduloulcerative purplish lesions on abdominal wall	St Judes stage III unspecified extracutaneous involvement	CD3, CD45, TdT	Not described	Not described
Chimenti et al. [17]	M/65y	Abdomen and extremities	BM	CD1a, CD3, CD43, CD99, TdT	Not described	Died 2 Mo after diagnosis
Sander et al. [9]	F/24y	Malar region, anterior chest wall, breasts	Submental LN, liver, BM	CD2, CD4, CD7, CD10, CD13, TdT	Cyclophosphamide, cytosine, arabinoside, teniposida, deoxycoformycin, vincristine	Died 21 Mo after diagnosis
Sander et al. [9]	M/25y	Scalp	Mediastinal mass, cervical, supraclavicular, axillary LN	CD1, CD2, CD3, CD4, CD5, CD7, CD8, CD10, TdT	Whole brain XRT, intrathecal MTX, cyclophosphamide, doxorubicin, vincristine, L-asparaginas, mercaptopurine	Complete remission

M: male; F: female; Mo: months; y: years; LN: lymph node; BM: bone marrow; MTX: methotrexate; XRT: radiation therapy; DHAP: cytosine arabinoside, cisplatin, and dexamethasone; ProMACE-cytaBOM: cyclophosphamide, methotrexate, vincristine, etoposide, epirubicin, bleomycin, and cytarabine; ABSCT: autologous bone marrow stem cell transplant.

They suggested gain of 1p36.33-p22.1 to be an interesting marker in PC-T-LBL, as it was noted to be present in early stages and persisted through later stages of the disease. Although we do not have the microarray analysis on initial presentation for our patient, microarray-based gene expression profiling done at later stages of the disease did not show presence of gain of 1p36.33-p22.1. Rather a loss at 1p36.33-p36.32 was noted in addition to multiple other genetic abnormalities along with retention of CDKN2A deletion and three intact copies of ABL1 +9q34, present at initial presentation (Figure 2). Therefore, based on different sets of genetic mutations seen in these two cases, we cannot make a conclusion of any specific genetic mutation to be associated with PC-T-LBL.

Treatment of LBL with regimens typically used for non-Hodgkin lymphoma is associated with poor outcomes with only 58% complete remission (CR) rate and a 5-year disease-free survival (DFS) rate of 36% [18]. ALL-based regimens provide a better long-term outcome with CR rates between 55% and 100% and 5-year DFS rates between 45% and 65% [18]. Because of high risk of relapse, hematopoietic stem cell transplantation is often considered as consolidative/ potentially curative strategy in first remission or at relapse [19]. However, the exact role of transplantation in T-LBL is not clear because of paucity of large body of data. Moreover, prognostic indicators that can identify patients who are most likely to benefit from transplant have not been defined.

Our case is extremely rare as we found only one previously reported case of primary cutaneous T-LBL. Vezolli et al. described a case of a 29-year-old female with multiple, red-violaceous ulcerated nodules on the left breast that was initially misdiagnosed as PTL-NOS [5]. Similar to our case, diagnosis was changed to T-LBL after positive immunostaining on the initial and relapsed skin specimen with TdT. This highlights the importance of keeping lymphoblastic lymphoma on the differential diagnosis of cutaneous lymphoma like lesions. Staining with TdT and/or other immature T-cell markers should be performed to avoid misdiagnosing T-LBL as other high-grade cutaneous T-cell lymphomas. We believe that this presentation of T-LBL is underreported, and many patients are likely misdiagnosed as having high-grade cutaneous T-cell lymphomas and inappropriately treated with non-Hodgkin's lymphoma-(NHL-) type regimens. Delay in diagnosis and inappropriate treatment will adversely affect the outcome of this aggressive disease. With this case report and literature review, we therefore would like to increase awareness of cutaneous only presentation of T-LBL.

Authors' Contributions

S. K. and M. B. wrote the manuscript; L. J. edited the case description and obtained the images; and E. A. and V. R. edited and finalized the manuscript.

References

[1] E. J. Jabbour, S. Faderl, and H. M. Kantarjian, "Adult acute lymphoblastic leukemia," *Mayo Clinic Proceedings*, vol. 80, no. 11, pp. 1517–1527, 2005.

[2] W. J. Lee, H. R. Moon, C. H. Won et al., "Precursor B- or T-lymphoblastic lymphoma presenting with cutaneous involvement: a series of 13 cases including 7 cases of cutaneous T-lymphoblastic lymphoma," *Journal of the American Academy of Dermatology*, vol. 70, no. 2, pp. 318–325, 2014.

[3] A. Maitra, R. W. McKenna, A. G. Weinberg, N. R. Schneider, and S. H. Kroft, "Precursor B-cell lymphoblastic lymphoma," *American Journal of Clinical Pathology*, vol. 115, no. 6, pp. 868–875, 2001.

[4] F. Millot, A. Robert, Y. Bertrand et al., "Cutaneous involvement in children with acute lymphoblastic leukemia or lymphoblastic lymphoma," *Pediatrics*, vol. 100, no. 1, pp. 60–64, 1997.

[5] P. Vezzoli, F. Novara, D. Fanoni et al., "Three cases of primary cutaneous lymphoblastic lymphoma: microarray-based comparative genomic hybridization and gene expression profiling studies with review of literature," *Leukemia and Lymphoma*, vol. 53, no. 10, pp. 1978–1987, 2012.

[6] R. L. Siegel, K. D. Miller, and A. Jemal, "Cancer statistics, 2018," *CA: A Cancer Journal for Clinicians*, vol. 68, no. 1, pp. 7–30, 2018.

[7] S. D. Esparza and K. M. Sakamoto, "Topics in pediatric leukemia—acute lymphoblastic leukemia," *MedGenMed*, vol. 7, no. 1, p. 23, 2005.

[8] I. M. Schmitt, L. Manente, A. Di Matteo, F. Felici, M. Giangiacomi, and S. Chimenti, "Lymphoblastic lymphoma of the pre-B phenotype with cutaneous presentation," *Dermatology*, vol. 195, no. 3, pp. 289–292, 2009.

[9] C. A. Sander, L. J. Medeiros, L. V. Abruzzo, I. D. Horak, and E. S. Jaffe, "Lymphoblastic lymphoma presenting in cutaneous sites," *Journal of the American Academy of Dermatology*, vol. 25, no. 6, pp. 1023–1031, 1991.

[10] D. I. Marks, E. M. Paietta, A. V. Moorman et al., "T-cell acute lymphoblastic leukemia in adults: clinical features, immunophenotype, cytogenetics, and outcome from the large randomized prospective trial (UKALL XII/ECOG 2993)," *Blood*, vol. 114, no. 25, pp. 5136–5145, 2009.

[11] M. Sekimizu, S. Sunami, A. Nakazawa et al., "Chromosome abnormalities in advanced stage T-cell lymphoblastic lymphoma of children and adolescents: a report from Japanese Paediatric Leukaemia/Lymphoma Study Group (JPLSG) and review of the literature," *British Journal of Haematology*, vol. 154, no. 5, pp. 612–617, 2011.

[12] M. Schraders, S. V. van Reijmersdal, E. J. Kamping et al., "High-resolution genomic profiling of pediatric lymphoblastic lymphomas reveals subtle differences with pediatric acute lymphoblastic leukemias in the B-lineage," *Cancer Genetics and Cytogenetics*, vol. 191, no. 1, pp. 27–33, 2009.

[13] C. Nascimbeni, S. Chantepie, C. Brugiere, F. Comoz, V. Salaun, and L. Verneuil, "Cutaneous involvement in T-lymphoblastic lymphoma," *Annales de Dermatologie et de Vénéréologie*, vol. 144, no. 4, pp. 268–274, 2017.

[14] E. Ginoux, F. Julia, B. Balme, L. Thomas, and S. Dalle, "T-lymphoblastic lymphoma with cutaneous involvement," *World Journal of Clinical Cases*, vol. 3, no. 8, p. 727, 2015.

[15] R. Yaar, R. Karen, and M. Mahalingam, "When dead cells tell tales-cutaneous involvement by precursor T-cell acute lymphoblastic lymphoma with an uncommon phenotype," *American Journal of Dermatopathology*, vol. 32, no. 2, pp. 183–186, 2010.

[16] P. G. Prasad, S. Cyriac, T. G. Sagar, and K. Rathnam, "T-lymphoblastic lymphoma relapsing in skin—a rare clinical scenario," *Indian Journal of Hematology and Blood Transfusion*, vol. 26, no. 1, pp. 19-20, 2010.

[17] S. Chimenti, R. Fink-Puches, K. Peris et al., "Cutaneous involvement in lymphoblastic lymphoma," *Journal of Cutaneous Pathology*, vol. 26, no. 8, pp. 379–385, 1999.
[18] S. Cortelazzo, M. Ponzoni, A. J. M. Ferreri, and D. Hoelzer, "Lymphoblastic lymphoma," *Critical Reviews in Oncology/Hematology*, vol. 79, no. 3, pp. 330–343, 2011.
[19] S. Lepretre, C. Graux, A. Touzart, E. Macintyre, and N. Boissel, "Adult T-type lymphoblastic lymphoma: treatment advances and prognostic indicators," *Experimental Hematology*, vol. 51, pp. 7–16, 2017.

39

Paraneoplastic Pemphigus: A Striking Complication of Undiagnosed Lymphoma

Blake O. Adnani,[1] **Kathleen O' Brien**,[2] **Zaw W. Myint**,[3] **and Brandon L. Adler**[2]

[1]*Department of Internal Medicine, Keck School of Medicine, University of Southern California, Los Angeles, USA*
[2]*Department of Dermatology, Keck School of Medicine, University of Southern California, Los Angeles, USA*
[3]*Department of Hematology, Keck School of Medicine, University of Southern California, Los Angeles, USA*

Correspondence should be addressed to Blake O. Adnani; omidadnani@gmail.com

Academic Editor: Gergely Feher

A 49-year-old male with no past medical history presented with acute-onset painful mucosal erosions along with flaccid bullae on his trunk, scalp, and intertriginous areas. The patient initially underwent a skin biopsy which demonstrated suprabasilar acantholysis and lichenoid interface dermatitis. This was followed by a computed tomography scan which identified a large abdominal lymph node. Core needle biopsy of this node demonstrated follicular lymphoma. Lastly, indirect immunofluorescence (IIF) in rat bladder was positive (titer 1 : 10,240). This finding confirmed the diagnosis of paraneoplastic pemphigus (PNP) in the setting of follicular lymphoma. The patient's cutaneous disease was treated with a combination of intravenous immunoglobulin and methylprednisolone, along with intravenous rituximab, with a resolution of his cutaneous symptoms. His lymphoma was treated with six cycles of rituximab, cyclophosphamide, doxorubicin, vincristine, and prednisone (R–CHOP), with an interval decrease in his tumor burden. PNP is an autoimmune-mediated mucocutaneous disease associated with underlying neoplasm, most commonly non-Hodgkin lymphoma or chronic lymphocytic leukemia. Affected patients develop variable autoantibodies to antigens on keratinocytes and the basement membrane zone. Severe intractable stomatitis is characteristic, in addition to polymorphous cutaneous eruptions including bullae and erosions. Mortality rates can reach up to 90% due to malignancy, sepsis, or bronchiolitis obliterans, an irreversible and often lethal cause of pulmonary insufficiency. We highlight PNP manifesting in a patient with lymphoma, who responded well to the skin- and malignancy-directed treatments. PNP is an exceedingly rare diagnosis that should be considered in a patient with intractable stomatitis.

1. Case Presentation

A 49-year-old male presented with acute-onset painful oral, genital, and ocular erosions along with dusky erythema and flaccid bullae on his trunk, scalp, and intertriginous areas (Figures 1 and 2). Ten days prior to presentation, the patient noted bilateral eye pain and redness. Two days after these initial symptoms, he developed dysphagia and painful oral lesions, which made it difficult for him to ingest food and water. The following day, he developed tender, painful perianal lesions. He denied any past medical history, recent travel, medication or illicit drug use, or infectious symptoms. Physical exam was notable for prominent bilateral conjunctival injection, bilateral periorbital erythema and ulcerations, perioral hemorrhagic crusting, tender perianal ulcerations, and a diffuse macular rash on the trunk along with multiple nontender papules in the bilateral axilla. Initial labs (including complete blood count, comprehensive metabolic panel, and peripheral blood cultures) were unremarkable.

Dermatology was consulted, and a skin biopsy demonstrated suprabasilar acantholysis with lichenoid interface dermatitis. Serologic studies, including enzyme-linked immunosorbent assays (ELISA), showed autoantibodies to bullous pemphigoid antigen 1 along with desmogleins 1 and 3. Computerized tomography (CT) demonstrated an eleven-centimeter preaortic lymph node in the abdomen (Figures 3 and 4), along with scattered retroperitoneal and mesenteric

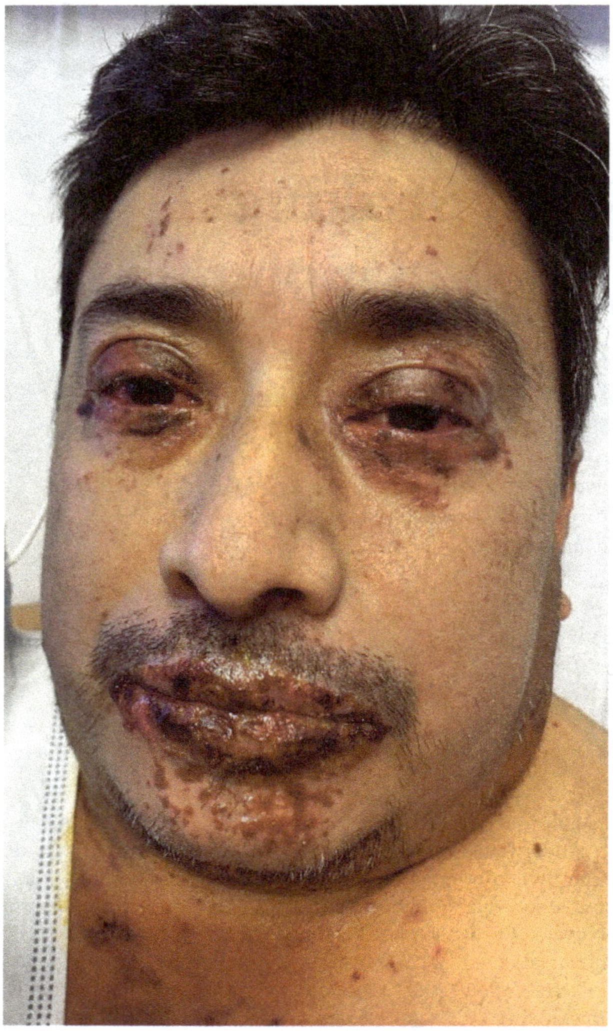

FIGURE 1: Mucocutaneous involvement in the initial presentation.

lymphadenopathy, Positron emission tomography (PET-CT) confirmed increased fluorodeoxyglucose (FDG) uptake in these areas. Core needle biopsy of the enlarged preaortic node revealed follicular lymphoma (CD10+, CD20+, BCL2+, and BCL6+ by immunohistochemistry). A paraneoplastic pemphigus panel displayed positive indirect immunofluorescence (IIF) on rat bladder (titer 1 : 10,240), mouse bladder (titer 1: 2,560), mouse heart (intercalating disks, titer 1 : 80), and monkey esophagus (cell surface). These findings confirmed the diagnosis of paraneoplastic pemphigus (PNP).

The patient's cutaneous disease was treated with 1 mg/kg/day of intravenous immunoglobulin for three days, 2 mg/kg/day of intravenous methylprednisolone for two weeks (followed by a two-month oral prednisone taper), and four doses of weekly 375 mg/m2 intravenous rituximab. He had a resolution of his skin lesions after two months of treatment (Figure 5), but his oral lesions persisted. His lymphoma was treated with six cycles of rituximab, cyclophosphamide, doxorubicin, vincristine, and prednisone (R-CHOP), with an interval decrease in his tumor burden. His oral lesions ultimately resolved about four months after the initiation of treatment (Figure 6).

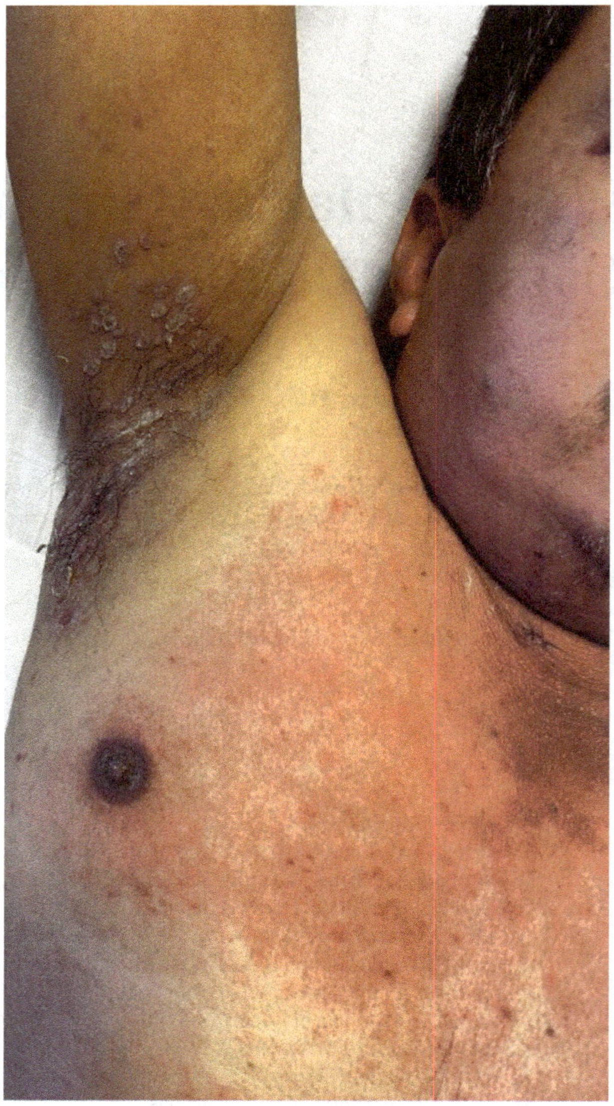

FIGURE 2: Axillary involvement in the initial presentation.

2. Discussion

PNP is an autoimmune-mediated mucocutaneous disease associated with underlying neoplasm, most commonly non-Hodgkin lymphoma or chronic lymphocytic leukemia. Affected patients develop variable autoantibodies to antigens on keratinocytes and the basement membrane zone [1]. Severe intractable stomatitis is characteristic, in addition to polymorphous cutaneous eruptions including bullae and erosions. Approximately one-third of patients with PNP present with new mucocutaneous lesions prior to diagnosis of their underlying neoplasia [1].

IIF using rat bladder is specific for PNP and differentiates it from pemphigus vulgaris [2]. However, previous studies have shown that IIF can be positive in roughly 20% of patients with pemphigus vulgaris and pemphigus foliaceus [3]. Mortality rates can reach up to 90% due to malignancy, sepsis, or bronchiolitis obliterans, an irreversible and often lethal cause of pulmonary insufficiency [4–6].

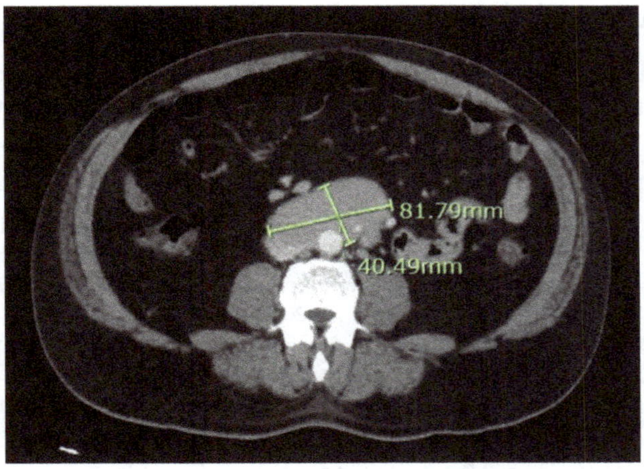

FIGURE 3: CT Abdomen and Pelvis with contrast showing enlarged preaortic lymph node (measured as 8×4 cm on axial view).

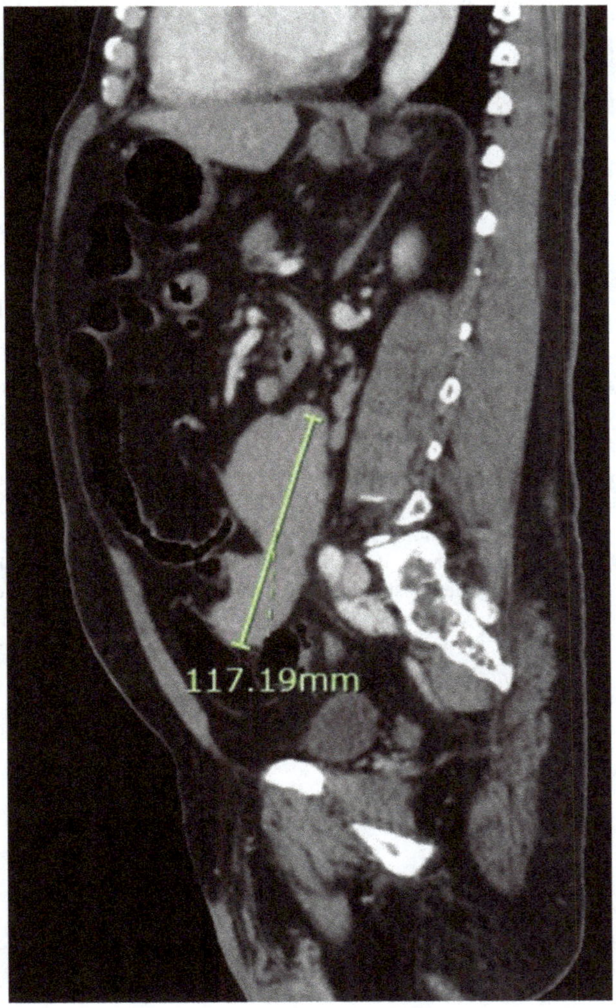

FIGURE 4: The same mass that was visualized in Figure 3, measured as 11.7 cm on sagittal view of CT.

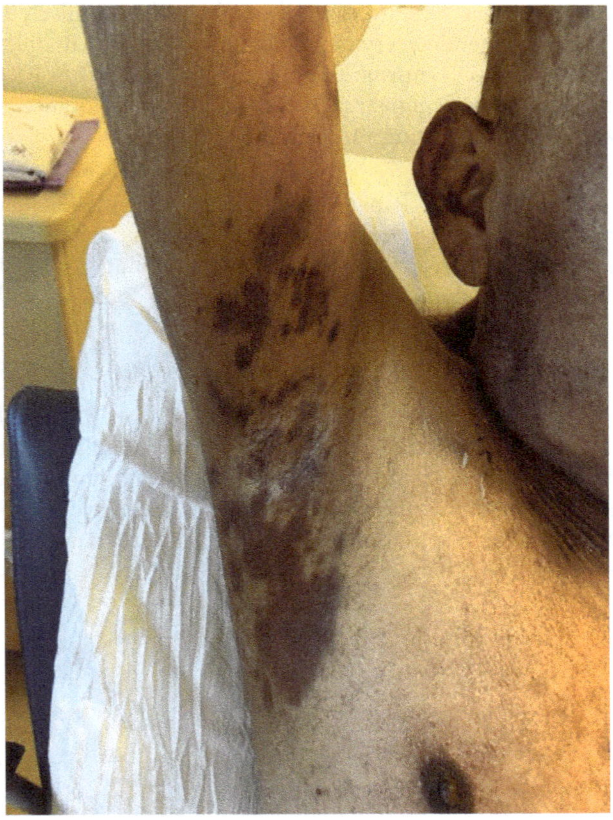

FIGURE 5: Resolution of axillary involvement after two months of treatment.

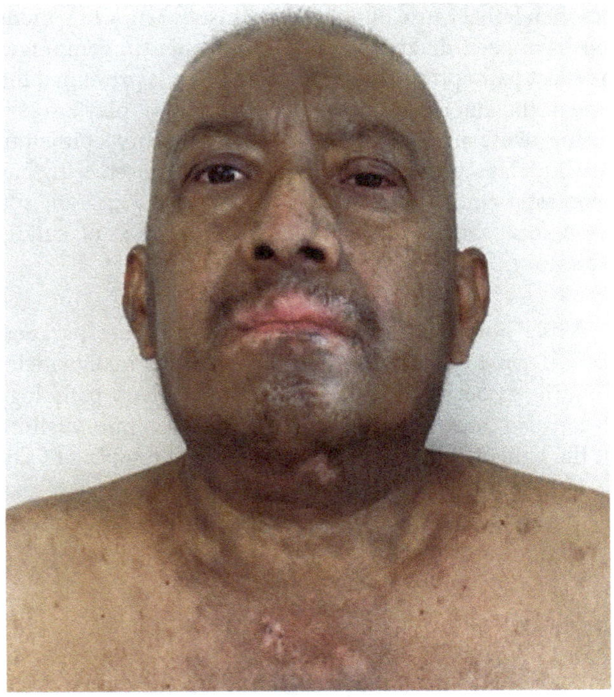

FIGURE 6: Resolution of oral and mucocutaneous involvement after four months of treatment.

PNP should not be confused with other paraneoplastic dermatoses, such as paraneoplastic dermatomyositis (PND) or necrolytic migratory erythema (NME). NME is characterized by peripheral vesicles and crusts, with central pigmentation in an annular pattern. It is often associated with glucagonomas and inflammatory bowel disease [7]. In contrast, PND presents as a heliotrope rash with splinter hemorrhages and is often associated with lung, breast, and ovarian cancer. The Sweet syndrome presents similarly to PND, with tender, erythematous papules and nodules. However, Sweet syndrome can be differentiated from PND through biopsy demonstrating a large proportion of mature neutrophils infiltrating the dermis [8, 9].

We highlight PNP manifesting in a patient with follicular lymphoma, who responded well to the skin- and malignancy-directed treatments. PNP is an exceedingly rare diagnosis that should be considered in a patient with intractable stomatitis.

2.1. Clinical Question. A 44-year-old male presents with sudden-onset intractable mucositis and flaccid bullae on his trunk. He is ultimately diagnosed with lymphoma and initiated on the appropriate treatment, but later develops acute hypoxic respiratory failure of unclear origin. What is the most likely diagnosis?

Stevens–Johnson syndrome (SJS)
Paraneoplastic pemphigus (PNP)
Pemphigus vulgaris
Sweet syndrome
Necrolytic migratory erythema (NME)

2.2. Answer. The correct answer, in this case, is paraneoplastic pemphigus. Bronchiolitis obliterans is an irreversible and often lethal cause of pulmonary insufficiency in patients who have been diagnosed with paraneoplastic pemphigus. The exact pathophysiology is unclear, but it is presumed that some of the autoantibodies generated by PNP play a role in causing acute inflammation of the respiratory epithelium [8]. Clinicians taking care of patients diagnosed with paraneoplastic pemphigus should have a high degree of suspicion for bronchiolitis obliterans in the case of sudden respiratory decline.

While both NME and Sweet syndrome are paraneoplastic dermatoses associated with underlying malignancies, neither is associated with significant pulmonary pathology. SJS can also cause lung disease leading to respiratory failure, but the patient's history of malignancy in the setting of skin erosions should lead you to consider the diagnosis of paraneoplastic pemphigus.

Consent

Written consent for publication was obtained directly from the patient.

Authors' Contributions

All authors were involved in the care of the patient, and the writing and approval of the manuscript.

Acknowledgments

The authors would like to thank Dr. Scott Worswick and Dr. Julian Mclain who were involved in the care of this patient.

References

[1] G. Paolino, D. Didona, G. Magliulo et al., "Paraneoplastic pemphigus: insight into the autoimmune pathogenesis, clinical features and therapy," *International Journal of Molecular Sciences*, vol. 18, no. 12, p. 2532, 2017.

[2] A. Y. Liu, R. Valenzuela, T. N. Helm, C. Camisa, A. L. Melton, and W. F. Bergfeld, "Indirect immunofluorescence on rat bladder transitional epithelium: a test with high specificity for paraneoplastic pemphigus," *Journal of the American Academy of Dermatology*, vol. 28, no. 5, pp. 696–699, 1993.

[3] D. G. Ortolan, D. P. Souza, V. Aoki et al., "Analysis of the reactivity of indirect immunofluorescence in patients with pemphigus foliaceus and pemphigus vulgaris using rat bladder epithelium as a substrate," *Clinics*, vol. 66, no. 12, pp. 2019–2023, 2011.

[4] K. Watanabe, K. Yoshifuji, T. Saito et al., "Follicular lymphoma accompanied by paraneoplastic pemphigus and bronchiolitis obliterans: a case report," *Rinsho Ketsueki*, vol. 60, no. 1, pp. 7–11, 2019.

[5] M. Rivas-Calderon, M. A. Yamazaki-Nakashimada, L. Orozco-Covarrubias et al., "Bronchiolitis obliterans with anti-epiplakin antibodies in a boy with paraneoplastic pemphigus," *Pediatrics*, vol. 149, no. 3, 2022.

[6] M. Takahashi, Y. Shimatsu, T. Kazama, K. Kimura, T. Otsuka, and T. Hashimoto, "Paraneoplastic pemphigus associated with bronchiolitis obliterans," *Chest*, vol. 117, no. 2, pp. 603–607, 2000.

[7] M. G. Foss and S. J. Ferrer-Bruker, "Necrolytic migratory erythema," 2021, https://www.ncbi.nlm.nih.gov/books/NBK532872/.

[8] P. R. Cohen, "Sweet's syndrome--a comprehensive review of an acute febrile neutrophilic dermatosis," *Orphanet Journal of Rare Diseases*, vol. 2, p. 34, 2007.

[9] D. Didona, L. Fania, B. Didona, R. Eming, M. Hertl, and G. Di Zenzo, "Paraneoplastic dermatoses: a brief general review and an extensive analysis of paraneoplastic pemphigus and paraneoplastic dermatomyositis," *International Journal of Molecular Sciences*, vol. 21, no. 6, 2020.

Arsenic Trioxide Treatment during Pregnancy for Acute Promyelocytic Leukemia in a 22-Year-Old Woman

Claire Cochet,[1] Marion Simonet,[2] Julie Cattin,[1] Jean-Patrick Metz,[1] Ana Berceanu,[2] Eric Deconinck,[2,3] Etienne Daguindau,[2] Françoise Schillinger,[4] Pierre Fenaux,[5] Nicolas Mottet,[1] and Yohan Desbrosses[2]

[1]*University Hospital of Besancon, Department of Obstetrics, Besançon F-25000, France*
[2]*University Hospital of Besancon, Department of Hematology, Besançon F-25000, France*
[3]*University Bourgogne Franche-Comté, INSERM, EFS BFC, UMR 1098, Interactions Hôte-Greffon Tumeur/Ingénierie Cellulaire et Génique, Besançon F-25000, France*
[4]*Etablissement Français du Sang Bourgogne Franche Comté, Laboratoire d'hématologie-Immunologie-Biologie Moléculaire, Besançon F-25020, France*
[5]*Saint Louis Hospital, Paris Diderot University, Paris F-75010, France*

Correspondence should be addressed to Claire Cochet; clairecccht@gmail.com

Academic Editor: Kazunori Nakase

Acute leukemia during pregnancy is rare (1 for 100000 pregnancies). The association of arsenic trioxide (ATO) and all-trans retinoic acid (ATRA) is known as the best therapy in standard-risk acute promyelocytic leukemia (APL). We describe the first case of a pregnancy with ATRA and ATO reported in the literature. In March 2018 at the University Hospital of Besançon, a 22-year-old woman was diagnosed with APL at 14 weeks of gestation (WG). She received a total of 2160 mg of ATRA and 930 mg of ATO between 14 and 35 WG. The mother's cytological remission was very fast. No maternal or fetal complications occurred during pregnancy. The pediatrics outcomes were good. Many case reports about ATRA exposure during the second and third trimesters report no serious adverse effect for pregnancy. ATO is teratogenic, genotoxic, and carcinogenic and passes through the placenta. Fetal exposure seems to be associated with bad pregnancy outcomes (preterm delivery, decreased birth weight, and fetal loss) and with lung diseases in young adults. No clinical trial is obviously possible, and the only data available are environmental exposure or animal studies. This case report may help medical teams to make hard decision for a treatment of APL during pregnancy.

1. Introduction

Acute promyelocytic leukemia (APL) is a sub-type of acute myeloid leukemia. It is characterized by a translocation between chromosomes 15 and 17 t(15:17), which leads to the fusion between the promyelocytic leukemia protein (PML) gene and the retinoic acid receptor α (RARα). The association of arsenic trioxide (ATO) and all-trans retinoic acid (ATRA) is known as the best therapy in standard-risk APL compared to the combination of ATRA and anthracycline-based chemotherapy [1–3].

Acute leukemia during pregnancy is rare (1 for 100000 pregnancies) [4]. APL is curable, but it can have dramatical issues for the mother and the fetus. Its treatment is an emergency. It is associated with ethical questions about the pregnancy outcomes since arsenic is known to be teratogenic. Almost 30 cases of pregnancies with ATRA during the 2nd and/or 3rd trimester are reported, but none with ATO according to the French teratogen agents reference center (CRAT). We describe the case of a treatment of APL in pregnancy with ATRA and ATO in the University Hospital of Besançon.

2. Case Description

In March 2018, the patient, a 22-year-old woman with no medical history, was 14 weeks of gestation (WG). She was diagnosed with APL on a blood test, revealing a pancytopenia and a minimal diffuse intravascular coagulopathy (white blood cells (WBC) count 4.2 × 10^9/L with 6% of circulating hypergranular blasts with bilobed nuclear, neutrophil cells count 2 × 10^9/L, hemoglobin rate 11.6 g/dL, and platelet count 8 × 10^9/L). Bone marrow aspiration confirmed the diagnosis: 82% of hypergranular blasts with bundles of Auer rods and a translocation t(15;17) on cytogenetic analyses (Figure 1). The ratio PML-RARα was 0.47.

ATRA (45 mg/m^2/day per os) was introduced immediately after the APL suspicion. The couple was informed about the unknown consequences of the recommended treatment for APL and the absence of malformation risk after 10 WG. There was no pregnancy termination demand.

We started a complete induction-treatment and added ATO 0.15 mg/kg/day with ATRA (45 mg/m^2/day) until the hematological complete remission (Figure 2). Dexamethasone 10 mg twice daily was administered to prevent ATRA differentiation syndrome. Heparin (50 UI/kg) was also introduced to prevent thrombotic events. The induction-treatment ended after 4 weeks. The tolerance was good. We quickly obtained a complete cytological remission with minimal residual disease (MRD) (PML-RARα = 7.4×10^{-4}).

The consolidation-treatment consisted in ATRA (45 mg/m^2/day) 7 cycles of 2 weeks each 4 weeks and 4 cycles of ATO of 4 weeks each 8 weeks. The MRD became undetectable after the first consolidation-treatment's cycle.

Pregnancy monitoring consisted in monthly ultrasound scans and medical examinations. Sonographies showed no fetal abnormality especially concerning neurological, renal, and cardiac development. Fetus vitality was normal, and its growth reached the 50th percentile. No maternal complication occurred: no bleeding, tension disorder, or preterm birth threat. Clinical examinations and biological observations showed no particularity. No additional treatment was necessary. The hemoglobin rate remained >10 g/dL during the pregnancy.

Since the patient's biological response was total, the consolidation-treatment was suspended after 2 cycles (around 35 WG) in anticipation of the delivery, to avoid perinatal fetal exposure of arsenic. Pregnancy progress was still totally normal, and no induction of labor was necessary.

At 40 + 6 WG, our patient gave birth to a healthy girl of 3330 g with an Apgar score of 10 at 5 minutes. The delivery process was normal. The blood sample was proceeded on the new born cord to monitor the hepatic and renal functions. Two electrocardiograms and two blood samples at day 1 and day 4 did not show any cardiac or electrolytic complication. Breast feeding was forbidden.

The consolidation-treatment was resumed 2 months after the delivery.

After the complete treatment, the cytological remission was complete with an undetectable MRD. The patient confessed she did not follow the medical prescription and never took the ATRA during the prenatal consolidation-treatment phase. The patient received a total of 2160 mg of ATRA and 930 mg of ATO while she was pregnant.

The pediatric control 3 months and 9 months after birth showed no complication. The baby's growth and development were normal.

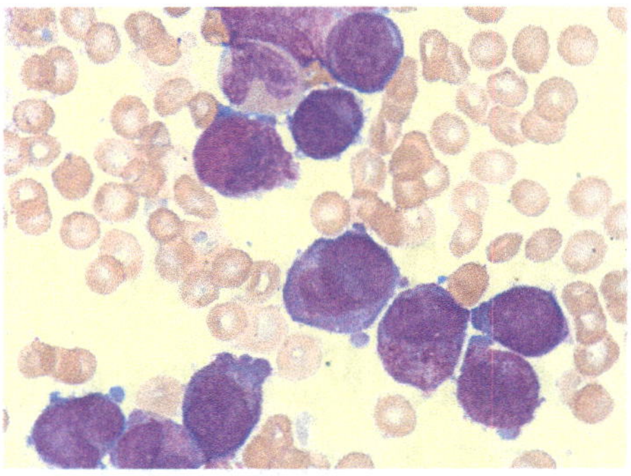

Figure 1: Medullary smear: presence of 82% of hypergranular blasts with bundles of Auer rods.

3. Results and Discussion

Cancers during pregnancy represent clinical and ethical dilemmas for medical teams. So far, evidences on pediatric outcomes after most of maternal cancer's treatment during pregnancy are reassuring [5]. APL is an oncologic emergency known to increase the risk of abortion, perinatal mortality, preterm delivery, and intrauterine growth restriction during pregnancy [6].

The combination of ATO and ATRA without chemotherapy significantly improved survival and relapse risk in patients with newly diagnosed standard-risk APL [1–3]. The French-Belgian-Swiss APL group proved in APL 2006 trial that ATO, added to a "classical" ATRA and anthracycline-based chemotherapy regimen, reduces the incidence of relapse in standard-risk APL [7]. Since the superiority of this treatment is proved, medical teams will have to deal with the question of arsenic use in pregnant women with APL. Our case confirms ATO's relevance since the patient confessed she did not take her ATRA-based treatment during the consolidation phase.

ATRA is teratogenic when given during organogenesis. When used during the 2nd or 3rd trimester of pregnancy in human, fetal arrhythmia and retarded-fetal growth have been described [8]. In our case, there was no teratogenic risk since the treatment began after the organogenesis period (4–10 WG). Many cases of pregnancies with ATRA during the second and third trimesters are reported in the literature with no serious adverse outcomes [6, 9–11].

ATO is teratogenic, genotoxic, and carcinogenic. No case report on ATO's use during pregnancy in human are available in the literature, but it passes through the placenta [12]. Animal studies proved the carcinogenic effect of high doses of arsenic (up to 10 mg/kG/day) [12, 13]. There is a variation of sensibility to arsenic exposure due to the rate of methylation, which is very different between species. Human sensibility is still unknown [14]. The only data available on intrauterine arsenic exposure effects are environmental studies. It seems to be associated with malignant and nonmalignant lung diseases in young adults through epigenetic effects [15]. Studies in Bangladesh and Taiwan showed that arsenic environmental fetal exposure is associated with decreased birth weight and preterm delivery [16, 17]. A Bangladesh cohort study also showed that there is

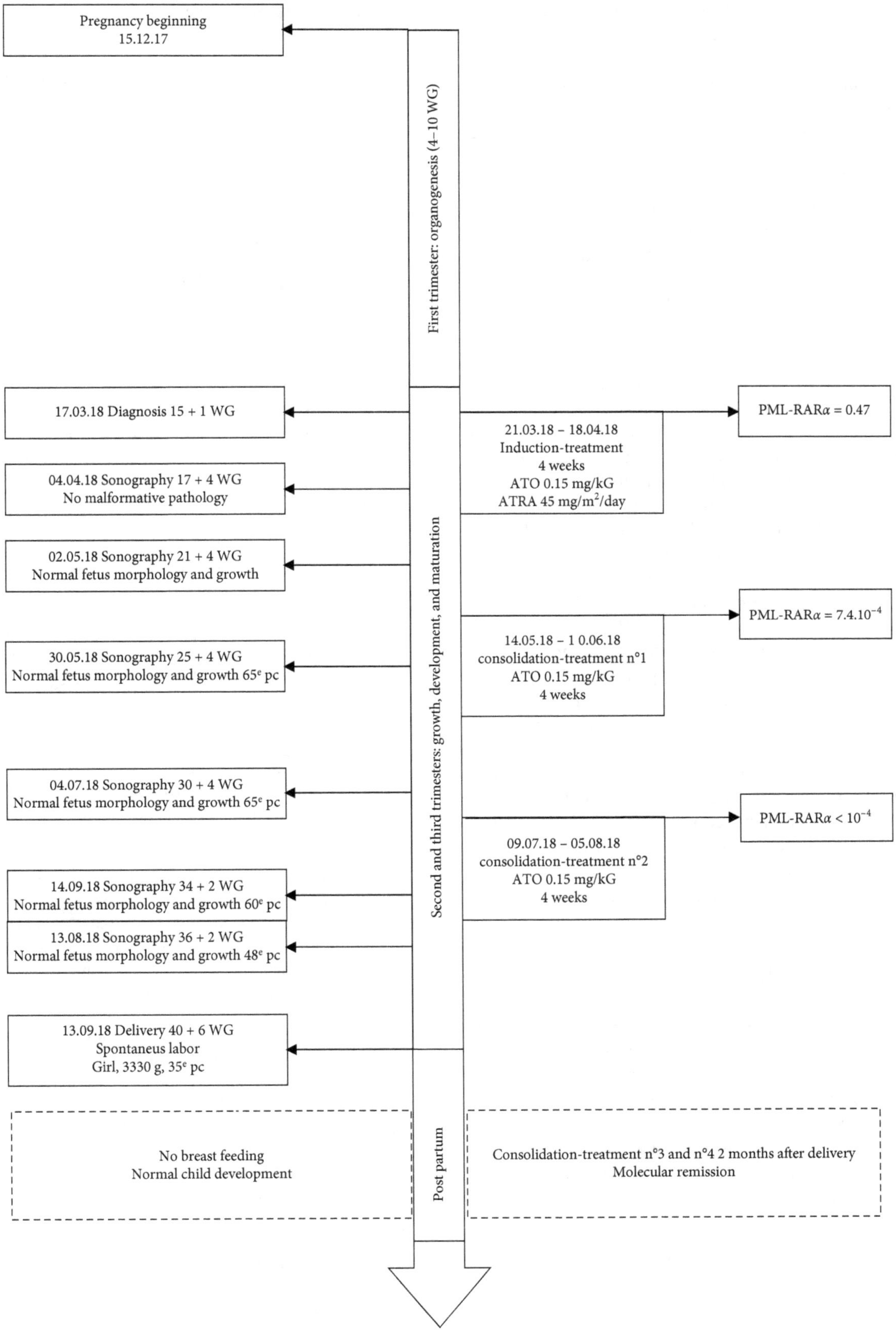

Figure 2: Chronology of treatment received, assessment of disease response, and pregnancy control.

a bigger risk of fetal loss and infant death for women who drink water with more than 50 microgram of arsenic per liter. It also seems to be a dose effect [16]. All those studies are observational and retrospective. The exact dose of arsenic maternal exposure is difficult to weight. Moreover, the environmental exposure also affects the periconceptional period and first trimester of pregnancy. In our case, the patient received more than 900 mg of arsenic trioxide. It is far more than in environmental studies. However, this exposure was limited to the second and third trimesters of pregnancy with a therapeutic window for the delivery. Since no clinical trials are obviously possible on pregnant women, the generalization of our case is difficult.

Regarding the treatment choice, it is important to highlight that any delay can compromise the remission in APL. At time of diagnosis, a medical termination of pregnancy was impossible because our patient had cytopenia and a minimal diffuse intravascular coagulopathy. Despite the limited clinical experience, ATRA was introduced immediately. This treatment seemed reasonably safe when used in patients with APL in second and third trimesters of pregnancy. Indeed, recommendations from the European LeukemiaNet published in 2009 recommend the use of ATRA and chemotherapy in these patients and an induction of labor between cycles of chemotherapy [18]. The update of these recommendations in 2019 did not make any change in the management of APL during pregnancy [19]. Anthracycline-based chemotherapy can increase the risk of abortion, prematurity, low weight, neonatal neutropenia, and sepsis [18]. For these reasons, we were reluctant to use chemotherapy during pregnancy. Moreover, anthracycline-based chemotherapy induces a long aplasia which can cause infections and hemorrhagic complications. The expected response rate with ATRA alone is not significantly different from ATRA plus chemotherapy in terms of complete remission rate, but it can have unfavorable impact on the risk of relapse [18]. Therefore, after a multidisciplinary consultation, we decided to use ATRA and ATO treatment with stringent fetal monitoring.

In our case, no adverse fetal outcome occurred. The mother's response was very fast, and it seems that pregnancy did not have effect on treatment efficiency. It will take time to assess the long-term effect on the child development of prenatal ATO exposure. Nevertheless, this unique case report may help medical teams to make hard decision for treatment of acute promyelocytic leukemia during pregnancy, whose best option is nowadays known to be ATRA and ATO.

Consent

The patient gave her consent for the publication of her medical information.

Authors' Contributions

C. C. and M. S. wrote the manuscript and prepared the figures; JP. M., A. B., and J. C. provided helpful advises with the manuscript; F. S. provided additional information and medullary smear picture; P. F., Y. D., E. D., and N. M. reviewed the manuscript.

Acknowledgments

The authors thank their colleagues of Hematology and Obstetrics Department of University Hospital of Besançon for collaboration on the care of this patient.

References

[1] F. Lo-Coco, G. Avvisati, M. Vignetti et al., "Retinoic acid and arsenic trioxide for acute promyelocytic leukemia," *New England Journal of Medicine*, vol. 369, no. 2, pp. 111–121, 2013.

[2] U. Platzbecker, G. Avvisati, L. Cicconi et al., "Improved outcomes with retinoic acid and arsenic trioxide compared with retinoic acid and chemotherapy in non-high-risk acute promyelocytic leukemia: final results of the randomized Italian-German APL0406 trial," *Journal of Clinical Oncology*, vol. 35, no. 6, pp. 605–612, 2017.

[3] A. K. Burnett, N. H. Russell, R. K. Hills et al., "Arsenic trioxide and all-trans retinoic acid treatment for acute promyelocytic leukaemia in all risk groups (AML17): results of a randomised, controlled, phase 3 trial," *The Lancet Oncology*, vol. 16, no. 13, pp. 1295–1305, 2015.

[4] U. Abadi, G. Koren, and M. Lishner, "Leukemia and lymphoma in pregnancy," *Hematology/Oncology Clinics of North America*, vol. 25, no. 2, pp. 277–291, 2011.

[5] T. Vandenbroucke, M. Verheecke, M. Fumagalli, C. Lok, and F. Amant, "Effects of cancer treatment during pregnancy on fetal and child development," *The Lancet Child & Adolescent Health*, vol. 1, no. 4, pp. 302–310, 2017.

[6] Y. Chelghoum, N. Vey, E. Raffoux et al., "Acute leukemia during pregnancy," *Cancer*, vol. 104, no. 1, pp. 110–117, 2005.

[7] L. Adès, X. Thomas, A. G. Bresler et al., "Arsenic trioxide is required in the treatment of newly diagnosed acute promyelocytic leukemia. Analysis of a randomized trial (APL 2006) by the French Belgian Swiss APL group," *Haematologica*, vol. 103, no. 12, pp. 2033–2039, 2018.

[8] Y. Terada, T. Shindo, A. Endoh, M. Watanabe, T. Fukaya, and A. Yajima, "Fetal arrhythmia during treatment of pregnancy-associated acute promtelocytic leukemia with all-trans retinoic acid and favorable outcome," *Leukemia*, vol. 11, no. 3, pp. 454-455, 1997.

[9] S. Valappil, M. Kurkar, and R. Howell, "Outcome of pregnancy in women treated with all-trans retinoic acid; a case report and review of literature," *Hematology*, vol. 12, no. 5, pp. 415–418, 2007.

[10] D. Yang and L. Hladnik, "Treatment of acute promyelocytic leukemia during pregnancy," *Pharmacotherapy*, vol. 29, no. 6, pp. 709–724, 2009.

[11] K. Agarwal, M. Patel, and V. Agarwal, "A complicated case of acute promyelocytic leukemia in the second trimester of pregnancy successfully treated with all-trans-retinoic acid," *Case Reports in Hematology*, vol. 2015, Article ID 634252, 4 pages, 2015.

[12] Report NRC (US) S to U the 1999, *A in DW. Experimental Studies*, National Academies Press, Washington, DC, USA, 2001.
[13] M. P. Waalkes, J. M. Ward, and B. A. Diwan, "Induction of tumors of the liver, lung, ovary and adrenal in adult mice after brief maternal gestational exposure to inorganic arsenic: promotional effects of postnatal phorbol ester exposure on hepatic and pulmonary, but not dermal cancers," *Carcinogenesis*, vol. 25, no. 1, pp. 133–141, 2004.
[14] M. Vahter, "Methylation of inorganic arsenic in different mammalian species and population groups," *Science Progress*, vol. 82, no. Pt 1, pp. 69–88, 1999.
[15] M. Vahter, "Health effects of early life exposure to arsenic," *Basic & Clinical Pharmacology & Toxicology*, vol. 102, no. 2, pp. 204–211, 2008.
[16] K. L. Huyck, M. L. Kile, G. Mahiuddin et al., "Maternal arsenic exposure associated with low birth weight in Bangladesh," *Journal of Occupational and Environmental Medicine*, vol. 49, no. 10, pp. 1097–1104, 2007.
[17] C.-Y. Yang, C.-C. Chang, S.-S. Tsai, H.-Y. Chuang, C.-K. Ho, and T.-N. Wu, "Arsenic in drinking water and adverse pregnancy outcome in an arseniasis-endemic area in northeastern Taiwan," *Environmental Research*, vol. 91, no. 1, pp. 29–34, 2003.
[18] M. A. Sanz, D. Grimwade, M. S. Tallman et al., "Management of acute promyelocytic leukemia: recommendations from an expert panel on behalf of the European LeukemiaNet," *Blood*, vol. 113, no. 9, pp. 1875–1891, 2009.
[19] M. A. Sanz, P. Fenaux, M. S. Tallman et al., "Management of acute promyelocytic leukemia: updated recommendations from an expert panel of the European LeukemiaNet," *Blood*, vol. 133, no. 15, pp. 1630–1643, 2019.

41

Myeloid Sarcomas Causing Unilateral Cranial Nerve Palsies in a Patient with Relapsed Acute Myeloblastic Leukemia

A. Mendez-Hernandez,[1] X. A. Andrade,[2] S. Upadhyay,[1] L. M. Parra-Rodriguez,[1] E. Caldeira,[3] L. H. Paz,[4] H. Mann,[5] M. Zia,[6] and L. Sumoza[7]

[1]*Department of Medicine, John H. Stroger Jr. Hospital of Cook County, Chicago, IL, USA*
[2]*Department of Hematology and Oncology, Mayo Clinic, Rochester, MN, USA*
[3]*Department of Medicine, Advocate Illinois Masonic Medical Center, Chicago, IL, USA*
[4]*Department of Cardiology, North Shore University Hospital, Evanston, IL, USA*
[5]*Department of Hematology and Oncology, Tufts Medical Center, Boston, MA, USA*
[6]*Department of Hematology and Oncology, John H. Stroger Jr. Hospital of Cook County, Chicago, IL, USA*
[7]*Department of Hematology and Oncology, Alton Memorial Hospital, Alton, IL, USA*

Correspondence should be addressed to A. Mendez-Hernandez; amendez@cookcountyhhs.org

Academic Editor: Stephen E. Langabeer

Myeloid sarcomas (MS) are a rare manifestation of myeloid malignancies and can often be misdiagnosed, leading to a delay in treatment. The objective of this clinical case is to highlight the challenges of the clinical presentation and to emphasize the importance of this manifestation ensuring timely diagnosis and therapy. Here, we present a 43-year-old man who was diagnosed with acute myeloblastic leukemia (AML) after being evaluated for unintentional weight loss, subcutaneous nodules, thrombocytopenia, and anemia. The patient underwent chemotherapy with complete remission and presented 4 months later with dysphagia and cranial nerve palsies. Appropriate imaging and biopsy led to a diagnosis of myeloid sarcoma, and a decision was made to begin reinduction chemotherapy for AML achieving a second complete remission although his neurological deficits did not improve. Our case illustrates the protean presentation of myeloid sarcomas; clinicians should have a high suspicion for MS and remain vigilant when unexplained signs and symptoms arise in the background of a myeloid malignancy although challenges still remain when presentation is de novo. Advancements in understanding the pathophysiology of MS have been performed but remain not completely understood. High clinical suspicion, appropriate imaging, biopsy techniques, and expertise are paramount for timely diagnosis and treatment.

1. Introduction

Myeloid sarcomas (MS) are extramedullary tumors composed of malignant immature myeloid cells and represent a rare complication of myeloid malignancies. In patients with acute myeloblastic leukemia (AML), the prevalence of MS ranges from 3 to 9%, but certain AML subtypes may have a higher prevalence. Common sites of involvement are skin, soft tissue, bone, and lymph nodes. Clinical presentation depends fundamentally on the size and location of the mass and mechanical compression of nearby structures. MS are commonly diagnosed concurrently with a primary myeloid malignancy; however, they can occur in the absence of bone marrow involvement by myeloid neoplasms which makes diagnosis challenging.

We present a case of a patient with a diagnosis of AML who presented with numerous myeloid sarcomas at the time of the first relapse.

2. Case Description

The patient is a 43-year-old man who underwent evaluation for unintentional weight loss and several abdominal subcutaneous nodules. Initial laboratory workup showed an elevated LDH level (1,165 UI/L) and the presence of anemia, thrombocytopenia, and circulating myeloid blasts in

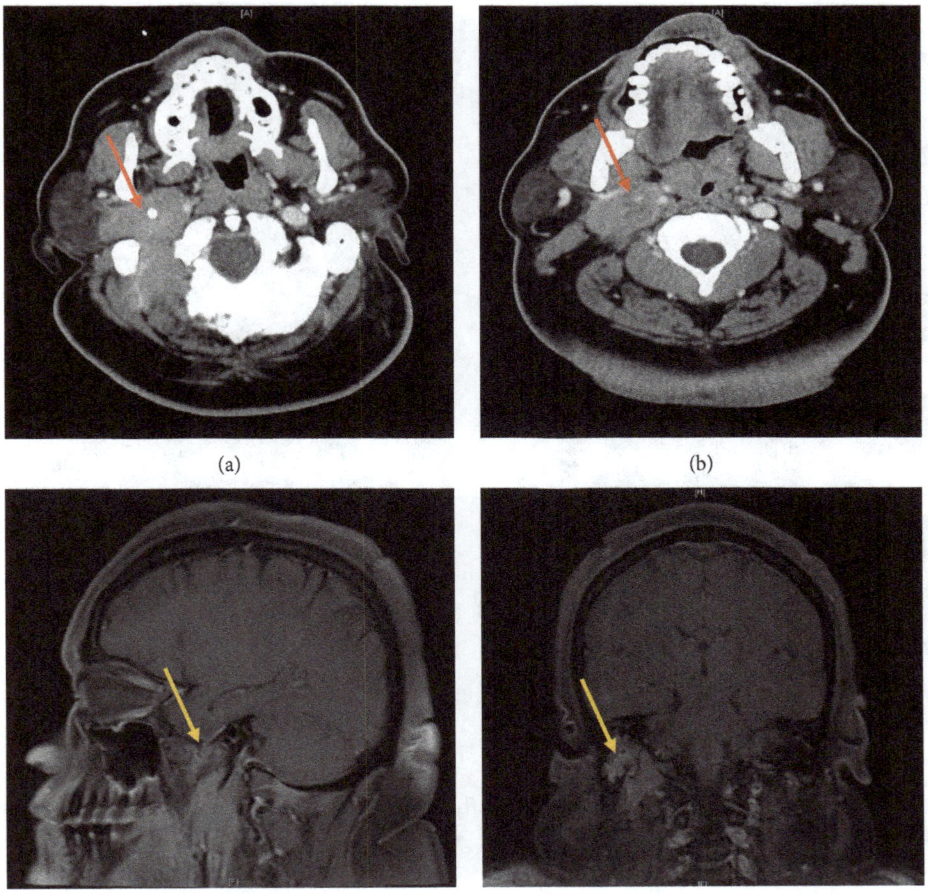

(a) (b) (c) (d)

FIGURE 1: CT scan of the neck and soft tissue showing and infiltrative mass on the right skull base extending to the right jugular and stylomastoid foramen (a) encasing and occluding the right jugular vein (b). MRI confirms a soft-tissue mass on the skull base without intracranial involvement (c and d).

peripheral blood. Initial bone marrow aspiration and biopsy showed infiltration by 47% myeloid blasts with an abnormal karyotype (46, XY t(2; 21; 8) (p13; q22; q22), del(9)(q13q22)) and positive for *AML1-ETO* fusion gene and *c-kit* mutation. Further molecular studies for CEBPA, FLT3, NPM, PML RARA, and BCR/ABL were negative for mutations, and myeloid immunophenotype was positive for CD34, MPO, CD117, and CD56. Computerized tomography (CT) of the chest, abdomen, and pelvis showed numerous soft-tissue masses involving anterior mediastinum, pericardium, and subcutaneous tissue in the abdomen and pelvis.

The patient was diagnosed with acute myeloblastic leukemia with t(8; 21) variant and extramedullary involvement. He underwent induction and consolidation chemotherapy attaining a complete remission.

Four months after completion of therapy, the patient developed acute oropharyngeal dysphagia and right facial asymmetry. On physical examination, there was a right parotid gland enlargement and a palpable left axillary four-centimeter mass. Neurological exam was relevant for palsies of cranial nerves VII, X, and XII. Laboratory results were unremarkable, and a peripheral blood smear did not show leukemic blasts. CT and magnetic resonance imaging (MRI) of the neck and soft tissue showed an infiltrative soft-tissue right skull base mass extending into the inferior margin of the right jugular foramen, right stylomastoid foramen, deep and superficial lobes of the right parotid gland, the right temporomandibular junction, and styloglossus muscle also causing displacement of the internal carotid artery, encasing the internal jugular vein to the point of occlusion. Figure 1.

CT scan of the chest, abdomen, and pelvis showed multiple soft-tissue masses in the anterior mediastinum (4×1.5 cm), left renal hilum (1.7×1.9 cm), left paraspinal area (3.6×4 cm), and subcutaneous tissue in the abdomen and pelvis Figure 2. Biopsy of the bone marrow and subcutaneous left axillary mass confirmed a relapse of acute myeloblastic leukemia and myeloid sarcoma, respectively. Figures 3 and 4. The patient underwent reinduction chemotherapy attaining a second complete response of medullary and extramedullary disease and is currently receiving consolidation chemotherapy. Despite the complete remission of his leukemia, his neurological deficits did not resolve.

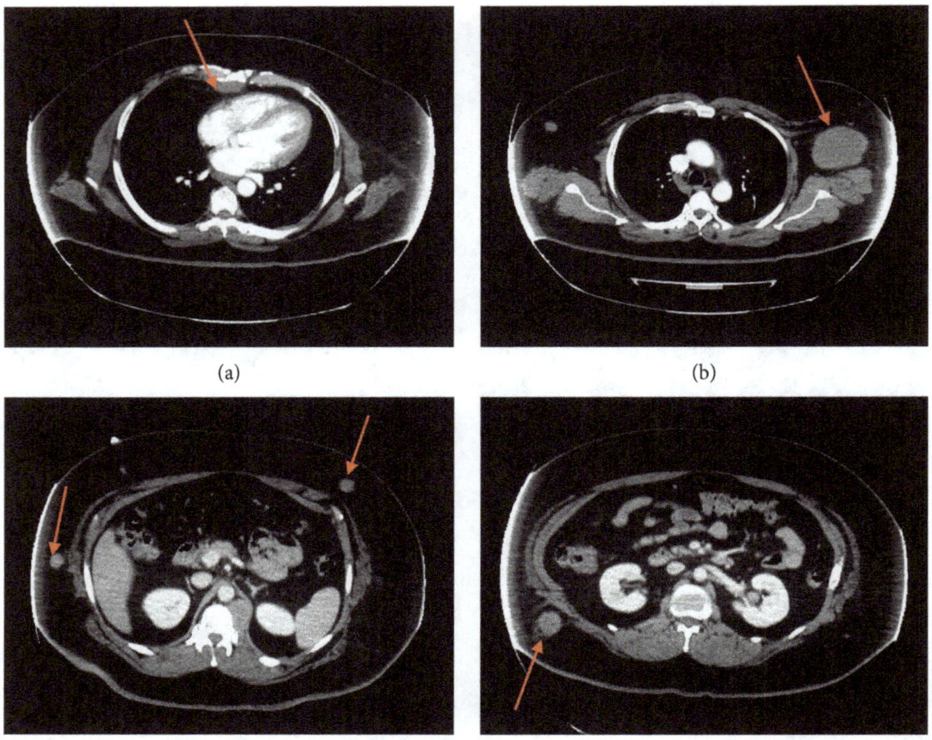

(a) (b) (c) (d)

FIGURE 2: CT scan of the chest and abdomen showing multiple soft-tissue masses involving the anterior mediastinum (a), left axillary, (b) and abdominal subcutaneous tissue (c and d).

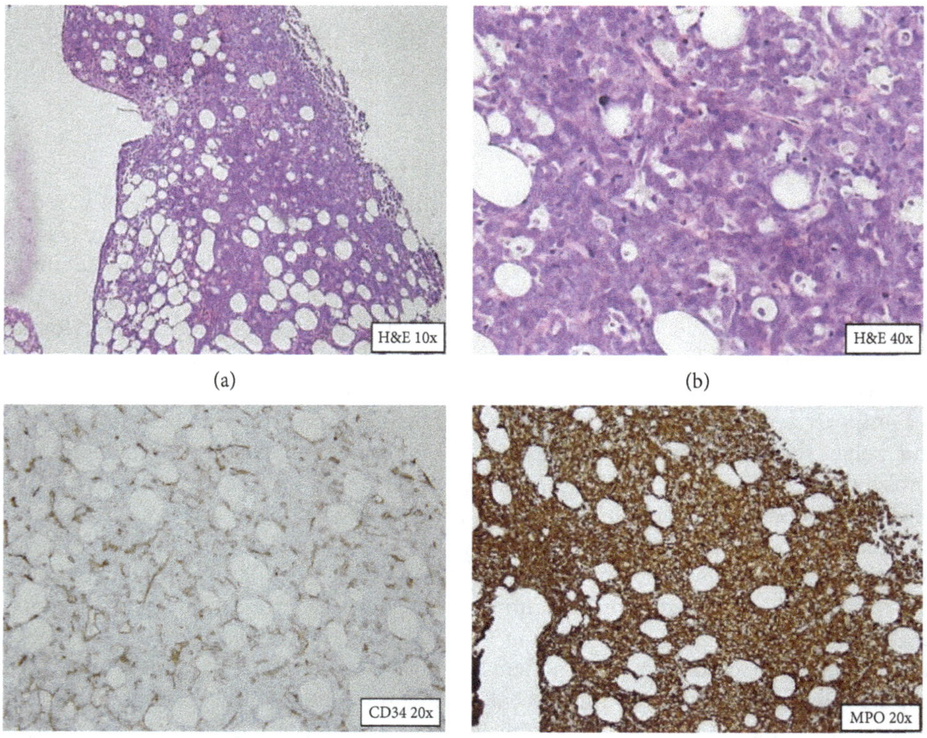

(a) (b) (c) (d)

FIGURE 3: Bone marrow biopsy showed a hypercellular bone marrow with a diffuse infiltrate of large myeloid blast cells staining positive for CD34 and MPO markers in immunohistochemistry studies.

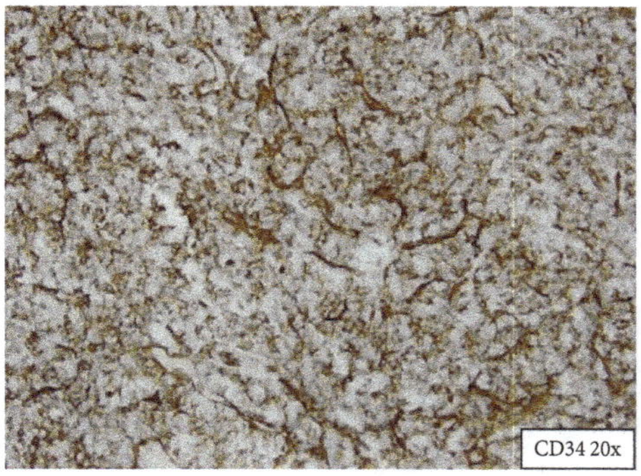

(a)

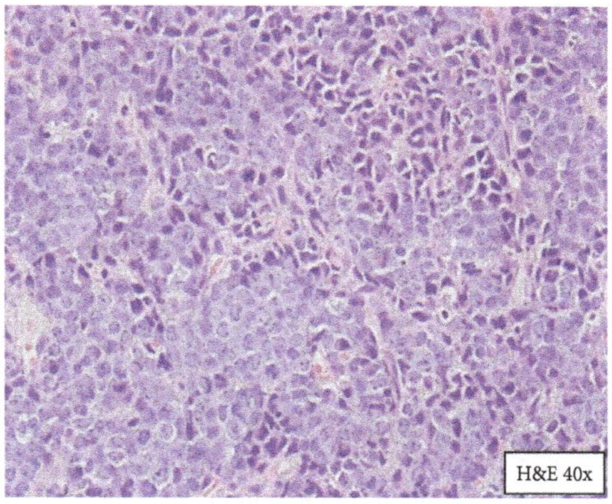

(b)

FIGURE 4: Core-needle biopsy shows a large atypical monomorphous infiltrate staining strongly for CD34 and MPO diffusely.

3. Discussion

MS is a rare extramedullary tumor of immature granulocytic cells or myeloblasts, frequently associated with myeloid hematological malignancies. In patients with AML, the prevalence of MS ranges from 2% to 8% of cases, either as a single or as a multifocal tumor [1, 2]. Interestingly, MS can precede AML by months or years in 25%, appear concomitantly in 15–35%, or follow AML in 50% of patients [1].

Patients with AML may have a different prevalence of MS based on French-American-British (FAB) classification subgroups. In large case series, the most common FAB subtype associated with MS was M5 (14%) [3], possibly demonstrating a relationship between morphologic phenotype, underlying cytogenetic and molecular abnormalities frequently associated with MS.

Cytogenetic and molecular abnormalities are present in 55% of cases of MS [4, 5, 6], the most common being t(8; 21), inv(16), and trisomy 8 [7]. Interestingly, patients with AML and t(8; 21) have a high prevalence of MS ranging from 2–30% among different studies [3, 5, 8]. C-kit proto-oncogene mutations are also common, appearing up to 87% of cases of MS [6] The clinical relevance of cytogenetic and molecular aberrancies is still under investigation.

Pathogenesis of MS is not completely understood; however, molecular interactions between malignant cells and their microenvironment is thought to be the main component. Animal studies in murine models by Stefanidakis et al. suggest a mechanism involving a supramolecular complex of matrix metalloproteinases and integrins (MMP-integrin), referred to as "*invadosome*" [9]. The interaction between the invadosome and leukocyte surface B2 integrin could mediate pericellular proteolysis and migration of AML-derived cells into extramedullary tissues [9]. Other adhesion molecules as CD56 have also been associated with higher frequency of MS; however, the exact mechanism involving this molecule is not fully understood [10, 11].

Clinical presentation depends on size and location of MS; signs and symptoms develop mainly from compression of adjacent structures due to mass effect, distorting normal organ architecture and causing pain and/or organ dysfunction. In a large case series by Pileri et al., the most commonly involved sites were the skin (28.2%), lymph nodes (16.3%), testis (6.5%), and intestines (6.5%) [3].

Patients with myeloid hematological malignancies presenting with soft-tissue masses can present a diagnostic challenge given the broad differential diagnoses including MS, infectious causes, and second primary malignancies such as melanoma or Hodgkin's lymphoma [12]. Unfortunately, up to 56% of patients of AML-related MS and up to 40% of de novo MS are misdiagnosed [2, 13]. Common misdiagnoses are diffuse large B-cell lymphoma (20%), myeloid metaplasia (4%), and small lymphocytic lymphoma (4%) [3]. Examination by an experienced pathologist and immunohistochemistry testing is paramount for accurate diagnosis.

Standard induction chemotherapy is the largely accepted treatment for AML-related MS. However, there is much debate regarding patients with isolated MS. There are currently no guidelines, but it is agreed that patients with isolated MS should receive chemotherapy given that they almost always progress to AML in a median of 5–12 months [10, 13]. Treatment strategies for relapsed AML presenting as MS vary depending on prior chemotherapy. Overall, current expert opinion recommends reinduction chemotherapy and radiation therapy if relapse occurs after chemotherapy alone [10]. Consolidation treatment with allogeneic bone marrow transplant has shown to prolong survival and may be recommended in relapsed patients [3]. The prognostic relevance of MS remains unclear, but it is widely considered as a poor prognostic factor in patients with AML [10, 14].

Future directions in patients with MS include investigation of the molecular mechanisms of disease and development of risk-stratification models to guide decisions regarding risk-adapted treatment interventions including bone marrow transplantation.

Acknowledgments

The author acknowledges the previous presentation of this case in the form of a poster in the Illinois Chapter Northern

Region from ACP performed on November 8, 2017, at the University of Illinois at Chicago.

References

[1] B. Avni and M. Koren-Michowitz, "Myeloid sarcoma: current approach and therapeutic options," *Therapeutic Advances in Hematology*, vol. 2, no. 5, pp. 309–316, 2011.

[2] J. Y. Lee, H. Chung, H. Cho et al., "Clinical characteristics and treatment outcomes of isolated myeloid sarcoma without bone marrow involvement: a single-institution experience," *Blood Research*, vol. 52, no. 3, pp. 184–192, 2017.

[3] S. A. Pileri, S. Ascani, M. C. Cox et al., "Myeloid sarcoma: clinico-pathologic, phenotypic and cytogenetic analysis of 92 adult patients," *Leukemia*, vol. 21, no. 2, pp. 340–350, 2007.

[4] P. Djurdjevic, D. Jovanovic, and D. Antic, "Isolated myeloid sarcoma of the neck and chest: differential diagnosis and therapeutic approach," *Open Medicine*, vol. 10, no. 1, pp. 34–38, 2014.

[5] W.-Y. Chen, C.-W. Wang, C.-H. chang et al., "Clinicopathologic features and responses to radiotherapy of myeloid sarcoma," *Radiation Oncology (London, England)*, vol. 8, no. 1, p. 245, 2013.

[6] J. Chen, R. R. Yanuck, S. L. Abbondanzo, W. S. Chu, and N. S. Aguilera, "C-kit (CD117) reactivity in extramedullary myeloid tumor/granulocytic sarcoma," *Archives of Pathology & Laboratory Medicine*, vol. 125, no. 11, pp. 1448–1452, 2001.

[7] H. Al-Khateeb, B. Ahmed, H. Haddad, L. Marei, and S. Abbasi, "Myeloid sarcoma: clinicopathologic, cytogenetic, and outcome analysis of 21 adult patients," *Leukemia Research and Treatment*, vol. 2011, Article ID 523168, 4 pages, 2011.

[8] J. C. Byrd, R. B. Weiss, D. C. Arthur et al., "Extramedullary leukemia adversely affects hematologic complete remission rate and overall survival in patients with t(8;21)(q22;q22): results from cancer and leukemia group B 8461," *Journal of Clinical Oncology*, vol. 15, no. 2, pp. 466–475, 1997.

[9] M. Stefanidakis, K. Karjalainen, D. E. Jaalouk et al., "Role of leukemia cell invadosome in extramedullary infiltration," *Blood*, vol. 114, no. 14, pp. 3008–3017, 2009.

[10] R. L. Bakst, M. S. Tallman, D. Douer, and J. Yahalom, "How I treat extramedullary acute myeloid leukemia," *Blood*, vol. 118, no. 14, pp. 3785–3793, 2011.

[11] X. Wang, W.-S. Li, Y. Zheng et al., "The progression of CD56+ myeloid sarcoma: a case report and literature review," *Oncology Letters*, vol. 11, no. 5, pp. 3091–3096, 2016.

[12] P. A. Hagen, C. Singh, M. Hart, and A. H. Blaes, "Differential diagnosis of isolated myeloid sarcoma: a case report and review of the literature," *Hematology Reports*, vol. 7, no. 2, 2015.

[13] D. Mitkowski and L. Gil, "Isolated myeloid sarcoma as the first manifestation of acute myeloid leukemia: a case study," *Clinical Case Reports*, vol. 5, no. 11, pp. 1802–1806, 2017.

[14] G. Goyal, A. C. Bartley, M. M. Patnaik, M. R. Litzow, A. Al-Kali, and R. S. Go, "Clinical features and outcomes of extramedullary myeloid sarcoma in the United States: analysis using a national data set," *Blood Cancer Journal*, vol. 7, no. 8, e592 pages, 2017.

42

Biological versus Clinical Risk Factors in Acute Myeloid Leukemia: Is There a Winner?

M. Malagola,[1] N. Polverelli,[1] V. Cancelli,[1] E. Morello,[1] A. Turra,[1] E. Borlenghi,[2] F. Cattina,[1] B. Rambaldi,[1] S. Bernardi,[1,3] C. Zanaglio,[1,3] Elif Dereli Eke,[1,3] L. Gandolfi,[1] M. Farina,[1] and D. Russo[1]

[1]*Chair of Hematology, Department of Clinical and Surgical Sciences, University of Brescia, Bone Marrow Transplant Unit, ASST-Spedali Civili, Brescia, Italy*
[2]*Unit of Hematology, ASST-Spedali Civili, Brescia, Italy*
[3]*Centro di Ricerca Ematologica-Oncologia AIL (CREA), ASST-Spedali Civili, Brescia, Italy*

Correspondence should be addressed to M. Malagola; michelemalagola@yahoo.it

Academic Editor: Håkon Reikvam

We present a case of a patient with a three-month history of peripheral blood cytopenia without a confirmed diagnosis of myelodysplastic syndrome, who developed a favourable-risk acute myeloid leukemia (AML), according to the European Leukemia Net (ELN) criteria. The patient achieved a complete remission with incomplete platelet recovery (CRi) after induction. The patient achieved the morphological CR after the first consolidation and completed the first-line treatment with a syngeneic stem cell transplantation (SCT). A disease relapse occurred after one year of CR (blast cell count in the bone marrow 15%), and the patient was offered a haplo-SCT, which he refused due to personal reasons. In this paper, we discuss the interplay between clinical and biological risk factors in non-high-risk AML patients and speculate that some old clinical risk factors (e.g., age of the patient, achievement of CR after induction, and previous history of myelodysplastic syndrome) may still impact on the treatment decision algorithm of some of these patients.

1. Introduction

The treatment algorithm of newly diagnosed AML patients is currently driven by ELN criteria [1]. ELN classification is based on the presence of specific mutations on target genes, with the identification of peculiar clinical-biological entities (e.g., AML with FlT3-ITD mutation or NPM-1A mutation, variably combined together). According to these criteria, allogeneic stem cell transplantation (allo-SCT) should be offered to those patients aged less than 65 years, who have less than 20–30% of expected long-term overall survival with conventional chemotherapy (usually accounting for 40–50% of the cases). Favourable and intermediate risk patients, who may be cured in 50 to 80% of the cases with conventional chemotherapy, are usually excluded from first-line allo-SCT. In this setting, there is still a debate on the role of some clinical risk factors (e.g., patient's age, previous history of myelodysplastic syndrome, and CR achievement after induction), and the management of these patients is still largely dependent on single-center internal guidelines.

2. Case Presentation

Recently, a 67-year-old man with acute myeloid leukemia (AML) was referred to our Transplant Center for salvage treatment in overt relapse. He was diagnosed with a primary AML in December 2017. A three-month history of peripheral blood cytopenia before AML diagnosis was present, without a confirmed diagnosis of myelodysplastic syndrome. The cytogenetics was normal; Flt3-ITD and point mutation and NPM mutation were absent; the only molecular lesion as detected by RT-qPCR was a biallelic CEBP-alpha mutation. This lesion was absent in the germinal DNA. Thus, the disease risk was classified as favourable according to the recently published European Leukemia Net (ELN) criteria [1]. The patient received an induction with a conventional idarubicine, cytarabine, and etoposide combination and achieved a complete remission with incomplete platelet recovery (CRi). Subsequently, 3 cycles of high-dose cytarabine was administered. Considering the standard risk of the disease at diagnosis, the availability of a homozygous twin, and the expected low transplant-related mortality (TRM) of syngeneic allo-SCT, the latter was performed for intensification. The conditioning regimen was adapted to the patient's age (busulfan 6.4 mg/kg total dose and fludarabine 160 mg/sqm total dose). A complete hematological recovery was obtained after the first consolidation cycle and maintained since November 2018, when peripheral blood cytopenia occurred, with a bone marrow leukemic infiltration of 15%. Thus, the patient was referred for salvage treatment with haplo-SCT from his son. Unfortunately, the patient refused the procedure due to personal reason and is currently lost to follow-up.

3. Discussion

In the nineties, the prognosis of AML was mainly influenced by cytogenetics and by clinical risk factors, mainly represented by the age, the achievement of CR after the first induction cycle, and a previous history of myelodysplastic syndrome [2]. In those years, the decision of whether or not to perform an allo-SCT was relatively easy to take, and 60–70% of the cases were addressed to allo-SCT as soon as possible. In the subsequent years, the biological characterization of AML underwent a rapid and progressive evolution, and now, more than 25 genes have been clearly identified as crucial for AML onset, progression, and prognosis [3]. Among these genes, the most important ones for disease-risk identification are Flt3, NPM-1, IHD-1, IDH-2, CEBP-alpha, GATA-1, ASXL1, and P53 [3]. As a consequence, the recently published ELN criteria for AML risk stratification in AML include some of these genes and identify peculiar biological entities, with different prognosis and for which different therapeutic strategies are suggested [1]. Moreover, minimal residual disease (MRD), either by flow cytometry or by RT-PCR on target genes, has been integrated in the dynamic assessment of treatment response, thus refining risk allocation [4–9]. A recent paper published by Chen and colleagues suggested that both MRD and the type of response after induction chemotherapy (CR vs CRi) are independent prognostic factors for outcome in patients achieving remission [6]. Minetto and colleagues addressed the issue of the best time-point of MRD assessment by flow cytometry. In a cohort of AML patients treated with a fludarabine-based induction regimen, they showed that early MRD assessment (after induction) is the strongest predictor of outcome [8]. Moreover, they confirmed their previous observation that the integration MRD monitoring by flow cytometry and molecular biology on WT1 leads to an improvement in prognostic stratification. This was previously demonstrated in their paper on the impact of MRD status before allo-SCT. Thanks to the combination of the high positive predictive value of WT1 MRD and the high negative predictive value of flow cytometry MRD, three cohorts of patients could be identified according to MRD status before transplant, showing worsening outcome: negative by WT1 and flow cytometry, positive by flow cytometry and negative by WT1, and positive by WT1 and flow cytometry [8]. In this complex scenario, allo-SCT should be offered to those patients who have less than 20–30% of expected long-term overall survival with conventional chemotherapy (usually high-risk AML) [7]. In the favourable/intermediate-risk group, the old clinical prognostic factors should be considered in the treatment algorithm, with particular regard to allo-SCT indication. In this setting, it is unquestionable that a 35-year-old man with a primary resistant AML should be addressed to allo-SCT as soon as a CR is achieved, but the agreement among hematologists of whether or not to perform an allo-SCT front-line in a patient as the one reported here is probably less evident (67-year-old patient, with favourable risk AML, with CRi after induction, and with a previous history of peripheral blood cytopenia). This fact may reflect the enthusiasm of hematologists in the era of molecular markers of AML that put a shadow on the role of the old clinical factors. In the clinical case presented, the choice to perform a syngeneic SCT was made, considering the safety of the procedure even though it is well known that the lack of graft versus leukemia (GVL) effect in this transplant is the cause of its failure in the great majority of patients. Moreover, the reduction of the conditioning intensity, which was necessary for the patient's age, is often performed in the setting of allo-SCT, where the GVL effect is present. In the setting of syngeneic SCT, the reduction of conditioning intensity put the patient at risk of disease recurrence, for incomplete leukemia eradication. How could we improve the risk definition of the patient presented in this case? The recent development of the next generation sequencing (NGS) technology has dramatically expanded the genes that can be studied and analyzed both in the diagnostic phase and in the MRD monitoring [10]. An extensive study of the genes involved in leukemogenesis and with known prognostic impact could help in better depicting the complexity of the leukemic transformation and could give clear prognostic information. Focusing on this clinical case, if we had found mutations in genes such as p53 or DNMT3A or ASXL1 at diagnosis, we would have considered the patient at high risk of disease recurrence, thus with a strong indication of front-line allo-SCT. The extensive and routine use of NGS technology in the incoming future will be a useful tool to improve the prognostic classification of AML.

In 2011, we published a simple and reproducible prognostic score for cytogenetically normal AML (CN-AML) [11]. This score was created in 337 patients with CN-AML (training set) and then validated in a cohort of 197 CN-AML (validation set). The variables that were independent prognostic factors for event-free survival (EFS) and overall survival (OS) in the training set were: age ≥ 50 years, secondary AML, and white blood cell count (WBC) $\geq 20 \times 10^9$/L. The patients of the training set were stratified into three groups: low, intermediate, and high risk. The median EFS was 25, 12, and 7 months in the low-,

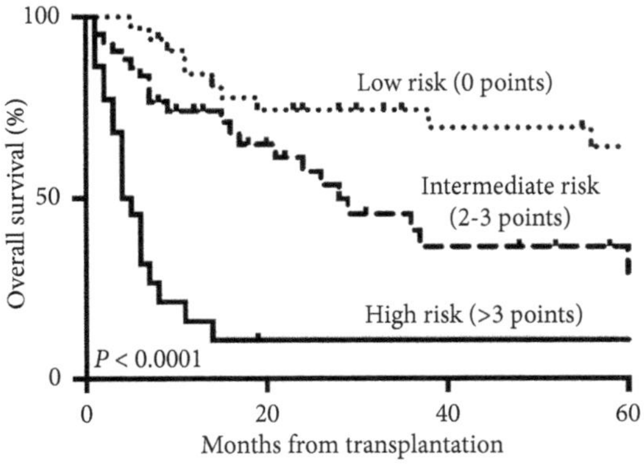

FIGURE 1: OS of the 101 patients with AML submitted to allo-SC, according to the PIS.

intermediate-, and high-risk groups ($p < 0.0001$), respectively. The median OS was not reached in the low-risk group and was 19 and 10 months in the intermediate- and high-risk groups ($p < 0.0001$). Very similar results were obtained in the validation set. We concluded that the score was useful for dissecting patients with CN-AML and different prognosis and that it could be integrated with the biological markers that, in those years, were still not completely validated.

We recently retrospectively collected the data on 101 AML patients submitted to allo-SCT in our Center, between 2010 and 2017. In about 50% of the cases, the median age was greater than 55 years and 79% of the patients had a primary AML. Focusing on ELN risk, 60% and 40% had an unfavorable and a favourable/intermediate-risk AML, respectively. The patients with favourable/intermediate-ELN risk were addressed to allo-SCT because of primary refractory AML in 69% of the cases and for other clinical risk factors in 31% of the cases. 53% of the patients were allo-transplanted in first CR, 55% received a myeloablative conditioning regimen, and 73% received peripheral blood stem cells. 43% and 44% of them received a matched sibling and a matched unrelated donor, respectively. At the time of allo-SCT, the HCT-CI index according to the published criteria [12] was <3 in 36% of the cases and the performance status according to the Karnofsky index was 100% in 40%, between 80 and 90% in 51%, and less than 70% in 9% of the cases. By univariate analysis, the factors significantly influencing OS were age >55 years at transplant ($p = 0.037$; HR 1.77; 95% CI 1.04–3.01), induction refractoriness ($p = 0.003$; HR 2.47; 95% CI 1.37–4.44), morphological CR at allo-SCT ($p < 0.001$; HR 0.25; 95% CI 0.14–0.45), and Karnofsky PS < 90% ($p < 0.001$; HR 3.59; 95% CI 2.96–6.26). By multivariate analysis, the independent factors associated with OS were age >55 years at transplant ($p = 0.03$; HR 2.3; 95% CI 1.33–4.00), morphological CR at allo-SCT ($p = 0.039$; HR 0.45; 95% CI 0.21–0.96), and Karnofsky PS < 90% ($p = 0.01$; HR 2.56; 95% CI 1.22–5.36). A prognostic index score (PIS) was calculated by totaling the score derived from the regression coefficients of each clinical variable significantly associated with prognosis by multivariate analysis. In particular, the following scores were associated to the single variables: 2 for age >55 years, 3 for Karnofsky <90%, and 2 for no CR at the time of allo-SCT. Patients were grouped in low-risk (PIS = 0), intermediate-risk (PIS 2-3), and high-risk (PIS > 3) groups. Figure 1 reports the OS of patients in the three cohorts. The OS at 5 years was 65%, 35%, and 10% in the low-, intermediate- and high-risk groups, respectively ($p < 0.0001$).

Our data, both in patients with CN-AML [11] and in patients submitted to allo-SCT (unpublished), strongly suggest that clinical factors still have an impact on the outcome of AML. We think that these factors should still be accurately integrated in the risk assessment of AML. In the era of the next generation sequencing, many more data on molecular markers of AML will be available [10]. Moreover, the dynamic monitoring of MRD either by flow cytometry or by molecular biology is becoming a useful tool for early allocation of patients in different risk categories and, for example, for addressing patients who do not clear MRD to intensive treatments or new target drugs before allo-SCT [8, 9]. As a consequence, clinicians have to be very skillful in combining these data with the clinical prognostic factors. In other words, we think that there is no winner between biology and clinic, but a strong integration between these two elements is helpful to choose the best treatment program for our patients.

Authors' Contributions

MM, PN, and CV analyzed the data and drafted the article. CV, CF, BR, GL, and FM collected the data. EM, TA, BE, BS, CZ, EDE, and DR revised the paper. All the authors gave their final approval to the manuscript before submission.

References

[1] H. Döhner, E. Estey, D. Grimwade et al., "Diagnosis and management of AML in adults: 2017 ELN recommendations from an international expert panel," *Blood*, vol. 129, no. 4, pp. 424–447, 2017.

[2] G. Visani, P. Bernasconi, M. Boni et al., "The prognostic value of cytogenetics is reinforced by the kind of induction/consolidation therapy in influencing the outcome of acute myeloid leukemia—analysis of 848 patients," *Leukemia*, vol. 15, no. 6, pp. 903–909, 2001.

[3] L. Bullinger, K. Döhner, and H. Döhner, "Genomics of acute myeloid leukemia diagnosis and pathways," *Journal of Clinical Oncology*, vol. 35, no. 9, pp. 934–946, 2017.

[4] J. A. L. Yin, M. A. O'Brien, R. K. Hills, S. B. Daly, K. Wheatley, and A. K. Burnett, "Minimal residual disease monitoring by quantitative RT-PCR in core binding factor AML allows risk stratification and predicts relapse: results of the United Kingdom MRC AML-15 trial," *Blood*, vol. 120, no. 14, pp. 2826–2835, 2012.

[5] E. Abdelhamid, C. Preudhomme, N. Helevaut et al., "Minimal residual disease monitoring based on FLT3 internal tandem duplication in adult acute myeloid leukemia," *Leukemia Research*, vol. 36, no. 3, pp. 316–323, 2012.

[6] X. Chen, H. Xie, B. L. Wood et al., "Relation of clinical response and minimal residual disease and their prognostic impact on outcome in acute myeloid leukemia," *Journal of Clinical Oncology*, vol. 33, no. 11, pp. 1258–1264, 2015.

[7] M. Malagola, C. Skert, E. Borlenghi et al., "Postremission sequential monitoring of minimal residual disease by WT1 Q-PCR and multiparametric flow cytometry assessment predicts relapse and may help to address risk-adapted therapy in acute myeloid leukemia patients," *Cancer Medicine*, vol. 5, no. 2, pp. 265–274, 2016.

[8] P. Minetto, F. Guolo, M. Clavio et al., "Early minimal residual disease assessment after AML induction with fludarabine, cytarabine and idarubicin (FLAI) provides the most useful prognostic information," *British Journal of Haematology*, vol. 184, no. 3, pp. 457–460, 2019.

[9] F. Guolo, P. Minetto, M. Clavio et al., "Combining flow cytometry and WT1 assessment improves the prognostic value of pre-transplant minimal residual disease in acute myeloid leukemia," *Haematologica*, vol. 102, no. 9, pp. e348–e351, 2017.

[10] M. Malagola, C. Skert, M. Vignetti et al., "A simple prognostic scoring system for newly diagnosed cytogenetically normal acute myeloid leukemia: retrospective analysis of 530 patients," *Leukemia & Lymphoma*, vol. 52, no. 12, pp. 2329–2335, 2011.

[11] G. Visani, F. Loscocco, A. Isidori, and P. P. Piccaluga, "Genetic profiling in acute myeloid leukemia: a path to predicting treatment outcome," *Expert Review of Hematology*, vol. 11, no. 6, pp. 455–461, 2018.

[12] M. L. Sorror, M. B. Maris, R. Storb et al., "Hematopoietic cell transplantation (HCT)-specific comorbidity index: a new tool for risk assessment before allogeneic HCT," *Blood*, vol. 106, no. 8, pp. 2912–2919, 2005.

43

Primary Cutaneous Diffuse Large B-Cell Lymphoma of the Upper Limb: Double Hit/ Double Expressor with CNS Involvement: From Hospice to Remission

Brenda S. Castillo,[1] Maria L. Rodriguez,[2] Ju-Hsien John Chao,[3] and Behyar Zoghi[3]

[1]*Texas Tech University Health Sciences Center Paul L. Foster School of Medicine, El Paso, Texas, USA*
[2]*Brown University, Providence, RI, USA*
[3]*Methodist Hospital, Texas Transplant Institute, San Antonio, Texas, USA*

Correspondence should be addressed to Behyar Zoghi; behyar.zoghi@mhshealth.com

Academic Editor: Kiyotaka Kawauchi

We report a patient with diffuse large B-cell lymphoma of skin, nongerminal center type double hit double expressor, with an initial presentation as a left forearm mass. The patient underwent chemotherapy after initial diagnosis. After chemotherapy regimen, she developed a second mass, followed by CNS involvement with neurological defects. At this time, a three line of chemotherapy was used with minimal effects. The patient was deemed terminal and was recommended hospice care. The patient decided to continue with skin and crainospinal radiotherapy and intrathecal chemotherapy; she achieved complete remission. After achieving complete remission, the patient underwent an autologous stem cell transplant with minimal transplant-related toxicity.

1. Introduction

Diffuse large B-cell lymphoma (DLBCL) is the most common type of non-Hodgkin lymphoma (NHL), accounting for 30–58% of all cases [1]. High-grade B-cell lymphoma (HGBL) is a new World Health Organization classification of high-risk DLBCL, characterized by double hit (DH) or triple hit MYC and BCL2 and/or BCL6 rearrangement [2]. Different types of chemotherapy regimens such as R-CHOP (rituximab, cyclophosphamide, doxorubicin, vincristine, and prednisone) and DA-R-EPOCH (dose adjusted rituximab, etoposide, prednisone, cyclophosphamide, and doxorubicin) have been used with less response [3]. The nongerminal center subtype of HGBL-DH occurs in 1.7% of all DLBCL patients, and it presents with MYC/BCL6 rearrangements more often than MYC/BCL2 rearrangements [4]. There are no significant prognostic differences between MYC/BCL2 and MYC/MCL6 outcomes, and there is no established difference or similarity between each subtype of HGBL-DH [5]. Given the high risk of relapse of disease, maintenance therapy using lenalidomide or venetoclax was attempted and has had positive results, but there is no recommended primary therapy as of yet [6].

We present a case with characteristics of DLBCL with primary skin involvement. There are five types of primary cutaneous B-cell lymphoma: marginal zone primary cutaneous B-cell lymphoma, centrofollicular primary cutaneous lymphoma, diffuse large B-cell primary cutaneous lymphoma-leg type, large B-cell primary cutaneous lymphoma (NOS), and intravascular large B-cell primary cutaneous lymphoma [7]. The case we present behaves like cutaneous DLBCL leg type, which is the most aggressive subtype, with MYC and BCL2/BCL6 expression. DLBCL leg type presents with red to bluish nodules or tumors on one or both lower legs. Only about 10% to 15% of these patients are noted to develop lesions outside of the lower extremities, as was the case with our patient, who presented with a left arm nodule [4]. DLBCL leg type tumors are more aggressive with worse outcomes, since they frequently disseminate to lymph nodes. Given the relapse and progression of the disease, which was initially noted in the skin and immunohistochemistry analysis, our case behaved as DLBCL leg type. Lymph node involvement was secondary since the only lymph nodes involved are the axillary lymph nodes, the most proximal to the cutaneous involvement. Chemotherapy by itself had minimal effect in controlling the disease. Only after the addition of radiation therapy was complete remission achieved. The patient subsequently received autologous stem cell transplant as consolidation therapy.

2. Case Presentation

In 2016, a 39-year-old healthy woman began having night sweats, and within the next month, she discovered an erythematous, round skin lesion in her left, middle forearm. She presented to her primary care provider with a progressively growing erythematous nodule and was treated with antibiotics (Figure 1(a)). While the initial lesion continued to grow, a second lesion appeared next to the first (Figure 1(b)). The patient was evaluated by a dermatologist, and two biopsies were obtained. The patient was diagnosed with DLBCL non-GC subtype (Figures 1(c)–1(e)). CT showed left axillary lymphadenopathy with lymphoma confined to the left forearm. Bone marrow biopsy showed no lymphoma. PET scan showed lymphoma in the left forearm and left axilla.

The patient began R-CHOP regimen on April 2017. Following three cycles of R-CHOP, the tumor continued to grow (Figure 2). In addition to the R-CHOP regimen, radiotherapy to the left forearm begun in May 2017. After the fifth R-CHOP cycle and radiotherapy completion, the tumor began to shrink (Figure 3).

Unfortunately, one month later, the patient noted a nodule on her left upper arm (Figure 4(a)). Two more cycles of R-CHOP were administered. In the next month, restaging PET/CT showed an increase in nodularity of the left forearm, indicating progressive lymphoma. Fine-needle aspiration (FNA) of the left forearm lesion was positive for DLBCL non-GC subtype. The R-CHOP regimen was stopped, and the patient received one cycle of E-SHAP (etoposide, methylprednisolone, and cytarabine). Skin masses and nodules in her left upper arm continued to grow fast within 3 months (Figure 4(b)). The regimen was changed to rituximab, gemcitabine, and oxaliplatin with no response. The patient was evaluated by the bone marrow transplant team at the Methodist hospital and was referred to MD Anderson Cancer Center (MDACC) to participate in a chimeric antigenic receptor (CAR) T-cell clinical trial.

Lymph node (left axilla) needle biopsy at MDACC was diagnostic for DLBCL non-GC subtype immunophenotype. The neoplasm showed a diffuse pattern composed predominantly of large cells with immunoblastic cytological features. Immunohistochemical studies were reviewed, and the neoplastic cells were positive for CD19, CD20, PAX-5, BCL2, BCL6, and MUM-1/IRF4. Ki-67 showed a proliferation rate of 70–80%, negative for Epstein–Barr virus-encoded small RNA (EBER). Immunohistochemistry using c-MYC antibody showed 70–80% of neoplastic cells weakly to moderately positive for MYC. Combined with the BCL2 result, the neoplasm was a double expressor immunophenotype (Figure 5). MYC FISH analysis showed a positive result for MYC gene rearrangement. IGH BCL2 FISH was negative for IGH/BCL-2 gene rearrangement. BCL6 FISH was positive for BCL6 gene rearrangement with 70% of the interphase indicating BCL6 rearrangement.

Although the patient's stem cells were collected in November 2017 and only CD4 cells were amplified, she did not receive the infusion. She developed Bell's palsy of the right side of her face that was attributed to a viral illness for which she received treatment. She also developed double vision. Lumbar puncture showed atypical lymphoid cells, consistent with involvement by patient's lymphoma. CSF analysis by flow cytometry was positive for large number of aberrant B cells with partial CD10 expression. Aberrant cell phenotype was positive for CD10, CD19, CD20, and CD22. At the beginning of December, the left upper arm mass had continued to grow (Figure 6(a)). She received high-dose methotrexate. Days later, a third nodule was present in the patient's left forearm (Figure 6(b)). At the end of the month, she was admitted to MDACC ER, was unable to walk, and had generalized weakness.

Brain MRI showed no acute intracranial abnormality or intracranial metastasis. Lumbar puncture CSF showed large malignant cells, consistent with involvement by the patient's known DLBCL. Cervical, thoracic, and lumbar MRI showed C5 metastasis that extended into the right C4-C5 and C5-C6 foramina. No spinal cord compression was observed. Days later, lumbar puncture CSF showed large malignant lymphoid cells, morphologically consistent with involvement by patient's known DLBCL. CSF flow cytometry was positive for lymphoma with aberrant cell phenotype positive for CD19, CD20, CD22, CD38, CD43, CD79b, and CD200. Cervical, thoracic, and lumbar MRI showed an enhancing mass involving the right C5 vertebral body with extension into the right C4-C5 foramina (Figures 7(a) and 7(b)) and epidural extension of tumor along the right aspect of the spinal canal touching the right aspect of the cord and leptomeningeal metastasis (Figure 7(c)). She received Ferreri regimen (high dose of methotrexate with high-dose cytarabine) followed by intrathecal methotrexate. Lumbar puncture CSF showed rare atypical cells, suspicious for involvement by patient's known large B-cell lymphoma. The patient was told that was terminal and advised to seek comfort measures.

She decided to continue treatment and radiotherapy to the left arm, 3000 cGy for 10 cycles. After beginning left arm radiotherapy, she received craniospinal radiation 2000 cGy for 4 cycles. She began to walk again, and at the time, her left forearm tumor had subsided. Lumbar puncture CSF in the middle of January showed no malignant cells.

In February 2018, the patient had a left upper arm mass infection, treated with IV antibiotics, and the left arm tumor mass was excised (Figure 8). She received a skin graft from her left thigh (Figure 9). Biopsy showed no evidence of lymphoma.

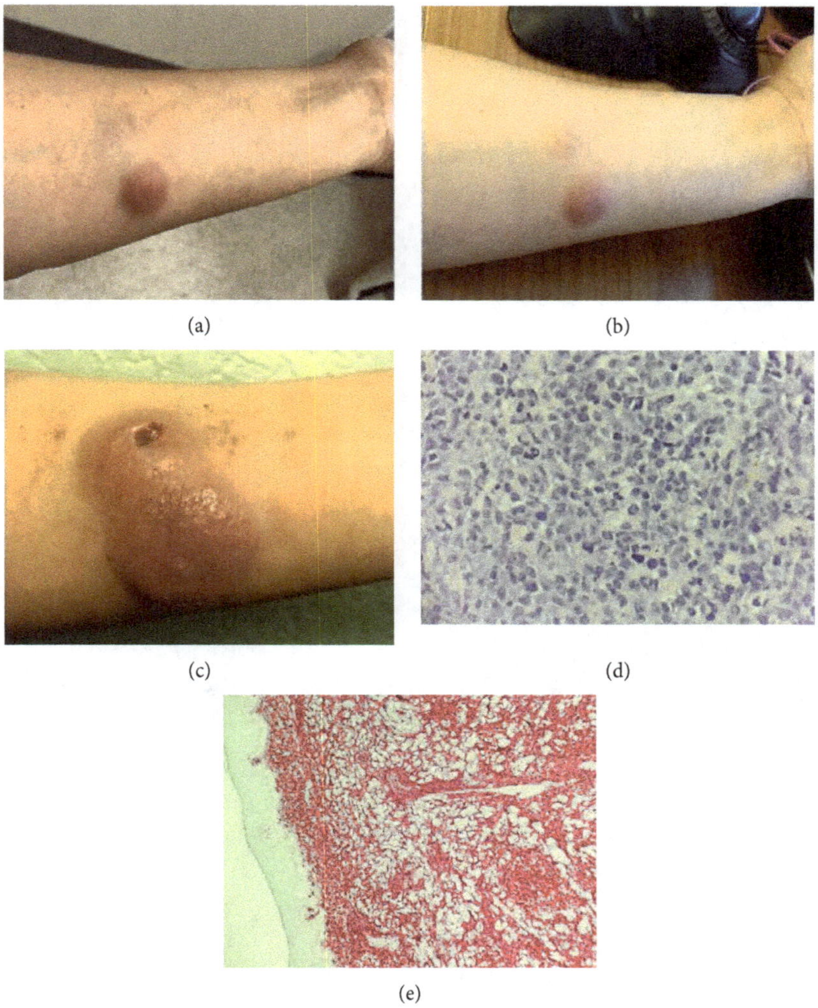

FIGURE 1: Left forearm masses. (a) Initial mass at time of antibiotic treatment on 03/03/17. (b) Appearance of the second lesion on 03/08/17. (c) Lesion appearance on 03/30/17. Skin biopsy representing cutaneous (d) DLBCL and (e) CD20 staining.

A month later, CSF showed revealed no lymphoma. PET/CT, skull base to midthigh, showed soft nodular recurrence in the patient's left arm, as well as asymmetric uptake in the patient's right shoulder musculature. She was reevaluated by MDACC in order to continue her involvement in CAR T-cell clinical trial. The patient had regained the ability to walk, and talk without limitation, but had a residual left facial droop. Tumor status was as assessed as complete remission by PET; external CSF reports are negative for lymphoma. After evaluation, it was confirmed that she was in remission. In May 2018, CSF revealed no lymphoma. Bone marrow biopsy showed no blasts or lymphoma, and it showed hypocellular 35–40% marrow with active progressive trilineage hematopoiesis. Her left forearm and left upper arm skin had healed (Figure 8). She received consolidation therapy with autologous bone marrow transplant, with conditioning regimen of rituximab, thiotepa, and carmustine. The patient was engrafted by day 12 and had a readmission shortly for *C. diff* diarrhea which was treated appropriately. The patient was subsequently discharged and is followed as an outpatient.

3. Discussion

The standard therapy for patients with DLBCL non-GC subtype is R-CHOP. Our patient presented with DLBCL non-GC subtype on the left forearm and was initially treated with R-CHOP. Her condition deteriorated, and treatment regimen was switched to E-SHAP, then to rituximab, gemcitabine, oxaliplatin, and high-dose methotrexate, showing no resolution. Her disease progressed to involve the CNS, leaving her unable to walk. Upon treatment with radiotherapy, she went into remission. Immunohistochemistry and cytogenetic analysis of the patient revealed expression of MYC and BCL2, along with MYC and BCL6 gene rearrangements. The use of radiotherapy caused left forearm, left upper arm, and CNS lymphoma eradication. Immunohistochemistry and cytogenetic analysis should be considered when deciding on treatment modalities, given that expression of MYC and BCL2 (double hit lymphoma) and MYC and BCL6 gene rearrangement, make disease progression not only more aggressive in course, and higher risk to involve the CNS, but it is also associated with poor outcomes using the R-CHOP regimen [3]. Radiotherapy should be considered as a first-line

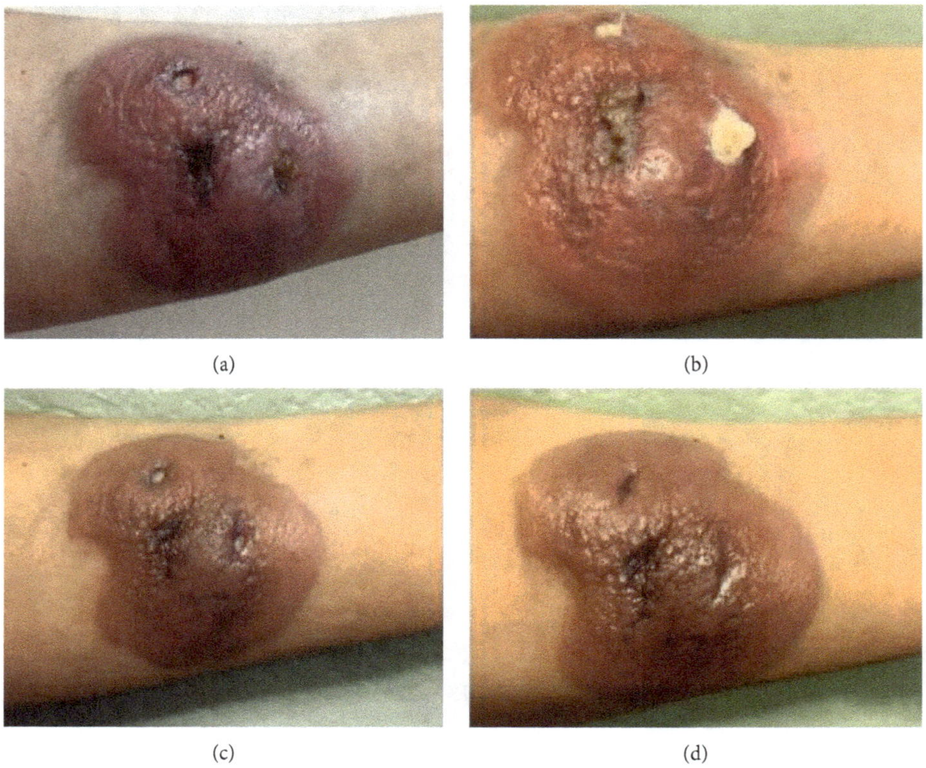

Figure 2: Left forearm tumor. (a) Before receiving first R-CHOP regimen on 04/19/17. (b) After the first R-CHOP cycle on 04/22/17. (c) After the second R-CHOP cycle on 05/11/17. (d) Left forearm at the end of the third cycle on 07/14/17 R-CHOP cycle on 06/01/17.

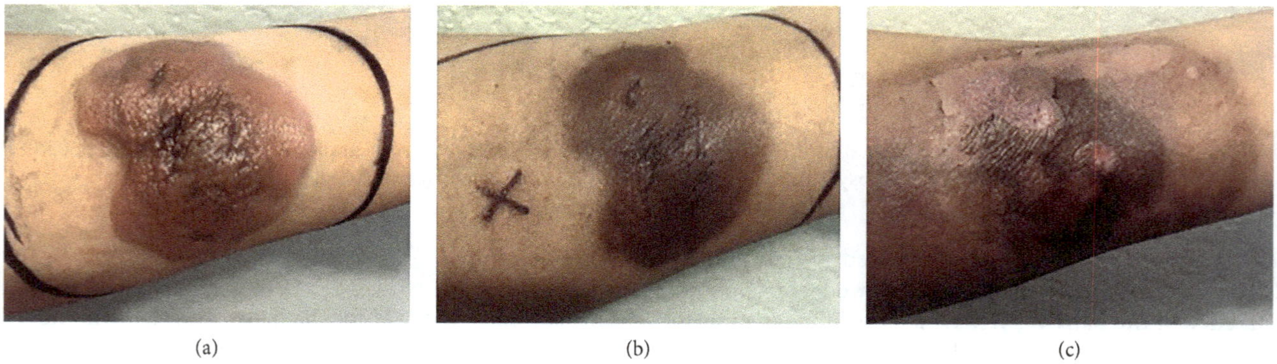

Figure 3: Left forearm during radiotherapy. (a) Left forearm at the beginning of radiotherapy on 06/05/17. (b) Left forearm at the end of radiotherapy on 06/25/17. (c) Left forearm at the end of the fifth R-CHOP cycle on 07/14/17.

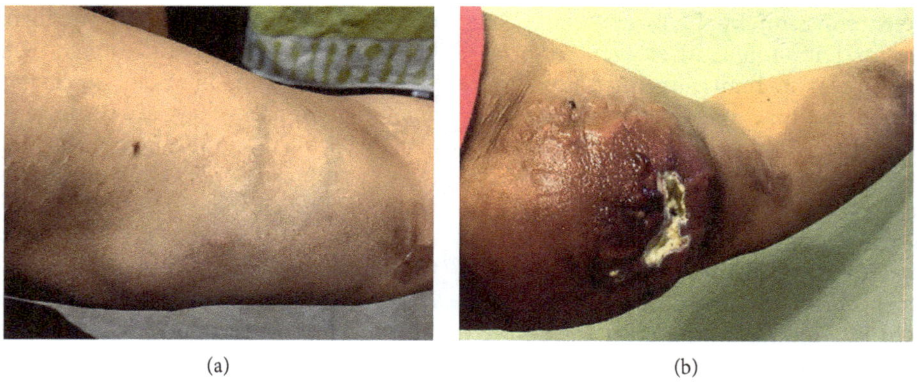

Figure 4: (a) Left upper arm mass on 08/11/17. (b) Left upper arm mass on 11/05/17.

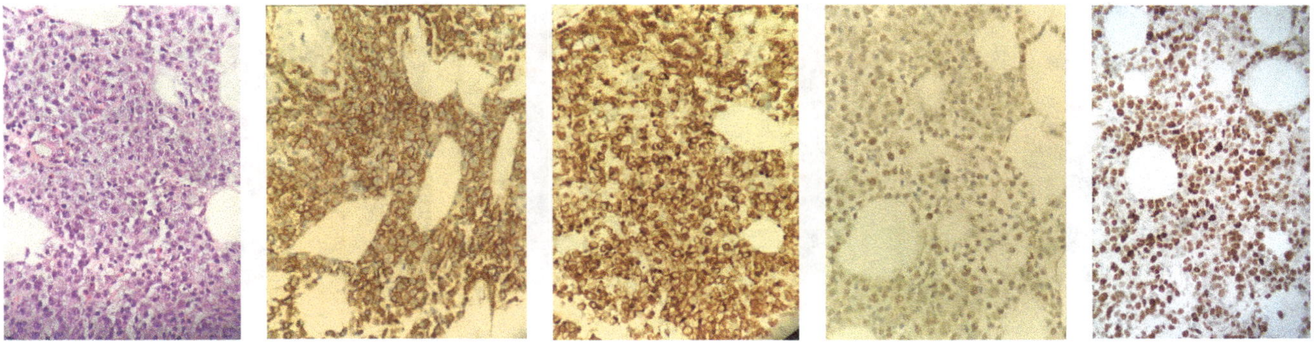

(a) (b) (c) (d) (e)

FIGURE 5: (a) H&E staining of diffuse large B-cell lymphoma; (b) CD20 immunostaining; (c) BCL2 immunostaining; (d) BCL6 immunostaining; (e) MYC immunostaining.

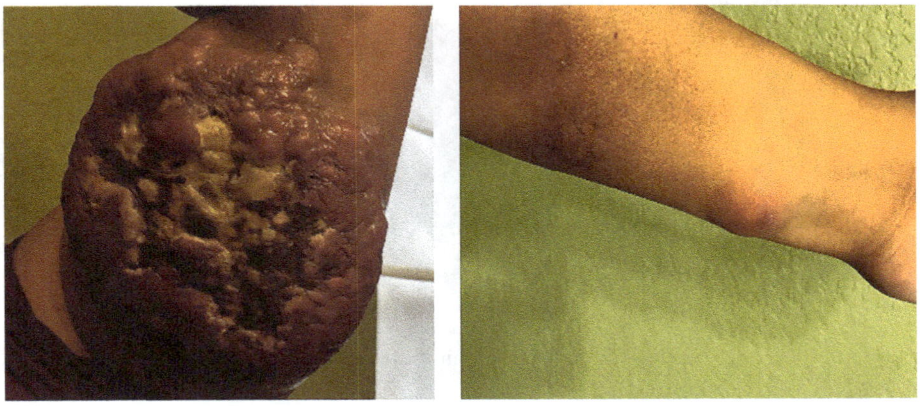

(a) (b)

FIGURE 6: (a) Left upper arm mass 12/04/17. (b) Third nodule appearance on left forearm 12/18/17.

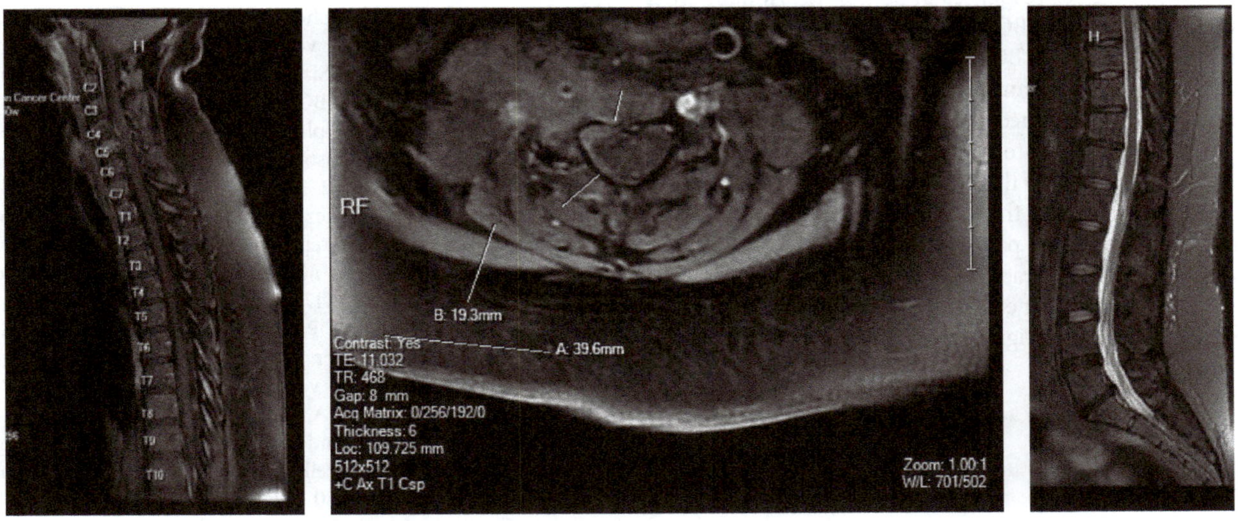

(a) (b) (c)

FIGURE 7: (A and B) MRI cervical and thoracic showed C5 metastasis that extended into the right C4-C5 and C5-C6 foramina (C) with leptomeningeal metastasis.

treatment combined with chemotherapy. Other alternatives include intensifying current therapies using dose-adjusted DA-R-EPOCH, which has been associated with better outcome for double hit DLBCL that can be substituted for R-CHOP [5]. The use of BCL2 inhibitors, such as venetoclax, could serve as an agent for maintenance therapy. A potent,

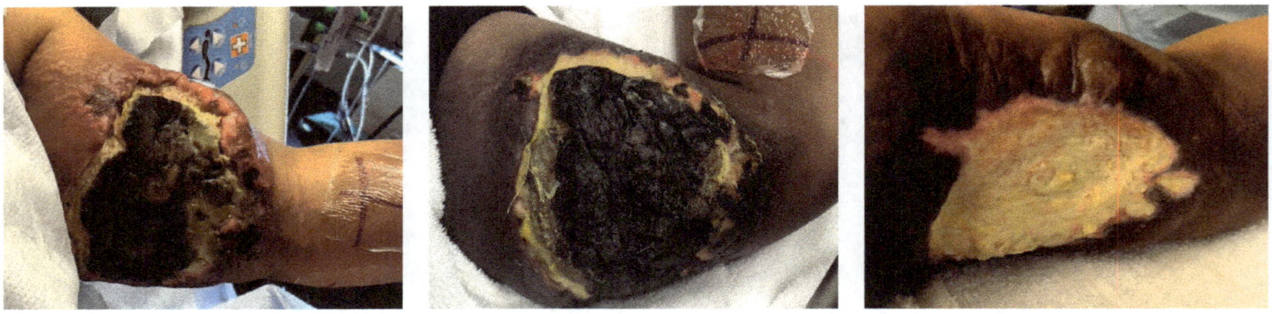

FIGURE 8: Left upper arm during radiotherapy. (a) Left upper arm at the beginning of radiotherapy on 01/07/18. (b) Left upper arm after completing radiotherapy on 01/11/18. (c) Left upper arm after excision of mass on 02/27/18.

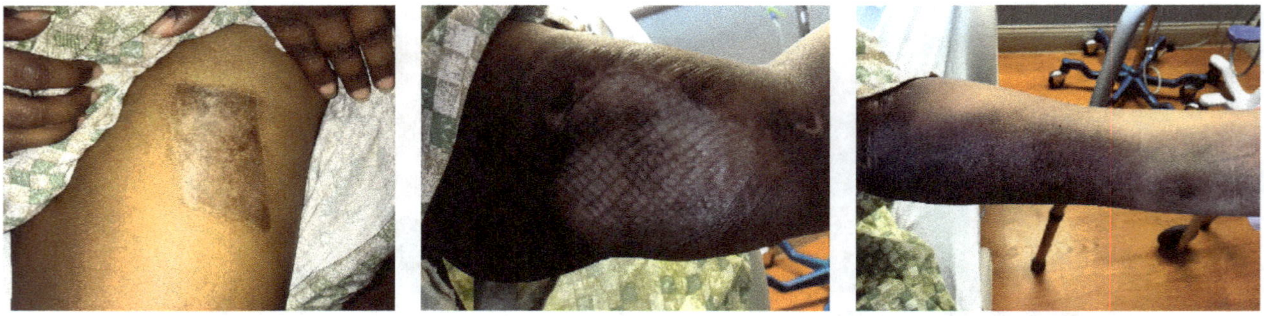

FIGURE 9: (a) Region of left thigh where skin graft was obtained. (b) Left upper arm with skin graft. (c) Left forearm.

selective, and orally bioavailable agent, venetoclax, has been used in clinical trials to evaluate its efficacy in relapsed or refractory cases of NHL [6]. In addition, lenalidomide has been shown to induce responses in both nongerminal center and germinal center DLBCL, showing superior responses in nongerminal center DLBCL [4]. Our patient experienced further tumor reduction and CNS involvement with the use of radiotherapy. She regained the ability to walk, attained remission, and received autologous stem cell transplant. Given very aggressive mature of this type of lymphoma and high risk of relapse, maintenance therapy around day 100 posttransplant is suggested after patient full engraftment. This case shows that radiation therapy should be incorporated early on as it showed a significant effect in achieving remission in our patient. This case should ignite a new standard of care for this type of lymphoma.

Acknowledgments

The authors would like to thank our patient for sharing her unique story and pictures with them, in the hope of helping others. The authors also would like to thank Dr. Thomas J Casey MD and Dr. Alan Brown MD from the Department of Pathology at Methodist Hospital, Ms. Angelica M. Olivarez from the research team, and Leticia M. Soliz for their help.

References

[1] A. Rosenthal and A. Younes, "High grade B-cell lymphoma with rearrangements of MYC and BCL2 and/or BCL6: double hit and triple hit lymphomas and double expressing lymphoma," *Blood Reviews*, vol. 31, no. 2, pp. 37–42, 2016.

[2] N. A. Johnson, G. W. Slack, K. J Savage et al., "Concurrent expression of MYC and BCL2 in diffuse large B-cell lymphoma treated with rituximab plus cyclophosphamide, doxorubicin, vincristine, and prednisone," *Journal of Clinical Oncology*, vol. 30, no. 28, pp. 3452–3459, 2012.

[3] Y. Khelfa and Y. Lebowicz, "Cutaneous presentation of double hit lymphoma: a case report with review of the literature," *Journal of Investigative Medicine High Impact Case Reports*, vol. 4, no. 2, article 232470961664259, 2016.

[4] M. Gopal and A. Malik, "Primary cutaneous diffuse large B-cell lymphoma of the upper limb: a fascinating entity," *Indian Journal of Dermatology*, vol. 58, no. 5, pp. 366–368, 2013.

[5] D. W. Scott, R. L. King, A. M. Staiger et al., "High-grade B-cell lymphoma with MYC and BCL2 and/or BCL6 rearrangements with diffuse large B-cell lymphoma morphology," *Blood*, vol. 131, no. 12, pp. 2060–2064, 2018.

[6] J. F. Gerecitano, A. W. Roberts, J. F. Seymour et al., "A phase 1 study of venetoclax (ABT-199/GDC-0199) monotherapy in patients with relapsed/refractory non-hodgkin lymphoma," *Blood*, vol. 126, no. 23, p. 254, 2015.

[7] P. Mondello, N. Steiner, W. Willenbacher et al., "Lenalidomide in relapsed or refractory diffuse large B-cell lymphoma: is it a valid treatment option?," *Oncologist*, vol. 21, no. 9, pp. 1107–1112, 2016.

44

Central Nervous System Involvement by Waldenstrom Macroglobulinemia: A Case Report of the Bing–Neel Syndrome

Ananth Arjunan[1] **and Hema Rai**[2]

[1]*University of Pittsburgh Medical Center, Division of Hematology/Oncology, UPMC Cancer Pavilion, 5150 Centre Avenue, Room 463, Pittsburgh, PA 15232, USA*
[2]*VA Pittsburgh Healthcare System, Division of Hematology/Oncology, University Drive C, 8th Floor, Pittsburgh, PA 15240, USA*

Correspondence should be addressed to Hema Rai; hema.rai@va.gov

Academic Editor: Tomás J. González-López

Bing–Neel syndrome (BNS) is a rare complication of Waldenstrom macroglobulinemia (WM) defined by a lymphoplasmacytic infiltration of the central nervous system (CNS). Patients present with a range of neurologic symptoms of variable severity. Diagnosis requires a low threshold of suspicion and is considered in WM patients with unexplained neurologic symptoms. It can occur in the presence of quiescent serum markers of WM. Direct CNS tissue biopsy should be pursued if feasible and remains the gold standard for diagnosis. No standard of care treatment exists, but expert guidelines suggest intravenous chemotherapy in standard dose or high-dose regimens or use of oral ibrutinib. Consideration is also made for intravenous rituximab, intrathecal therapies, and autologous stem cell transplantation. Patient factors and tolerability should drive decisions regarding treatment choice in this arena, given a lack of data for standard frontline therapy.

1. Introduction

Waldenstrom macroglobulinemia (WM) is a B-cell lymphoproliferative disorder characterized by a monoclonal lymphoplasmacytic infiltrate in the bone marrow with production of circulating monoclonal IgM antibody. WHO classification designates WM as a lymphoplasmacytic lymphoma (LPL) [1]. WM is rare with less than 1500 cases diagnosed yearly in the United States [2]. Bone marrow evaluation shows an intertrabecular infiltrate of small lymphocytes, plasmacytoid lymphocytes, and plasma cells. Over 90% of patients exhibit the *MYD88*^{L265P} activating somatic mutation which leads to NF-κB-dependent survival of LPL cells [3]. WM is incurable with median survival of 5 to 10 years. Clinical manifestations of WM result from either marrow infiltration by the LPL tumor cells or peripheral effects of the circulating monoclonal IgM. Marrow infiltration by the tumor cells leads to myelophthisic anemia and thrombocytopenia. Circulating IgM exerts deleterious effects through several mechanisms: (i) increased serum viscosity, (ii) deposition in end organs, and (iii) auto-antibody activity.

Neurologic manifestations are fairly common in WM. Hyperviscosity due to IgM-related erythrocyte agglutination can lead to stroke, confusion, headache, vision changes, and intracranial hemorrhage. Peripheral sensory neuropathy can result from IgM deposition in the peripheral nerves or from auto-antibody activity of IgM against myelin-associated glycoprotein in the peripheral nerve sheath [4]. An infrequent and poorly characterized neurologic disorder in WM patients, known as Bing–Neel syndrome, can be diagnosed when the dura, meninges, brain, or CSF are infiltrated by LPL tumor cells.

2. Case Presentation

A 60-year-old male presented with fatigue, sensory neuropathy, and lab findings of anemia and elevated albumin-globulin gap. Serum protein electrophoresis (SPEP) with immunofixation detected an IgM-kappa monoclonal protein quantitated at 3.9 g/dL. Free kappa-lambda light chain ratio was >390. Bone marrow evaluation revealed 70% marrow cellularity with kappa light chain restriction on staining.

Bone marrow core biopsy evaluation showed 14% plasmacytes and plasmacytoid lymphocytes. A diagnosis of WM was made after serum IgM returned elevated at 12,500 mg/dL. The patient underwent plasmapheresis after developing hyperviscosity symptoms of blurred vision and headache. Subsequently, he received several lines of systemic therapy including rituximab-based and bortezomib-based treatment as well as ibrutinib. He was eventually hospitalized for fevers and altered mental status. Infectious work up, brain MRI, and routine CSF studies were unrevealing and he spontaneously improved. Several weeks later, he was hospitalized again with confusion and falls. Despite treatment of identified bacteremia and urinary tract infections, his mental status progressively worsened. Exam was notable for bilateral paratonia with sustained leg flexion, decorticate posture of right upper extremity, bilateral patellar hyperreflexia, and complete disorientation. MRI brain showed left cerebellar signal hyperintensity on T2 FLAIR sequence. Serum viscosity was within the normal range. EEG revealed no epileptiform activity. CSF had elevated protein and normal glucose levels, and all CSF infectious studies were negative. Cell counts showed only 2 WBC/mm^3, and cytology and flow cytometry were limited by a paucity of cells. Paraneoplastic panels in serum and CSF were unrevealing. Immunofixation of CSF revealed a kappa-restricted IgM. Serum levels of IgM, free light chains, and beta-2 glycoprotein all were stable to improved.

Given the cerebellar enhancement noted on MRI and monoclonal IgM noted in the CSF, concern was raised for infiltration of CNS by his WM. Brain biopsy was offered but declined by the patient's family, given his overall clinical deterioration. A trial of empiric high-dose corticosteroid failed to yield improvement, and he was transitioned to hospice care.

3. Discussion

First described in 1936, involvement of the CNS by WM is eponymously titled as the Bing–Neel syndrome (BNS) [5]. BNS is relatively infrequent and is likely underrecognized. Fewer than 200 cases have been reported in our review of the literature. One review of 44 French patients with BNS showed median age at diagnosis of 63 years with 80% of patients of male sex. BNS was the first manifestation of WM in 36%. In the remaining patients, BNS was found at a median of 9 years after initial WM diagnosis with a median of 2 prior systemic therapies. Presenting symptoms were heterogeneous and included paresis, seizure, cord compression, confusion, and psychiatric derangements [6].

Direct biopsy of brain or meningeal tissue to assess for lymphoplasmacytic infiltrate is the gold standard and strongly recommended when it can be safely performed. CSF cytology and multidetector flow cytometry for immunophenotyping is advised. The culprit LPL cells always express CD19, CD20, CD52, and Ig-light chain and a majority express CD79b, CD11c, CD25, and surface IgM. CD5 and CD10 are usually negative [7]. Repeat CSF sampling increases diagnostic yield if initial cytology or flow cytometry are unrevealing. Quantitative PCR of CSF fluid to look for the *MYD88*^{L265P} mutation can be helpful [8]. Electrophoresis and immunofixation to identify monoclonal IgM in CSF can raise suspicion for BNS but are insufficient to confirm a diagnosis on their own. While monoclonal IgM in CSF may be from infiltrating LPL tumor cells, a disruption in the blood-brain barrier can allow peripheral IgM to enter the CNS. MRI imaging, preferably of the entire neuraxis, should be performed to assess for suspicious infiltrative lesions and rule out other causes. Findings on MRI may be described as diffuse infiltrative (leptomeningeal or periventricular white matter involvement) or tumoral (discrete lesions) but there are no established diagnostic radiologic criteria [9]. Brain MRI detects abnormalities in 78% of patients with this disorder; however, an absence of findings on MRI does not exempt the patient from an evaluation for BNS. Serum markers of WM may be stable or improved in patients with BNS and should not lower clinical suspicion for this entity.

Given the infrequency of BNS, there are no gold standard treatments and the opportunity for prospective trials is limited. A range of therapies have been utilized historically including intravenous and intrathecal chemotherapy, intravenous and intrathecal rituximab, radiation, and autologous stem cell transplantation. Oral ibrutinib has been shown in a recent case report to have CSF penetration with partial remission maintained in at 23 months of therapy [10]. One previously proposed treatment strategy established a dichotomy based on the degree of CNS involvement [11]. Group A was defined by direct CNS involvement and felt to benefit from chemotherapy and radiotherapy. Group B was defined by low CSF involvement (<5 cells/mm^3) with symptoms driven by IgM deposition and thus plasmapheresis the mainstay of therapy. A concerted effort was recently made by the 8th International Workshop on WM (IWWM-8) to produce diagnostic and therapeutic guidelines for BNS [12]. Several options proposed for symptomatic BNS include: (1) purine analogues, (2) bendamustine, (3) ibrutinib, or (4) high-dose methotrexate or cytarabine-based chemotherapy with potential additions of rituximab, intrathecal therapy, and autologous stem cell transplantation. Radiotherapy is effective in some case reports, but more data are needed to define its utility.

4. Conclusion

BNS is an infrequent complication of WM defined by CNS infiltration by lymphoplasmacytic cells. The median time from onset of symptoms to the diagnosis of BNS is 4 months [9]. The delay in achieving a diagnosis may be reflective of lack of uniformity in neurologic symptoms, lack of awareness of the disease state, and symptoms being incorrectly attributed to other WM-related neurologic disorders. BNS should be considered in WM patients with unexplained neurologic symptoms. Efforts should be made to obtain an MRI scan of the entire neuraxis, CSF sampling, and direct CNS tissue biopsy. Recent guidelines from IWWM-8 suggest use of a variety of cytotoxic chemotherapies or ibrutinib in the initial setting. Given a lack of clear standard of care therapy, emphasis should be placed on patient factors and tolerability in selection of a specific treatment regimen.

References

[1] E. Campo, S. H. Swerdlow, N. L. Harris, S. Pileri, H. Stein, and E. S. Jaffe, "The 2008 WHO classification of lymphoid neoplasms and beyond: evolving concepts and practical applications," *Blood*, vol. 117, no. 19, pp. 5019–5032, 2011.

[2] J. Sekhar, K. Sanfilippo, Q. Zhang, K. Trinkaus, R. Vij, and D. Morgensztern, "Waldenström macroglobulinemia: a surveillance, epidemiology, and end results database review from 1988 to 2005," *Leukemia and Lymphoma*, vol. 53, no. 8, pp. 1625-1626, 2012.

[3] Z. R. Hunter, L. Xu, G. Yang et al., "The genomic landscape of Waldenstrom macroglobulinemia is characterized by highly recurring MYD88 and WHIM-like CXCR4 mutations, and small somatic deletions associated with B-cell lymphomagenesis," *Blood*, vol. 123, no. 11, pp. 1637–1646, 2014.

[4] K. Viala, T. Stojkovic, A.-V. Doncker et al., "Heterogeneous spectrum of neuropathies in Waldenström's macroglobulinemia: a diagnostic strategy to optimize their management," *Journal of the Peripheral Nervous System*, vol. 17, no. 1, pp. 90–101, 2012.

[5] J. Bing and A. Neel, "Two cases of hyperglobulinaemia with affection of the central nervous system on a toxi-infectious basis," *Acta Medica Scandinavica*, vol. 88, no. 5-6, pp. 492–506, 1936.

[6] L. Simon, A. Fitsiori, R. Lemal et al., "Bing-Neel syndrome, a rare complication of Waldenstrom macroglobulinemia: analysis of 44 cases and review of the literature. A study on behalf of the French Innovative Leukemia Organization (FILO)," *Haematologica*, vol. 100, no. 12, pp. 1587–1594, 2015.

[7] S. Konoplev, L. J. Medeiros, C. E. Bueso-Ramos, J. L. Jorgensen, and P. Lin, "Immunophenotypic profile of lymphoplasmacytic lymphoma/Waldenström macroglobulinemia," *American Journal of Clinical Pathology*, vol. 124, no. 3, pp. 414–420, 2005.

[8] C. Jiménez, E. Sebastián, M. C. Chillón et al., "MYD88 L265P is a marker highly characteristic of, but not restricted to, Waldenström's macroglobulinemia," *Leukemia*, vol. 27, no. 8, pp. 1722–1728, 2013.

[9] H.-J. Kim, S.-I. Suh, J. H. Kim, and B.-J. Kim, "Brain magnetic resolution imaging to diagnose Bing-Neel syndrome," *Journal of Korean Neurosurgical Society*, vol. 46, no. 6, pp. 588–91, 2009.

[10] C. Mason, S. Savona, J. N. Rini et al., "Ibrutinib penetrates the blood brain barrier and shows efficacy in the therapy of Bing Neel syndrome," *British Journal of Haematology*, vol. 179, no. 2, pp. 339–341, 2017.

[11] K. I. Ly, F. Fintelmann, R. Forghani, P. W. Schaefer, E. P. Hochberg, and F. H. Hochberg, "Novel diagnostic approaches in Bing-Neel syndrome," *Clinical Lymphoma Myeloma and Leukemia*, vol. 11, no. 1, pp. 180–183, 2011.

[12] M. C. Minnema, E. Kimby, S. D'Sa et al., "Guideline for the diagnosis, treatment and response criteria for Bing-Neel syndrome," *Haematologica*, vol. 102, no. 1, pp. 43–51, 2017.

45

A Case Report of Leptomeningeal Myelomatosis and Rapid Improvement with Regimen Consisting of Daratumumab, Pomalidomide, Vincristine, Procarbazine, and Dexamethasone

Jew Win Kuan,[1] Sing Ling Chai,[2] Pathmanathan Rajadurai,[3] Lee Gong Lau,[4] Joseph Uchang,[4] and Sharifah Noor Akmal Syed Husain[5]

[1]*Department of Medicine, Universiti Malaysia Sarawak, Kota Samarahan, Sarawak, Malaysia*
[2]*Timberland Medical Centre, Kuching, Sarawak, Malaysia*
[3]*Subang Jaya Medical Centre, Subang Jaya, Selangor, Malaysia*
[4]*Borneo Medical Centre, Kuching, Sarawak, Malaysia*
[5]*Pantai Premier Pathology Sdn Bhd, Kuala Lumpur, Malaysia*

Correspondence should be addressed to Jew Win Kuan; kuanjewwin@gmail.com

Academic Editor: Massimo Breccia

Central nervous system (CNS) involvement in multiple myeloma (MM) (MM-CNS) in the form of leptomeningeal myelomatosis or brain parenchyma plasmacytoma is rare, causing challenges in clinical diagnosis and treatment. We would like to report a case of leptomeningeal myelomatosis and illustrated the challeges. A 61-year-old man was diagnosed with MM with left paravertebral plasmacytoma, R-ISS II with high suspicion of double-hit MM, either biallelic aberrancy of TP53 or del(17p) and IGH aberrancy depending on the definition chosen, treated with lenalidomide-bortezomib-dexamethasone and local radiotherapy, later developed systemic relapse and progression to MM-CNS in the form of leptomeningeal myelomatosis. A modified CNS-based treatment not reported before, consisting of daratumumab, pomalidomide, vincristine, procarbazine, and dexamethasone, brought a rapid clinical improvement and warrants a further study. Incorporation of intrathecal thiotepa into the regimen would likely increase the efficacy.

1. Introduction

Central nervous system (CNS) is much less involved in multiple myeloma (MM) (MM-CNS) compared to other haematological neoplasms like acute leukaemia and lymphoma. Cranium osseous or osteodural plasmacytoma that usually results from the spread of contiguous bone lesion should be separated from MM-CNS because it is common and has a better prognosis than MM-CNS (median overall survival (OS): 25 months ($n = 38$) versus 6 months ($n = 12$)) [1].

MM-CNS could be in the form of leptomeningeal myelomatosis (usually with cerebral spinal fluid (CSF) plasmatocytosis) or, rarer, brain parenchyma plasmacytoma (usually without CSF plasmacytosis). It can present at diagnosis or relapse/progression of MM, rarer in the former—16% at diagnosis [2]. This rarity could be an underestimation because CNS assessment is not a routine MM diagnostic workout unless there was CNS symptom, which if present, might also be overlooked because the treating physician might attribute the CNS symptom to the localised bony lesion, hypercalcaemia, uraemia, paraproteinaemia, concomitant disease e.g. psychological disorder, and adverse effects of MM or non-MM drugs.

2. Case Presentation

A 61-year-old man with underlying hypertension and anxiety disorder presented with backache and left lower chest pain since end of year 2020 and later was diagnosed with MM with left T8-T11 paravertebral plasmacytoma in March 2021. There was no bone marrow examination because patient refused. CT-guided biopsy of left lower thoracic paravertebral mass showed plasmacytoma with lambda light chain restriction (Figure 1). MRI thoracic spine showed left T8-T11 posterior mediastinal soft tissue mass, with a size of $6.8 \times 3.8 \times 10.0$ cm, with intra-spinal extension and infiltration into left posteromedial segment of 10th and 11th rib (Supplementary Data (available here)). Serum protein electrophoresis (SPE) and immunofixation (IF) showed IgA lambda of 10 g/L without immunoparesis, while urine protein electrophoresis (UPE) and IF did not show evidence of paraprotein. Serum free light chain (sFLC) showed reduced kappa:lambda ratio of 0.10 (13.2 mg/L: 132.7 mg/dL). Other investigations were normal—beta2-microglobulin 1.7 mg/L, albumin 42 g/L, Hb 15.7 g/dL, TWC 4.547×10^9/L, PLT 219.9×10^9/L, creatinine 83 μmol/L, eGFR 87 mL/min/1.73 m^2, corrected Ca 2.37 mmol/L, and LDH 172 μ/L within normal range.

Patient developed major depressive disorder since the diagnosis of MM on top of the preexisting anxiety disorder. Despite psychological therapy, both conditions waxed and waned following the condition of MM. Hence, throughout the follow-up, it is difficult to manage this patient, especially on the evaluation of certain subjective symptoms.

Dexamethasone was started at the end of March 2021 while waiting for the results of the investigations above. Bortezomib-dexamethasone plus zoledronic acid (VD + *Z*) was started in the middle of April 2021 instead of the usual triplet with addition of cyclophosphamide, thalidomide, or lenalidomide (*R*) due to patient's concern on potential adverse effect of all drugs and to keep the number of drug minimum with intention to increase to triplet once proven he was tolerable to VD + *Z*. In early May 2021, MRI thoracic spine showed progression of the paravertebral plasmacytoma, with a size of $8.2 \times 5.8 \times 15$ cm, without significant change in the involvement at T9/10 and T10/11 foramina and intraspinal extension (Supplementary Data). In the middle of May 2021, local radiotherapy to the left paraspinal plasmacytoma, 30 Gy in10 fractions, was completed, while systemic MM treatment was changed to RVD + *Z*. Retrospective investigation of the initial paravertebral plasmacytoma sample revealed that about 30% of the tumour cells showed aberrant nuclear p53 protein expression (Figure 1), positivity for fluorescent in situ hybridisation (FISH) TP53 deletion (nuc ish (DLEU × 2,TP53 × 1)(200)) (Figure 1), and positivity for FISH IGH rearrangement (nuc ish (IGH × 3,BCL × 2)(51/200)) (Figure 1).

After 2nd cycle of RVD + *Z* at the end of June 2021, patient achieved at least a partial response (PR) [3]. SPE showed IgA lambda of <1 g/L. UPE showed a faint band at fast moving gamma region. sFLC showed normal ratio of 1.04 (18.8 mg/L:18.0 mg/L). MRI and PETCT showed reduction of the paravertebral mass (Supplementary Data).

After 4th cycle of RVD + *Z* in the middle of August 2021, patient achieved a very good PR (VGPR) or near complete response (CR) [3]. SPE and IF were negative, while UPE showed a faint restriction band at fast moving gamma region for which IF did not reveal any abnormality. sFLC showed normal ratio of 1.22 (15.4 mg/L:12.6 mg/L). MRI and PETCT showed further reduction of the paravertebral mass (Supplementary Data).

The patient was a heavy smoker. During treatment of MM, imaging showed occurrence of lung changes which were progressive (Supplementary Data). He was investigated and treated as smear-negative pulmonary tuberculosis (PTB) due to clinical suspicion and endemicity of PTB in the region. Anti-TB was started in August 2021, while MM treatment was changed to lenalidomide maintenance. The lung changes improved with anti-TB (Supplementary Data).

In November 2021, SPE/IF, UPE/IF, and sFLC remained negative and PETCT showed stable left paraspinal mass. His anti-TB was continued until the diagnosis of leptomeningeal myelomatosis in February 2022.

His backache and peripheral sensory neuropathy worsened around December 2021. He was diagnosed with sciatica due to nerve root compression and received a steroid injection to left L4/4 facet joint at the end of December 2021, but the injection did not improve his condition. Lenalidomide maintenance was off in the middle of January because worsening drug-induced peripheral neuropathy was suspected while anti-TB, which could also cause drug-induced peripheral neuropathy, was continued to ascertain the main causative agent and in view of the importance of complete anti-TB regimen. However, symptoms were not improved and motor weakness at right wrist and fingers appeared in February 2022. MRI brain and whole spine in the middle of February 2022 showed multiple nodular lesions at leptomeningeal at the cerebrum, cerebellum, spinal cord, cauda equina, and bilateral internal auditory canals (Supplementary Data). CSF analysis showed protein 1.83 g/L, glucose 3.3 mmol/L, cell count 113×10^6/L with all mononuclear cells, cytology of abundant large atypical plasmacytoid cells in loose clusters along with singly dispersed cells, and immunophenotyping of lambda-restricted plasma cells (Figure2). SPE showed reappearance of M-protein <1 g/L. He was treated as MM-CNS at relapse/progression in this case given the tempo of the worsening CNS symptoms which appeared more than a year after initial diagnosis of MM, although MM-CNS at diagnosis could not be confidently ruled out because no CNS assessment was done.

After the diagnosis of leptomeningeal myelomatosis, he received intravenous methylprednisolone 1 g daily for three days which improved the symptoms partially. He decided to take traditional treatment, which did not improve the symptoms further instead the symptoms started to worsen after a week. At the end of March 2022, he and his family members agreed for chemotherapy. Before the start of chemotherapy, he was wheelchair and bed bound with lower limbs' power of grade 3 at the right and 4 at the left and upper limbs' power of 3-4 at the right and 4-5 at the left. Finger-nose test was positive. He was delirious and had visual and auditory hallucination. MRI showed worsening of leptomeningeal lesions (Figure 3). Dara-PVPD (daratumumab, pomalidomide, vincristine, procarbazine, and dexamethasone) was started. His condition was rapidly improved. He was able to stand and walk with walking frame after two cycles of treatment. At the time of writing, he completed the 4th cycle in the middle of May 2022. Between the 2nd and 3rd cycle, he developed an abscess at left gluteal ischial tuberosity region which resolved with antibiotic and local surgical drainage but resulted a week delay to the commencement of the 3^{rd}cycle.

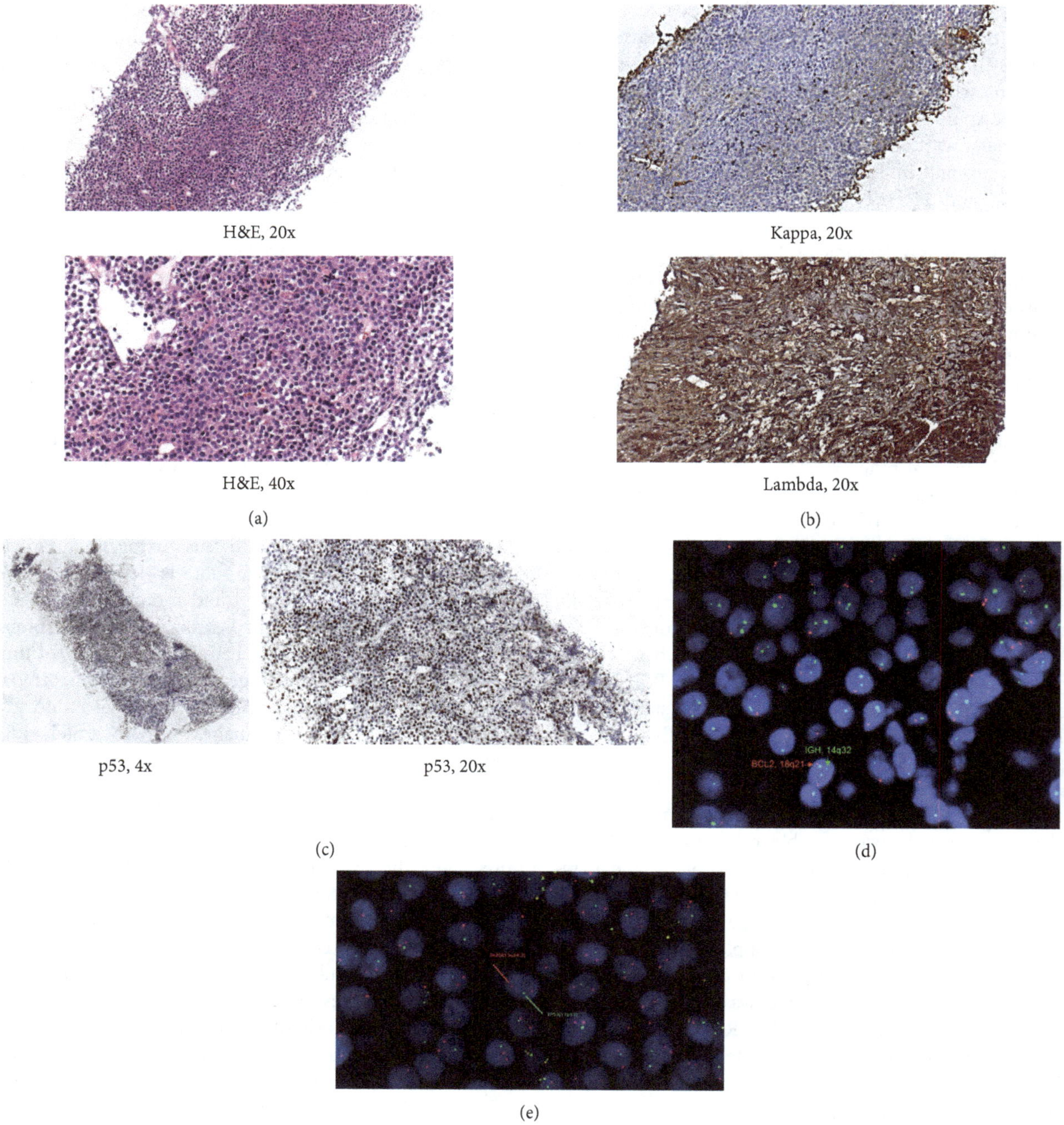

FIGURE 1: Left paravertebral plasmacytoma biopsy on (a) haematoxylin and eosin (H&E) stain, (b) immunohistochemical (IHC) stain of kappa and lambda light chain, (c) IHC stain of p53, (d) FISH of IGH breakapart, and (e) FISH of TP53 deletion.

The peripheral sensory neuropathy worsened from fingertips to whole palms and soles after the 2nd cycle needing dose modification. The detail of Dara-PVPD given from the 1st to 4th cycle is shown in Supplementary Data.

He achieved a VGPR[3] after the 4th cycle. CSF analysis in the middle of the 4th cycle showed protein 0.58 g/L, glucose 3.2 mmol/L, cell count 6×10^6/L, cytology of low cellularity with no malignant cell seen, and immunophenotyping of no evidence of clonal plasma cells and myeloma involvement. MRI showed disappearance of leptomeningeal lesion in the cerebrum, cerebellum, spinal cord, and cauda equina, except PR at left internal auditory canal and left external capsule (Supplementary Data).

He completed 6th cycle in the middle of June 2022. Assessment post-6th cycle showed further CNS improvement—CR with CSF and other MRI lesions except stable external capsule lesion as compared to MRI post-4th cycle. At the time of writing, he was undergoing peripheral blood haematopoietic stem cell collection and planned for thiotepa-based autologous haematopoietic stem cell transplantation in the middle of July 2022.

3. Discussion

This case illustrated the diagnostic difficulty of leptomeningeal myelomamastosis like the other reported cases,

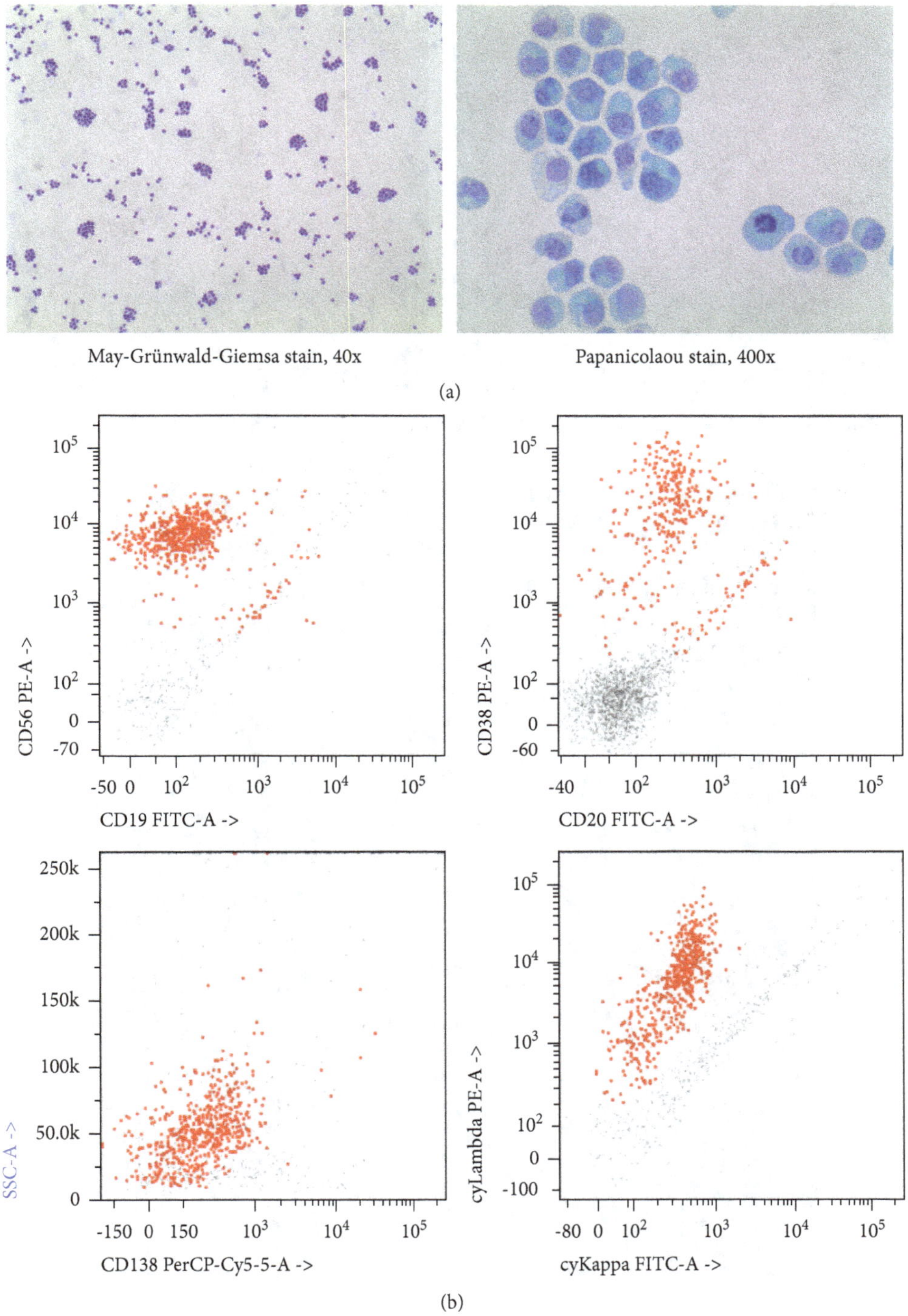

FIGURE 2: Cerebrospinal fluid examination at diagnosis (February 2022): (a) cytology and (b) immunophenotyping (the neoplastic plasma cells CD38+/CD56+/CD138-/lambda-restricted were gated red).

but further complicated by the psychological disorders and neurotoxicity effect of anti-TB. The MM drugs which commonly cause CNS adverse effects and were used in this patient are bortezomib, lenalidomide, and dexamethasone. Bortezomib causes peripheral neuropathy 28-41%, neuralgia/pain in limb 8-34%, paresthesia and dysesthesia 9-16%, headache 4-13%, and dizziness 3-5% more than the control group [4]. Lenalidomide causes peripheral neuropathy (3–5%), neuralgia/pain in limb (3–11%), paresthesia and dysesthesia (3–7%), headache (5–20%), dizziness (4–20%), muscle cramp (12–18%), back pain (7–21%), and bone pain (2%) [5]. We are aware of the potential CNS and musculoskeletal adverse effects of Dara-PVPD. However, after diagnosis of leptomeningeal myelomatosis was made, more objective assessments like CSF analysis and imaging would greatly assist in evaluation of symptoms.

Revised International Staging System (R-ISS) is a widely used risk stratification approach in MM which incorporates high risk chromosomal abnormalities (CAs)—del(17p), t(4; 14), or t(14; 16), but not 1 q gain or mutated TP53 as the data

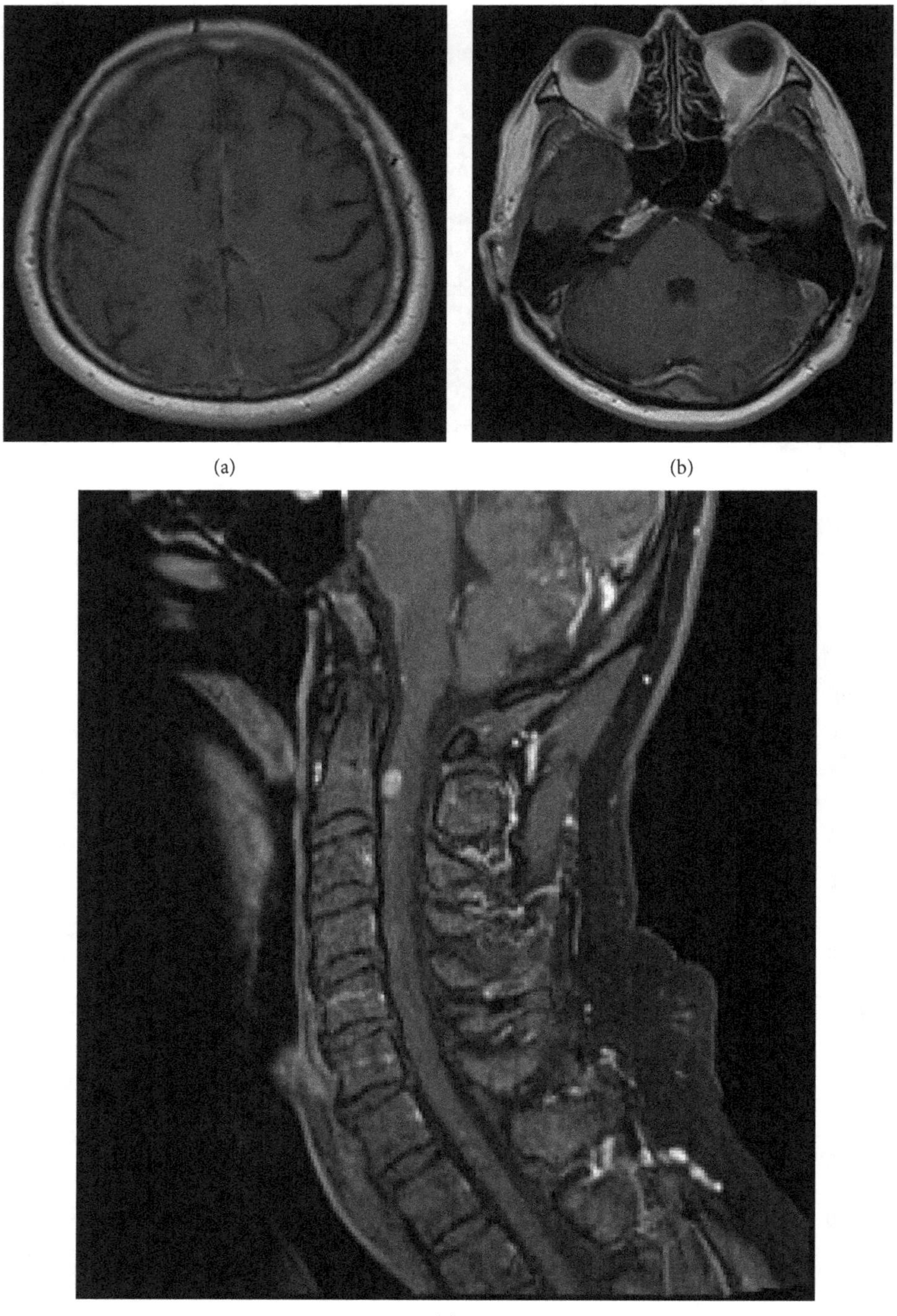

(a) (b) (c)

FIGURE 3: MRI of leptomeningeal myelomatosis at progression of leptomeningeal myelomatosis (March 2022): (a) T1 with contrast, vertex level, (b) T1 with contrast, level at bilateral IAC lesions, and (c) T1 with contrast, cerebellum and cervical spine.

were not available [6]. Walker et al. identified a group (6.1%) in newly diagnosed MM with the highest risk, labelled as double-hit which was defined as having either biallelic inactivation of TP53 (at chromosome 17p) or ISS stage III with CKS1B (at chromosome 1 q) amplification [7]. Mayo Clinic proposed double or triple hit MM as having two or three of the CAs—t (4; 14), t (14; 16), t (14; 20), del 17p, p53 mutation, gain 1 q, and del (1p), respectively [8]. FISH can detect del(17p), t(4;14), t(14;16), t(14;20), gain 1q, and del(1p) with high sensitivity and specificity in MM if the sample has high number of plasma cell or was CD138+ cells sorted or if the test has simultaneous CD138 immunofluorescence.However, FISH cannot detect TP53 mutation and CKS1B amplification which are detected using next generation sequencing that is not readily available in our setting. Our patient was likely to have biallelic TP53 aberrancy because his paravertebral plasmacytoma clearly had TP53 deletion at one allele and probably TP53 mutation at the other allele on the argument that MM patients with del17p are likely to have biallelic TP53 aberrancy [9,10] and about 30% of the tumour cells showed aberrant nuclear p53 protein expression. The half-life of the mutated p53 protein is longer compared to the wild type p53 protein which facilitates its detection. Presence of nuclear p53 protein, except nonsense mutation, is highly concordant with TP53 mutation in acute myeloid leukaemia, acute lymphoid leukaemia, myelodysplastic syndrome, or chronic lymphocytic leukaemia [11], less in lymphoma [12–14], and probably also in MM [15]. Nonetheless, p53 nuclear expression correlates with hemizygous TP53 deletion [16, 17] and predicts an adverse outcome [15, 17]. Our patient also had IGH (at chromosome 14q) aberrancy although could not ascertain the aberrancy was t(4;14), t(14;16), or t(14;20). Could there be a discrepancy of result if bone marrow sample was available? We would not be able to answer the question but certainly the sample with highest number of neoplastic plasma cells should be chosen, like the paravertebral plasmacytoma in this case when simultaneous CD138 immunofluorescence was not available.

There is no standard treatment for MM-CNS. Given the poor reported median OS after diagnosis of MM-CNS, 3.5 months ($n = 9$) [18], 4.6 months ($n = 37$) [19], 6 months ($n = 12$) [1], and 6.7 months ($n = 172$) [20], the treatment regimen, Dara-PVPD, was built after consideration of myeloma-effective drugs with CNS penetration. Dara-PVPD was based on a 2-weekly immunochemotherapy regimen used in Primary Diffuse Large B-cell Lymphoma of the CNS, R-MPV (rituximab, methotrexate, procarbazine, vincristine, dexamethasone, intrathecal (IT) or intra-Ommya methotrexate) (Supplementary Data) which was evolved from an established chemotherapy regimen, DeAngelis Protocol21 (Supplementary Data) [21] [22, 23].

Daratumumab, which takes the place of rituximab, has been used in combination with pomalidomide and dexamethasone, first in systemic relapsed and/or refractory MM treatment [24]. Both drugs have CNS penetration [25–27], although daratumumab is likely to have a suboptimal penetration given a case report of leptomeningeal myelomatosis which occurred while on daratumumab maintenance [26]. Daratumumab has been used at a shorter interval, weekly in cycle 1 and 2 of some regimens [24, 28]. Methotrexate was omitted because of its low efficacy in myeloma, while vincristine and procarbazine were retained because of their anti-myeloma activity [29]. IT methotrexate was omitted, again, for the same reason. Other IT agents commonly used in lymphoma were cytarabine and dexamethasone. However, cytarabine is ineffective against myeloma although there was a case report which might support its use [26], while dexamethasone has a doubtful effect as a single agent. IT thiotepa is probably a better choice as a case series reported a median OS of 17 months ($n = 13$) [30]. Thus, IT thiotepa was incorporated in Dara-PVPD but not given during 1st to 6th cycle because the patient was not cooperative for the procedure during the first two cycles and was waiting for import permit and arrival of the drug.

In summary, this case underlined the difficulties to identify CNS involvement in MM in clinical practice and treat the patient in the optimal way. The proposed daratumumab-based regimen could represent a new strategy to treat MM-CNS. Large prospective studies are warranted to identify the optimal therapy for MM-CNS.

Authors' Contributions

Jew Win Kuan was responsible for conceptualization and writing. Other authors were responsible for figures and reviewing.

Acknowledgments

We would like to thank UNIMAS for the publication support.

References

[1] A. Gozzetti, A. Cerase, F. Lotti et al., "Extramedullary intracranial localization of multiple myeloma and treatment with novel agents: a retrospective survey of 50 patients," *Cancer*, vol. 118, no. 6, pp. 1574–1584, 2012.

[2] P. A. Egan, P. T. Elder, W. I. Deighan, S. J. O'Connor, and H. D. Alexander, "Multiple myeloma with central nervous system relapse," *Haematologica*, vol. 105, no. 7, pp. 1780–1790, 2020.

[3] S. Kumar, B. Paiva, K. C. Anderson et al., "International Myeloma Working Group consensus criteria for response and minimal residual disease assessment in multiple myeloma," *The Lancet Oncology*, vol. 17, no. 8, pp. e328–e346, 2016.

[4] U.S. Food and Drug Administration, *VELCADE (Bortezomib) for Injection*, U.S. Food and Drug Administration, Silver Spring, MA, USA, 2008.

[5] U.S. Food and Drug Administration, *REVLIMID (Lenalidomide) Capsules, for Oral Use*, U.S. Food and Drug Administration, Silver Spring, MA, USA, 2019.

[6] A. Palumbo, H. Avet-Loiseau, S. Oliva et al., "Revised international staging system for multiple myeloma: a report from international myeloma working group," *Journal of Clinical Oncology*, vol. 33, no. 26, pp. 2863–2869, 2015.

[7] B. A. Walker, K. Mavrommatis, C. P. Wardell et al., "A high-risk, Double-Hit, group of newly diagnosed myeloma identified by genomic analysis," *Leukemia*, vol. 33, no. 1, pp. 159–170, 2019.

[8] M. Baysal, U. Demirci, E. Umit et al., "Concepts of double hit and triple hit disease in multiple myeloma, entity and prognostic significance," *Scientific Reports*, vol. 10, no. 1, p. 5991, 2020.

[9] L. Lodé, M. Eveillard, V. Trichet et al., "Mutations in TP53 are exclusively associated with del (17p) in multiple myeloma," *Haematologica*, vol. 95, no. 11, pp. 1973–1976, 2010.

[10] S. Thanendrarajan, E. Tian, P. Qu et al., "The level of deletion 17p and bi-allelic inactivation of TP53 has a significant impact on clinical outcome in multiple myeloma," *Haematologica*, vol. 102, no. 9, pp. e364–e367, 2017.

[11] P. Lepelley, C. Preudhomme, M. Vanrumbeke, B. Quesnel, A. Cosson, and P. Fenaux, "Detection of p53 mutations in hematological malignancies: comparison between immunocytochemistry and DNA analysis," *Leukemia*, vol. 8, no. 8, pp. 1342–1349, 1994.

[12] R. Villuendas, M. A. Piris, P. Algara et al., "The expression of p53 protein in non-Hodgkin's lymphomas is not always dependent on p53 gene mutations," *Blood*, vol. 82, no. 10, pp. 3151–3156, 1993.
[13] A. Y. Matsushima, E. Cesarman, A. Chadburn, and D. M. Knowles, "Post-thymic T cell lymphomas frequently overexpress p53 protein but infrequently exhibit p53 gene mutations," *American Journal Of Pathology*, vol. 144, no. 3, pp. 573–584, 1994.
[14] G. Z. Rassidakis, A. Thomaides, S. Wang et al., "p53 gene mutations are uncommon but p53 is commonly expressed in anaplastic large-cell lymphoma," *Leukemia*, vol. 19, no. 9, pp. 1663–1669, 2005.
[15] G. Pruneri, N. Carboni, L. Baldini et al., "Cell cycle regulators in multiple myeloma: prognostic implications of p53 nuclear accumulation," *Human Pathology*, vol. 34, no. 1, pp. 41–47, 2003.
[16] H. Chang, J. Yeung, C. Qi, and W. Xu, "Aberrant nuclear p53 protein expression detected by immunohistochemistry is associated with hemizygous P53 deletion and poor survival for multiple myeloma," *British Journal of Haematology*, vol. 138, no. 3, pp. 324–329, 2007.
[17] M.-H. Chen, C. X. Y. Qi, M. N. Saha, and H. Chang, "p53 nuclear expression correlates with hemizygous TP53 deletion and predicts an adverse outcome for patients with relapsed/refractory multiple myeloma treated with lenalidomide," *American Journal of Clinical Pathology*, vol. 137, no. 2, pp. 208–212, 2012.
[18] N. Majd, X. Wei, A. Demopoulos, A. Hormigo, and A. Chari, "Characterization of central nervous system multiple myeloma in the era of novel therapies," *Leukemia and Lymphoma*, vol. 57, no. 7, pp. 1709–1713, 2016.
[19] C. I. Chen, E. Masih-Khan, H. Jiang et al., "Central nervous system involvement with multiple myeloma: long term survival can be achieved with radiation, intrathecal chemotherapy, and immunomodulatory agents," *British Journal of Haematology*, vol. 162, no. 4, pp. 483–488, 2013.
[20] A. Jurczyszyn, N. Grzasko, A. Gozzetti et al., "Central nervous system involvement by multiple myeloma: a multi-institutional retrospective study of 172 patients in daily clinical practice," *American Journal of Hematology*, vol. 91, no. 6, pp. 575–580, 2016.
[21] L. M. DeAngelis, W. Seiferheld, S. C. Schold, B. Fisher, and C. J. Schultz, "Combination chemotherapy and radiotherapy for primary central nervous system lymphoma: radiation Therapy Oncology Group Study 93-10," *Journal of Clinical Oncology*, vol. 20, no. 24, pp. 4643–4648, 2002.
[22] P. G. Morris, D. D. Correa, J. Yahalom et al., "Rituximab, methotrexate, procarbazine, and vincristine followed by consolidation reduced-dose whole-brain radiotherapy and cytarabine in newly diagnosed primary CNS lymphoma: final results and long-term outcome," *Journal of Clinical Oncology*, vol. 31, no. 31, pp. 3971–3979, 2013.
[23] A. Omuro, D. D. Correa, L. M. DeAngelis et al., "R-MPV followed by high-dose chemotherapy with TBC and autologous stem-cell transplant for newly diagnosed primary CNS lymphoma," *Blood*, vol. 125, no. 9, pp. 1403–1410, 2015.
[24] A. Chari, A. Suvannasankha, J. W. Fay et al., "Daratumumab plus pomalidomide and dexamethasone in relapsed and/or refractory multiple myeloma," *Blood*, vol. 130, no. 8, pp. 974–981, 2017.
[25] M. Vercruyssen, G. El Hachem, and M. Maerevoet, "The daratumumab crosses the blood brain barrier," *Clinical Lymphoma, Myeloma & Leukemia*, vol. 18, p. S289, 2018.
[26] M. Zajec, K. A. Frerichs, M. M. van Duijn et al., "Cerebrospinal fluid penetrance of daratumumab in leptomeningeal multiple myeloma," *Hemasphere*, vol. 4, no. 4, p. e413, 2020.
[27] A. Mussetti, S. Dalto, and V. Montefusco, "Effective treatment of pomalidomide in central nervous system myelomatosis," *Leukemia and Lymphoma*, vol. 54, no. 4, pp. 864–866, 2013.
[28] G. Palladini, E. Kastritis, M. S. Maurer et al., "Daratumumab plus CyBorD for patients with newly diagnosed AL amyloidosis: safety run-in results of ANDROMEDA," *Blood*, vol. 136, no. 1, pp. 71–80, 2020.
[29] E. Nagura, A. Ichikawa, O. Kamiya et al., "A randomized study comparing VMCP and MMPP in the treatment of multiple myeloma," *Cancer Chemotherapy and Pharmacology*, vol. 39, no. 4, pp. 279–285, 1997.
[30] A. Claudel, A. Talbot, S. Harel et al., "Thiotepa intrathecal injections for myelomatous central nervous system involvement," *British Journal of Haematology*, vol. 193, no. 2, pp. e9–e12, 2021.

46

Primary Bone Lymphoma: A Case Series and Review of Literature

Poorva Bindal,[1] Aakash Desai,[2] Lukas Delasos ,[2] Sudhanshu Mulay,[3] and James Vredenburgh[3]

[1]*Department of Hematology and Oncology, Beth Israel Deaconess Medical Center, Boston, MA, USA*
[2]*Department of Internal Medicine, University of Connecticut Health Center, Farmington, CT, USA*
[3]*Department of Hematology and Oncology, Smilow Cancer Hospital at St. Francis, Hartford, CT, USA*

Correspondence should be addressed to Lukas Delasos; delasos@uchc.edu

Academic Editor: Tomás J. González-López

Primary bone lymphoma (PBL) is a subtype of lymphoma that exclusively affects skeletal tissue. Despite the relatively common involvement of skeletal structures as a manifestation of non-Hodgkin's lymphoma (NHL), primary and exclusive involvement of the skeletal system is rare. The prevalence of PBL is estimated to be 3–7% amongst primary bone tumors and less than 2% amongst all lymphomas in adults. However, the definition of primary bone lymphoma has been inconsistent over time. Within our institution, we identified four cases of primary bone lymphoma based on diagnostic criteria formed from the general consensus of multiple organizations, including the World Health Organization (WHO) and International Extranodal Lymphoma Study Group (IELSG). Here, we discuss the distinct characteristics amongst these cases in addition to performing a systematic review of current literature regarding this lymphoproliferative entity.

1. Introduction

Primary bone lymphoma (PBL) is a subtype of lymphoma that exclusively affects skeletal tissue. Despite the relatively common involvement of skeletal structures as a manifestation of non-Hodgkin's lymphoma (NHL), primary and exclusive involvement of the skeletal system is rare [1]. The prevalence of PBL is estimated to be 3–7% amongst primary bone tumors and less than 2% amongst all lymphomas in adults [2].

The definition of primary bone lymphoma has been inconsistent over time. The previous World Health Organization (WHO) classification of soft tissues and bone tumors defined PBL as either single osseous lesions without regional lymph node involvement, or tumor involvement of multiple osseous sites without associated visceral or lymph node disease [3]. However, there is no clearly defined criteria for this malignancy outlined in newer WHO classifications. In the retrospective study conducted by the International Extranodal Lymphoma Study group (the IELSG 14 study), authors defined that only cases with a clear bone origin are classified as primary bone lymphomas, i.e., either a single bony lesion, with or without involvement of regional lymph nodes or multiple bony lesions without nodal or visceral disease, defined as "multifocal osseous lymphoma" or "polyostotic lymphoma". This definition corroborates with the prior WHO classification; thus, the general consensus amongst clinicians seems to be in line with these criteria.

Here, we describe a case series of four patients from our institution diagnosed with primary bone lymphoma based on the aforementioned diagnostic criteria, in addition to discussing distinct characteristics amongst these cases.

1.1. Case Series

1.1.1. Case 1. A 60-year-old female presented to the clinic with complaints of progressive swelling and dull aching pain over the mid-tibia in her left lower extremity. Of note, she had a past medical history of bilateral breast carcinoma in 2003 (Stage I, Grade III invasive ductal carcinoma of the left breast and carcinoma in situ of the right breast) that was estrogen receptor (ER) positive, progesterone receptor (PR) positive, and HER2 negative with absence of BRCA mutation treated with bilateral mastectomies and hormonal therapy.

A plain radiograph of the left leg (Figure 1) demonstrated increased lucency in the medullary canal extending from the proximal diaphysis of the mid-shaft with normal cortical appearance and no periosteal reaction or evidence of fractures. Magnetic resonance imaging (MRI) of the left leg revealed findings consistent with diffuse intramedullary metastasis involving the left tibia, visualized distal left femur, and proximal/mid-right tibia (Figure 2). Computed tomography (CT) scans of the chest, abdomen, and pelvis did not show any evidence of metastatic disease but demonstrated a few scattered nonspecific small mediastinal lymph nodes measuring up to 11 mm, which were likely reactive. The patient subsequently underwent an open tibial bone biopsy with tumor debulking and resection, along with prophylactic intramedullary nail placement of the left lower extremity. Pathology results of the bone biopsy were consistent with aggressive large B-cell non-Hodgkin's lymphoma (NHL). Neoplastic cells were found to be positive for CD3, Pax-5, CD20, MUM1, and BLC-2, while negative for CD10 and BLC-6. Ki-67 expression was high at greater than 95%. Following this new diagnosis, she underwent a positron emission tomography with computed tomography (PET/CT) scan which reported extensive disease involvement in both tibias, left humerus, and likely left mandible, as well as extensive adenopathy which extended from the supraclavicular region to the distal left external iliac system, believed to be due to her lymphoma (Figure 3).

1.1.2. Case 2. A 51-year-old female presented to the emergency department with gradually progressive right knee pain in the summer of 2014. Plain radiography of her right femur showed a mottled appearance of the cortex and intramedullary spaces which was concerning for malignancy. MRI of the right femur showed an abnormal intramedullary signal and enhancement involving the distal femur with associated abnormal periosteal soft tissue, suggestive of an underlying lymphoma.

She underwent an open biopsy of the right distal femur and had pathology results consistent with kappa-restricted B-cell non-Hodgkin's lymphoma with high-grade features and significant necrosis. Neoplastic cells were positive for CD19, CD 20, PAX 5, and CD 10 and negative for CD23, CD5, and CD103. The Ki-67 index was more than 80%. Bone marrow aspiration and biopsy showed mild hypercellularity with trilineage hematopoiesis, but there was no evidence of lymphoma infiltration. PET/CT imaging demonstrated intense metabolic activity in the distal part of the right femur measuring 13.7 × 9.4 × 8.6 cm and a maximum standardized uptake value (SUV) of 21.3. There was also noted uptake in the medial aspect of the right thigh as well as intense metabolic activity in the right breast. Further investigation with MRI revealed suspicious lesions of the right breast at 8 o' clock and 11 o' clock positions, measuring 1.2 and 1.9 cm, respectively. She underwent ultrasound-guided biopsy of these lesions and had pathology results consistent with high grade B-cell non-Hodgkin lymphoma (NHL). CD20, PAX 5, and B-cell markers were strongly positive. Ki-67 showed a very high nuclear proliferative index with positive staining in 80–90% of the cells. The staining pattern for BCL-6, CD10, and MUM1 suggested a nongerminal center subtype. Fluorescent in situ hybridization (FISH) showed evidence of cMYC mutation, but t(14;18) was not observed.

The patient completed 6 cycles of dose-adjusted chemotherapy with rituximab, etoposide phosphate, prednisone, vincristine sulfate, cyclophosphamide, and doxorubicin (i.e., R-EPOCH). Restaging CT scans had demonstrated complete remission. She is currently under active surveillance with no evidence of disease recurrence since completing her chemotherapy regimen more than 3 years ago.

1.1.3. Case 3. A 45-year-old male presented with right knee pain that was gradual in onset and not associated with any previous trauma. He was evaluated by orthopedic surgery and found to have a large effusion of the right knee. The patient subsequently underwent an MRI of the involved extremity that showed a diffuse heterogeneous marrow signal in the visualized distal femoral diaphysis extending to the femoral condyles with associated periosteal inflammation. Also noted was a fairly large soft tissue mass extending along the lateral and posterior aspects of the distal femoral diametaphysis. There was heterogeneous enhancement of the marrow process and a soft tissue mass which raised concern for an underlying neoplasm. CT scan of the chest did not show evidence of lymphadenopathy but did reveal a large mass extending from the posterior mediastinum around the right paraspinal soft tissues. Bone scan showed intense abnormal activity in the right distal femur. He underwent an open excisional biopsy of the right femoral mass which revealed kappa-restricted large B-cell NHL with high-grade features. Ki-67 expression was estimated to be between 80% and 90%. Cells partially expressed CD20 with loss of CD19. Immunohistochemical stains showed an expanded population of cells that were positive for CD45, CD20, PAX 5, CD10, and MUM1. Bone marrow biopsy and aspirate showed normocellular bone marrow without evidence of lymphoma through morphology or flow cytometry testing. Biopsy of the paraspinal mass revealed lambda-restricted B-cell NHL. The cytologic features in the paraspinal mass (predominance of small cells) and light chain restriction (lambda monotypia) were different than those observed in the right thigh mass (kappa-restricted large B-cell lymphoma). After confirmation with flow cytometry, he was diagnosed with unrestricted B-cell NHL and started treatment with a dose-adjusted R-EPOCH regimen. He completed 6 cycles of chemotherapy with partial response. His treatment course was complicated by avascular necrosis of the right distal femur. Although there has been persistence of the right paraspinal mass, he has had no evidence of disease progression close to 2 years after completion of chemotherapy.

1.1.4. Case 4. A 28-year-old female had developed progressive right hip pain which acutely worsened after

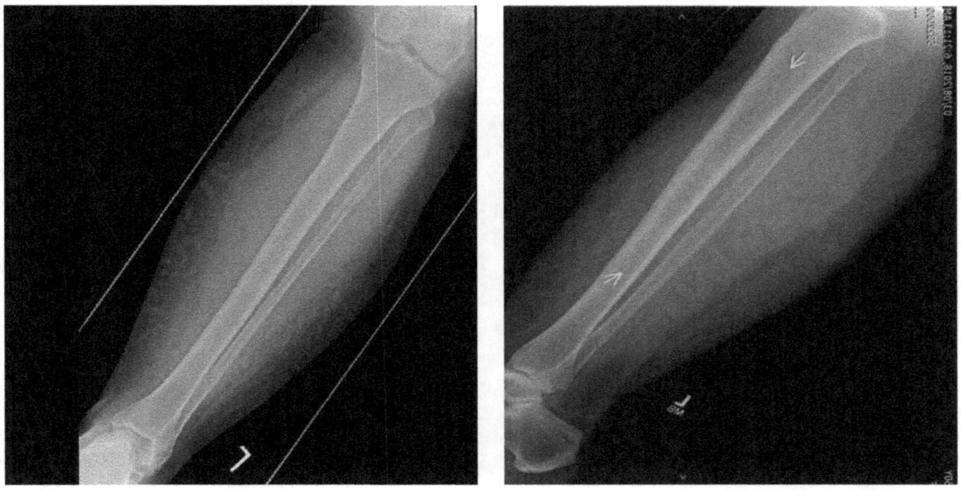

(a) (b)

FIGURE 1: X-ray of the tibia fibula. (a) Antero-posterior (AP) view. (b) lateral view.

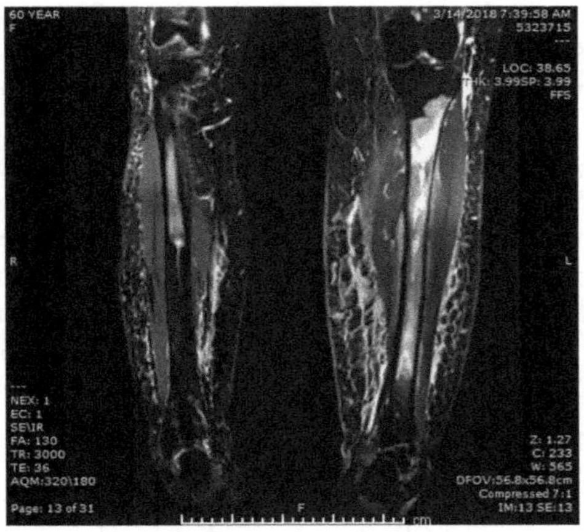

FIGURE 2: MRI of left tibia with/without IV contrast.

sustaining a fall while exiting her car and prompted her to go to the emergency department. Plain radiographs showed an impacted subcapital right hip fracture with multiple ill-defined lytic lesions throughout the femoral neck and intertrochanteric region, thus raising concern for a pathologic hip fracture. MRI of the hip showed areas of marrow replacement with enhancement throughout the proximal right femur as well as marrow enhancement within the superior and inferior pubic ramus, right sacrum, right iliac bone, and pubic symphysis. A bone scan was done that showed numerous foci of increased radiotracer activity in the right femur, left tibia, sternum, skull, and lumbar spine suggestive of metastatic disease. CT scan of the chest, abdomen, and pelvis demonstrated osseous destructive lesions with pathologic fractures at L2 and L4, as well as ill-defined hypodensities within the spleen. There was absence of lymphadenopathy noted on the CT scan. She underwent a total right hip replacement as well as biopsy of the bone lesion. Pathology results were consistent with diffuse large B-cell lymphoma with aggressive features and a germinal center subtype histology. The neoplastic cells demonstrated a lymphoid phenotype and expressed CD20 and PAX-5, as well as BCL-6, but were negative for CD10 and MUM1. Ki-67 staining was noted in more than 95% of the viable specimen. Tumor cells were negative for BCL-2 and cMYC. Core biopsy of the bone marrow demonstrated 95% cellularity with extensive diffuse pattern proliferation of neoplastic lymphocytes, consistent with large B-cell lymphoma infiltration of the bone marrow.

2. Discussion

The exact definition of PBL has remained a controversial topic throughout medical literature. The general consensus based on old WHO classifications and recommendations provided by the abovementioned IELSG 14 study has been to classify patients with osseous lesions that have no evidence of regional lymph node or distal visceral involvement within the category of PBL. There are currently no clearly defined risk factors associated with the development of this malignancy. Although there have been identified correlations between PBL and other bone disorders (e.g., Paget's disease and hereditary exostoses), infectious processes (e.g., human immunodeficiency virus (HIV) and osteomyelitis), and autoimmune disorders (e.g., sarcoidosis), none of these associations are well established as risk factors for the development of this disease [4–7].

2.1. Clinical Features. The median age range for patient's diagnosed with PBL varies between 45 and 60 years old, with fewer cases reported in the pediatric population [8]. The disease shows a male preponderance with a male-to-female ratio ranging from 1.2 to 1.8 [9]. There is insufficient data to provide any racial or geographical distribution of the disease. Pain (82–92%) and swelling (34–45%) of the involved site are two of the most common clinical manifestations of this disease [10]. Other less common presentations include pathological fractures and systemic "B-type" symptoms such as fevers, weight loss, and night sweats. Any skeletal site can be involved by PBL, but there is a higher rate of axial

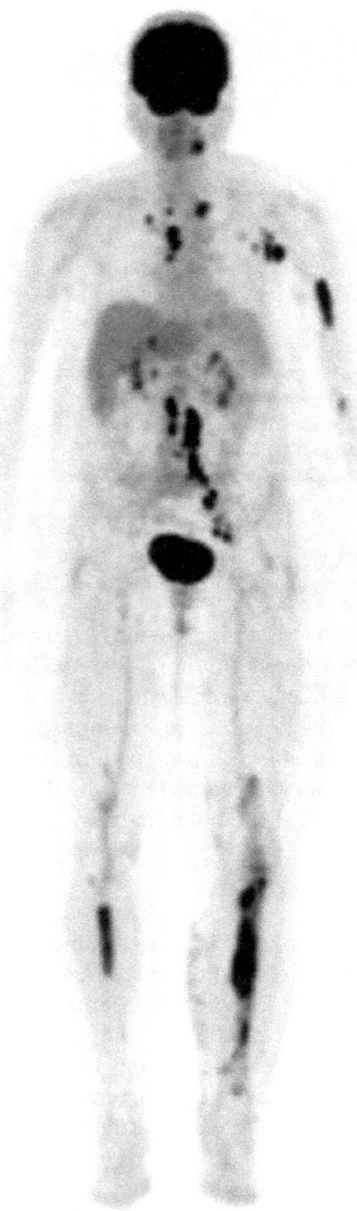

Figure 3: Whole body PET/CT scan.

involvement as compared to the appendicular skeleton. When there is appendicular skeletal involvement, the femurs have proven to be most commonly affected, consisting of approximately 20–38% of cases [10]. Spread to lymph nodes and bone marrow occurs in about 28% and 35% of cases, respectively. Spinal cord compression is the most dreaded complication associated with this malignancy, occurring in almost 16% of patients. Osteolysis and resultant hypercalcemia is another major complication observed in approximately 5–10% of patients upon their initial presentation. It is absolutely pertinent that these medical emergencies are not overlooked within this patient population and that they are identified in a timely manner in order to prevent further complications.

2.1.1. Diagnosis. Laboratory results are usually unremarkable and do not aid in the diagnosis of PBL. Initial diagnostic workup includes radiographic imaging of the affected area. However, radiographic findings for cases of PBL can be difficult to distinguish from other primary bone tumors such as osteosarcoma, Ewing's sarcoma, and chondrosarcoma. Plain X-ray films are the initial diagnostic test of choice. PBL most commonly presents as osteolytic or osteoblastic lesions with disease involvement of the cortex and reactive periosteal changes [11]. CT scan can be used to further delineate these lesions and remains the primary modality for staging, restaging, and follow-up of PBL. CT can accurately define the tumor boundaries and detect evidence of extraosseous extension as well as cortical breakthrough [12]. MRI further assists in diagnosis by revealing the extent of disease in greater detail through demonstration of abnormal signal intensity areas on T1- and T2-weighted images with minimal contrast enhancement. When comparing this imaging modality to PET/CT, MRI has proven to be equally effective at monitoring tumor response to treatment [13]. However, functional assessment of bone lesions using fluorodeoxyglucose (FDG)-PET imaging continues to play an important role. Studies have shown that FDG-PET displays a higher specificity and sensitivity than conventional bone scintigraphy in identifying lymphomatous infiltration of skeletal tissue [14]. In addition, sensitivity, specificity, and accuracy rates for staging of extranodal lymphomas with PET-CT have been reported to be 97%, 100%, and 98%, respectively, as compared to rates of 87%, 85%, and 84% using conventional CT imaging [15]. Despite the minimal availability of data, PET-CT is recommended as a standard tool for the initial evaluation, staging, and response assessment of FDG-avid lymphomas by the recent Lugano Classification System [16].

2.1.2. Microscopy. Clinical and radiological suspicion for PBL should be further assessed by pathology via bone biopsy. It is recommended to avoid excisional biopsies and minimize the amount of resected tissue in order to reduce the risk of pathological fractures in these cases. The majority of PBL cases are diagnosed as diffuse large B-cell lymphoma (DLBCL) and less commonly as follicular lymphoma, small lymphocytic lymphoma, and marginal zone lymphoma [9].

Upon morphological inspection, tumor cells are large in size and appear consistent with follicle center or centroblastic cell types [17]. Flow cytometry demonstrates immunoreactivity for B-cell markers including CD45, CD20, CD21, CD45, and CD79a, with variable immunoreactivity for CD75 and CD10 [18, 19]. T-cell markers are usually negative using this technique, except for occasional small CD3 positivity. Available data on primary bone T-cell lymphomas are currently lacking with most reported cases being anaplastic large-cell lymphoma (CD3 +; CD43+; CD30+), which are often associated with *t* (2; 5) (p23; q35) and ALK-1 expression [20].

BCL2 and MYC rearrangements play an important role in tumor mechanisms. A study by Li et al., which studied the gene expression signatures of PBL, reported 6 out of 8 cases with BCL2 rearrangement while an additional 5 out of 17 cases were found to have MYC rearrangements. A case of dual MYC and BCL-2 gene rearrangements has also been reported. Thus far, BCL-6 rearrangements have not been shown to occur in patients with PBL [21].

2.1.3. Staging and Prognostic Factors. Staging of PBL is required in order to provide appropriate therapy and avoid excessive treatment with antineoplastic agents which would potentiate the risk of developing serious adverse effects. The most commonly used staging criteria for PBL has been proposed by the Lugano Classification System [16]. Stage IE represents disease confined to an extranodal site, such as a solitary bone lesion. If there is evidence of regional lymph node involvement with a single bone lesion, the disease is then classified as stage IIE. Multifocal disease that is strictly limited to the skeletal system is classified as stage IV [22].

The prognosis of patients with primary bone DLBCL is directly correlated to the stage of disease. 5-year overall survival (OS) varies from 82% for patients with stage IE disease to 38% for cases of disseminated DLBCL with skeletal involvement. Conventional prognostic factors, such as the International Prognostic Index (IPI), have proven to be ineffective in predicting the prognosis for PBL since staging and the number of extranodal sites have no variability in PBL [23]. Importantly, however, the IELSG14 study revealed that patient age, functional performance status, and serum lactate dehydrogenase (LDH) levels are independently associated with OS in each subgroup of PBL. Furthermore, the germinal center (GC) phenotype with certain molecular features (i.e., CD10 expression, BCL-6 mutations, translocations involving 3q27) are associated with favorable outcomes in primary bone DLBCL [24]. On the other hand, non-GC signatures and related features (i.e., immunoblastic variant, MUM1 expression) are unfavorable predictors of survival in DLBCL of the bone [25]. Additionally, there is a worse prognosis associated with primary bone T-cell lymphomas as compared to primary bone B-cell lymphomas, especially in cases of CD56-positive anaplastic large-cell lymphomas in particular [26].

2.1.4. Treatment. Given the rarity of this disease process, randomized-controlled clinical trials addressing treatment alternatives for PBL are not readily available. Therefore, current treatment recommendations are largely based upon data collected from retrospective studies. In the past, PBL was treated with radiation therapy alone which achieved appropriate localized disease control, but was associated with high relapse rates. Due to the elevated rate of disease recurrence, chemotherapy was introduced for the treatment of this malignancy [27]. Currently, there exist multiple treatment modalities for PBL including chemotherapy, localized radiation therapy, and surgical intervention. A retrospective multicenter Rare Cancer Network study involving 116 patients with stage IE (80% of cases) or IIE PBL demonstrated multiple factors associated with improved 5-year survival. These include an IPI score of less than 2, radiation dose greater than 40 Gy, and the administration of at least 6 cycles of chemotherapy [28]. The role of surgery is often limited to surgical biopsy with or without debulking and plays little role in cases of advanced disease. In some cases, patients with involvement of the weight-bearing bones may require internal stabilization or bracing until treatment and subsequent bone healing occur.

Most of PBLs have characteristics consistent with DLBCL; hence, chemotherapeutic regimens usually consist of anthracycline-based combination therapies such as cyclophosphamide, doxorubicin, vincristine, and prednisone (CHOP) with or without rituximab (R-CHOP). Of note, in a study involving 131 PBL patients treated with either CHOP or R-CHOP, Ramadan et al. demonstrated that R-CHOP was superior to CHOP with 3-year progression-free survival (PFS) rates of 88% as compared to 52%, respectively [29]. Treatment with radiation therapy dates to an era without the addition of rituximab to chemotherapy; thus, its use remains a topic of much debate. Prior to the introduction of rituximab, combination chemotherapy and radiotherapy was the treatment regimen of choice. In patients with unifocal disease, consolidative involved-field radiotherapy provides an adequate response. A dose of 30–36 Gy has been found to be effective, with higher doses (e.g., 40 Gy) offered to patients with an indeterminate response to radiation. However, attention should be drawn to the specific areas of disease involvement before pursuing treatment with radiotherapy. Radiation applied to skeletal structures involved in a significant amount of bone marrow production, such as the pelvis, should be cautiously considered in order to avoid complications with hematopoiesis.

Even with the limited data available, chemotherapy has proven to be more effective than radiation therapy for the treatment of PBLs with 10-year overall survival rates of 56% as compared to 25%, respectively. Yet, several studies have demonstrated improved overall survival when using combined chemoradiation rather than chemotherapy or radiation alone [30]. For example, a prospective study conducted by Christie et al. involving cases of PBL treated with three cycles of CHOP followed by 45 Gy of involved field radiation listed 5-year local control rates of 72% and overall survival rates of 90% [31]. Therefore, it is currently recommended that patients with diagnosed PBL receive treatment with combined chemoradiation in order to best achieve remission. Nevertheless, with the increasing development of novel systemic therapies, further research is warranted for the identification of treatment regimens that will improve progression-free and overall survival rates for patients suffering from PBL.

References

[1] P. Dubey, C. S. Ha, P. C. Besa et al., "Localized primary malignant lymphoma of bone," *International Journal of Radiation OncologyBiologyPhysics*, vol. 37, no. 5, pp. 1087–1093, 1997.

[2] D. Limb, C. Dreghorn, J. K. Murphy, and R. Mannion, "Primary lymphoma of bone," *International Orthopaedics*, vol. 18, pp. 180–183, 1994.

[3] K. K. Unni and P. C. W. Hogendoorn, "Malignant lymphoma," in *Pathology and Genetics of Tumours of Soft Tissue and Bone*, C. D. M. Fletcher, K. K. Unni, and F. Mertens, Eds., IARC Press World Health Organization Classification of Tumours, Lyon, France, 2002.

[4] N. V. Sipsas, A. Kontos, G. D. Panayiotakopoulos et al., "Extranodal non-Hodgkin lymphoma presenting as a soft tissue mass in the proximal femur in a HIV (+) patient," *Leukemia & Lymphoma*, vol. 43, no. 12, pp. 2405–2407, 2002.

[5] H. Kobayashi, Y. Kato, M. Hakamada et al., "Malignant lymphoma of the bone associated with systemic sarcoidosis," *Internal Medicine*, vol. 40, no. 5, pp. 435–438, 2001.

[6] G. Christopher Stephens, W. J. Lennington, and H. S. Schwartz, "Primary lymphoma and Paget's disease of the femur," *American Journal of Clinical Pathology*, vol. 101, no. 6, pp. 783–786, 1994.

[7] K. Neben, M. Werner, L. Bernd, V. Ewerbeck, G. Delling, and A. Ho, "A man with hereditary exostoses and high-grade non-Hodgkin's lymphoma of the bone," *Annals of Hematology*, vol. 80, no. 11, pp. 682–684, 2001.

[8] A. Qureshi, A. Ali, N. Riaz, and S. Pervez, "Primary non-Hodgkin's lymphoma of bone: experience of a decade," *Indian Journal of Pathology and Microbiology*, vol. 53, no. 2, p. 267, 2010.

[9] M. U. Jawad, M. M. Schneiderbauer, E. S. Min, M. C. Cheung, L. G. Koniaris, and S. P. Scully, "Primary lymphoma of bone in adult patients," *Cancer*, vol. 116, no. 4, pp. 871–879, 2010.

[10] C. Messina, D. Christie, E. Zucca, M. Gospodarowicz, and A. J. M. Ferreri, "Primary and secondary bone lymphomas," *Cancer Treatment Reviews*, vol. 41, no. 3, pp. 235–246, 2015.

[11] H. Shoji and T. R. Miller, "Primary reticulum cell sarcoma of boneSignificance of clinical features upon the prognosis," *Cancer*, vol. 28, no. 5, pp. 1234–1244, 1971.

[12] M. E. Mulligan and M. J. Kransdorf, "Sequestra in primary lymphoma of bone: prevalence and radiologic features," *American Journal of Roentgenology*, vol. 160, no. 6, pp. 1245–1248, 1993.

[13] K. M. Garrett, H. K. Kim, J. Stanek, and K. H. Emery, "MR findings of primary bone lymphoma in a 15-year-old girl: emphasis on diffusion-weighted imaging," *Pediatric Radiology*, vol. 41, no. 5, pp. 658–662, 2011.

[14] F. Moog, J. Kotzerke, and S. N. Reske, "FDG PET can replace bone scintigraphy in primary staging of malignant lymphoma," *Journal of Nuclear Medicine*, vol. 40, no. 40, pp. 1407-13, 1999.

[15] F. M. Paes, D. G. Kalkanis, P. A. Sideras, and A. N. Serafini, "FDG PET/CT of extranodal involvement in non-Hodgkin lymphoma and Hodgkin disease," *Radiographics*, vol. 30, no. 1, pp. 269–291, 2010.

[16] B. D. Cheson, R. I. Fisher, S. F. Barrington et al., "Recommendations for initial evaluation, staging, and response assessment of Hodgkin and non-Hodgkin lymphoma: The Lugano classification," *Journal of Clinical Oncology*, vol. 32, no. 27, pp. 3059–3067, 2014.

[17] D. E. Dosoretz, A. K. Raymond, G. F. Murphy et al., "Primary lymphoma of bone the relationship of morphologic diversity to clinical behavior," *Cancer*, vol. 50, no. 5, pp. 1009–1014, 1982.

[18] U. Gianelli, C. Patriarca, A. Moro et al., "Lymphomas of the bone: a pathological and clinical study of 54 cases," *International Journal of Surgical Pathology*, vol. 10, no. 4, pp. 257–266, 2002.

[19] D. Huebner-Chan, B. Fernandes, G. Yang, and M. S. Lim, "An immunophenotypic and molecular study of primary large B-cell lymphoma of bone," *Modern Pathology*, vol. 14, no. 10, pp. 1000–1007, 2001.

[20] R. Ali, F. Ö iMed/Cro, T. Ö iMed/, Üz Ozan, V. Ö aned/Cr, and A. Tunali, "Primary non-Hodgkin's T-cell lymphoma of bone," *Leukemia & Lymphoma*, vol. 45, no. 8, pp. 1719-1720, 2004.

[21] F. P. Lima, M. Bousquet, A. Gomez-Brouchet et al., "Primary diffuse large B-cell lymphoma of bone displays preferential rearrangements of the c-MYCorBCL2Gene," *American Journal of Clinical Pathology*, vol. 129, no. 5, pp. 723–726, 2008.

[22] C. Messina, A. J. M. Ferreri, S. Govi et al., "Clinical features, management and prognosis of multifocal primary bone lymphoma: a retrospective study of the international extranodal lymphoma study group (the IELSG 14 study)," *British Journal of Haematology*, vol. 164, no. 6, pp. 834–840, 2014.

[23] G. Held, S. Zeynalova, N. Murawski et al., "Impact of rituximab and radiotherapy on outcome of patients with aggressive B-cell lymphoma and skeletal involvement," *Journal of Clinical Oncology*, vol. 31, no. 32, pp. 4115–4122, 2013.

[24] F. H. Heyning, P. C. W. Hogendoorn, M. H. H. Kramer, C. T. Q. Holland, E. Dreef, and P. M. Jansen, "Primary lymphoma of bone: extranodal lymphoma with favourable survival independent of germinal centre, post-germinal centre or indeterminate phenotype," *Journal of Clinical Pathology*, vol. 62, no. 9, pp. 820–824, 2009.

[25] F. Heyning, P. Hogendoorn, M. Kramer et al., "Primary non-Hodgkin's lymphoma of bone: a clinicopathological investigation of 60 cases," *Leukemia*, vol. 13, no. 12, pp. 2094–2098, 1999.

[26] P.-P. Hsieh, H.-H. Tseng, S.-T. Chang, T.-Y. Fu, C.-L. Lu, and S.-S. Chuang, "Primary non-Hodgkin's lymphoma of bone: a rare disorder with high frequency of T-cell phenotype in southern Taiwan," *Leukemia & Lymphoma*, vol. 47, no. 1, pp. 65–70, 2006.

[27] R. K. Fairbanks, J. A. Bonner, C. Y. Inwards et al., "Treatment of stage IE primary lymphoma of bone," *International Journal of Radiation OncologyBiologyPhysics*, vol. 28, no. 2, pp. 363–372, 1994.

[28] L. Cai, M. C. Stauder, Y.-J. Zhang et al., "Early-stage primary bone lymphoma: a retrospective, multicenter Rare Cancer Network (RCN) Study," *International Journal of Radiation OncologyBiologyPhysics*, vol. 83, no. 1, pp. 284–291, 2012.

[29] K. M. Ramadan, T. Shenkier, L. H. Sehn, R. D. Gascoyne, and J. M. Connors, "A clinicopathological retrospective study of 131 patients with primary bone lymphoma: a population-based study of successively treated cohorts from the British Columbia Cancer Agency," *Annals of Oncology*, vol. 18, no. 1, pp. 129–135, 2007.

[30] M. B. Ventre, A. J. Ferreri, M. Gospodarowicz et al., "Clinical features, management, and prognosis of an international series of 161 patients with limited-stage diffuse large B-cell lymphoma of the bone (the IELSG-14 study)," *The Oncologist*, vol. 19, pp. 291–298, 2014.

[31] D. Christie, K. Dear, T. Le et al., "Limited chemotherapy and shrinking field radiotherapy for osteolymphoma (primary bone lymphoma): results from the trans-Tasman Radiation Oncology Group 99.04 and Australasian Leukaemia and Lymphoma Group LY02 prospective trial," *International Journal of Radiation OncologyBiologyPhysics*, vol. 80, no. 4, pp. 1164–1170, 2011.

47

Plasmablastic Lymphoma or Plasmablastic Myeloma: A Case of Post-Transplant Lymphoproliferative Disorder

Poornima Ramadas[1,2] **Michael Williams,**[1] **and David B. Duggan**[1]

[1]*SUNY Upstate Medical University, 750 East Adams Street, Syracuse, New York 13210, USA*
[2]*LSU Health Sciences Center, 1501 Kings Hwy, Shreveport, LA 71103, USA*

Correspondence should be addressed to Poornima Ramadas; poornimaramadas@gmail.com

Academic Editor: Salah Aref

Plasmablastic lymphomas and plasmablastic myelomas are malignancies with overlapping clinical and pathological features which pose a diagnostic dilemma and are known to be aggressive with a poor outcome. CD38 is a common immunophenotypic maker for both these malignancies and provides a rationale for using daratumumab-based regimes. We describe a 57-year-old male with a history of end-stage renal disease who underwent a deceased-donor renal transplant maintained on chronic immunosuppression who presented with ascites and was found to have abdominal adenopathy and a lytic lesion in the humerus and diagnosed with a post-transplant lymphoproliferative disorder with features intermediate between plasmablastic lymphoma and plasmablastic myeloma. The patient was subsequently treated with a daratumumab-based regime with an excellent response. This case highlights a rare scenario that poses a diagnostic and therapeutic challenge. As there is no standard of care for the treatment of both these malignancies, this case report also describes the use of daratumumab with a good long-term outcome, especially when the pathological distinction between the two entities is difficult.

1. Introduction

Post-transplant lymphoproliferative disorder (PTLD) is the most common malignancy that occurs in recipients of solid organ transplants and occurs because of immunosuppression (IS) [1]. Monomorphic PTLD includes lymphomas and plasma cell neoplasms. Plasmablastic lymphoma (PBL) is a rare aggressive lymphoma that is usually associated with IS with no definite standard of care and a poor outcome [2]. Plasmablastic myeloma (PBM) is a rare morphological variant of plasma cell neoplasm which is also known to be extremely aggressive with poor survival [3]. Both these malignancies have overlapping clinical and pathological features which pose a diagnostic dilemma [4]. In addition, treatment options are not well defined for either of these and are decided based on institutional/physician preferences and the clinical scenario. CD38 is a common immunophenotypic marker for both these diseases. This provides a good rationale for using daratumumab-based regimes in management, especially when the pathological distinction between the two entities is difficult.

In this case report, we describe a patient with PTLD with features intermediate between PBL and PBM, with clinical features more consistent with PBL, and with an excellent response to a daratumumab-based regimen.

2. Case Presentation

A 57-year-old male who underwent a deceased-donor renal transplant in 1993, maintained on chronic IS with tacrolimus, mycophenolate mofetil, and prednisone, presented with abdominal distention for 2 weeks. He had a history of end-stage renal disease due to hypertension, renal cell carcinoma status post-right-sided nephrectomy, andright lower extremity deep vein thrombosis (DVT) in 2012 and left lower extremity DVT in 2013 and was on anticoagulation. Initial labs showed hemoglobin of 11.4 g/dL (similar to baseline), WBC count of 16,700/uL, platelets of

313,000/uL, with creatinine of 3.13 mg/dL (baseline around 2.5 mg/dL), and corrected calcium of 9.3 mg/dL. CT abdomen pelvis showed a moderate to a large amount of ascites with multiple small, enlarged lymph nodes within the abdomen and pelvis along with the nodularity of the mesentery within the anterior abdomen. He underwent paracentesis, and cytology was reported as plasma cell neoplasm. Immunophenotype showed bright positivity for CD45, moderate positivity for CD138, lambda-restriction, and was also positive for CD19, CD38, and CD56, and negative for CD20 (Figure 1). Cytogenetics showed 5% of nuclei with three copies of 1q and 2 copies of 1p with no evidence for gains or losses of chromosome 5; deletions of 13q14.2, 14q32.3 (IgH), or 17p13 (TP53); or an IgH rearrangement. Given cytology findings, serum protein electrophoresis and immunofixation were obtained which showed a small IgA lambda paraprotein of 570 mg/dL and total IgA of 740 mg/dL. Urine protein electrophoresis was normal. Serum free light chains showed lambda light chains of 163 mg/L, kappa light chains of 58 mg/L, and a normal kappa lambda ratio of 0.36. Uric acid was 11.1 mg/dL and LDH was 634 U/L. CT thorax and soft tissue neck showed small to moderate bilateral pleural effusions and a 1.7 × 3.3 cm lymph node in the superior diaphragmatic region. Over the next few days, he was noted to have worsening renal failure with oliguria and underwent biopsy of the transplanted kidney, and pathology was suggestive of calcineurin inhibitor toxicity with no evidence of rejection or light chain deposition. He also underwent biopsy of the node in the diaphragmatic region, and pathology was consistent with plasma cell myeloma with anaplastic morphology with an immunophenotype like the ascitic fluid (Figure 2). Bone marrow biopsy showed normocellular marrow with no evidence of plasma cell neoplasm. He started having right arm pain and underwent a CT scan which showed intramedullary soft tissue density within the mid-humeral diaphysis with a central lytic lesion and associated areas of cortical breakthrough. He was diagnosed with PTLD with intermediate features between PBL and PBM.

Immunosuppression was tapered and stopped per recommendations from transplant nephrology. He was transferred to hematology service and started on cyclophosphamide, bortezomib, and dexamethasone along with daratumumab. He also started having right foot pain, and CT scan showed midfoot patchy demineralization and mild fragmentation, possibly an acute lytic process. He had ascitic fluid accumulation again and underwent repeat paracentesis 11 days after the initial procedure. He was continued on weekly cyclophosphamide, bortezomib, dexamethasone, and daratumumab. He underwent radiation treatment to the right arm to a dose of 2400 cGy in 6 fractions and the right ankle to a dose of 2400 cGy in 6 fractions. Ascitic fluid accumulation started improving on treatment. He received 4 weekly treatments during the initial inpatient stay and was discharged once stable. He was readmitted 6 days later with a pathologic fracture of the right humerus for which he underwent open reduction internal fixation. He resumed treatment as an outpatient. Cytoxan, bortezomib, and dexamethasone (CyBorD) were continued weekly (days 1, 8, 15, and 22 of 28-day cycles), and daratumumab was given per the standard de-escalation schedule (weekly for 8 doses followed by 2 weekly doses). After around 5 months since the initial diagnosis, he underwent repeat CT scans which showed significant overall improvement in the abdominal ascites and mesenteric lymphadenopathy. He also underwent a SPECT-CT which only showed some uptake in the right humerus but no other areas of uptake. He started developing severe neuropathy, and bortezomib was held from cycle 6 day 15. In addition, he started developing generalized bone pain with no etiology on imaging, and this was thought to be related to daratumumab. He completed a total of 6 cycles of treatment, which included 14 doses of daratumumab. Given multiple adverse effects and good response to treatment, the decision was made to stop treatment and monitor the patient closely. He is currently 18 months post his initial diagnosis and continues to be in remission. It was decided not to resume immunosuppression for renal transplant, and he has been initiated on hemodialysis.

3. Discussion

PBL is a rare subtype of diffuse large B-cell lymphoma (DLBCL) with plasmacytic differentiation. Around 70% is associated with HIV positivity, and the remaining 30% is seen in HIV-negative patients, of which iatrogenic immunosuppression is a common etiology. It also has a strong association with Epstein–Barr virus (EBV) infection and may be positive in around 80% of the cases [5]. Immunophenotype shows an absent expression of CD45, CD20, CD79a, and PAX5 and strong expression of plasma cell markers, CD38, CD138, and MUM1, along with high Ki67 expression [6]. Rearrangements in MYC oncogene were seen in around 50% of the cases and more often seen in EBV positive tumors [7]. The oral cavity and gastrointestinal tract are the most commonly involved sites in both HIV-positive and HIV-negative patients, but any other site including CNS and bone marrow can be involved [5]. Treatment involves multiagent chemotherapy, and intensive regimens like infusional EPOCH, HyperCVAD, or CODOX-M/IVAC are recommended over cyclophosphamide, doxorubicin, vincristine, and prednisone (CHOP), though it is unclear if these regimes offer a survival benefit [8]. Bortezomib and lenalidomide have also been studied, especially in refractory cases [9]. Though an aggressive disease, treatment with chemotherapy improves survival as reported in a SEER database analysis published in August 2020 which showed a 5-year overall survival of 52.8% in treated PBL patients [10]. The presence of a MYC rearrangement has been reported to have a poor prognosis [7].

PBM is a subtype of multiple myeloma (MM) comprising plasmablasts, which are immature plasma cells with clear round nuclei, nucleoli, and small amounts of cytoplasm. Immunophenotype shows positive CD38 and CD138 along with light chain restriction [4]. In a population-based study, patients with plasmablastic morphology had unfavorable clinical features, extensive marrow infiltration, and

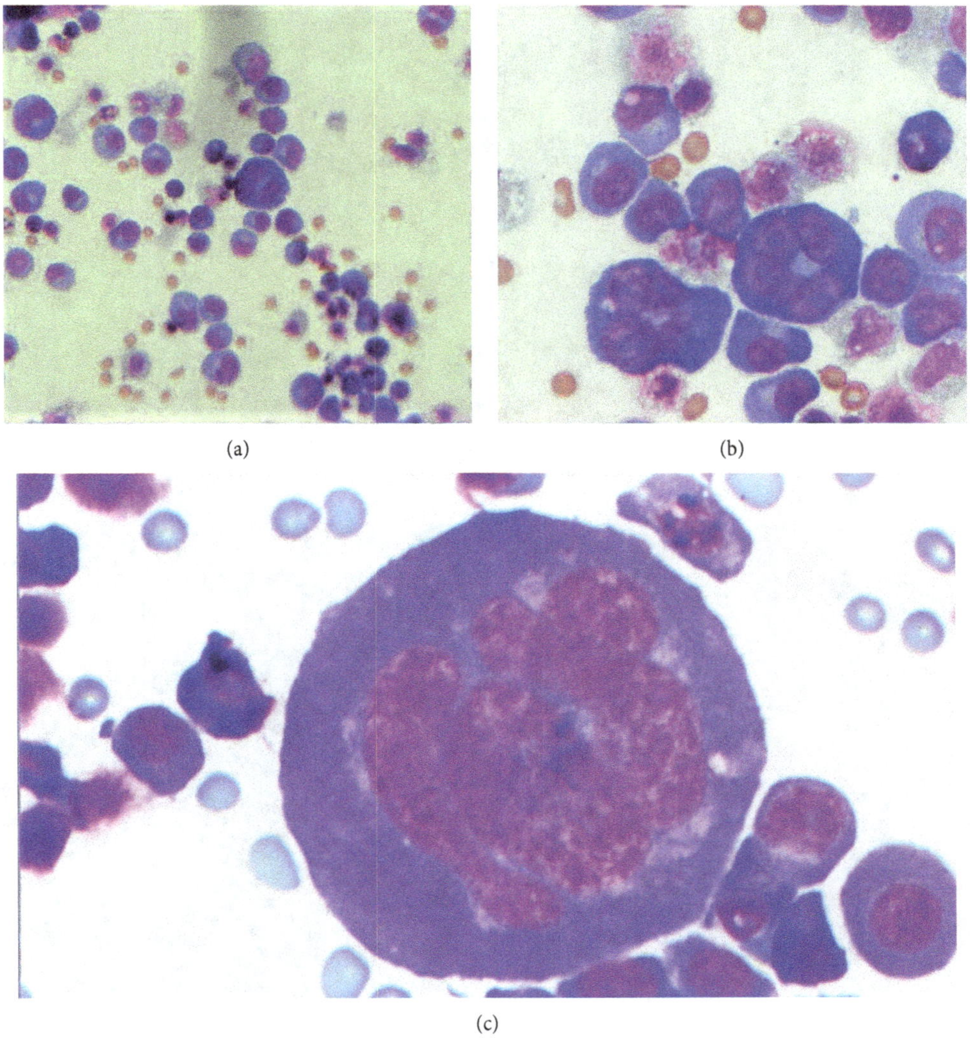

(a) (b) (c)

FIGURE 1: Ascitic fluid cytology showing large immature cells, some of which are multinucleated and admixed with smaller mature looking plasma cells. (a) 200X magnification. (b) 500X magnification. (c) 500X magnification showing large cell with multilobed nucleus.

high Ki67 but did not correlate with poor-risk cytogenetics [11]. Treatment involves myeloma regimes. PBM is also known to be an independent predictor of poor survival after autologous stem cell transplantation [12].

The distinction between PBL and PBM can be a diagnostic dilemma. The immunophenotype of these is remarkably similar, and all patients with PBL and PBM show positivity for CD38, CD138, and MUM1 with high Ki67 and are negative for CD20. CD56 can be positive in PBM, and EBER can be positive in PBL [13]. A study published in March 2017 identified the clinical and pathological features between the two entities and proposed a diagnostic algorithm [14]. The truly borderline cases also pose a challenge in making a treatment decision. Our patient had intermediate features between PBL and PBM. The presence of a paraprotein with lambda restriction on pathology, lytic lesion, and negativity for EBER supported PBM. However, the clinical presentation with the extramedullary disease with nodal involvement and ascites with no evidence of marrow involvement and the mixed immunophenotypic features supported PBL.

Daratumumab is an IgG1κ human monoclonal antibody against CD38 and inhibits the growth of tumor cells with CD38 expression by inducing apoptosis. Daratumumab is well studied in multiple myeloma although the data with PBM have only been reported in case reports [15]. In PBL, a feasibility multicenter study has been proposed, but most of the studies which reported the use of daratumumab are case reports and have been used in relapsed refractory disease [16, 17]. Given that CD38 is a common immunophenotypic marker for both these diseases, the use of daratumumab-based regimes can be considered in borderline cases. As our patient had intermediate features, the decision was made to use daratumumab up front, and given his overall functional status, we did not believe that he could tolerate a more intensive lymphoma regime.

In conclusion, this case report highlights a rare scenario of PTLD where the distinction between PBL and PBM was a diagnostic challenge and describes the use of daratumumab with good long-term outcome. Daratumumab should be considered in the initial treatment of CD38-positive PTLD when the pathological features

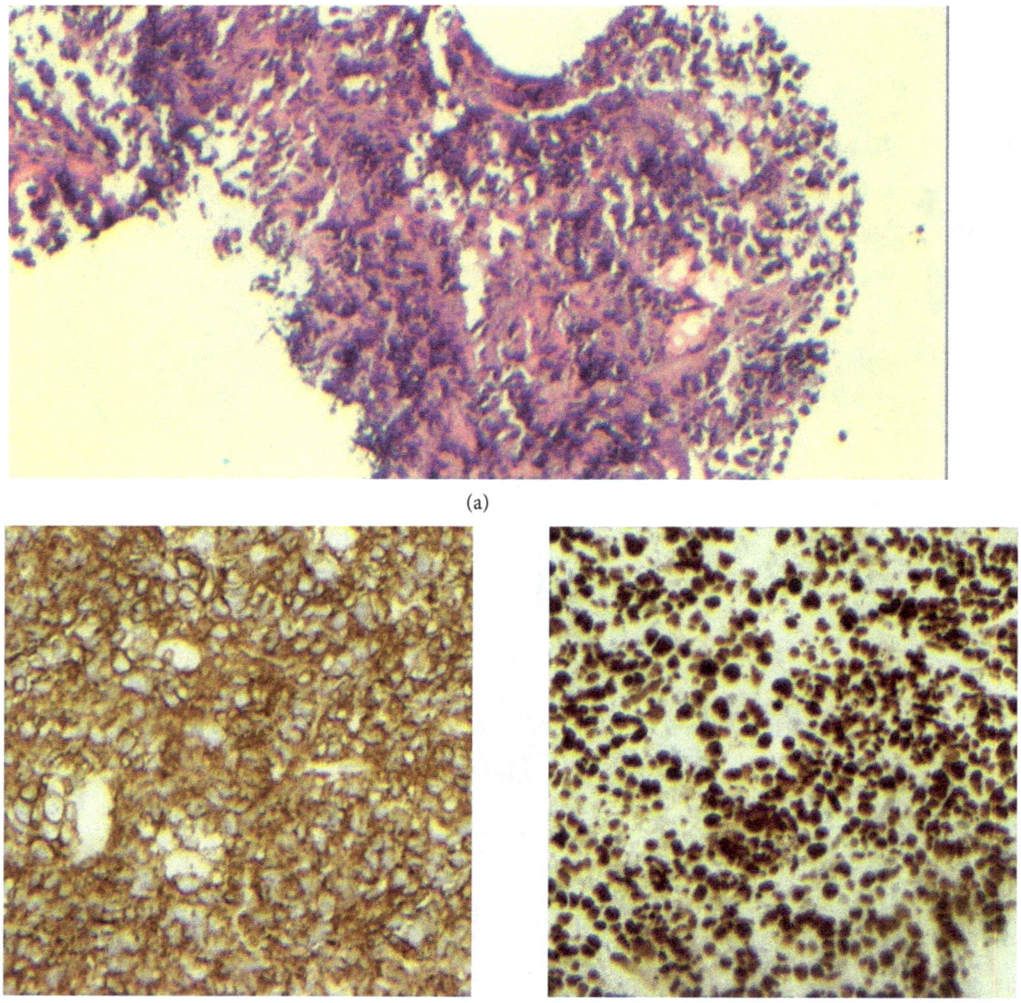

(a)

(b)

(c)

Figure 2: Lymph node biopsy. (a) 4X magnification showing infiltration of the node with abnormal uniform looking cells. (b) 200X magnification for Ki67 highlighting >90% of cells. (c) 200X magnification of CD138 stain.

overlap. Further studies are needed in exploring the use of daratumumab in PBL.

References

[1] I. Penn, "Cancers complicating organ transplantation," *New England Journal of Medicine*, vol. 323, no. 25, pp. 1767–1769, 1990.

[2] J. J. Castillo, M. Bibas, and R. N. Miranda, "The biology and treatment of plasmablastic lymphoma," *Blood*, vol. 125, no. 15, pp. 2323–2330, 2015.

[3] P. R. Greipp, T. Leong, J. M. Bennett et al., "Plasmablastic morphology-an independent prognostic factor with clinical and laboratory correlates: eastern cooperative oncology group (ECOG) myeloma trial e9486 report by the ECOG myeloma laboratory group," *Blood*, vol. 91, no. 7, pp. 2501–2507, 1998.

[4] G. Monohan, "Plasmablastic myeloma versus plasmablastic lymphoma: different yet related diseases," *IJHT*, vol. 6, pp. 25–28, 2018.

[5] J. J. Castillo, E. S. Winer, D. Stachurski et al., "Clinical and pathological differences between human immunodeficiency virus-positive and human immunodeficiency virus-negative patients with plasmablastic lymphoma," *Leukemia and Lymphoma*, vol. 51, no. 11, pp. 2047–2053, 2010.

[6] G. S. Folk, S. L. Abbondanzo, E. L. Childers, and R. D. Foss, "Plasmablastic lymphoma: a clinicopathologic correlation," *Annals of Diagnostic Pathology*, vol. 10, no. 1, pp. 8–12, 2006.

[7] A. Valera, O. Balagué, L. Colomo et al., "IG/MYC rearrangements are the main cytogenetic alteration in plasmablastic lymphomas," *The American Journal of Surgical Pathology*, vol. 34, no. 11, pp. 1686–1694, 2010.

[8] J. J. Castillo, E. S. Winer, D. Stachurski et al., "Prognostic factors in chemotherapy-treated patients with HIV-associated plasmablastic lymphoma," *The Oncologist*, vol. 15, no. 3, pp. 293–299, 2010.

[9] K. Ando, Y. Imaizumi, Y. Kobayashi et al., "Bortezomib- and lenalidomide-based treatment of refractory plasmablastic lymphoma," *Oncology research and treatment*, vol. 43, no. 3, pp. 112–116, 2020.

[10] J. A. Florindez, J. P. Alderuccio, I. M. Reis, and I. S. Lossos, "Survival analysis in treated plasmablastic lymphoma patients: a population-based study," *American Journal of Hematology*, vol. 95, no. 11, pp. 1344–1351, 2020.

[11] H. E. Møller, B. S. Preiss, P. Pedersen et al., "Clinicopathological features of plasmablastic multiple myeloma: a pop-

ulation-based cohort," *Apmis*, vol. 123, no. 8, pp. 652–658, 2015.

[12] S. V. Rajkumar, R. Fonseca, M. Q. Lacy et al., "Plasmablastic morphology is an independent predictor of poor survival after autologous stem-cell transplantation for multiple myeloma," *Journal of Clinical Oncology*, vol. 17, no. 5, p. 1551, 1999.

[13] F. Vega, C.-C. Chang, L. J. Medeiros et al., "Plasmablastic lymphomas and plasmablastic plasma cell myelomas have nearly identical immunophenotypic profiles," *Modern Pathology*, vol. 18, no. 6, pp. 806–815, 2005.

[14] J. S. Ahn, R. Okal, J. A. Vos, M. Smolkin, A. S. Kanate, and F. G. Rosado, "Plasmablastic lymphoma versus plasmablastic myeloma: an ongoing diagnostic dilemma," *Journal of Clinical Pathology*, vol. 70, no. 9, pp. 775–780, 2017.

[15] J. A. Suarez-Londono, A. Rohatgi, C. Antoine-Pepeljugoski, and M. J. Braunstein, "Aggressive presentation of plasmablastic myeloma," *BMJ Case Reports*, vol. 13, no. 4, 2020.

[16] C. R. Tan, S. K. Barta, S. Y. Lensing, and A. Noy, "A multicenter, open-label feasibility study of daratumumab with dose-adjusted EPOCH in newly diagnosed plasmablastic lymphoma," *AIDS Malignancy Consortium*, vol. 105, 2021.

[17] M. Kathrotiya, V. S. Radhakrishnan, S. J. Bhave et al., "Relapsed plasmablastic lymphoma in a HIV-negative patient: pushing the envelope," *Clinical Case Reports*, vol. 9, no. 2, pp. 873–877, 2021.

Use of KRD-PACE as Salvage Therapy in Aggressive, Relapsed/Bortezomib-Refractory Extramedullary Multiple Myeloma: A Report of Two Cases and Literature Review

Ricardo D. Parrondo[1] **Vivek Roy**[1] **Taimur Sher**[1] **Victoria Alegria,**[1]
Asher A. Chanan-Khan,[1,2] **and Sikander Ailawadhi**[1]

[1]*Department of Hematology-Oncology, Mayo Clinic Florida, Jacksonville, FL, USA*
[2]*Department of Hematology-Oncology, St. Vincent's Riverside, Jacksonville, FL, USA*

Correspondence should be addressed to Sikander Ailawadhi; ailawadhi.sikander@mayo.edu

Academic Editor: Sylvain Choquet

Extramedullary multiple myeloma is defined by the presence of plasma cell infiltration outside of the bone marrow. It is associated with a poor prognosis and resistance to therapy and is often associated with high-risk cytogenetics. Aggressive relapsed and refractory extramedullary multiple myeloma is often treated with salvage infusional chemotherapy to achieve rapid disease control. Commonly used regimens include DCEP, CVAD, and VTD-PACE. While VTD-PACE contains bortezomib and thalidomide which have potent antimyeloma activity, the advent of novel agent therapy with proteasome inhibitors and immunomodulatory agents being used in the first-line setting has resulted in many patients being refractory to bortezomib by the time they are treated with VTD-PACE. Herein, we discuss two cases of aggressive relapsed, high-risk, bortezomib-refractory extramedullary multiple myeloma treated with KRD-PACE and review the available clinical data on salvage chemotherapy regimens used in relapsed refractory myeloma.

1. Introduction

Multiple myeloma (MM) is a plasma cell neoplasm that accounts for 1% of all cancers and approximately 10% of all hematologic malignancies [1]. MM is defined by the presence of ≥10% of clonal plasma cells in the bone marrow (or a biopsy proven extramedullary plasmacytoma) and by end-organ damage attributable to the MM such as anemia, lytic bone lesions, renal failure, and hypercalcemia [1]. Approximately, 1% to 2% of patients have extramedullary disease (EMD) upon initial diagnosis and 8% develop EMD later on in the disease course, typically after multiple relapses [2]. EMD is defined by the presence of soft-tissue plasmacytomas or plasma cell infiltration outside of the bone marrow [3]. The presence of high-risk cytogenetics (particularly del(17p) and amp [1q21]) is associated with development of EMD [4]. EMD is associated with an adverse prognosis in newly diagnosed and in relapsed MM patients and tends to be resistant to proteasome inhibitors, immunomodulatory agents, and even novel agents such as daratumumab [5–7]. As such, infusional "traditional" chemotherapy agents are used in the treatment of patients with relapsed/refractory MM (RRMM) as a means of rapid tumor debulking or as a bridge to high-dose therapy and stem cell transplant. Several such intensive infusional chemotherapy regimens are currently used.

In a population of patients with RRMM, hyperfractionated cyclophosphamide, vincristine, doxorubicin, and dexamethasone (CVAD) has been reported to produce an overall response rate (ORR) of 40% and a median overall survival (OS) of 15 months [8]. Dexamethasone with continuous-infusion cyclophosphamide, etoposide, and cisplatin (DCEP) demonstrated an ORR of 58% and a median response duration of 9 months in a population of RRMM patients [9]. In patients with RRMM, DT-PACE (thalidomide, dexamethasone, and 4-d continuous infusions of cisplatin, doxorubicin, cyclophosphamide, and etoposide) produced an ORR of 61% [10]. Bortezomib (V) is frequently administered with DT-PACE [11]. In RRMM, the proteasome inhibitor carfilzomib (K) has proven to produce superior response rates, progression-free survival (PFS), and OS compared to V [12]. Likewise, the addition of K to lenalidomide (R) and D produces superior response rates and PFS compared to RD in RRMM [13]. Furthermore, the overlapping toxicity of peripheral neuropathy by bortezomib and thalidomide makes them less desirable to combine in a regimen [14].

As a majority of patients may be heavily pretreated and refractory to V by the time they are considered for salvage infusional chemotherapy, we wanted to examine the efficacy of KRD-PACE as the salvage therapy for RRMM. Herein, we describe the efficacy and clinical course of two patients with aggressive, V-refractory, extramedullary, RRMM with high-risk cytogenetics who were treated with KRD-PACE and provide a succinct review of the literature.

2. Discussion

2.1. Patient 1. A 32-year-old male was diagnosed with a solitary plasmacytoma of the left T4 paraspinal area extending into the T4 vertebral body in the July of 2016. A CT-guided biopsy of the T4 lesion was performed which revealed sheets of kappa-restricted plasma cells. A bone marrow biopsy did not reveal a clonal plasma cell population. Serum protein electrophoresis revealed an M spike of 0.7 g/dL, and immunofixation revealed an IgG kappa monoclonal protein. The patient subsequently received radiation therapy (RT) consisting of 360 cGy in 2 fractions. Prior to receiving a 3rd fraction of RT, the patient developed acute onset severe back pain with bilateral lower extremity paresthesias and weakness. An MRI of the spinal canal revealed a persistent paraspinal mass and a new fracture of the T4 vertebrae. The patient subsequently underwent surgical resection of the plasmacytoma with reconstruction spinal fusion. Pathology revealed kappa-restricted plasma cells arising in sheets. The patient then underwent postoperative RT to the tumor bed receiving 3960 cGy in 22 fractions. In the May of 2018, the patient developed back pain, and an MRI of the back revealed a 5 cm × 5.7 cm mass on the left T4 hemivertebra with extra vertebral extension along the posterior left chest wall. In the June of 2018, a biopsy of this lesion revealed kappa-restricted plasma cells in sheets. Fluorescence *in situ* hybridization (FISH) of the lesion revealed monosomies 1, 8, 13, 14, and 17, which includes loss of the TP53 gene region. Restaging workup is shown in Table 1. The patient was not a candidate for additional RT or surgery to the spine, and thus was started on V-cyclophosphamide-D (CyBorD) for relapsed, extramedullary multiple myeloma. After receiving one cycle of CyBorD, the patient continued to complain of back pain and developed worsening paresthesias of the thighs bilaterally and lower extremity weakness. An MRI of the thoracic spine revealed an increase in the size of the lateral aspect of the left-sided paraspinal mass with severe cord compression from T3 through T5, and 18F FDG PET-CT images are shown in Figure 1(a). Given the patient's poor response to CyBorD and urgency of cord compression, it was decided to start the patient on salvage carfilzomib (K), lenalidomide (R), dexamethasone (D), cisplatin (P), doxorubicin (A), cyclophosphamide (C), and etoposide (E); KRD-PACE. KRD-PACE was dosed at K (20 mg/m^2 on days 1 and 2 followed by 56 mg/m^2 on days 8,9,15, and 16), R (25 mg daily on days 1–21), D (40 mg orally on days 1–4) with P (10 mg/m^2/day), A (10 mg/m^2/day), C (400 mg/m^2/day), and E (40 mg/m^2/day) given as a continuous intravenous infusion over 24 hours on days 1–4 (Table 2). The patient tolerated two cycles of KRD-PACE well without the need for extended hospitalization, dose reductions, transfusion, or growth factor support. He did not develop febrile neutropenia. The patient had a very good partial response (VGPR) to therapy (Table 1) with near resolution of the paraspinal plasmacytoma (Figure 1(b)). He subsequently went on to stem cell mobilization and collection followed by a melphalan 200 mg/m^2 salvage autologous stem cell transplant (ASCT) after which he obtained a complete response. He is currently on maintenance therapy with lenalidomide 10 mg on days 1–21 and ixazomib 2 mg weekly, 13 months after KRD-PACE.

2.2. Patient 2. A 56-year-old male developed temporal-occipital headaches in the April of 2017. In the November of 2017, an MRI brain was done which revealed an enlarging enhancing skull base lesion involving the clivus, right temporal bone, right petrous apex, and bilateral occipital condyles with the involvement of the right hypoglossal canal. The MRI brain also picked up bilateral upper cervical lymphadenopathy. A subsequent skeletal survey revealed multiple poorly defined lytic lesions throughout the axial and appendicular skeleton. A CT of the chest, abdomen, and pelvis revealed left axillary, right retrocrural, and left pericardial lymphadenopathy. The patient had a multiple myeloma workup (Table 1) which revealed a high-risk, revised international scoring system (R-ISS) III IgA kappa myeloma. A biopsy of one of the aforementioned cervical lymph nodes revealed sheets of kappa-restricted plasma cells, and FISH revealed a duplication 1q consistent with extramedullary disease at diagnosis. Bone marrow cytogenetics revealed a 1q duplication as well as trisomy 6, 11, and 15 and monosomy 13. The patient was subsequently started on VRD in the December of 2017 and achieved a partial response after 4 cycles. The patient had progressive disease in the April of 2018 as evidenced by a pathologic right humerus midshaft fracture. He then had surgical fixation of the fracture (pathology revealed a plasmacytoma with kappa-restricted plasma cells) and was started on daratumumab (Dara)-R-D in the May of 2018. After 4 cycles of Dara-R-D, restaging labs and an 18F FDG PET-CT revealed stable disease. After 6 cycles of Dara-R-D, the patient developed disease progression manifested by back pain for which thoracic and lumbar CT scans revealed a pathologic fracture of L5 and multiple pathologic nondisplaced fractures of the rib cage. Extramedullary disease was noted on 18F FDG PET-CT

TABLE 1: Response measurement and hematologic toxicity/recovery time after 2 cycles of KRD-PACE.

	Patient 1			Patient 2	
Parameter	Staging studies at relapse before KRD-PACE	Staging studies after 2 cycles of KRD-PACE	Parameter	Staging studies at relapse before KRD-PACE	Staging studies after 2 cycles of KRD-PACE
ISS score (at diagnosis)	I	—	ISS score (at diagnosis)	III	—
Revised-ISS score (at diagnosis)	II	—	Revised-ISS Score (st diagnosis)	III	—
Cytogenetics/ FISH (at diagnosis)	Monosomies 1, 8, 13, 14 and 17, which includes loss of the TP53 gene region	—	Cytogenetics/ FISH (at diagnosis)	1q duplication. In addition, trisomy 6, 11, and 15, monosomy 13	—
Hgb	14.2 g/dL	11.1 g/dL	Hgb	13.0 g/dL	11.1 g/dL
Plt	172×10^9/L	312	Plt	169×10^9/L	68×10^9/L
Cr	0.86 mg/dL	0.74 mg/dL	Cr	0.96 mg/dL	1.06 mg/dL
LDH	635 U/L	184 U/L	LDH	235 U/L	159 U/L
B_2-microglobulin	1.55 mcg/mL	1.27 mcg/mL	B_2-microglobulin	9.41 mcg/mL	2.37 mcg/mL
M-spike	0.9 g/dL	0.1 g/dL	M-spike	0.2 g/dL	0.1 g/dL
IFE	IgG kappa	IgG kappa	IFE	IgA kappa	No monoclonal protein
IgG	1410 mg/dL	544 mg/dL	IgG	257 mg/dL	294 mg/dL
IgA	155 mg/dL	92 mg/dL	IgA	584 mg/dL	9 mg/dL
IgM	80 md/dL	24 mg/dL	IgM	24 md/dL	9 mg/dL
Lambda	0.738 mg/dL	0.283 mg/dL	Lambda	0.248 mg/dL	0.042 mg/dL
Kappa	22.9 mg/dL	0.701 mg/dL	Kappa	1.25 mg/dL	<0.030 mg/dL
K/L ratio	31.02	2.48	K/L Ratio	5.04	<0.712
Bone marrow biopsy	2-3% kappa-restricted atypical plasma cells.	—	Bone marrow biopsy	—	No atypical plasma cells detected.
Response	—	Very good partial response	Response	—	Complete response
Plt nadir/time to recovery	—	69×10^9/L/7 days	Plt nadir/time to recovery	—	8×10^9/L/45 days
ANC nadir/time to recovery	—	1.18×10^9/L	ANC nadir/time to recovery	—	0.04×10^9/34 days
Hgb nadir/time to recovery	—	11.2 g/dL	Hgb nadir/time to recovery	—	6.3 g/dl/48 days

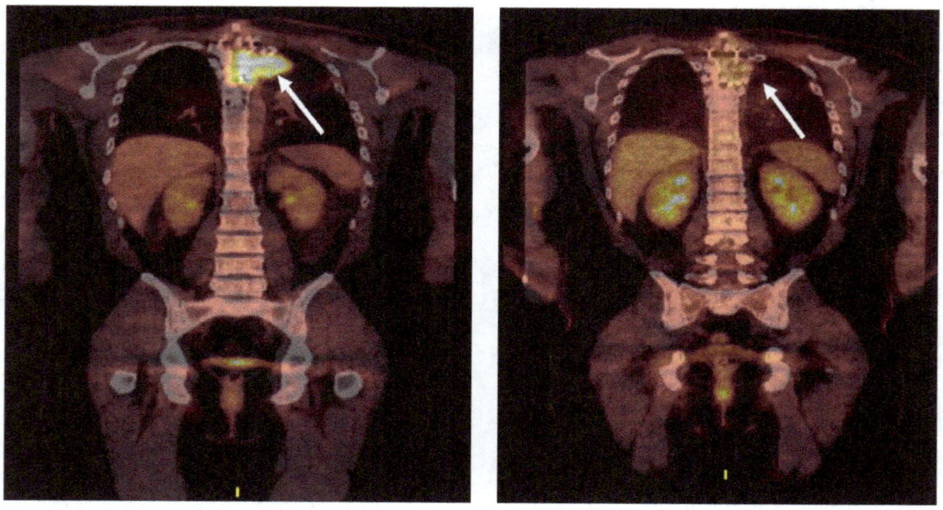

(a) (b)

FIGURE 1: (a) 18F FDG PET-CT at relapse showing large soft-tissue mass replacing the T4 vertebral body (white arrow). (b) 18F FDG PET-CT after 2 cycles of KRD-PACE showing near-complete resolution of the extraosseous soft-tissue component involving patient's known T4 vertebral body lesion (white arrow).

Table 2: KRD-PACE dosing schedule for patient 1 and KRD-PACE dosing schedule for patient 2.

28d cycle	K	R	D	P	A	C	E
A: Patient 1, KRD-PACE schedule							
Dose	20 mg/m^2 (day 1) then 56 mg/m^2 thereafter	25 mg	40 mg	10 mg/m^2	10 mg/m^2	400 mg/m^2	40 mg/m^2
Schedule	Days 1, 2, 8, 9, 15, 16	Days 1–21	Days 1–4	Days 1–4	Days 1–4	Days 1–4	Days 1–4
B: Patient 2, KRD-PACE schedule							
Dose	20 mg/m^2 (day 1) then 27 mg/m^2	15 mg	40 mg	10 mg/m^2	10 mg/m^2	400 mg/m^2	40 mg/m^2
Schedule	Days 1,2	Days 1–21	Days 1–4	Days 1–4	Days 1–4	Days 1–4	Days 1–4

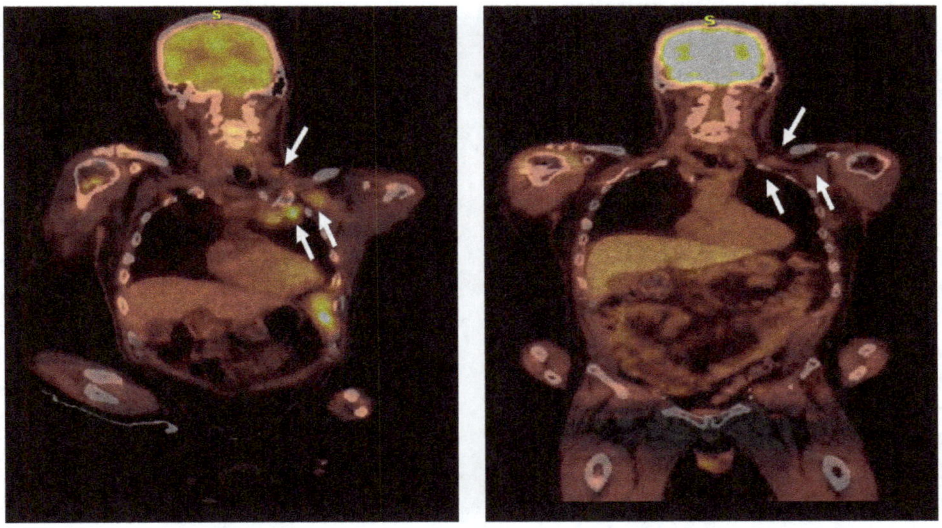

(a) (b)

Figure 2: (a) 18F FDG PET-CT at relapse showing left cervical and supraclavicular adenopathy and numerous left subpectoral, axillary, and internal mammary adenopathy (white arrows). (b) 18F FDG PET-CT after 2 cycles of KRD-PACE revealing complete resolution of adenopathy.

(Figure 2(a)). Restaging studies are given in Table 1. Peripheral flow cytometry did not real evidence of plasma cell leukemia. The patient was subsequently started on KRD-PACE salvage therapy with the following dosing schedule: K (20 mg/m^2 on day 1 followed by 27 mg/m^2 on day 2 of each cycle), R (15 mg daily on days 1–21), D (40 mg orally on days 1–4) with P (10 mg/m^2/day), A (10 mg/m^2/day), C (400 mg/m^2/day), and E(40 mg/m^2/day) given as a continuous intravenous infusion over 24 hours on days 1–4 (Table 2). He ultimately received 2 cycles of KRD-PACE. The patient developed grade 3 mucositis and anemia, grade 4 thrombocytopenia and neutropenia requiring transfusion (a total of 8 units of packed red cells and 10 units of platelets), and growth factor support (three 6 mg filgrastim injections), as well as a right upper extremity deep venous thrombosis (Table 1). He did not develop neutropenic fever. The patient was only hospitalized for 4 days during each cycle of KRD-PACE and was never rehospitalized. Transfusional and growth factor support was managed in the outpatient setting. The patient had a complete response (CR) to therapy (Table 1) with a resolution of lymphadenopathy (Figure 2(b)). He went on to stem cell mobilization but was unable to collect an adequate number of stem cells on two occasions. He remained in CR of therapy but developed an extramedullary relapse 6 months after completion of KRD-PACE and is now being considered for enrollment in an anti-B-cell maturation antigen (BCMA) chimeric antigen receptor T-cell (CAR-T) therapy trial.

3. Conclusion

We describe two cases of aggressive, relapsed, bortezomib-refractory extramedullary MM with high-risk cytogenetics who achieved deep responses with KRD-PACE salvage therapy. One of the patients, a 32-year-old male with minimal MM bone marrow involvement and less prior treatment, tolerated 2 cycles of KRD-PACE without any complications or need for transfusional support. He achieved a VGPR and proceeded to high-dose therapy and ASCT to which he achieved a CR. The 56-year-old patient had extensive bone marrow involvement and 2 prior lines of treatment. He tolerated 2 cycles of KRD-PACE without the need for extended hospitalization, but developed profound cytopenias which required 34–48 days to recover and multiple red cell and platelet transfusions as well as granulocyte colony stimulating factor support. He achieved a complete response which lasted for 6 months without additional therapy.

DCEP, CVAD, and VTD-PACE-like regimens are the most commonly used infusional salvage chemotherapy regimens in patients with RRMM. In a retrospective analysis of 107 patients with RRMM, the ORR, PFS, and OS were 52%, 3.8 months, and 8.9 months for DCEP; 49%, 5.8 months, and 8.3 months for CVAD; and 73%, 4.5 months, and 8.5 months for VTD-PACE, respectively [15]. There were no significant differences in response rates or survival benefit amongst the three regimens [15]. Patients received a median number of 2 cycles, >70% were refractory to V and >60% were refractory to R [15]. Successful autologous transplant after salvage chemotherapy was associated with superior PFS (HR, 0.25; 95% CI, 0.14–0.45) and OS (HR 0.19, 95% CI, 0.12–0.30) [15]. High-risk cytogenetics ($P = 0.05$) and EMD ($P = 0.006$) were the factors associated with inferior OS in the study population [14]. Common adverse effects were increased transfusion requirements (62%), febrile neutropenia (37%), delays in treatment (36%), rehospitalization (34%), venous thromboembolism (6%), dose reductions due to adverse events (5%), and treatment-related mortality (7%) [15]. There was a trend toward more febrile neutropenia with VTD-PACE and prolonged hospitalization among patients treated with CVAD, but there were no statistically significant differences in adverse events among the 3 regimens [15]. In a retrospective study of 141 patients with RRMM treated with VTD-PACE-like regimens, ORR was 54%, OS was 8.1 months, and PFS was 3.1 months [16]. Most patients received 1–2 cycles of a VTD-PACE-like regimen, 85% were refractory to V, and 60% were refractory to R. Patients required a median of 4 packed red cell transfusions and 4 platelet transfusions during cycle 1 [16]. Median time to recovery of absolute neutrophil count and platelet count from initiation of a VTD-PACE-like regimen was 18 (range, 12–44) and 21(range 11–45) days, respectively [16]. Age ≥60 (HR 2.28, 95% CI, 1.41–3.70) and R-ISS III (HR 2.38, 95% CI, 1.35–4.04) predicted shortened OS [16]. Presence of EMD and high-risk cytogenetics, and being refractory to proteasome inhibitors or immunomodulatory agents were not associated with shortened OS [16].

Salvage chemotherapy regimens, including the most intensive regimen, VTD-PACE, confer a median OS of 8 months and a median PFS of 3–4 months for RRMM patients based on the current published studies [15,16]. OS and PFS are even shorter for patients with high-risk cytogenetics and EMD. Given that over 60% of patients in the aforementioned studies were refractory to V and R when they received salvage regimens, substitution of VT for KR to make KRD-PACE is a plausible alternative. A study by Cowan et al. examined the use of KRD-PACE for chemomobilization in 20 patients with RRMM [17]. 15 patients received 1 cycle of KRD-PACE, and 5 patients received 2 cycles. The ORR was 25% with 75% achieving stable disease. 100% of patients underwent ASCT. No patients experienced cardiac toxicity. Following transplant, the median time to neutrophil engraftment was 18 days and the median time to platelet engraftment was 13 days. The PFS at 6 months was 63% (95% CI, 0.382–1), and the OS at 6 months was 91% (95% CI, 0.754–1) [17]. Harrell et al. reported a retrospective study of 52 patients with RRMM who were treated with KD-PACE-like regimens [18]. In this study, 54% of patients had high-risk cytogenetics and had received a median of 3 prior lines of therapy and 64% had KD-PACE together with an immunomodulatory agent. Grade 3/4 toxicities included neutropenia (93%), thrombocytopenia (87%), and anemia (37%). Febrile neutropenia occurred in 35%. The overall response rate (≥PR) was 77% including CR (12%), VGPR (23%), and PR (42%). Median PFS was 4.6 mo (95% CI 3.2–7.5 mo) and median OS 11.2 mo (95% CI 6.1–14.5 mo) [18].

Relapsed refractory extramedullary MM with high-risk cytogenetics is a highly aggressive, treatment-refractory disease state with a dismal prognosis. Salvage chemotherapy followed by ASCT is one of the few treatment options that can prolong survival and act as a bridge to a clinical trial. While most patients are refractory to V by the time they are treated with salvage regimens, KRD-PACE offers an efficacious option for treatment that introduces a novel agent (K) highly active in RRMM. In the ASPIRE and ENDEAVOR trials, K has proven to produce superior ORR, OS, and PFS compared to V-based or R-based regimens in RRMM [12,13]. Furthermore, in the ASPIRE trial, KRD was superior to RD for PFS across high-risk cytogenetic risk groups, suggesting that this combination partly abrogates the negative impact of t(4; 14) and del(17p) [13]. Prospective trials evaluating the safety and efficacy of salvage KRD-PACE in RRMM, especially patients with high-risk myeloma and those with EMD, are warranted.

References

[1] S. V. Rajkumar, M. A. Dimopoulos, A. Palumbo et al., "International myeloma working group updated criteria for the diagnosis of multiple myeloma," *The Lancet Oncology*, vol. 15, no. 12, pp. e538–e548, 2014.

[2] K. D. Short, S. V. Rajkumar, D. Larson et al., "Incidence of extramedullary disease in patients with multiple myeloma in the era of novel therapy, and the activity of pomalidomide on extramedullary myeloma," *Leukemia*, vol. 25, no. 6, pp. 906–908, 2011.

[3] M. Weinstock and I. M. Ghobrial, "Extramedullary multiple myeloma," *Leukemia & Lymphoma*, vol. 54, no. 6, pp. 1135–1141, 2013.

[4] X. Qu, L. Chen, H. Qui et al., "Extramedullary manifestation in multiple myeloma bears high incidence of poor cytogenetic aberration and novel agents resistance," *BioMed Research International*, vol. 2015, Article ID 787809, 7 pages, 2015.

[5] N. Gagelmann, D.-J. Eikema, S. Iacobelli et al., "Impact of extramedullary disease in patients with newly diagnosed multiple myeloma undergoing autologous stem cell transplantation: a study from the chronic malignancies working party of the EBMT," *Haematologica*, vol. 103, no. 5, pp. 890–897, 2018.

[6] S. Z. Usmani, C. Heuck, A. Mitchell et al., "Extramedullary disease portends poor prognosis in multiple myeloma and is over-represented in high-risk disease even in the era of novel agents," *Haematologica*, vol. 97, no. 11, pp. 1761–1767, 2012.

[7] M. Pick, V. Vainstein, N. Goldschmidt et al., "Daratumumab resistance is frequent in advanced-stage multiple myeloma patients irrespective of CD38 expression and is related to dismal prognosis," *European Journal of Haematology*, vol. 100, no. 5, pp. 494–501, 2018.

[8] M. A. Dimopoulos, D. Weber, H. Kantarjian, K. B. Delasalle, and R. Alexanian, "HyperCVAD for VAD-resistant multiple myeloma," *American Journal of Hematology*, vol. 52, no. 2, pp. 77–81, 1996.

[9] M. Dadacaridou, X. Papanicolaou, D. Maltesas et al., "Dexamethasone, cyclophosphamide, etoposide and cisplatin (DCEP) for relapsed or refractory multiple myeloma patients," *Journal of Balkan Union of Oncology*, vol. 12, no. 1, pp. 41–44, 2007.

[10] B. Barlogie, E. Anaissie, F. van Rhee et al., "Incorporating bortezomib into upfront treatment for multiple myeloma: early results of total therapy 3," *British Journal of Haematology*, vol. 138, no. 2, pp. 176–185, 2007.

[11] C.-K. Lee, B. Barlogie, N. Munshi et al., "DTPACE: an effective, novel combination chemotherapy with thalidomide for previously treated patients with myeloma," *Journal of Clinical Oncology*, vol. 21, no. 14, pp. 2732–2739, 2003.

[12] M. A. Dimopoulous, P. Moreau, A. Palumbo et al., "Carfilzomib and dexamethasone versus bortezomib and dexamethasone for patients with relapsed or refractory multiple myeloma (ENDEAVOR): a randomised, phase 3, open-label, multicentre study," *The Lancet Oncology*, vol. 17, no. 1, pp. 27–38, 2016.

[13] A. K. Stewart, S. V. Rajkumar, M. A. Dimopoulos et al., "Carfilzomib, lenalidomide, and dexamethasone for relapsed multiple myeloma," *New England Journal of Medicine*, vol. 372, no. 2, pp. 142–152, 2015.

[14] M. Pineda-Roman, M. Zangari, F. van Rhee et al., "VTD combination therapy with bortezomib-thalidomide-dexamethasone is highly effective in advanced and refractory multiple myeloma," *Leukemia*, vol. 22, no. 7, pp. 1419–1427, 2008.

[15] P. T. Griffin, V. Q. Ho, W. Fulp et al., "A comparison of salvage infusional chemotherapy regimens for recurrent/refractory multiple myeloma," *Cancer*, vol. 121, no. 20, pp. 3622–3630, 2015.

[16] A. Lakshman, P. P. Singh, S. V. Rajkumar et al., "Efficacy of VDT PACE-like regimens in treatment of relapsed/refractory multiple myeloma," *American Journal of Hematology*, vol. 93, no. 2, pp. 179–186, 2018.

[17] A. J. Cowan, M. Karami, E. N. Libby et al., "Outcome of multiple myeloma patients treated with carrd-PACE chemomobilization: a single-center experience," *Blood*, vol. 128, no. 22, p. 3377, 2016.

[18] S. Harrell, M. Khan, B. Dhakal, H. Parameswaran, and R. Cornell, "KD-PACE salvage therapy for aggressive relapsed multiple myeloma," *Clinical Lymphoma Myeloma and Leukemia*, vol. 19, no. 10, pp. e252–e253, 2019.

An Unusually Short Latent Period of Therapy-Related Myeloid Neoplasm Harboring a Rare MLL-EP300 Rearrangement: Case Report and Literature Review

Reina Takeda[1,2] **Kazuaki Yokoyama**[1] **Seiichiro Kobayashi,**[3] **Toyotaka Kawamata,**[1,3] **Sousuke Nakamura,**[3] **Tomofusa Fukuyama,**[1,2] **Mika Ito,**[3] **Nozomi Yusa,**[4] **Eigo Shimizu,**[5] **Nobuhiro Ohno,**[1,3] **Rui Yamaguchi**[5] **Seiya Imoto**[6] **Satoru Miyano,**[5,6] **Kaoru Uchimaru,**[1,7] **and Arinobu Tojo**[1,3]

[1]*Department of Hematology/Oncology, Research Hospital, The Institute of Medical Science, The University of Tokyo, Tokyo 108-8639, Japan*
[2]*Division of Cellular Therapy, The Institute of Medical Science, The University of Tokyo, Tokyo 108-8639, Japan*
[3]*Division of Molecular Therapy, The Institute of Medical Science, The University of Tokyo, Tokyo 108-8639, Japan*
[4]*Department of Applied Genomics, Research Hospital, Institute of Medical Science, The University of Tokyo, Tokyo 108-8639, Japan*
[5]*Laboratory of DNA Information Analysis, Human Genome Center, Institute of Medical Science, The University of Tokyo, Tokyo 108-8639, Japan*
[6]*Division of Health Medical Data Science, Health Intelligence Center, Institute of Medical Science, The University of Tokyo, Tokyo 108-8639, Japan*
[7]*Laboratory of Tumor Cell Biology, Department of Computational Biology and Medical Science, Graduate School of Frontier Sciences, The University of Tokyo, Tokyo 108-8639, Japan*

Correspondence should be addressed to Kazuaki Yokoyama; k-yoko@ims.u-tokyo.ac.jp

Academic Editor: Kiyotaka Kawauchi

Therapy-related myeloid neoplasm (t-MN) is a late and lethal complication induced by chemotherapy and/or radiation therapy. Hematological malignancy is one of the most common primary diseases in patients with t-MN. However, the occurrence of t-MN in adult T-cell leukemia/lymphoma (ATL) patients is rarely reported, possibly due to the dismal prognosis of ATL per se. Here, we report a 62-year-old female who developed t-MN only three months after the completion of conventional chemotherapy and anti-CCR4 antibody for ATL acute type. The patient presented with persistent fever and monocytosis without any evidence of infectious diseases. Bone marrow examinations revealed chronic myelomonocytic leukemia-like disease with a chromosomal translocation of t(11;22)(q23;q13) as a solo cytogenetic abnormality, resulting in the diagnosis of t-MN. Next-generation sequencing analysis identified a rare chimeric transcript, MLL-EP300, without any additional somatic mutations. Although the patient underwent allogenic hematopoietic stem cell transplantation, she died of viral encephalomyelitis at 7 months after diagnosis of t-MN. Since recent therapeutic advances have extended the survival of patients with ATL, further evaluation of the long-term risks of developing t-MN in these patients is warranted.

1. Introduction

Therapy-related myeloid neoplasm (t-MN) is a late complication induced by chemotherapy and/or radiation therapy for both malignant diseases and nonmalignant diseases [1]. Typically, t-MN has a latency period of at least a few years following exposure to therapeutic agents [2]. Median survival time after diagnosis of t-MN is 8 months, and five-year overall survival is less than 10% [2]. As well as breast cancer, hematological malignancy including non-Hodgkin's lymphoma, Hodgkin's lymphoma, and multiple myeloma is observed as the most common primary disease in patients with t-MN [1–3]. However, there have been only a few reports on t-MN developing in adult T-cell leukemia/lymphoma (ATL) patients [4–8]. The incidence risk of t-MN in ATL patients was estimated as 2.1% [4], which is much lower than that of non-Hodgkin's lymphoma (5–10%) [3, 9]. This is possibly due to the dismal survival outcomes of ATL per se [4, 5]. In particular, the acute type of ATL has a median survival time of only 8.3 months despite intensive therapies [10]. Thus, patients with ATL rarely survive long enough to develop secondary malignancies. Recent introduction of an anti-CCR4 antibody called mogamulizumab has improved prognosis in ATL patients [11, 12]. Here, we report a case of t-MN developing shortly after intensive chemotherapy combined with a humanized anti-CCR4 antibody, mogamulizumab, for ATL, along with the results of molecular investigation using next-generation sequencing and literature review.

2. Case Presentation

A 62-year-old female patient with the acute type of ATL received five sessions of mLSG-15 therapy combined with mogamulizumab [12]. A dose-intensified chemotherapy called mLSG-15 therapy is commonly used as an initial treatment for aggressive ATL and consists of VCAP (vincristine, cyclophosphamide, doxorubicin, and prednisone), AMP (doxorubicin, ranimustine, and prednisone), and VECP (vindesine, etoposide, carboplatin, and prednisone) [12]. She achieved a complete response (CR) from ATL. Three months later, she was referred to our hospital for allogeneic hematopoietic stem cell transplantation (alloHSCT). On admission, she had persistent fever accompanied by repetitive skin rash and arthralgia. The skin rash exhibited patches of 2-3 cm in diameter and sometimes harbored a subcutaneous mass with pain. Interestingly, these skin and joint symptoms always recovered spontaneously in a few days before recurring in different parts of the body. Peripheral blood (PB) examination showed WBC 4.9×10^9/L (neutrophils 32.5%, lymphocytes 15.0%, monocytes 48.5%, myeloblasts 0.0%, abnormal lymphocytes 0.5%, and monocytoid cells 3.5%), Hb 9.6 g/dL, and platelets 87×10^9/L. The absolute monocyte count in PB was 2.4×10^9/L. Monocytosis had been persistently observed, although ATL cells had hardly been detected in PB by either morphological or immunophenotypic analysis. Lactate dehydrogenase increased slightly (LDH: 247 IU/L, normal range 105–211 IU/L). C-reactive protein was highly elevated (CRP: 20.46 mg/dL). The proviral load (PVL) of HTLV-1 was only 0.45%. A systemic computed tomography scan indicated no hepatosplenomegaly or lymphadenopathy or other signs associated with malignant diseases, infectious diseases, or inflammatory diseases. Bone marrow (BM) examination revealed a slight hypocellularity with a predominance of differentiated monocytes (58% of nuclear cell count) without an increase of blast cells (2%) (Figure 1(a)). Screening analysis for the representative 11 leukemic chimera genes including BCR-ABL1 by polymerase chain reaction was negative. Flow cytometric analysis revealed that the monocytes increased in the BM were positive for CD45, CD33, CD4, CD14, and HLA-DR but negative for CD2, CD13, and CD56. Fluorescence in situ hybridization (FISH) analysis showed split mixed lineage leukemia (MLL) gene signals in 78% of the interphase cells (Figure 1(b)) but no rearrangement signals with regard to two genes: platelet-derived growth factor receptor alpha and beta. Karyotyping analysis using the G-band method detected the t(11;22)(q23;q13) translocation as a solo cytogenetic abnormality (Figure 1(c)). This chromosomal aberration was not observed at the onset of ATL. Human T-cell leukemia virus type 1 (HTLV-1) provirus DNA analysis (via inverse polymerase chain reaction) of CD14-sorted monocytes revealed no monoclonal integration (Figure 1(d)) [13].

Therefore, the patient was diagnosed with therapy-related myeloid neoplasm (t-MN), which phenotypically resembled chronic myelomonocytic leukemia (CMML)-1. The latent period between the initial therapy and the onset of t-MN was 10 months. On the contrary, ATL was confirmed as CR, in accordance with the response criteria for ATL [14]. Our case did not have clinical evidence of ATL disease such as increase of ATL cells in PB and BM, swollen lymph nodes, hepatosplenomegaly, and skin involvement of ATL cells. Additionally, the results from PVL and inverse PCR analysis were also consistent with the conclusion that her ATL had remained in CR (Figure 1(d)). She underwent alloHSCT but died of viral complications of encephalomyelitis at 4 months after transplantation (7 months after diagnosis of t-MN).

In order to identify the partner gene of MLL gene rearrangement in this case, we performed RNA sequencing analysis. Total RNA was extracted from the patient's BM sample using a QIAGEN RNeasy Mini Kit (QUIAGEN, Venlo, Netherlands). cDNA libraries for next-generation sequencing were constructed from 24 ng of total RNA using a Truseq RNA Access Library Prep Kit (Illumina, San Diego, CA, USA). Each paired-end indexed library was sequenced to a length of 75 nucleotides per mate (2×75 bp) on a Nextseq instrument (Illumina). Sequence reads were processed by our in-house Genomon-RNA pipeline [15, 16] (available at http://genomon.readthedocs.org/ja/latest/, http://genomon.hgc.jp/rna/). Fusion transcripts were detected by Genomon-fusion. The Integrative Genomics Viewer (IGV) version 2.3.57 (https://software.broadinstitute.org/software/igv/download) was used to visualize the fusion-sequence. For validation of the fusion transcripts, reverse transcription polymerase chain reaction (RT-PCR) and Sanger sequencing were performed. Total RNA was extracted from the patient's BM sample using a PAXgene blood RNA kit (QIAGEN) and QIAqube. The RNA was reverse transcribed into cDNA by using SuperScript™ IV VILO™ Master Mix (Thermo Fisher Scientific, Massachusetts, USA). DNA was amplified and sequenced using Platinum Taq HF (Thermo Fisher Scientific) and the following primers: primer F 5′-GTGTGGGAGATGGGAGGCT-3′ from MLL exon 10 and primer R 5′-CCTCCATCTTCACTTCCTGGG-3′ from EP300 exon 15.

Next, to explore the molecular mechanisms of leukemogenesis in this case, we performed a targeted deep

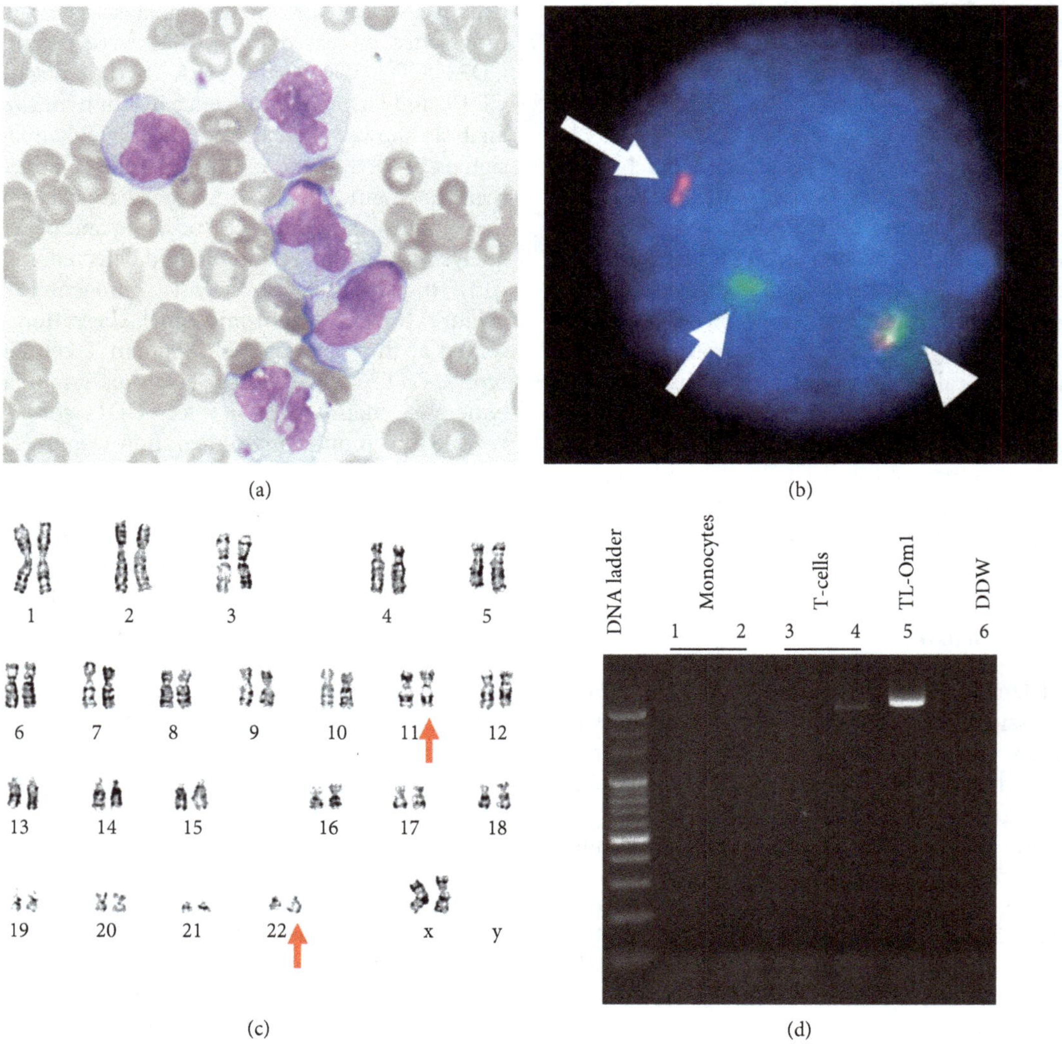

FIGURE 1: Characteristics of MLL-EP300-positive therapy-related myeloid neoplasm in the present case. (a) Bone marrow (BM) showed numerous differentiated monocytes without any increase in the number of myeloblasts or adult T-cell lymphoma/leukemia (ATL) cells (May–Giemsa stain, original magnification, 1,000x). Some monocytes exhibited slightly atypical nuclei. (b) Fluorescence in situ hybridization (FISH) analysis for gene rearrangements involving in the mixed lineage leukemia (MLL) gene at 11q23 was performed. The normal MLL gene exhibited a yellow signal (arrow head), whereas a split MLL gene exhibited as a pair of green and red signals (arrows). The BM sample from the present case showed that 78.5% of the interphase cells were positive for the split MLL gene signals. (c) G-banding of the BM material revealed 46,XX, t(11;22)(q23;q13)[17]/46,XX[3]. Red arrows indicate the abnormal chromosomes involving the translocation. (d) Human T-cell leukemia virus type 1 (HTLV-1) provirus DNA analysis was performed by using inverse polymerase chain reaction. CD14-sorted monocytes (lanes 1, 2) showed no bands. CD3-sorted T-cells (lanes 3, 4) failed to show a visible band with the reproducibility, indicating that the case was negative for a major ATL clone. TL-Om1 was an HTLV-1-infected cell line as positive control (lane 5), and distilled and deionized water (DDW) was used for negative control (lane 6).

sequencing analysis. Flow cytometric sorting of the CD14-positive monocytes and CD4-positive T-cells (control 1) from the patient's peripheral blood was performed using a FACS Aria II (BD Biosciences, San Jose, CA). Oral epithelial cells (control 2) were collected via buccal swab from the patient. Targeted sequencing was performed using 20 ng of DNA via the TruSight Myeloid Panel on the MiSeq platform (Illumina), which included the analysis of the following 54 genes related to myeloid malignancies: ABL1, ASXL1, ATRX, BCOR, BCORL1, BRAF, CALR, CBL, CBLB, CBLC, CDKN2A, CEBPA, CSF3R, CUX1, DNMT3A, ETV6/TEL, EZH2, FBXW7, FLT3, GATA1, GATA2, GNAS, HRAS, IDH1, IDH2, IKZF1, JAK2, JAK3, KDM6A, KIT, KRAS, MLL, MPL, MYD88, NOTCH1, NPM1, NRAS, PDGFRA, PHF6, PTEN, PTPN11, RAD21, RUNX1, SETBP1, SF3B1, SMC1A, SMC3, SRSF2, STAG2, TET2, TP53, U2AF1, WT1, and ZRSR2. T cells and oral epithelial cells served as a germline control in this case. Bioinformatic analysis was performed using standard procedures [17].

Cytogenetic and FISH analyses revealed that MLL on chromosome 11q23 was involved in gene rearrangement as the result of chromosomal translocation t(11;22)(q23;q13). RNA sequencing analysis followed by RT-PCR validation was performed to identify the partner gene of MLL rearrangement. RNA sequencing analysis detected a chimeric gene, MLL-EP300, formed by the in-frame fusion of MLL exon 10 to EP300 exon 15. The fusion gene was also confirmed by RT-PCR and Sanger sequencing (Figure 2) [18–20].

To seek the molecular details underlying leukemogenesis in this case, mutation screening analysis with a targeted deep sequencing method was performed. The panel was focused on myelodysplastic syndrome- (MDS-) and acute myeloid leukemia- (AML-) related genes. Among these 54 genes, SRSF2, TET2 and ASXL1 are frequently mutated in CMML patients [21]. However, any additional somatic mutations were not detected in our case (data not shown).

This study was approved by the Institutional Review Board of the Institute of Medical Science, the University of Tokyo, and informed consent was obtained from the patient in accordance with the Declaration of Helsinki.

3. Discussion

t-MN typically occurs as a late complication of chemotherapy and/or radiation administered for primary malignant diseases [1]. The most common subtype of t-MN is caused by alkylating agents and/or radiation after a long latency period of 5–7 years [1, 2]. This subtype is associated with the type of MDS that often progresses to AML and is frequently characterized by complete or partial deletion of chromosomes 5 and 7 [1, 2]. In contrast, the second major subtype caused by topoisomerase II inhibitors presents as overt AML with a shorter latent period of 2–3 years [1, 2, 22]. This topoisomerase II inhibitor-associated t-MN is associated with balanced translocation, such as chromosomal translocations involving the MLL at 11q23; the runt-related transcription factor 1 (RUNX1) at 21q22; and a promyelocytic leukemia-retinoic acid receptor alpha (PML-RARA) fusion resulting from the t(15; 17) [1, 2, 22]. Our present case had a therapeutic history of topoisomerase II inhibitors including etoposide and exhibited a balanced chromosomal translocation t(11;22)(q23;q13) resulting in MLL gene rearrangement. Collectively, these clinical features suggest that our case was consistent with t-MN induced by topoisomerase II inhibitors. Of note, our case had a shorter latency period of 10 months from the diagnosis of ATL.

The rare chimera MLL-EP300 has been reported in three different cases so far (Table 1) [16–18]. In all four cases including our case, MLL-EP300-positive leukemia emerged as t-MN following a medical history of malignancies. Although all the primary malignancies were treated with topoisomerase II inhibitors, other clinical features were quite varied. For example, there were variations in diagnostic ages, types of primary malignancies, latent periods, and locations of fusion breakpoints [18–20]. Intriguingly, only our case exhibited a phenotype of sustained monocytosis mimicking CMML-like disease, whereas the other three were acute myeloid leukemia (AML). In addition, the former three cases had one or more additional cytogenetic abnormalities other than t(11;22)(q23;q13), but only our case showed t(11;22)(q23;q13) as a solo cytogenic abnormality and had no additional cytogenetic abnormalities. Because only a limited number of cases were observed, it remains unclear whether and how differences of chromosomal breakpoints can affect leukemogenesis and the clinical features in MLL-EP300-positive leukemia. Molecular profiling by next-generation sequencing analysis is valuable to understand the pathogenesis and invent better therapeutic strategies. The genetic investigation with targeted deep sequencing demonstrated that our case had no additional somatic mutations, strongly implying that MLL-EP300 was a principal driver gene causing t-MN in this case.

EP300 is a rare fusion partner of MLL rearrangements among various translocations involving in MLL gene identified [18–20]. Interestingly, each MLL rearrangement can have different phenotypes and mechanisms for leukemogenesis, depending on the fusion partners [23]. Somatic mutations of EP300 gene have been found in hematological malignancies including MDS [24]. A recent study showed that loss of function of EP300 accelerates leukemic transformation of MDS cells [25]. On the contrary, it was reported that lysine acetyltransferase (KAT) activity of EP300 promotes leukemogenesis in AML by acetylating H3K18 [26]. In addition, a study showed that bromodomain of EP300 regulates functions of myeloid-derived suppressor cells via controlling H3K27 acetylation [27]. As shown in Figure 2, MLL-EP300 fusion protein in this case includes both KAT domain and bromodomain of EP300, indicating that this fusion protein could induce myeloid transformation via altering epigenetic modifications in hematopoietic cells. Functional analysis of MLL-EP300 fusion protein is necessary to elucidate leukemogenesis induced by this rare translocation.

In previous studies, t-MN developing after ATL had a devastating prognosis, regardless of primary ATL disease status [4–8]. Most of the patients died only a few months after diagnosis of t-MN [4–8]. Various cytogenetic abnormalities not limited to MLL rearrangements were detected in t-MN after ATL [4–8]. The risk of t-MN among ATL patients was estimated as 2.1% [4]. This is obviously lower than the incidence rate of t-MN in patients with non-Hodgkin's lymphoma (estimated as 5–10%) [1, 3, 9]. This is possibly due to the dismal survival outcomes of ATL per se [4, 5]. However, it is important to note that these previous studies on t-MN after ATL were published before the introduction of mogamulizumab, which has recently been reported to improve the prognosis of patients with aggressive ATL [11, 12]. Given such recent therapeutic progress, further evaluation of the long-term risks of t-MN in ATL patients should be warranted.

In conclusion, we present a case of t-MN, with a rare MLL-EP300 rearrangement and an unusually short latent period. Additionally, according to the previous literature of t-MN with MLL-EP300 rearrangement, only our case exhibited a phenotype of CMML. Based on the cytogenetic abnormality of balanced translocation, a topoisomerase II inhibitor was thought to be the causative factor for t-MN in this case. Because survival time increases for patients with ATL who had prior exposure to chemotherapeutic agents, the clinician must keep in mind the cumulative risk of t-MN in these patients as well.

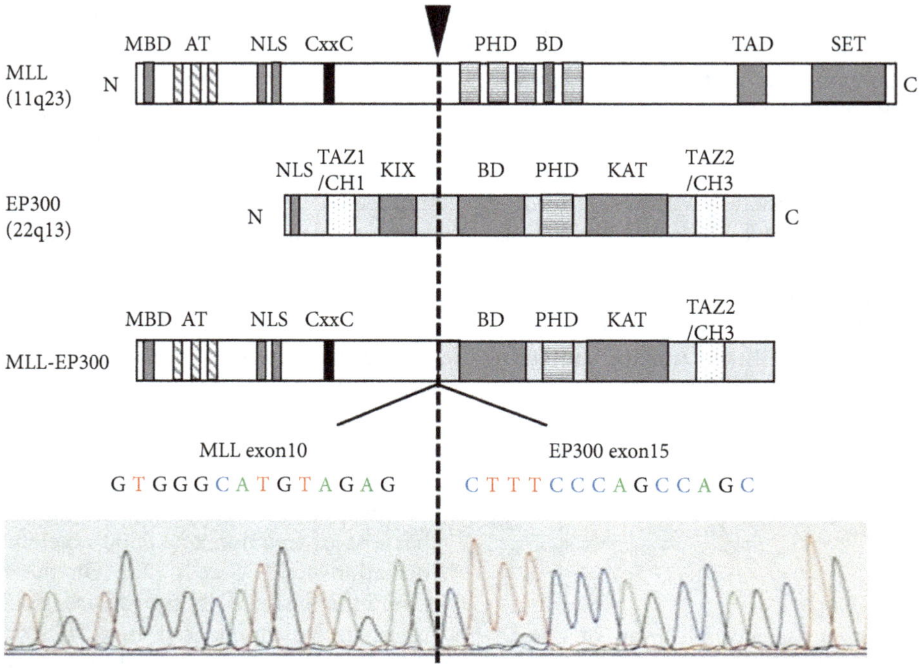

Figure 2: The structures of MLL, EP300, and MLL-EP300 fusion protein and the sequence of the fusion gene. RNA sequencing and RT-PCR followed by Sanger sequencing demonstrated that MLL exon 10 was fused in-frame to EP300 exon 15. The breakpoint is indicated by the arrow and dashed line. MBD, menin-binding domain; AT, AT hooks; NLS, nuclear localization signal; CxxC, motif recognizing unmethylated CpG dinucleotides; PHD, plant homeodomain fingers; BD, bromodomain; TAD, transactivation domain; SET, H3K4 histone methyltransferase domain; TAZ, transcriptional-adaptor zinc-finger domain; CH, cysteine/histidine-rich regions; KIX, kinase-inducible domain of the CREB-interacting domain; KAT, lysine acetyltransferase domain.

Table 1: A summary of cases of therapy-related MLL-EP300-positive leukemia (cases 1–4).

Case	Age/sex	Phenotype	Karyotype	MLL-EP300 breakpoint	Latent period (months)	Primary malignancy	Cytotoxic exposure	Reference
1	4/M	AML	48,XY, +8, +8, t(11;22)(q23;q13)	MLLexon9/EP300exon15	67	NHL	Chemo including ETP	[16]
2	5/F	AML	46,XX, t(1;22;11)(q44;q13;q23), t(10;17)(q22;q21)	MLLexon7/EP300exon15	36	Neuroblastoma	Chemo including THP,	[17]
3	66/M	AML	46,XY, t(11;22)(q23;q13). idem, +8	MLLexon10, 11/EP300exon13	16	PTCL NOS, AML with MDS	CBDCA, CPA CHOP-14, ESHAP	[18]
4	62/F	CMML	46,XX, t(11;22)(q23;q13)	MLLexon10/EP300exon15	10	ATL	mLSG+ mogamulizumab	Present case

CHOP-14 contains cyclophosphamide, doxorubicin, vincristine, and prednisolone. ESHAP consists of etoposide, methylprednisolone, cytarabine, and cisplatin. ETP, etoposide; THP, pirarubicin; CBDCA, carboplatin; CPA, cyclophosphamide. mLSG contains VCAP (vincristine, cyclophosphamide, doxorubicin, and prednisone), AMP (doxorubicin, ranimustine, and prednisone), and VECP (vindesine, etoposide, carboplatin, and prednisone). NHL, non-Hodgkin lymphoma; PTCL NOS, peripheral T-cell lymphoma not otherwise specified; ATL, adult T-cell leukemia/lymphoma.

Acknowledgments

The authors are very grateful to the physicians, nurses, and other care providers and staff at Research Hospital IMUST and especially the patients and their families. The authors have no funding support in this study to declare.

References

[1] M. E. McNerney, L. A. Godley, and M. M. Le Beau, "Therapy-related myeloid neoplasms: when genetics and environment collide," *Nature Reviews Cancer*, vol. 17, no. 9, pp. 513–527, 2017.

[2] S. M. Smith, M. M. Le Beau, D. Huo et al., "Clinical-cytogenetic associations in 306 patients with therapy-related myelodysplasia and myeloid leukemia: the University of Chicago series," *Blood*, vol. 102, no. 1, pp. 43–52, 2003.

[3] L. M. Morton, G. M. Dores, M. A. Tucker et al., "Evolving risk of therapy-related acute myeloid leukemia following cancer chemotherapy among adults in the United States, 1975-2008," *Blood*, vol. 121, no. 15, pp. 2996–3004, 2013.

[4] S. Owatari, M. Otsuka, K. Uozumi, T. Takeshita, and S. Hanada, "Two cases of secondary acute myeloid leukemia accompanying adult T-cell leukemia/lymphoma," *International Journal of Hematology*, vol. 85, no. 1, pp. 32–35, 2007.

[5] S. Owatari, A. Arai, T. Tsuruta, K. Haraguchi, M. Otsuka, and S. Hanada, "Acute myeloid leukemia diagnosed 5 Years after adult T-cell leukemia/lymphoma," *Journal of Clinical and Experimental Hematopathology*, vol. 55, no. 1, pp. 29–31, 2015.

[6] K. Tsukasaki, T. Koba, M. Iwanaga et al., "Possible association between adult T-cell leukemia/lymphoma and acute myeloid leukemia," *Cancer*, vol. 82, no. 3, pp. 488–494, 1998.

[7] H. Nakamura, T. Ishizaki, T. Itoyama et al., "Acute myeloid leukaemia with t(9;11)(p22;q23) in a patient treated for adult T cell leukaemia," *British Journal of Haematology*, vol. 86, no. 1, pp. 222–224, 1994.

[8] N. Shimada, N. Ohno, R. Tanosaki et al., "Therapy-related acute myeloid leukemia after the long-term administration of low-dose etoposide for chronic-type Adult T-cell leukemia-lymphoma: a case report and literature review," *Internal Medicine*, vol. 56, no. 14, pp. 1879–1884, 2017.

[9] J. O. Armitage, P. P. Carbone, J. M. Connors, A. Levine, J. M. Bennett, and S. Kroll, "Treatment-related myelodysplasia and acute leukemia in non-Hodgkin's lymphoma patients," *Journal of Clinical Oncology*, vol. 21, no. 5, pp. 897–906, 2003.

[10] H. Katsuya, K. Ishitsuka, A. Utsunomiya et al., "Treatment and survival among 1594 patients with ATL," *Blood*, vol. 126, no. 24, pp. 2570–2577, 2015.

[11] T. Ishida, T. Joh, N. Uike et al., "Defucosylated anti-CCR4 monoclonal antibody (KW-0761) for relapsed adult T-cell leukemia-lymphoma: a multicenter phase II study," *Journal of Clinical Oncology*, vol. 30, no. 8, pp. 837–842, 2012.

[12] T. Ishida, T. Jo, S. Takemoto et al., "Dose-intensified chemotherapy alone or in combination with mogamulizumab in newly diagnosed aggressive adult T-cell leukaemia-lymphoma: a randomized phase II study," *British Journal of Haematology*, vol. 169, no. 5, pp. 672–682, 2015.

[13] S. Kobayashi, E. Watanabe, T. Ishigaki et al., "Advanced human T-cell leukemia virus type 1 carriers and early-stage indolent adult T-cell leukemia-lymphoma are indistinguishable based on CADM1 positivity in flow cytometry," *Cancer Science*, vol. 106, no. 5, pp. 598–603, 2015.

[14] K. Tsukasaki, O. Hermine, A. Bazarbachi et al., "Definition, prognostic factors, treatment, and response criteria of adult T-cell leukemia-lymphoma: a proposal from an international consensus meeting," *Journal of Clinical Oncology*, vol. 27, no. 3, pp. 453–459, 2009.

[15] Y. Shiraishi, K. Kataoka, K. Chiba et al., "A comprehensive characterization of cis-acting splicing-associated variants in human cancer," *Genome Research*, vol. 28, no. 8, pp. 1111–1125, 2018.

[16] Y. Shiraishi, A. Fujimoto, M. Furuta et al., "Integrated analysis of whole genome and transcriptome sequencing reveals diverse transcriptomic aberrations driven by somatic genomic changes in liver cancers," *PLoS One*, vol. 9, no. 12, Article ID e114263, 2014.

[17] K. Yokoyama, E. Shimizu, N. Yokoyama et al., "Cell-lineage level-targeted sequencing to identify acute myeloid leukemia with myelodysplasia-related changes," *Blood Advances*, vol. 2, no. 19, pp. 2513–2521, 2018.

[18] K. Ida, I. Kitabayashi, T. Taki et al., "Adenoviral E1A-associated protein p300 is involved in acute myeloid leukemia with t(11;22)(q23;q13)," *Blood*, vol. 90, no. 12, pp. 4699–4704, 1997.

[19] H. Ohnishi, T. Taki, H. Yoshino et al., "A complex t(1;22;11)(q44;q13;q23) translocation causingMLL-p300fusion gene in therapy-related acute myeloid leukemia," *European Journal of Haematology*, vol. 81, no. 6, pp. 475–480, 2008.

[20] F. P. Duhoux, G. Ameye, J.-M. Libouton et al., "The t(11;19)(q23;p13) fusing MLL with MYO1F is recurrent in infant acute myeloid leukemias," *Leukemia Research*, vol. 35, no. 9, pp. e171-e172, 2011.

[21] C. C. Mason, J. S. Khorashad, S. K. Tantravahi et al., "Age-related mutations and chronic myelomonocytic leukemia," *Leukemia*, vol. 30, no. 4, pp. 906–913, 2016.

[22] J. D. Rowley and H. J. Olney, "International workshop on the relationship of prior therapy to balanced chromosome aberrations in therapy-related myelodysplastic syndromes and acute leukemia: overview report," *Genes, Chromosomes and Cancer*, vol. 33, no. 4, pp. 331–345, 2002.

[23] A. C. Winters and K. M. Bernt, "MLL-rearranged leukemias-an update on science and clinical approaches," *Frontiers in Pediatrics*, vol. 5, no. 4, 2017.

[24] E. Papaemmanuil, M. Gerstung, L. Malcovati et al., "Clinical and biological implications of driver mutations in myelodysplastic syndromes," *Blood*, vol. 122, no. 22, pp. 3616–3627, 2013.

[25] G. Cheng, F. Liu, T. Asai et al., "Loss of p300 accelerates MDS-associated leukemogenesis," *Leukemia*, vol. 31, no. 6, pp. 1382–1390, 2017.

[26] G. Giotopoulos, W.-I. Chan, S. J. Horton et al., "The epigenetic regulators CBP and p300 facilitate leukemogenesis and represent therapeutic targets in acute myeloid leukemia," *Oncogene*, vol. 35, no. 3, pp. 279–289, 2016.

[27] D. E. de Almeida Nagata, E. Y. Chiang, S. Jhunjhunwala et al., "Regulation of tumor-associated myeloid cell activity by CBP/EP300 bromodomain modulation of H3K27 acetylation," *Cell Reports*, vol. 27, no. 1, pp. 269–281, 2019.

50

Sarcoidosis and Multiple Myeloma: A Case Report and Literature Review

Joao Tiago Serra, Aurelia Martinho, Fernanda Paixao Duarte, and Fernando Aldomiro

Department of Internal Medicine II, Professor Doutor Fernando Fonseca Hospital, Amadora, Portugal

Correspondence should be addressed to Joao Tiago Serra; joao.t.serra@gmail.com

Academic Editor: Takashi Sonoki

The existence of a sarcoidosis-lymphoma syndrome has been previously proposed since the relation between sarcoidosis and an increased risk of lymphoproliferative disorders is well established. Multiple myeloma is a malignant multifocal proliferation of clonal plasma cells within the bone marrow, and its association with sarcoidosis has been rarely described. We present a concurrent diagnosis of sarcoidosis and multiple myeloma and make a brief analysis of the reported cases in the literature. A 65-year-old woman underwent surgery for the excision of a wrist mass that presented 3 years before. Histological analysis showed sarcoid-type epithelioid granulomas without necrosis, establishing soft tissue sarcoidosis. Further evaluation revealed marked interstitial lung parenchyma lesions and large intrathoracic adenopathies. Bronchofibroscopy with transbronchial biopsy confirmed lung sarcoidosis. In addition, blood analysis showed monoclonal IgG kappa gammopathy. A bone marrow biopsy confirmed hypercellularity with 60% plasma cells and plasmocyte infiltration. Thus, the diagnosis of systemic sarcoidosis and multiple myeloma was established simultaneously. In a brief review of the literature, we identified 33 reports of cases with both sarcoidosis and multiple myeloma. We point out the importance of a high level of suspicion for the association of sarcoidosis with malignant haematological diseases such as multiple myeloma.

1. Introduction

Sarcoidosis is a T-cell-mediated immunological response against an unknown environmental trigger in a susceptible host. Noncaseating granulomas, consisting of compact and centrally organized collections of CD4+ T cells, macrophages, and epithelioid cells, are the hallmark of sarcoidosis and the outcome of an unbalanced T-helper 1 immune response [1, 2]. Multiple myeloma (MM) is a malignant multifocal proliferation of clonal plasma cells within the bone marrow, associated with skeletal destruction, serum monoclonal gammopathy, and end-organ sequelae [3]. Brincker [4] described the sarcoidosis-lymphoma syndrome in 1986 for the particular association between sarcoidosis and lymphoproliferative disorders (LD); however, the association between sarcoidosis and MM has been rarely reported and the explanation for this relation remains unclear and controversial. We describe a case of sarcoidosis associated with MM and present a brief analysis of published cases in the literature.

2. Case Report

A 65-year-old Caucasian women, retired cook, was referred to our outpatient clinic due to a three-year history of a painless mass on the dorsal side of the right wrist. Her medical background was positive for type 2 diabetes mellitus, dyslipidaemia, bronchitis, and venous thrombosis of the right eye. The wrist lesion had been growing gradually and affected finger movement. There was no history of blunt or penetrating trauma.

An ultrasound, complemented with nuclear magnetic resonance, identified a lesion on the dorsal plane of the right wrist, extending to the inner face, but without vascular or tendinous invasion, measuring about $100 \times 60 \times 18$ mm in diameter and having well-defined limits (Figure 1). After surgery for lesion removal, histological analysis showed an extensive granulomatous process without necrosis, consisting of sarcoid-type epithelioid granulomas. The patient also complained of long-term intermittent nodular skin lesions on both legs, dry cough, and dyspnoea, for which she

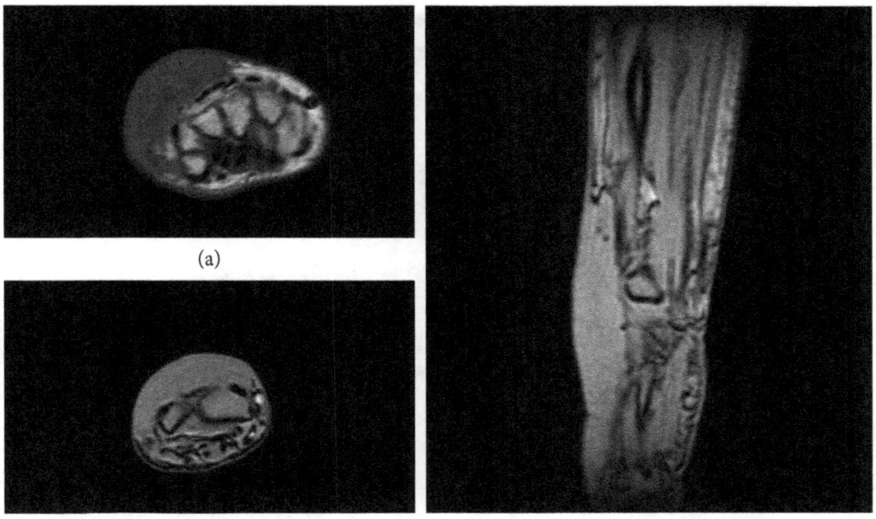

(a)

(b)

(c)

FIGURE 1: Magnetic resonance images in T1-weighted axial view (a), T2-weighted axial view (b), and T2-weighted sagital view (c), identifying a lesion on the dorsal plane of the right wrist, extending to the inner face but without vascular or tendinous invasion, measuring about $100 \times 60 \times 18$ mm in diameter, with well-defined limits.

had been previously prescribed bronchodilators with little symptomatic relief. Physical examination revealed painless bilateral supraclavicular lymphadenopathies, bibasilar coarse crackles, and nodular skin lesions scattered along both inferior limbs (*erythema nodosum*). There were no other palpable lymph nodes, hepatosplenomegaly, fever, night sweats, or constitutional symptoms.

Laboratory studies showed haemoglobin 9.7 g/dL (reference range 11.5–16.5 g/dL), white blood cells count of 4.6×10^9/L (reference range $4–11 \times 10^9$/L), C-reactive protein of 0.87 mg/dL (reference range <0.30 mg/dL), erythrocyte sedimentation rate of 83 mm (reference range <20 mm), serum angiotensin converting enzyme (ACE) of 141.28 U/L (reference range 12–68 U/L), albumin of 3.66 g/dL (reference range 3.97–4.94 g/dL), and total serum protein level of 8.40 g/dL (reference range 6.40–8.20 g/dL). Serum protein electrophoresis revealed a monoclonal band, confirmed by immunofixation to be immunoglobulin IgG kappa. Further quantification of serum immunoglobulins showed an elevated IgG level of 3120 mg/dL (reference range 70–1600 mg/dL), with normal IgM and IgA, and beta-2 microglobulin of 2.09 mg/dL (reference range 0.67–1.31 mg/dL). Mantoux assay and Bence Jones proteinuria quantification were negative, and both renal function and serum calcium were within the normal range. The screening for HIV and hepatitis B and C was negative.

A high-resolution computed tomography of the chest showed large mediastinal and axillary adenopathies with extensive conglomerates, associated with marked and diffuse permeability of the entire pulmonary parenchyma, thickening of the interlobular septa, and fine bronchovascular and subpleural micronodularity (Figure 2).

The patient's lung function testing revealed a mild restrictive pattern with decreased diffusion capacity. A bronchofibroscopy with transbronchial biopsy and bronchioalveolar lavage was performed. Respiratory tract fluid analysis showed an increased CD4/CD8 ratio of 9.02, and both acid-fast staining (Ziehl–Neelsen coloration) and mycobacterial culture were negative. Bronchial biopsy histological results revealed mild chronic inflammatory infiltrate with multiple nonnecrotizing sarcoid-type epithelioid granulomas and giant multinucleated Langerhans cells (Figures 3(a) and 3(b)). The patient also underwent a scintigraphy with gallium 67, which documented pathological uptake in the lungs, axillary and inguinal regions, and several cutaneous foci on the lower limbs. Ophthalmologic evaluation was consistent with ocular sarcoidosis. For further evaluation of serum monoclonal IgG kappa gammopathy, a bone marrow aspirate and biopsy were performed, showing a hypercellular bone marrow with 60% plasma cells and plasmocyte infiltration with K light chain restriction, respectively (Figures 3(c) and 3(d)).

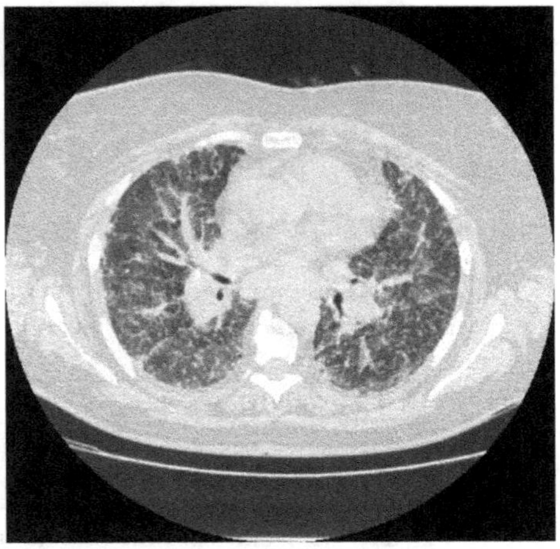

FIGURE 2: Chest high-resolution computed tomography image showing marked and diffuse alteration of pulmonary parenchyma permeability, thickening of the interlobular septa, and fine bronchovascular and subpleural micronodularity, associated with mediastinal lymphadenopathy.

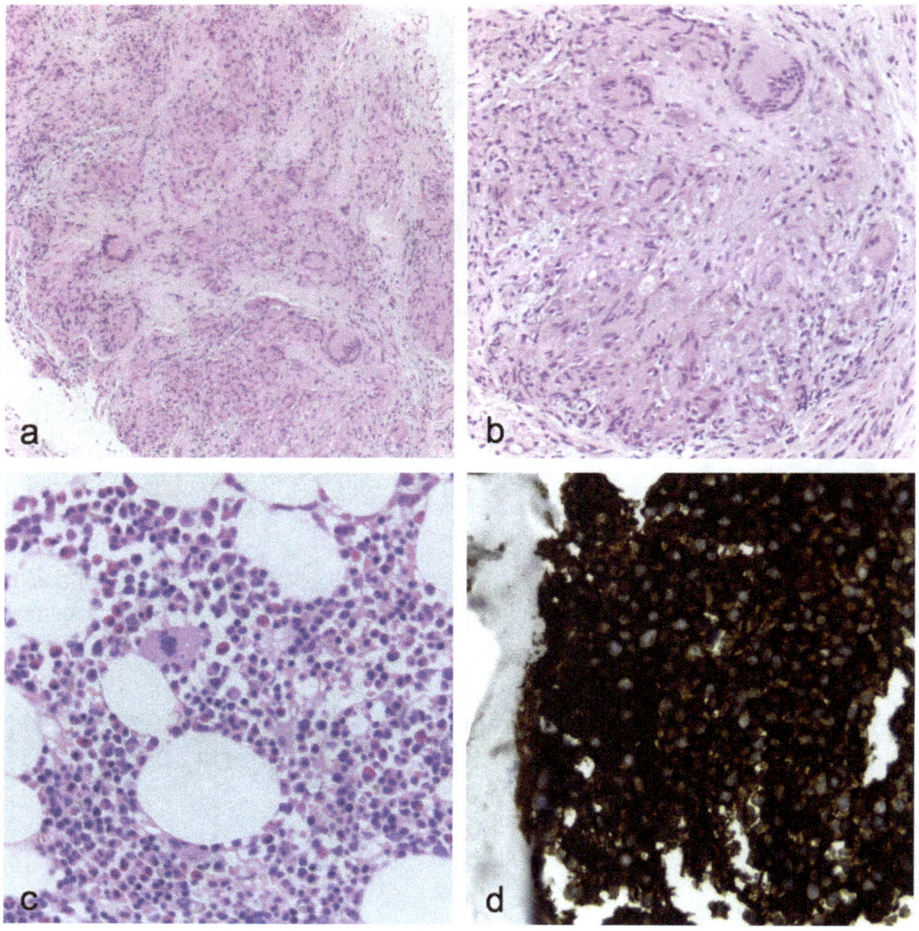

FIGURE 3: Histological analysis: transbronchial biopsy (a, b) revealing granulomatous inflammatory process compatible with lung sarcoidosis; bone marrow biopsy showing hypercellularity with plasmocyte infiltration (c) and kappa light chain restriction (d).

Hence, a simultaneous diagnostic of systemic sarcoidosis and multiple myeloma stage I according to the International Staging System was established. The patient was started on prednisolone 60 mg/day with clinical and biochemical improvement. Bone marrow plasma cell infiltration dropped to 28%, and IgG immunoglobulin and ACE returned to normal values. Although a slow reduction of steroid therapy (to 5 mg/day) was achieved in time, previous oral antidiabetic therapy became insufficient and prompted insulin introduction.

3. Discussion

Only few cases of sarcoidosis in association with MM have been reported in the literature, so there is not enough scientific evidence available to support a causal relation for the occurrence of these two diseases. Nonetheless, epidemiological data highlight the higher risk for lymphoproliferative disease development in sarcoidosis patients [5–8].

Brincker and Wilbek [5] published the first study regarding the association between sarcoidosis and malignant diseases in 1974. In a retrospective analysis of 2544 Danish sarcoidosis patients, the risk of lymphoproliferative diseases was found to be 11.5 times higher than expected, the most common being Hodgkin's disease. That same year, Selroos et al. [9] reported the first known case of sarcoidosis associated with MM, in a 56-year-old Finnish woman. Based on previous publications, Brincker [4] hypothesised the existence of a sarcoidosis-lymphoma syndrome, anchored on the following features: lymphoproliferative disorders always followed sarcoidosis, the median age of sarcoidosis diagnosis in patients with lymphoma was 10 years later than those with sarcoidosis diagnosed first, and B-cell Hodgkin's malignancy was more frequent then T-cell lymphomas.

In our review of the literature, 33 cases with both sarcoidosis and MM were identified although patient characteristics and diagnostic information were not available for all of them [4, 6–25]. Data analyses showed female gender predominance, with a median age at sarcoidosis diagnosis of 46 years (24–65). Despite being about 10 years lower than previous authors have reported, it is still higher than the median age for sarcoidosis diagnosis in the general population [3, 16, 19]. The median time interval between sarcoidosis and MM diagnosis was 8.2 years (0–27), but in 9 cases a simultaneous diagnosis of both diseases was reported. These data are in favour of Brincker's [4] hypothesis that malignant haematological diseases are associated with chronic active sarcoidosis in middle-aged patients. Also in accordance with this predisposing relation is the fact that in almost all patients, sarcoidosis preceded the diagnosis of

MM. With respect to MM, IgG was the most common monoclonal protein reported, followed by IgA and IgM.

The explanation for the relationship between sarcoidosis and lymphoproliferative disorders, particularly MM, is still controversial and unknown. One possible link between sarcoidosis and MM is the polyclonal hypergammaglobulinemia induced by sarcoidosis chronic inflammatory response. This continuous state of stimulation results in prolonged B cell and plasma cell half-life, which in addition to immune system imbalance in sarcoidosis patients, predisposes for genetic mutations and might lead to haematological malignancy development [16, 20]. Recent studies have highlighted the potential role of T_H17 cells and T_{reg} cells in sarcoidosis and MM immune mechanisms [1]. Despite MM being a primary B-cell malignancy, both quantitative and functional T-cell abnormalities have been demonstrated to occur in this disease.

In our case, sarcoidosis diagnosis was first made after a soft tissue lesion excision in a 65-year-old woman. Although both sarcoidosis and MM were diagnosed simultaneously, previous respiratory symptoms suggest that sarcoidosis pulmonary involvement was already present years before and misdiagnosed as bronchitis. This fact might also account for the older age at the time of the diagnosis of sarcoidosis. No usual abnormalities related to MM, such as lytic lesions or renal function impairment, were present at the time of diagnosis, and only the serum protein electrophoresis monoclonal band called the attention to a possible underlying disease other than sarcoidosis. We aim to call the attention to the possibility of LD development in patients with sarcoidosis. A high level of suspicion should always be present both at the time of diagnosis as well as during follow-up since LD seems to develop years after the diagnosis of sarcoidosis.

Consent

Written informed consent was obtained from the patient.

Authors' Contributions

Joao Tiago Serra wrote the manuscript and analysed the data. Aurelia Martinho provided the patient and analysed the data. Fernanda Paixao Duarte provided the patient and reviewed the manuscript. Fernando Aldomiro reviewed the manuscript. All authors read and approved the final manuscript.

References

[1] W. S. J. Loke, C. Herbert, and P. S. Thomas, "Sarcoidosis: immunopathogenesis and immunological markers," *International Journal of Chronic Diseases*, vol. 2013, Article ID 928601, 13 pages, 2013.

[2] M. C. Iannuzzi, B. A. Rybicki, and A. S. Teirstein, "Sarcoidosis," *New England Journal of Medicine*, vol. 357, no. 21, pp. 2153–2165, 2007.

[3] C. Röllig, S. Knop, and M. Bornhäuser, "Multiple myeloma," *The Lancet*, vol. 385, no. 9983, pp. 2197–2208, 2015.

[4] H. Brincker, "The sarcoidosis-lymphoma syndrome," *British Journal of Cancer*, vol. 54, no. 3, pp. 467–473, 1986.

[5] H. Brincker and E. Wilbek, "The incidence of malignant tumours in patients with respiratory sarcoidosis," *British Journal of Cancer*, vol. 29, no. 3, pp. 247–251, 1974.

[6] M. Karakantza, E. Matutes, K. MacLennan, N. T. O'Connor, P. C. Srivastava, and D. Catovsky, "Association between sarcoidosis and lymphoma revisited," *Journal of Clinical Pathology*, vol. 49, no. 3, pp. 208–212, 1996.

[7] P. Boffetta, C. S. Rabkin, and G. Gridley, "A cohort study of cancer among sarcoidosis patients," *International Journal of Cancer*, vol. 124, no. 11, pp. 2697–2700, 2009.

[8] N. Blank, H.-M. Lorenz, A. D. Ho, and M. Witzens-Harig, "Sarcoidosis and the occurrence of malignant diseases," *Rheumatology International*, vol. 34, no. 10, pp. 1433–1439, 2014.

[9] O. Selroos, L. Brander, and M. Virolainen, "Sarcoidosis and myeloma of lambda-type IgG," *Acta Medica Scandinavica*, vol. 195, no. 1–6, pp. 59–63, 1974.

[10] A. I. Schafer and J. B. Miller, "Association of IgA multiple myeloma with pre-existing disease," *British Journal of Haematology*, vol. 41, no. 1, pp. 19–24, 1979.

[11] T. Pettersson, E. Koivunen, M. Ilvonen, J. Jouppila, E. Aalto, and C. Wasastjerna, "Sarcoidosis and multiple myeloma: an association," *British Medical Journal*, vol. 295, no. 6604, p. 958, 1987.

[12] H. Uchiumi, H. Murakami, T. Matsushima et al., "Does sarcoidosis induce multiple myeloma?," *American Journal of Hematology*, vol. 44, no. 3, p. 220, 1993.

[13] R. D. Rakhit, G. J. Clesham, and J. G. F. Cleland, "Sarcoid, amyloid and heart failure," *International Journal of Cardiology*, vol. 41, no. 2, pp. 180–182, 1993.

[14] O. I. Kamaeva, N. M. Kostiagina, N. S. Pimenova, and I. N. Shestakova, "A case of a combination of sarcoidosis and myeloma," *Terapevticheskiĭ Arkhiv*, vol. 67, no. 12, pp. 57–59, 1995.

[15] C. Panizo Santos, J. Rifón Roca, N. Gómez Manero, O. Beloqui Ruiz, A. Panizo Santos, and E. Rocha Hernando, "Simultaneous presentation of multiple myeloma and sarcoidosis," *Sangre*, vol. 42, no. 5, pp. 411–413, 1997.

[16] F. Sen, K. P. Mann, and L. J. Medeiros, "Multiple myeloma in association with sarcoidosis," *Archives of Pathology & Laboratory Medicine*, vol. 126, no. 3, pp. 365–368, 2002.

[17] A. Özet, Ş. Güran, and M. Beksac, "Familial multiple myeloma associated with disorders of chronic inflammation: first report from Turkey," *Clinical Lymphoma and Myeloma*, vol. 8, no. 4, pp. 246–248, 2008.

[18] C. Gashti, A. Vijaykumar, and M. Larson, "Renal sarcoidosis and multiple myeloma," *The Internet Journal of Nephrology*, vol. 6, no. 1, pp. 1–4, 2009.

[19] G. Brown, L. G. Shapeero, B. M. Weiss, and M. Roschewski, "Multiple myeloma with lacrimal gland amyloidosis and sarcoidosis," *American Journal of Hematology*, vol. 85, no. 7, pp. 506–509, 2010.

[20] R. Dachs, A. Horn, H. Koornhof, L. de Jager, S. Maqungo, and S. Roche, "Double pathology, sarcoidosis associated with multiple myeloma: a case report," *Journal of Bone Oncology*, vol. 3, no. 2, pp. 61–65, 2014.

[21] Y. Elgaried, F. Alkhankan, and R. Wolfer, "727: systemic sarcoidosis and multiple myeloma, rare presentation," *Critical Care Medicine*, vol. 42, p. A1535, 2014.

[22] Y. Etman, M. Shalaby, L. Brown, R. Wolfer, and F. Alkhankan, "Sarcoidosis in association with multiple myeloma," *American Journal of Respiratory and Critical Care Medicine*, vol. 189, p. A2264, 2014.

[23] V. Nair, O. Jha, and D. Talwar, "Sarcoidosis and multiple myeloma: concurrent presentation of an unusual association," *Lung India*, vol. 33, no. 5, pp. 75–88, 2016.

[24] C. Terry, M. Luthra, and A. M. Esper, "Coexisting sarcoidosis and multiple myeloma presenting as acute leg weakness and chest pain," *American Journal of Respiratory and Critical Care Medicine*, vol. 195, p. A3367, 2017.

[25] K. Kusaba, K. Kojima, S. Naito et al., "Paraneoplastic sarcoidosis in multiple myeloma," *Internal Medicine*, vol. 56, no. 15, pp. 2049–2051, 2017.

Permissions

All chapters in this book were first published by Hindawi Publishing Corporation; hereby published with permission under the Creative Commons Attribution License or equivalent. Every chapter published in this book has been scrutinized by our experts. Their significance has been extensively debated. The topics covered herein carry significant findings which will fuel the growth of the discipline. They may even be implemented as practical applications or may be referred to as a beginning point for another development.

The contributors of this book come from diverse backgrounds, making this book a truly international effort. This book will bring forth new frontiers with its revolutionizing research information and detailed analysis of the nascent developments around the world.

We would like to thank all the contributing authors for lending their expertise to make the book truly unique. They have played a crucial role in the development of this book. Without their invaluable contributions this book wouldn't have been possible. They have made vital efforts to compile up to date information on the varied aspects of this subject to make this book a valuable addition to the collection of many professionals and students.

This book was conceptualized with the vision of imparting up-to-date information and advanced data in this field. To ensure the same, a matchless editorial board was set up. Every individual on the board went through rigorous rounds of assessment to prove their worth. After which they invested a large part of their time researching and compiling the most relevant data for our readers.

The editorial board has been involved in producing this book since its inception. They have spent rigorous hours researching and exploring the diverse topics which have resulted in the successful publishing of this book. They have passed on their knowledge of decades through this book. To expedite this challenging task, the publisher supported the team at every step. A small team of assistant editors was also appointed to further simplify the editing procedure and attain best results for the readers.

Apart from the editorial board, the designing team has also invested a significant amount of their time in understanding the subject and creating the most relevant covers. They scrutinized every image to scout for the most suitable representation of the subject and create an appropriate cover for the book.

The publishing team has been an ardent support to the editorial, designing and production team. Their endless efforts to recruit the best for this project, has resulted in the accomplishment of this book. They are a veteran in the field of academics and their pool of knowledge is as vast as their experience in printing. Their expertise and guidance has proved useful at every step. Their uncompromising quality standards have made this book an exceptional effort. Their encouragement from time to time has been an inspiration for everyone.

The publisher and the editorial board hope that this book will prove to be a valuable piece of knowledge for researchers, students, practitioners and scholars across the globe.

List of Contributors

Kim Uy, Elizabeth Levin and Surbhi Shah
University of Minnesota, Department of Medicine, Division of Hematology, Oncology and Transplantation, Minneapolis, MN, USA

Pawel Mroz and Faqian Li
University of Minnesota, Department of Laboratory Medicine and Pathology, Minneapolis, MN, USA

Kunhwa Kim, Harpreet Kaur and Matthew Chan
Department of Internal Medicine, Einstein Medical Center Philadelphia, Philadelphia, PA, USA

Manju Balasubramanian
Department of Pathology, Einstein Medical Center Philadelphia, Philadelphia, PA, USA

Sorab Gupta and Vinicius M. Jorge
Department of Hematology-Oncology, Einstein Medical Center Philadelphia, Philadelphia, PA, USA

Hesham Yasin, Tessa Laytem, Grerk Sutamtewagul and Sabarish Ayyappan
University of Iowa Health Care, Iowa City, Iowa, USA

Jack Lichy
The George Washington University, Department of Pathology, Washington, DC, USA
Veterans Health Administration, Department of Pathology, Washington, DC, USA

Francisco Mot Ara
Hospital J. M.de Los Rios, Department of Pathology, Caracas, Venezuela

Victor E. Nava
The George Washington University, Department of Pathology, Washington, DC, USA
Veterans Health Administration, Department of Pathology, Washington, DC, USA
Hospital J.M. de Los Rios, Department of Pathology, Caracas, Venezuela
Washington DC Veterans Affairs Medical Center, Washington, DC, USA

Maryam Mehdipour Dalivand and Parastou Tizro
The George Washington University, Department of Pathology, Washington, DC, USA

Julie Partain
Oregon Health and Science University, Portland, OR, USA

Anita Aggarwal
The George Washington University, Department of Medicine, Hematology and Oncology, Washington, DC, USA
Veterans Health Administration, Department of Internal Medicine, Oncology and Hematology, Washington, DC, USA
The George Washington University Medical Faculty Associates, Washington, DC, USA
Washington DC Veterans Affairs Medical Center, Washington, DC, USA

Kee Tat Lee, Nurul Akmar Misron, Chin Hau Wong and Hong Keng Liew
Department of Medicine, Hospital Sultanah Bahiyah, Langgar, Kedah, Malaysia

Norasmidar Abdul Aziz
Department of Pathology, Hospital Sultanah Bahiyah, Langgar, Kedah, Malaysia

Karuna Dewan
Department of Otolaryngology Head and Neck Surgery, Stanford University, Stanford, USA

John H. Baird
Division of Hematology, Department of Medicine, Stanford University, Stanford, USA

Courtney B. Shires
Department of Otolaryngology Head and Neck Surgery, The University of Tennessee Health Sciences Center, Memphis, USA

Matthew Lee
Internal Medicine Resident, Donald and Barbara Zucker School of Medicine at Hofstra/Northwell, 300 Community Dr, Manhasset, NY 11030, USA

Xinmin Zhang
Donald and Barbara Zucker School of Medicine at Hofstra/Northwell,Pathology Department at North Shore University Hospital-Long Island Jewish Medical Center, 300 Community Dr, Manhasset, NY 11030, USA

Vinh Nguyen
Donald and Barbara Zucker School of Medicine at Hofstra/Northwell, Radiology Department at North Shore University Hospital-Long Island Jewish Medical Center, 300 Community Dr, Manhasset, NY 11030, USA

Monique Hartley-Brown
Donald and Barbara Zucker School of Medicine at Hofstra/Northwell, Hematology-Oncology Department at North Shore University Hospital-Long Island Jewish Medical Center, 300 Community Dr, Manhasset, NY 11030, USA

Pier Paolo Piccaluga
Department of Experimental, Diagnostic and Speciality Medicine, University of Bologna, Bologna, Italy
Istituto Euro-Mediterraneo di Scienza e Tecnologia (IEMEST), Palermo, Italy
Jomo Kenyatta University of Agriculture and Technology, Juja, Kenya
S. Orsola-Malpighi Hospital, Hematology and Hematopathology Units, Bologna, Italy

Stefania Paolini and Nicola Vianelli
S. Orsola-Malpighi Hospital, Hematology and Hematopathology Units, Bologna, Italy

Cristina Campidelli
Azienda Ospedaliera Ospedali di Legnano, U. O. Anatomia Patologica, Legnao, Milan, Italy

Luigi Bolondi
Department of Medical and Surgical Sciences, University of Bologna, Bologna, Italy

Benjamin Heyman
Division of Regenerative Medicine, Department of Medicine, UC San Diego, Moores Cancer Center, San Diego, CA, USA

Chris R. Kelsey
Department of Radiation Oncology, Duke University, Durham, NC, USA

Anne Beaven
Division of Hematology/Oncology, Department of Medicine, University of North Carolina, Chapel Hill, NC, USA

Kazuaki Teshima, Ko Abe and Hideaki Ohyagi
Department of Hematology, Hiraka General Hospital, Yokote, Japan
Department of Hematology, Nephrology, and Rheumatology, Akita University Graduate School of Medicine, Akita, Japan

Masaaki Kume
Department of Hematology, Hiraka General Hospital, Yokote, Japan

Yasushi Kawaharada, Masashi Zuguchi, Yosuke Kubota, Yoshitaka Enomoto and Ken Saito
Department of Surgery, Hiraka General Hospital, Yokote, Japan

Takashi Saito
Department of Otolaryngology, Hiraka General Hospital, Yokote, Japan

Sho Ikeda and Naoto Takahashi
Department of Hematology, Nephrology, and Rheumatology, Akita University Graduate School of Medicine, Akita, Japan

Megumi Zuguchi
Department of Gastroenterology, Hiraka General Hospital, Yokote, Japan

Masahito Miura, Satsuki Takahashi and Masahiro Saito
Department of Diagnostic Pathology, Hiraka General Hospital, Yokote, Japan

Majd Al Shaarani, Rodney E. Shackelford, Yasir AlZubaidi and Eric X. Wei
Department of Pathology and Translational Pathobiology, Louisiana State University Health Sciences Center, Shreveport, LA, USA

Samip R. Master and Glenn M. Mills
Department of Hematology and Oncology, Louisiana State University Health Sciences Center, Shreveport, LA, USA

Ahmed Mamilly
Department of Radiology, Louisiana State University Health Sciences Center, Shreveport, LA, USA

Yuta Inagawa
Department of Hematology, Japan Community Healthcare Organization (JCHO) Tokyo Yamate Medical Center, Tokyo, Japan
Department of Internal Medicine, JCHO Tokyo Yamate Medical Center, Tokyo, Japan

Yukiko Komeno and Tomiko Ryu
Department of Hematology, Japan Community Healthcare Organization (JCHO) Tokyo Yamate Medical Center, Tokyo, Japan

Satoshi Saito and Yasumasa Hatada
Department of Gastroenterology, JCHO Tokyo Yamate Medical Center, Tokyo, Japan

Yuji Maenohara and Taku Saito
Department of Orthopaedic Surgery, Faculty of Medicine, The University of Tokyo, Tokyo, Japan

Tetsuro Yamagishi and Hiroyuki Kawashima
Division of Orthopedic Surgery, Department of Regenerative and Transplant Medicine, Niigata University Graduate School of Medicine and Dental Sciences, Niigata, Japan

Keiko Abe and Kuniko Iihara
Department of Pathology, JCHO Tokyo Yamate Medical Center, Tokyo, Japan

Zhi zhuo Du, Mi Zhou, Jing Ling, Lan Cao, Lingjun Kong, Shengqin Cheng, Peifang Xiao and Shaoyan Hu
Children's Hospital of Suzhou University, Suzhou, China

Ilina Micheva, Vladimir Gerov, Stela Dimitrova and Merlin Efraim
UMHAT "Sveta Marina" Medical University, Varna, Bulgaria

Teruhito Takakuwa, Ippei Otomaru, Taku Araki, Akiko Miura, Yotaro Fujitani and Ryosuke Yamamura
Department of Hematology, Osaka Saiseikai Nakatsu Hospital, Osaka, Japan

Yasuhide Mochizuki
Department of Cardiology, Osaka Saiseikai Nakatsu Hospital, Osaka, Japan

Yoshimi Miyagi and Hideto Senzaki
Department of Pathology, Osaka Saiseikai Nakatsu Hospital, Osaka, Japan

Nicolas Gallastegui and Jonathan H. Schatz
Division of Hematology, Department of Medicine, University of Miami Leonard M. Miller School of Medicine/Sylvester Comprehensive Cancer Center, Miami, FL, USA

Daniel P. Cassidy and Francisco Vega
Division of Hematopathology, Department of Pathology and Laboratory Medicine, University of Miami Leonard M. Miller School of Medicine/Sylvester Comprehensive Cancer Center, Miami, FL, USA

Deborah O. Heros
Division of Neuro-Oncology, Department of Neurology,University of Miami Leonard M. Miller School of Medicine/Sylvester Comprehensive Cancer Center, Miami, FL, USA

Stamatios Chrysochoou
GPR Gesundheits- und Pflegezentrum Rüsselsheim Gemeinnützige GmbH, August-Bebel-Straße 59, Rüsselsheim Am Main 65428, Germany

Andreas Kreft
Institute of Pathology, Johannes Gutenberg University, Langenbeckstraße 1, Mainz 55131, Germany

Eberhard Schneider
GPR Gesundheits- und Pflegezentrum Rüsselsheim Gemeinnützige GmbH, August-Bebel-Straße 59, Rüsselsheim Am Main 65428, Germany
Department of Biology, Julius Maximilians University, Am Hubland, Würzburg 97074, Germany

Sara Kristina Viberg Tjønnfjord
Department of Nephrology, Odense University Hospital, Odense Kløverværnget 6, 5000 Odense C, Denmark
Department of Haematology, Oslo University Hospital, 4950 Nydalen, No. 0424 Oslo, Norway

Eirik Brekka Tjønnfjord
Department of Haematology, Oslo University Hospital, 4950 Nydalen, No. 0424 Oslo, Norway

Zbigniew Konopski
Department of Gastroenterology, Oslo University Hospital, 4950 Nydalen, No. 0424 Oslo, Norway

Geir Erland Tjønnfjord
Department of Haematology, Oslo University Hospital, 4950 Nydalen, No. 0424 Oslo, Norway
KG Jebsen Centre for B-Cell Malignancies, Institute of Clinical Medicine, University of Oslo, 4950 Nydalen, No. 0424 Oslo, Norway

Sofia Chiatamone Ranieri, Stefania Trasarti, Maria Antonietta Arleo, Luisa Bizzoni, Maria Assunta Limongiello, Maria Grazia Nardacci, Giuseppe Gentile and Robin Foà
Department of Translational and Precision Medicine, University of Rome "Sapienza", Rome, Italy

Livia Bonanni
Department of Molecular Medicine, University of Rome "Sapienza", Rome, Italy

Valeria Di Battista
Department of Medicine, Center of Hemato-Oncology Research (C.R.E.O.), University of Perugia, Perugia, Italy

Jeremy T. Larsen
Division of Hematology and Medical Oncology, Mayo Clinic, Phoenix, Arizona, USA

Frederick D. Leonard
International Waldenstrom's Macroglobulinemia Foundation (IWMF), Sarasota, Florida, USA

Timothy S. Oh
Department of Medicine, Northwestern University Feinberg School of Medicine, Chicago, IL, USA

Madelyn Burkart
Division of Hematology/Oncology, Robert H. Lurie Comprehensive Cancer Center of Northwestern University, Northwestern University Feinberg School of Medicine, Chicago, IL, USA

Amir Behdad
Department of Pathology, Northwestern University Feinberg School of Medicine, Chicago, IL, USA

Hatice Savas
Department of Radiology, Northwestern University Feinberg School of Medicine, Chicago, IL, USA

Reem Karmali
Division of Hematology/Oncology, Robert H. Lurie Comprehensive Cancer Center of Northwestern University, Chicago, IL, USA

Nicole Yun
Department of Internal Medicine, Rush University Medical Center, 1717 W. Congress Parkway, 1042 Kellogg, Chicago, IL 60612, USA

James Coggan and Parameswaran Venugopal
Division of Hematology, Oncology and Cell Therapy, Rush University Medical Center, Chicago, IL, USA

Ira Miller
Department of Pathology, Rush University Medical Center, Chicago, IL, USA

Yoshiki Uemura
Department of Hematology, Chikamori Hospital, 1-1-16, Okawasuzi, Kochi-shi, Kochi-ken 780-8522, Japan

Risa Maeda
Department of Nephrology, Chikamori Hospital, 1-1-16, Okawasuzi, Kochi-shi, Kochi-ken 780-8522, Japan

Hiroyoshi Saegusa
Department of General Medicine, Chikamori Hospital, 1-1-16, Okawasuzi, Kochi-shi, Kochi-ken 780-8522, Japan

Mridul Gupta and Sandhya Kadiyam
Internal Medicine, Monmouth Medical Center, Long Branch, New Jersey, USA

Divita Singh
Ambulatory Care Pharmacy Resident, University of Florida, Gainesville, Florida, USA

Patrick Lee
Hematology and Oncology, Monmouth Medical Center, Long Branch, New Jersey, USA

Coen J. Lap and Samah Nassereddine
The George Washington University Medical Faculty Associates, Washington, DC, USA

Min-Ling Liu
Washington DC Veterans Affairs Medical Center, Washington, DC, USA

Jared Williams and Shingi Chiruka
Department of Haematology, Dunedin Hospital, 201 Great King Street, Dunedin 9016, New Zealand

Ming Y. Lim and Nigel S. Key
Department of Medicine, Division of Hematology/Oncology, University of North Carolina, Chapel Hill, NC, USA

Keith E. Volmar
Department of Pathology, UNC REX Healthcare, Raleigh, NC, USA

Maryam Barkhordar, Fatemeh Tajic Rostami, Marjan Yaghmaie, Mehrdad Abbaszadeh, Bahram Chahardouli and Seied Asadollah Mousavi
Hematology Oncology and Stem Cell Transplantation Research Center, Tehran University of Medical Sciences, Tehran, Iran

Mark G. Evans
Department of Hematopathology, Division of Pathology and Laboratory Medicine, The University of Texas MD Anderson Cancer Center, Houston, TX, USA

Sherif A. Rezk and Xiaohui Zhao
Department of Pathology and Laboratory Medicine, University of California Irvine (UCI) Medical Center, Orange, CA, USA

Lauren C. Pinter-Brown
Department of Medicine, Division of Hematology/Oncology, University of California Irvine (UCI) Medical Center, Orange, CA, USA

Shannon Zhang, Casey Charlton, Akshay Amaraneni and Keri Maher
University of Arizona, Tucson College of Medicine, Tucson, AZ, USA

Aaron M. Lee
Department of Medicine, Internal Medicine Residency Program, University of California San Diego, La Jolla, CA, USA

Aaron M. Goodman
Department of Medicine, Division of Blood and Marrow Transplantation, Moores Cancer Center, University of California San Diego, La Jolla, CA, USA

James K. Mangan
Department of Medicine, Division of Blood and Marrow Transplantation, Moores Cancer Center, University of California San Diego, La Jolla, CA, USA
Moores Cancer Center, University of California, San Diego, 3855 Health Sciences Drive, Mail Code 0960, La Jolla, CA 92093, USA

R. Palmieri, F. Esposito, F. Meconi, V. M. Rapisarda, L. Anemona, G. Paterno, S. Vaccarini, D. Nasso, L. Pupo and M. Cantonetti
Fondazione Policlinico Tor Vergata, Dipartimento di Biomedicina e Prevenzione, Rome, Italy

Alaina J. Kessler
Department of Medicine, Icahn School of Medicine at Mount Sinai, 1 Gustave L. Levy Place, New York, NY 10029, USA

Bridget K. Marcellino, Scot A. Niglio and Adriana K. Malone
Tisch Cancer Institute, Icahn School of Medicine at Mount Sinai, New York, NY, USA

Bruce E. Petersen
Department of Pathology, Icahn School of Medicine at Mount Sinai, New York, NY, USA

Yutaka Tsutsumi, Shinich Ito and Mirei Kobayashi
Department of Hematology, Hakodate Municipal Hospital, 1-10-1, Minato-cho, Hakodate 041-8680, Japan

Takanori Teshima
Department of Hematology, Hokkaido University Graduate School of Medicine, Sapporo, Japan

Christophe Angelo
Department of Intensive Care, Cliniques St-Luc, Universite Catholique de Louvain, 1200 Brussels, Belgium

Marie-Françoise Vincent
Department of Clinical Chemistry, Cliniques St-Luc, Universite Catholique de Louvain, 1200 Brussels, Belgium

Mina Komuta
Department of Pathology, Cliniques St-Luc, Universite Catholique de Louvain, 1200 Brussels, Belgium

Philippe Hantson
Department of Intensive Care, Cliniques St-Luc, Universite Catholique de Louvain, 1200 Brussels, Belgium
Louvain Centre of Toxicology and Applied Pharmacology, Universite Catholique de Louvain, 1200 Brussels, Belgium

Nicole Straetmans and Edwige Boulet
Department of Hematology, Cliniques St-Luc, Universite Catholique de Louvain, 1200 Brussels, Belgium

Louisa Shackleton, David O'Brien, C. Larry Bacon and Catherine M. Flynn
Department of Haematology, St. James's Hospital, Dublin 8, Ireland

Stephen E. Langabeer and Sarah L. McCarron
Cancer Molecular Diagnostics, St. James's Hospital, Dublin 8, Ireland

Bridgette Byrne
Maternal Medicine Service, Coombe Women and Infants University Hospital, Dublin 8, Ireland

Rupert Barry
Department of Dermatology, St. James's Hospital, Dublin 8, Ireland

Richard Flavin
Department of Histopathology, St. James's Hospital, Dublin 8, Ireland

Mina Shenouda, Jennifer Dotson, Hassaan Yasin and Yehuda Lebowicz
Marshall University, Department of Hematology and Oncology, 1400 Hal Greer Blvd, Huntington, WV 25701, USA

Madhulika Urella
Marshall University, Department of Internal Medicine, 1249 15th St., Suite 2000, Huntington, WV 25701, USA

Sharad Khurana, Manuel Beltran, Liuyan Jiang and Ernesto Ayala
Mayo Clinic, Jacksonville, FL, USA

Vivek Roy
Mayo Clinic, Jacksonville, FL, USA
Department of Hematology-Oncology, Mayo Clinic Florida, Jacksonville, FL, USA

Blake O. Adnani
Department of Internal Medicine, Keck School of Medicine, University of Southern California, Los Angeles, USA

Kathleen O' Brien and Brandon L. Adler
Department of Dermatology, Keck School of Medicine, University of Southern California, Los Angeles, USA

Zaw W. Myint
Department of Hematology, Keck School of Medicine, University of Southern California, Los Angeles, USA

Claire Cochet, Julie Cattin, Jean-Patrick Metz and Nicolas Mottet
University Hospital of Besancon, Department of Obstetrics, Besançon F-25000, France

Marion Simonet, Ana Berceanu, Etienne Daguindau and Yohan Desbrosses
University Hospital of Besancon, Department of Hematology, Besançon F-25000, France

Eric Deconinck
University Hospital of Besancon, Department of Hematology, Besançon F-25000, France
University Bourgogne Franche-Comte, INSERM, EFS BFC, UMR 1098, Interactions Hote-Greffon Tumeur/ Ingenierie Cellulaire et Genique, Besançon F-25000, France

Françoise Schillinger
Etablissement Français du Sang Bourgogne Franche Comt´e, Laboratoire d'hematologie-Immunologie-Biologie Moleculaire, Besançon F-25020, France

Pierre Fenaux
Saint Louis Hospital, Paris Diderot University, Paris F-75010, France

A. Mendez-Hernandez, S. Upadhyay and L. M. Parra-Rodriguez
Department of Medicine, John H. Stroger Jr. Hospital of Cook County, Chicago, IL, USA

X. A. Andrade
Department of Hematology and Oncology, Mayo Clinic, Rochester, MN, USA

E. Caldeira
Department of Medicine, Advocate Illinois Masonic Medical Center, Chicago, IL, USA

L. H. Paz
Department of Cardiology, North Shore University Hospital, Evanston, IL, USA

H. Mann
Department of Hematology and Oncology, Tufts Medical Center, Boston, MA, USA

M. Zia
Department of Hematology and Oncology, John H. Stroger Jr. Hospital of Cook County, Chicago, IL, USA

L. Sumoza
Department of Hematology and Oncology, Alton Memorial Hospital, Alton, IL, USA

M. Malagola, N. Polverelli, V. Cancelli, E. Morello, A. Turra, F. Cattina, B. Rambaldi, L. Gandolfi, M. Farina and D. Russo
Chair of Hematology, Department of Clinical and Surgical Sciences, University of Brescia, Bone Marrow Transplant Unit, ASST-Spedali Civili, Brescia, Italy

E. Borlenghi
Unit of Hematology, ASST-Spedali Civili, Brescia, Italy

S. Bernardi, C. Zanaglio and Elif Dereli Eke
Chair of Hematology, Department of Clinical and Surgical Sciences, University of Brescia, Bone Marrow Transplant Unit, ASST-Spedali Civili, Brescia, Italy
Centro di Ricerca Ematologica-Oncologia AIL (CREA), ASST-Spedali Civili, Brescia, Italy

Brenda S. Castillo
Texas Tech University Health Sciences Center Paul L. Foster School of Medicine, El Paso, Texas, USA

Maria L. Rodriguez
Brown University, Providence, RI, USA

Ju-Hsien John Chao and Behyar Zoghi
Methodist Hospital, Texas Transplant Institute, San Antonio, Texas, USA

Ananth Arjunan
University of Pittsburgh Medical Center, Division of Hematology/Oncology, UPMC Cancer Pavilion, 5150 Centre Avenue, Room 463, Pittsburgh, PA 15232, USA

Hema Rai
VA Pittsburgh Healthcare System, Division of Hematology/Oncology, University Drive C, 8th Floor, Pittsburgh, PA 15240, USA

Jew Win Kuan
Department of Medicine, Universiti Malaysia Sarawak, Kota Samarahan, Sarawak, Malaysia

Sing Ling Chai
Timberland Medical Centre, Kuching, Sarawak, Malaysia

Pathmanathan Rajadurai
Subang Jaya Medical Centre, Subang Jaya, Selangor, Malaysia

Lee Gong Lau and Joseph Uchang
Borneo Medical Centre, Kuching, Sarawak, Malaysia

Sharifah Noor Akmal Syed Husain
Pantai Premier Pathology Sdn Bhd, Kuala Lumpur, Malaysia

Poorva Bindal
Department of Hematology and Oncology, Beth Israel Deaconess Medical Center, Boston, MA, USA

Aakash Desai and Lukas Delasos
Department of Internal Medicine, University of Connecticut Health Center, Farmington, CT, USA

Sudhanshu Mulay and James Vredenburgh
Department of Hematology and Oncology, Smilow Cancer Hospital at St. Francis, Hartford, CT, USA

Poornima Ramadas
SUNY Upstate Medical University, 750 East Adams Street, Syracuse, New York 13210, USA
LSU Health Sciences Center, 1501 Kings Hwy, Shreveport, LA 71103, USA

Michael Williams and David B. Duggan
SUNY Upstate Medical University, 750 East Adams Street, Syracuse, New York 13210, USA

Ricardo D. Parrondo, Taimur Sher, Victoria Alegria and Sikander Ailawadhi
Department of Hematology-Oncology, Mayo Clinic Florida, Jacksonville, FL, USA

Asher A. Chanan-Khan
Department of Hematology-Oncology, Mayo Clinic Florida, Jacksonville, FL, USA
Department of Hematology-Oncology, St. Vincent's Riverside, Jacksonville, FL, USA

Reina Takeda and Tomofusa Fukuyama
Department of Hematology/Oncology, Research Hospital, The Institute of Medical Science, The University of Tokyo, Tokyo 108-8639, Japan
Division of Cellular Therapy, The Institute of Medical Science, The University of Tokyo, Tokyo 108-8639, Japan

Kazuaki Yokoyama
Department of Hematology/Oncology, Research Hospital, The Institute of Medical Science, The University of Tokyo, Tokyo 108-8639, Japan

Seiichiro Kobayashi, Sousuke Nakamura and Mika Ito
Division of Molecular Therapy, The Institute of Medical Science, The University of Tokyo, Tokyo 108-8639, Japan

Toyotaka Kawamata, Nobuhiro Ohno and Arinobu Tojo
Department of Hematology/Oncology, Research Hospital, The Institute of Medical Science, The University of Tokyo, Tokyo 108-8639, Japan
Division of Molecular Therapy, The Institute of Medical Science, The University of Tokyo, Tokyo 108-8639, Japan

Nozomi Yusa
Department of Applied Genomics, Research Hospital, Institute of Medical Science, The University of Tokyo, Tokyo 108-8639, Japan

Eigo Shimizu and Rui Yamaguchi
Laboratory of DNA Information Analysis, Human Genome Center, Institute of Medical Science, The University of Tokyo,Tokyo 108-8639, Japan

Seiya Imoto
Division of Health Medical Data Science, Health Intelligence Center, Institute of Medical Science, The University of Tokyo, Tokyo 108-8639, Japan

Satoru Miyano
Laboratory of DNA Information Analysis, Human Genome Center, Institute of Medical Science, The University of Tokyo,Tokyo 108-8639, Japan
Division of Health Medical Data Science, Health Intelligence Center, Institute of Medical Science, The University of Tokyo, Tokyo 108-8639, Japan

Kaoru Uchimaru
Department of Hematology/Oncology, Research Hospital, The Institute of Medical Science, The University of Tokyo, Tokyo 108-8639, Japan
Laboratory of Tumor Cell Biology, Department of Computational Biology and Medical Science, Graduate School of Frontier Sciences, The University of Tokyo, Tokyo 108-8639, Japan

Joao Tiago Serra, Aurelia Martinho, Fernanda Paixao Duarte and Fernando Aldomiro
Department of Internal Medicine II, Professor Doutor Fernando Fonseca Hospital, Amadora, Portugal

Index

A

Acute Lymphoblastic Leukemia, 13, 15, 17, 70, 72-73, 128, 169, 174, 176, 179, 181

Acute Myeloid, 9, 12, 15-16, 24-25, 27-28, 56, 65-66, 69, 136, 141, 145, 147-148, 151, 166, 169, 172, 196-197, 199-200, 215, 237, 239

Agranulocytosis, 1, 3-4, 119

Anemia, 4, 14-15, 32, 37, 39-40, 51, 57, 85-87, 93-95, 97-100, 118-122, 124, 133-135, 137-138, 151, 159, 192, 207, 228, 231

Antinuclear Antibodies, 86-87, 97

Aplasia, 1, 3-4, 93, 95, 97-98, 118-119, 190

Aplastic Anemia, 93, 95, 97-98, 133, 135

B

B-cell Lymphoma, 5-6, 8, 22, 36-38, 40-41, 46, 49, 52, 56-58, 83, 105, 110, 115, 117, 142-144, 146, 154-158, 161, 164, 195, 201-202, 205-206, 215, 218-220, 222, 224

Bone Marrow, 1-3, 6, 9, 14, 16, 19, 24-26, 30, 32, 34, 36-37, 39-41, 50-60, 62-67, 69, 71, 75, 77, 80-81, 86, 93-95, 99-101, 104, 107-108, 112, 115-116, 123-125, 130-131, 134, 136-140, 142-147, 151, 155-156, 159-160, 162-166, 169, 171, 174, 176-179, 188, 193-198, 202-203, 207-208, 215, 218-219, 221, 224, 228-229, 231, 234-236, 240-242

Bone Marrow Fibrosis, 59, 63, 65

C

Cavernous Sinus, 24-25

Cefepime, 9, 11

Central Nervous System, 36, 40, 51, 79-81, 83-84, 99, 103, 106, 156, 176, 207, 209-210, 216

Chloroma, 24, 28

Chronic Lymphocytic Leukemia, 13, 17, 58, 79, 83-84, 92, 118, 121-122, 183

Ciprofloxacin, 11, 37

Cyclosporine, 2, 4, 67, 95, 97-98, 121

Cytarabine, 9, 11, 14, 25-26, 57, 60-62, 64-65, 67, 103, 130, 138, 148, 160, 166-167, 174, 178, 198, 200, 202, 208, 215-216

Cytomegalovirus, 37, 97

Cytoplasm, 24-25, 50-51, 53, 56, 133, 142-143

D

Daunorubicin, 9, 11, 25, 61-62, 67, 138

Depressive Disorder, 51, 211

Dermatitis, 1, 10, 183

Diabetes Mellitus, 5, 51

Dyspnea, 26, 37, 39, 51, 74, 112, 158

E

Epstein-barr Virus, 19, 22, 37, 50-51, 58, 97, 108, 110, 165, 202, 224

F

Flow Cytometry, 1-2, 14, 24-25, 27, 30-31, 34, 42-43, 46-47, 56, 58, 80, 100, 112, 116, 118-119, 130, 134, 137, 159, 174, 177, 198-200, 202, 208, 218, 220, 231, 239

Fungal Infection, 1, 130

G

Good's Syndrome, 1, 3-4, 97-98

Granulated Cytoplasm, 24-25

Granulocytic Sarcoma, 24, 27-28, 196

H

Hodgkin Lymphoma, 81, 103, 107-110, 117, 124, 142, 181, 183-184, 201, 206, 218, 222

Human Immunodeficiency Virus, 22, 50, 57-58, 85, 88, 97, 158, 161, 226

Hypercellular Marrow, 24-25, 50-51, 60, 125, 142

Hyperplasia, 14, 51, 124-125, 134

Hypoalbuminemia, 37, 40, 85-86, 99-102

I

Immunoglobulin, 1, 3, 13-14, 16, 50, 52, 56, 62, 93, 97, 99, 113, 121, 163, 170-171, 183-184, 241-242

Immunohistochemistry, 14, 16, 19, 50, 55-56, 80, 82, 143, 159-160, 171, 184, 194, 202-203, 216

Immunomodulatory Agents, 216, 228

Infratemporal Fossa, 24-25

Intranasal Tumor, 46, 49

L

Leukemia, 9-10, 12-17, 22, 24-25, 27-28, 34-35, 40, 44, 50-51, 56, 58-60, 64-66, 68-73, 78-79, 81, 83-84, 92, 102, 118-119, 121-125, 127-128, 130-132, 136-141, 144-148, 151, 157, 161, 164-167, 169-170, 172-174, 176-179, 181, 183-184, 187, 190-193, 196-200, 209, 215-216, 222, 226, 231-237, 239

Leukopenia, 4, 40

Lymph Node, 6-7, 43, 52, 75-76, 85-86, 104-105, 107, 119, 124, 129, 133-134, 144, 163, 177, 179, 183, 185, 202, 217, 219, 224, 226

Lymphocyte, 3, 44, 66, 71, 76, 80, 94, 109, 114, 124, 129-130

Lymphocytic Lymphoma, 79, 118, 122, 195, 220

Lymphocytosis, 13-15, 89, 115

Lymphoid Tissue, 49, 98, 107, 111, 117

Lymphoma, 5-6, 8, 12-14, 18, 20, 22-23, 27, 30, 34-38, 40-42, 44-46, 49-52, 55-58, 64-66, 68-69, 73, 78-81, 83-87, 89, 92, 102-119, 122, 124, 128-132, 141-144, 146, 154-165, 169, 172, 176-179, 181-184, 186, 195, 200-203, 205-206, 209-210, 215-227, 232-237, 239-240, 242-243

Lymphoproliferative Disorder, 18, 85-86, 170, 223

M
Mantle Cell Lymphoma, 89, 103, 106, 129-131, 160

Mass Biopsy, 2, 18-20

Methylprednisolone, 60, 66, 141, 183-184, 211

Monocyte, 114, 141, 235

Multiple Myeloma, 29-30, 32-35, 64, 74, 78, 101-102, 111, 117, 147, 159-162, 164-166, 169, 210, 215-216, 224-229, 232-233, 235, 240, 242-244

Mycosis, 42, 45

Mycosis Fungoides, 42, 45

Myelodysplastic Syndrome, 95, 123, 127, 133, 145, 197, 215, 237

Myeloma, 14, 18, 29-30, 32-35, 45, 55, 57-58, 64, 69, 73-75, 78, 86, 101-102, 111, 117, 122, 131, 147, 157-166, 169, 172, 209-210, 212, 215-216, 223-229, 232-233, 235, 240, 242-244

N
Neoplasm, 1, 14, 26, 30, 50-51, 53, 55-56, 80, 93, 117, 123-125, 127-128, 145, 170, 183-184, 202, 218, 223-224, 228, 234-236

Neurological Symptoms, 29-30, 32, 34, 36, 39

Neutropenia, 1-3, 30, 33, 43, 65, 93, 95, 145, 150-151, 171, 190, 229, 231-232

P
Plasma Cells, 29-30, 32-33, 51, 53, 86-87, 112-113, 162-165, 211-213, 215, 224-225, 228-229, 240-241

Plasmablastic Lymphoma, 18, 22-23, 50-52, 57-58, 158-159, 161, 223, 226-227

Plasmacytomas, 29, 32-35, 228

Promyelocytic Leukemia, 12, 59-60, 65, 187, 190-191

R
Red Cell Aplasia, 1, 93, 97-98, 118-119

S
Sarcoidosis, 76, 219, 222, 240, 242-244

Sezary Syndrome, 42, 45

Sinus, 6, 8, 18, 24-26

Sphenoid Sinus, 24-25

Stem Cell, 22, 24, 27, 34, 65-66, 69-70, 73, 91-92, 95, 97-98, 103, 107, 123, 128, 130, 136, 140-141, 145-147, 155-156, 158, 161, 169, 175-176, 178, 181, 197, 201-202, 206-208, 212, 225, 228-229, 231-232, 234-235

Sweet's Syndrome, 9-12, 170-172, 186

Syncope, 5-6, 8

T
Thrombocytopenia, 15, 26, 33, 37, 39-40, 51, 65, 85-86, 93-95, 97, 99, 104, 118, 129-132, 134, 138, 145-147, 150-151, 163, 170-172, 175, 192, 207, 231-232

Thymocytes, 93

Thymoma, 1-4, 93, 95, 97-98

V
Vancomycin, 9, 11, 137, 167

W
White Cell, 1, 3-4, 171, 174

White Cell Aplasia, 1, 3-4

www.ingramcontent.com/pod-product-compliance
Lightning Source LLC
LaVergne TN
LVHW082122200926
848484LV00008B/1994